HIV/AIDS: Diagnosis and Management

HIV/AIDS: Diagnosis and Management

Editor: Ivy Monroe

FOSTER ACADEMICS

www.fosteracademics.com

www.fosteracademics.com

FOSTER ACADEMICS

Cataloging-in-Publication Data

HIV/AIDS : diagnosis and management / edited by Ivy Monroe.
p. cm.
Includes bibliographical references and index.
ISBN 978-1-63242-870-7
1. HIV infections. 2. AIDS (Disease). 3. HIV infections--Diagnosis. 4. AIDS (Disease)--Diagnosis.
5. HIV infections--Treatment. 6. AIDS (Disease)--Treatment. I. Monroe, Ivy.
RC606.6 .H58 2020
616.979 2--dc23

Foster Academics,
118-35 Queens Blvd., Suite 400,
Forest Hills, NY 11375, USA

ISBN 978-1-63242-870-7 (Hardback)

Contents

Preface

I am honored to present to you this unique book which encompasses the most up-to-date data in the field. I was extremely pleased to get this opportunity of editing the work of experts from across the globe. I have also written papers in this field and researched the various aspects revolving around the progress of the discipline. I have tried to unify my knowledge along with that of stalwarts from every corner of the world, to produce a text which not only benefits the readers but also facilitates the growth of the field.

HIV/AIDS is a spectrum of conditions that occur due to infection with HIV or human immunodeficiency virus. An infection with HIV progresses through three main stages- acute infection, clinical latency and AIDS. 40-90% of individuals develop influenza-like illness after around 2-4 weeks of the initial infection with HIV. This lasts usually between one and two weeks while others experience no significant signs at all. Fever, throat inflammation, large tender lymph nodes, headache, a rash and/or sores of the mouth and genitals may occur. After this stage, follows a period of clinical latency that lasts between three to over twenty years, without treatment. Once AIDS sets in, pneumocystis pneumonia, cachexia and esophageal candidiasis start to occur. Viral-induced cancers and opportunistic infections may also start affecting the individual. This book provides comprehensive insights into the diagnosis and management of HIV/AIDS. It presents researches and studies performed by experts across the globe. It is meant for students who are looking for an elaborate reference text on HIV/AIDS.

Finally, I would like to thank all the contributing authors for their valuable time and contributions. This book would not have been possible without their efforts. I would also like to thank my friends and family for their constant support.

Editor

1

The pattern and predictors of mortality of HIV/AIDS patients with neurologic manifestation in Ethiopia

Tesfaye Berhe[1], Yilma Melkamu[2] and Amanuel Amare[1*]

Abstract

Background: Even though the prevalence of HIV infection among the adult population in Ethiopia was estimated to be 2.2% in 2008, the studies on the pattern of neurological manifestations are rare. The aim of this retrospective study was to assess the pattern and predictors of mortality of HIV/AIDS patients with neurologic manifestations.

Methods: Medical records of 347 patients (age ≥13 years) admitted to Tikur Anbesa Hospital from September 2002 to August 2009 were reviewed and demographic and clinical data were collected.

Results: Data from 347 patients were analysed. The mean age was 34.6 years. The diagnosis of HIV was made before current admission in 33.7% and 15.6% were on antiretroviral therapy (ART). Causes of neurological manifestation were: cerebral toxoplasmosis (36.6%), tuberculous meningitis (22.5%), cryptococcal meningitis (22.2%) and bacterial meningitis (6.9%). HIV-encephalopathy, primary central nervous system (CNS) lymphoma and progressive multifocal leukoencephalopathy were rare in our patients. CD4 count was done in 64.6% and 89.7% had count below 200/mm3[mean = 95.8, median = 57] and 95.7% were stage IV. Neuroimaging was done in 38% and 56.8% had mass lesion. The overall mortality was 45% and the case-fatality rates were: tuberculous meningitis (53.8%), cryptococcal meningitis (48.1%), cerebral toxoplasmosiss (44.1%) and bacterial meningitis (33.3%). Change in sensorium and seizure were predictors of mortality.

Conclusions: CNS opportunistic infections were the major causes of neurological manifestations of HIV/AIDS and were associated with high mortality and morbidity. Almost all patients had advanced HIV disease at presentation. Early diagnosis of HIV, prophylaxis and treatment of opportunistic infections, timely ART, and improving laboratory services are recommended. Mortality was related to change in sensorium and seizure.

Keywords: Africa, Antiretroviral therapy, Cryptococcus, Opportunistic infection, Toxoplasmosis, Tuberculosis

Introduction

Symptomatic neurologic dysfunction develops in more than 50% of individuals infected with human immunodeficiency virus (HIV) [1] and about 10% experience neurologic symptoms as the initial manifestation of acquired immunodeficiency syndrome (AIDS) [2]. Neurologic disorders associated with HIV infection include central nervous system (CNS) infections, neoplasms, vascular complications, peripheral neuropathies and myopathies [3]. Neurologic dysfunction is an important cause or a strong marker of poor prognosis in late HIV infection [4].

Studies done in developing countries showed that the major causes of neurologic disorders in HIV/AIDS patients are CNS opportunistic infections [5-12]. In Ethiopia, the adult prevalence of HIV infection was estimated to be 2.2% in 2008 [13] but data on the pattern of neurological complications of HIV/AIDS are rare. This study was designed to assess the clinical presentation, cause, treatment, outcome and predictors of mortality in HIV/AIDS patients with neurological complications who were admitted to Tikur Anbesa Hospital (TAH), the main teaching hospital of Addis Ababa University.

* Correspondence: amanuelaw@yahoo.com
[1]Department of Neurology, Addis Ababa University, Addis Ababa, Ethiopia

Patients and methods

In this retrospective study, HIV infected patients aged ≥ 13 years who were admitted with neurological manifestations of HIV/AIDS to TAH from September 2002 to August 2009 were included. Medical records of patients were retrieved and data sheets were used to collect the following data: age, sex, address, occupation, marital status, presenting symptoms and signs, investigations, treatment, duration of hospital stay, treatment outcome at hospital discharge.

Confidentiality was assured by giving each patient a unique number. The study was started after getting ethical approval from the appropriate body of the medical faculty of the university. Patients excluded from the study were: patients age < 13 years, patients who were not admitted, who had wrong diagnosis, or there were insufficient data for diagnosis.

Clinical staging of HIV/AIDS was made based on World Health Organization (WHO) staging system for HIV infection and disease [14]. The most recent CD4 count was taken into consideration. Poor outcome at hospital discharge was defined as patients who remained in the same clinical condition or deteriorated without death. Improved patients were patients who showed partial or complete recovery. The presumptive diagnosis of the neurological manifestations of HIV/AIDS was made as follows:

Cerebral toxoplasmosis

Presumed diagnosis based on some or all of the following: i) headache, fever, change in sensorium ii) focal neurologic deficit iii) seropositivity for anti-toxoplasma immunoglobulin G(IgG), iv) ring enhancing brain lesion (s) on computerized tomography(CT)/magnetic resonance imaging(MRI), v) low CD4 count(< 200/mm3), and vi) response to toxoplasma treatment.

Tuberculous meningitis

Based on some or all of the following: i) headache, fever, neck rigidity, change in mentation ii) cerebrospinal fluid (CSF) lymphocytosis iii) Acid-fast bacilli(AFB) on CSF smear iv) evidence of active tuberculosis in other part of the body (milliary tuberculosis, pulmonary tuberculosis etc.) v) CT/MRI showing meningeal enhancement vi) response to tuberculosis treatment.

Tuberculoma

i) headache, change in sensorium ii) focal deficit iii) CT/MRI contrast enhancing lesion, and iv) response to tuberculosis treatment.

Cyptococcal meningitis

CSF India ink positivity.

Bacterial meningitis

i) acute onset headache, fever, change in mentation, neck rigidity ii) CSF polymorph predominant pleocytosis iii) CSF culture and Gram stain showing bacteria iv) response to antibiotics.

Neurosyphilis

CSF Venereal Disease Research Laboratory (VDRL) reactive.

Stroke

Sudden onset of neurologic deficit which persisted for > 24 h of presumed vascular origin.

Guillian-Barre syndrome (GBS)/chronic inflammatory demyelinating polyneuropathy(CIDP)

Progressive weakness, paresthesias, areflexia, high CSF protein with pleocytosis, evidence of demyelination on nerve conduction studies.

Primary CNS lymphoma

i) headache, change in sensorium, focal neurologic deficit ii) low CD4 count (< 200/mm3) iii) CT/MRI enhancing mass lesion iv) no response to toxoplasmosis and tuberculosis treatment

Progressive multifocal leukoencephalopathy (PML)

i) multifocal progressive focal deficits, ii) CT/MRI multiple non-enhancing white matter lesions without edema or mass effect.

Neurocyticercosis

multiple cerebral calcified lesions on CT scan.

HIV encephalopathy

i) cognitive and motor abnormalities ii) CT/MRI showing brain atrophy iii) other opportunistic infections ruled out.

Pseudotumor cerebri

i) clinical evidence of increased intracranial pressure ii) normal CT/MRI

The data was analysed using SPSS 13.0 for Windows (SPSS, Chicago IL, USA). Logistic regression was used to assess each possible prognostic factor. Odds ratios and significant levels were calculated along with 95% confidence interval. A p-value of less than 0.05 was considered significant. A multivariate logistic regression analysis was performed to determine which prognostic factors, when considered together, were the best predictors of hospital death.

Results

Data from 347 patients were analysed. The mean age was 34.6 years (range 14-65) and 50.7% were males.

Their marital status was married (52.2%), single (31.4%), widowed (7.8%), divorced (6.3%) and unknown (2.3%). The occupation was known for 305(87.9%) patients: housewives 86(24.8%), office employees 74(21.3%), car driver 36(10.4%), unemployed 31(8.9%), merchant 28 (8.1%), daily laborer 21(6.1%), student 5(1.4%) and others 24 (6.9%).

Twenty-five percent (25%) came from outside Addis Ababa and the mean duration of symptoms was 30.6 days (range 1-240). The mean duration of symptoms for the major neurologic disorders identified was cerebral toxoplasmosis (25 days, median 14 days), tuberculous meningitis (34 days), cryptococcal meningitis (26 days) and bacterial meningitis (10 days). The diagnosis of HIV was made in 117 patients before current hospital admission and there was no statistically significant difference in case-fatality between patients who were diagnosed before and after admission (p = 0.315). The mean duration between diagnosis of HIV and current hospital admission was known for108 patients, and ranged between 1 and 120 months (mean 14.8 months). History of treatment with antiretroviral therapy (ART) was identified in 54(15.6%) patients with mean duration of treatment of 7.2 months (median 5 months, range1-29). ART was discontinued before hospital admission in 5 cases (They went to holy water). Co-trimoxazole prophylaxis was given to 15 cases before current admission and 2(13.3%) of these developed cerebral toxoplasmosis (p-value = 0.230).

The mean hospital stay was 21.9 days (range1-120). The mean hospital stay in days for improved and deceased patients was 26.4 (range 7-120) and 16.9 (range 1-91), respectively. The clinical manifestation of patients with neurological disorders is shown in Table 1 and the neurologic manifestation of HIV/AIDS in relation to outcome status is shown in Table 2. Herpes Zoster scar was identified in 67(19.3%) of cases. Co-morbidities identified at admission were pulmonary tuberculosis 18(5.2%) and pneumonia 18(5.2%). Some patients (n = 7, 2%) had more than one neurologic complications of HIV/AIDS: cryptococcal meningitis and neurosyphilis (n = 3), cryptococcal meningitis and GBS (n = 1), neurosyphilis and GBS (n = 1), tuberculous meningitis and tuberculoma (n = 1), cerebral toxoplasmosis and neurosyphilis (n = 1). The Glasgow coma scale (GCS) was recorded in 85(24.5%) of cases and 35 (41.2%) had score of ≤ 8. The Case-fatality of patients with GCS score of ≤ 8 and > 8 was not different (p-value = 0.936). The WHO clinical staging of HIV/AIDS patients showed that majority (n = 332, 95.7%) were stage IV and the remaining were stage III (n = 15, 4.3%) cases.

Investigations

CD4 count was done in 224(64.6%) cases and 201 (89.7%) had count of below 200/mm3. The mean and median CD4 count per mm3 was 95.8 and 57, respectively. The mean CD4 count per mm3 for the major neurologic disorders identified was: cryptococcal meningitis = 55.5, cerebral toxoplasmosis = 66.3, tuberculous meningitis = 113.8 and bacterial meningitis = 204.4. Lumbar puncture was done in 226(65.1%) and the mean cell count was 467.3(range 1-8400). The mean differential count of neutrophil and lymphocyte was 39.2% (range 0-98) and 60.4%(range2-100), respectively. India ink was done in 216(62.2%) and was positive in 77 (35.6%) cases. Out of 213(61.4%) patients tested for CSF VDRL, 9(4.2%) cases were reactive. Serology for toxoplasmosis (IgG) was done in 65(18.7%) and was positive in 44(67.7%) patients (titer was not done). CSF Gram stain and Acid fast stain showed organisms in 2 and 1 cases, respectively. Neuroimaging was done in 132(38%): CT-scan = 127, CT-scan and MRI = 2 and MRI = 3. The findings were: mass lesion (abscess and tumor) = 75(56.8%), normal = 30(22.7%), infarction = 13, meningeal enhancement = 5, brain atrophy = 5, non-enhancing white matter lesions = 2 and intracerebral hemorrhage = 2. Of the 75 patients with mass lesion on neuroimaging 60(80%) cases were diagnosed to have toxoplasmosis.

Treatment

Toxoplasmosis was treated with sulfadoxine-pyrimethamine [pyrimethamine-sulfadiazine was not available]. Tuberculosis was treated with combination of Isoniazid, rifampin, pyrazinamide, ethambutol or streptomycine

Table 1 Clinical presentations of HIV/AIDS patients with neurological disorders

Sign/symptom	Cerebral toxoplasmosis(127)	Tuberculos meningitis(78)	Cryptococcal meningitis(77)	Bacterial meningitis(24)
Headache(212)	60(47.2%)	51(65.4%)	71(92.2%)	16(66.7%)
Altered sensorium(187)	74(58.3%)	57(73.1%)	28(36.4%)	18(75%)
Meningeal sign(136)	17(13.4%)	45(57.7%)	49(63.6%)	19(79.2)
Seizure(119)	54(42.5%)	27(34.6%)	21(27.3%)	6(25%)
Focal deficit(117)	83(65.4%)	9(11.5%)	5(6.5%)	1(4.2%)
Fever(108)	25(19.7%)	31(39.7%)	30(39%)	14(58.3%)

Table 2 Neurologic manifestations of HIV/AIDS in relation to outcome in 347 patients

Diagnosis	n(%)	Dead(156) n(%)	Poor outcome(21) n(%)	Improved(170) n(%)
cerebral toxoplasmosis	127(36.6)	56(44.1)	9(7.1)	62(48.8)
Tuberculosis meningitis	78(22.5)	42(53.8)	2(2.6)	34(43.6)
Cryptococcal meningitis	77(22.2)	37(48.1)	3(3.8)	37(48.1)
Bacterial meningitis	24(6.9)	8(33.3)	2(8.3)	14(58.3)
Tuberculoma	10(2.9)	4(40)	1(10)	5(50)
Neurosyphilis	9(2.6)	0	1(11.1)	8(88.9)
Stroke	8(2.3)	3(37.5)	0	5(62.5)
GBS	5(1.4)	1(20)	0	4(80)
Tuberculos spondylitis	5(1.4)	1(20)	2(40)	2(40)
Primary CNS lymphoma	3(0.9)	3(100)	0	0
CIDP	3(0.9)	0	0	3(100)
PML	2(0.6)	1(50)	0	1(50)
Others	3(0.9)	0	2(66.7)	1(33.3)

Note: *GBS* Guillain-Barre syndrome, *CNS* central nervous system, *CIDP* chronic inflammatory demyelinating polyneuropathy, *PML* progressive multifocal leukoencephalopathy, Others = pseudotumor cerebri (n = 1), neurocycticercosis (n = 1), HIV-encephalopathy (n = 1). Stroke: ischemic (n = 6), Hemorrhagic (n = 2).

with pyridoxine. Cryptococcal meningitis was treated with oral fluconazole (n = 45) or Amphotericin B (n = 32). Seizure was treated with phenytoin in almost all patients. Dexamethasone intravenously was given (n = 182, 52.4%) and prednisolone used in 26(7.5%) cases. One or more intravenous antibiotics (ceftriaxone, crystalline penicillin, gentamycine etc.) was given to 212 (61.1%) cases. ART was started after admission in 135 (70.7% of cases discharged alive).

Outcome

The case-fatality was 45%(n = 156) and the number of patients with poor outcome (discharged in the same clinical condition or deteriorated without death) was 6.1%(n = 21). In almost all patients, the immediate cause of death was attributable to the identified neurologic disorder(s).

Both univariate and multivariate logistic regression analysis (Table 3) showed that address from Addis Ababa, altered sensorium and seizure were predictors of mortality.

Discussion

The objectives of our study were to assess the clinical presentation, cause, treatment, outcome and predictors of mortality in patients with HIV/AIDS with neurologic complications admitted to the largest referral hospital in Ethiopia. Both sexes were equally affected unlike other studies [7,8,10,11] where males outnumbered females. Majority of our patients were young (mean age 34.6 years) which is similar to other studies [7-11]. There was delay at presentation (mean duration of symptoms prior to presentation was 30.6 days). The mean duration of symptoms prior to presentation for patients with cerebral toxoplasmosis (25 days) and cryptococcal meningitis (26 days) was similar to another study [2]. Majority (66.3%) of cases were known to have HIV infection after current hospital admission. Almost all patients had advanced HIV disease at presentation (4.3% stage III and 95.7% stage IV) which is consistent with another study [8].

The occurrence of seizure in cerebral toxoplasmosis in other studies [2,3] was 25% and 29%, respectively, which was lower compared to our finding. In another study [12], seizure occurred in 40% of patients with cerebral toxoplasmosis which was similar to our study. In a study [12] the occurrence of seizure in tuberculous meningitis (28%) and cryptococcal meningitis (50%) was lower and higher, respectively, compared with findings in our study. The common neurologic disorders identified in our cases were: cerebral toxoplasmosis (36.6%), tuberculous meningitis (22.5%) and cryptococcal meningitis (22.2%), and the frequencies were similar to other studies [5,6,11,12,15]. In contrary to our findings, tuberculous meningitis and bacterial meningitis were rare findings in patients with neurologic manifestations of HIV/AIDS in the United States [2]. In a study from India [12], cerebral toxoplasmosis was detected in 8.8% (5/57) which is very low compared to our finding. The number of patients with presumed diagnosis of primary CNS lymphoma was very low in our cases probably due to failure to do brain biopsy when empiric therapy for toxoplasmosis failed.

Stoke was identified in 2.3% of our patients which is low compared to a finding in another study [2] which was 12%. The low number of patients (2%) with

Table 3 Risk factor for case-fatality: logistic regression analysis

Factor		n	%	Unadjusted OR(95% CI)	Adjusted OR(95% CI)
Age(year)	< 40	113	44.3	1.00	1.00
	≥ 40	43	46.7	1.10(0.684-1.779)	1.033(0.529-2.018)
Sex	Male	77	43.8	1.00	1.00
	female	79	46.2	1.10(0.723-1.686)	1.033(0.566-1.887)
Address	Addis Ababa	133	50.8	1.00	1.00
	Outside Addis Ababa	23	27.1	0.360(0.210-0.615)	0.282(0.127-0.630)
History of ART treatment	Yes	21	38.9	1.00	1.00
	No	135	46.1	1.343(0.742-2.430)	1.1(0.506-2.393)
Cotrimoxazole (prophylaxis)	Yes	8	53.3	1.00	1.00
	No	148	44.6	0.704(0.249-1.986)	0.992(0.266-3.705)
Altered sensorium	Yes	99	52.9	1.00	1.00
	No	57	35.6	0.492(0.319-0.758)	0.514(0.288-0.916)
Seizure	Yes	65	54.6	1.00	1.00
	No	91	39.9	0.552(0.353-0.863)	0.519(0.288-0.935)
Clinical stage of HIV infection	Stage iii	3	20	1.00	1.00
	Stage iv	153	46.1	3.419(0.947-12.339)	2.069(0.370-11.562)
CD_4 count(/mm^3)	< 200	85	42.3	1.00	1.00
	≥ 200	6	26.1	0.482(0.182-1.273)	0.572(0.205-1.595)

ART antiretroviral treatment, *HIV* human immunodeficiency virus *CD_4* cluster of differentiation 4

multiple neurologic disorders compared to 13.5% in another study [2] probably shows the limited investigations available in our set up. Unlike other studies [2,16,17] HIV-encephalopathy was diagnosed in only one of our patients (0.28%).

Majority of our patients (89.7%) had a CD4 count below 200/mm3 which is consistent with another study [12]. Note that adult healthy Ethiopians have a mean absolute CD4 T-cell count of 775 cell/μL(range 366-1,235) in one study [18]. Neuroimaging studies in our cases showed focal lesions in 56.8% which is higher when compared to 25.5% obtained in another study [2]. The commonest (80%) cause of mass lesion on imaging studies in our patients was cerebral toxoplasmosis which is similar to other studies [1-3,5-7] but contrary to a study done in South Africa [9] where tuberculosis predominates as a cause of focal brain lesion(69%). In our study, normal neuroimaging finding and cerebral atrophy were detected in22.7% and 3.9%, respectively which is lower compared to another study [2]. These might be explained by the limited access to neuroimaging studies and the low incidence of HIV-encephalopathy, which is the main cause of brain atrophy in HIV/AIDS patients, in our cases. A study [19] on HIV-related neuropathology showed that the incidence of HIV-encephalopathy rises as patients survive longer after initiation of antiretroviral therapy and is the most common neurologic complications of HIV/AIDS in such set up [2]. In a study from Nigeria [10] which included ART naive patients only, HIV-encephalopathy was found in 12% (19/154) of cases which is higher when compared to our study. These show that history of treatment with ART alone does not explain the low incidence of HIV-encephalopathy in our patients. Our patients were highly selected group of patients with advanced disease stage in whom the neurologic symptoms might be overshadowed by overwhelming systemic illness. In addition, lack of adequate screening techniques and readily available imaging studies might contribute.

Amphotericin B was not readily available and treatment of cryptococcal meningitis was either Amphotericin B (n = 32) or oral fluconazole only (n = 45) [There was no significant difference in mortality, p-value = 0.260]. The limited availability of standard therapy might explain partly the higher case-fatality of cryptococcal meningitis (48.1%) in our cases compared to 32.4% in another study [2]. Sulfadiazine-pyrimethamine was not available and patients with cerebral toxoplasmosis were treated with pyrimethamin-sulfadoxin. This might partly explain the higher mortality in our set up (44.1%) compared to 30.2% in patients who were treated with standard treatment [2].

The overall hospital mortality was 45% which is high compared to other studies. In a study done in Nigeria

[10] which included outpatients and inpatients, an overall 6-month mortality of 45% was found. In another study from India [11], a mortality of 34% was recorded. The in-hospital mortality of patients with neurologic manifestations of AIDS in Brazil [7] was 32%. The case-fatality for the major neurologic disorders in our study was: tuberculous meningitis (53.8%), cryptococcal meningitis (48.1%), cerebral toxoplasmosiss (44.1%) and bacterial meningitis (33.3%). In a study done in Cambodia [15], the case-fatality rates of tuberculous meningitis and cryptococcal meningitis was similar to our study which were 57% and 49%, respectively. In studies done in South Africa [20] and Nigeria [10] the case-fatality of HIV associated tuberculous meningitis was 71.8% and 77.5%, respectively, which is higher compared to our finding.

Both univariate and multivariate logistic regression analysis showed that address from Addis Ababa, altered sensorium and seizure were predictors of mortality. The unexpected relatively lower mortality of patients from outside the city of Addis Ababa might be partly explained by selection bias of cases who were relatively stable and able to travel to the city for better health care services. History of ART at admission was not found to improve mortality significantly.

This unexpected finding might be due to the relatively short period of treatment (mean 7 months, median 5 months), noncompliance (5 patients discontinued ART and of these 3 died) and only 15.6% of our cases were on ART. In patients with history of ART the common neurologic complications identified were: cerebral toxoplasmosis (n = 13), cyptococcal meningitis (n = 12), tuberculous meningitis (n = 10), bacterial meningitis (n = 9), stroke (n = 4) and others (n = 10). Further study is recommended to identify other possible reasons for the failure of ART in our patients.

There were several limitations to this study. Patients who were treated as outpatient only were not included and therefore the whole spectrum of neurologic manifestation might not be addressed. The absence of certain neurologic disorders in our study (myelopathy, peripheral neuropathy other than inflammatory demyelinating polyneurpathy, myopathy, etc.) might be partly explained by inclusion of inpatients only. Our hospital is a tertiary hospital and the chance of admitting selectively critically sick patients is high due to referral from other hospitals. The retrospective nature of the study might have caused unrecoverable missing data in some cases. There was no autopsy, biopsy, viral load and polymerase chain reaction done. CSF glucose and protein determination was done in minority of patients.

To improve care of patients with neurologic manifestations of HIV/AIDS, early diagnosis of HIV infection, patient education, starting prophylaxis when needed (e.g. INH and cotrimoxazole prophylaxis, BCG vaccination to decrease incidence of tuberculous meningitis), starting ART timely, making standard therapy for opportunistic infections readily available(e.g. sulfadiazine-pyremethamin with leucovorin and Amphotericin B), improving availability and quality of laboratory investigations and neuroimaging studies are very important.

In conclusion, most of our patients with neurologic manifestations of HIV/AIDS had advanced disease at presentations which was evidenced by: almost all were in stage IV, majority had low CD4 count and most had opportunistic CNS infections as the leading etiologies. Majority of patients were diagnosed to have HIV infection at admission and only a few patients were on ART and cotrimoxazole prophylaxis. Etiological diagnosis was difficult in some patients because of limited availability of laboratory services and lack of facilities for neuroimaging studies. Seizure and change in sensorium at presentation were independent predictors of mortality. To improve the high mortality and morbidity observed in our study, prevention of HIV infection, and when it occurs early diagnosis and appropriate prophylaxis and treatment of opportunistic infections and timely ART are recommended.

Author details

[1]Department of Neurology, Addis Ababa University, Addis Ababa, Ethiopia.
[2]School of Public Health, Addis Ababa University, Addis Ababa, Ethiopia.

Authors' contributions

AA wrote the first draft of the paper and all authors contributed comments and suggestions to various draft versions. TB participated in study design and data collection. YM participated in study design and coordinated the study. All authors have seen and approved the final manuscript.

Competing interests

The authors declare that they have no competing interests.

References

1. Weisberg LA: **Neurologic abnormalities in human immunodeficiency virus infection.** *South Med J* 2001, **94**:266-275.
2. Levy RM, Bredesen DE: **Central nervous system dysfunction in acquired immunodeficiency syndrome.** *J Acquir Immune Defic Syndr* 1988, **1**:41-64.
3. Simpson DM, Tagliati M: **Neurologic manifestations of HIV infection.** *Ann Intern Med* 1994, **121**:769-785.
4. Price RW, Yiannoutsos CT, Clifford DB, Zaborski L, Tselis A, Sidtis JJ, Cohen B, Hall CD, Erice A, Henry K: **Neurological outcomes in late HIV infection: adverse impact of neurological impairment on survival and protective effect of antiviral therapy.** *AIDS* 1999, **13**:1677-85.
5. Almeida SM, Ribeiro CE, Pessa LC, Moreira SD, Vidal LR, Nogueira MB, Raboni SM: **Incidence of neurological manifestations as AIDS defining clinical conditions in Brazil.** *BMC Proc* 2008, **2(Suppl I)**:45.
6. Bhigjee AI, Naidoo K, Patel VB, Govender D: **Intracranial mass lesions in HIVpostive patients-the KwaZulu/Natal experience.** *Neuroscience AIDS Research Group S Afr Med J* 1999, **89**:1284-8.
7. Fragoso YD, Mendes V, Adamo AM, Bosco LP, Tavares CF: **Neurologic manifestations of AIDS: a review of fifty cases in Santos, Brazil.** *Sao Paulo Med J* 1998, **116**:1715-1720.

8. Isezuo SA, Sani AZ, Ezunu E, Maiyaki S, Njoku CH, Obembe A: **Clinical neuropathy in HIV/AIDS: an eight-year review of hospitalized patients in Sokoto, northwestern Nigeria.** *Trop Doct* 2009, **39**:133-35.
9. Modi M, Mochan A, Modi G: **Management of HIV-associated focal brain lesions in developing countries.** *Q J Med* 2004, **97**:413-21.
10. Ogun SA, Ojini FI, Okubadejo N, Danesi M, Kolapo K, Osalusi B, Boyle B: **Pattern and outcome of Neurological manifestations of HIV/AIDS-a review of 154 cases in a Nigerian University Teaching Hospital- A preliminary report.** *Afr J Neuro Sci* 2005, **24**:29-36.
11. Satishchandra P, Nalini A, Gourie-devi M, Khanna N, Santosh V, Ravi V, Chandramuki AD, Jayakumar PN, Shankar SK: **Profile of neurologic disorders associated with HIV/AIDS from Bangalore, south India (1989-96).** *Indian J Med Res* 2000, **111**:14-23.
12. Satya AV, Kumar GA, Pratap SV, Vivekananda VD, Madhukar R, Shyam S: **Neurological manifestations of HIV- infected patients around Varanasi, India.** *Afr J Neuro Sci* 2006, **25**:33-40.
13. FMOH of Ethiopia: **Implementation guidelines for TB/HIV collaborative Activities in Ethiopia.** 2008, 2-3.
14. **WHO case definitions of HIV for Surveillance and revised clinical staging and immunological classification of HIV-related disease in adults and children.** 2007, 10-38.
15. Chhin S, Rozycki G, Pugatch D, Harwell JI: **Aetiology of meningitis in HIV-infected patients in a referral hospital in Phnom Penh, Cambodia.** *Int J STD AIDS* 2004, **15**:48-50.
16. Perriens JH, Mussa M, Luabeya MK, Kayembe K, Kapita B, Brown C, Piot P, Janssen R: **Neurological complications of HIV-1-Seropositive Internal Medicine Inpatients in Kinshasa, Zaire.** *J Acquir Immune Defic Syndr* 1992, **5**:333-340.
17. Portegies P, Enting RH, Gans J, Algra PR, Derix MA, Lange JA, Goudsmit J: **Presentation and course of AIDS dementia complex:10 years of follow-up in Amsterdam, The Netherlands.** *AIDS* 1993, **7**:669-75.
18. Tsegaye A, Messele T, Tilahun T, Hailu E, Sahlu T, Doorly R, Fontanet AL, Rinke de Wit TF: **Immunohematological reference ranges for adult Ethiopians.** *Clin Diagn Lab Immunol* 1999, **6(3)**:410-414.
19. Neuenburg JK, Brodt HR, Herndier BG, Bickel M, Bacchetti P, Price RW, Grant RM, Schlote W: **HIV-related neuropathology, 1985 to 1999; rising prevalence of HIV encephalopathy in the Era of highly active antiretroviral therapy.** *J Acquir Immune Defic Syndr* 2002, **31**:171-177.
20. Karstaedt AS, Valtchanova S, Barriere R, Crewe-brown HH: **Tuberculous meningitis in South African urban Adults.** *Q J Med* 1998, **91**:743-747.

2

Women and HIV in Sub-Saharan Africa

Gita Ramjee[1,2*] and Brodie Daniels[1]

Abstract

Thirty years since the discovery of HIV, the HIV pandemic in sub-Saharan Africa accounts for more than two thirds of the world's HIV infections. Southern Africa remains the region most severely affected by the epidemic. Women continue to bear the brunt of the epidemic with young women infected almost ten years earlier compared to their male counterparts. Epidemiological evidence suggests unacceptably high HIV prevalence and incidence rates among women. A multitude of factors increase women's vulnerability to HIV acquisition, including, biological, behavioral, socioeconomic, cultural and structural risks. There is no magic bullet and behavior alone is unlikely to change the course of the epidemic. Considerable progress has been made in biomedical, behavioral and structural strategies for HIV prevention with attendant challenges of developing appropriate HIV prevention packages which take into consideration the socioeconomic and cultural context of women in society at large.

Keywords: HIV incidence, Sub-Saharan Africa, Adherence, Prevention

Introduction

Sub-Saharan Africa (SSA) remains the region most affected by the HIV epidemic. Almost three quarters (69%) of the 23.5 million people infected worldwide reside in this region [1]. Most countries in SSA report a generalized epidemic (infection rates of > 1%) with pockets of concentrated epidemics in key populations [1]. South Africa remains the country with over 6 million people reported to be infected with HIV [2]. Swaziland has the highest adult prevalence rate of 26.5% followed by South Africa, Namibia and Mozambique at 17.9%, 13.3% and 11.1% respectively [2]. Transmission is mainly through heterosexual sex, with women disproportionately infected compared to their male counterparts. It is reported that every minute one young woman becomes infected with HIV [3]. The purpose of this review is to discuss the HIV epidemic among women in SSA, associated risks for HIV acquisition, and to provide a brief update on HIV prevention options which may collectively impact on reducing incidence of HIV infection.

HIV and women in Africa

In SSA, women bear the brunt of the HIV epidemic [2]. In 2011, 92% of pregnant women who were HIV positive were living in this region [4]. Most countries in SSA report the state of the epidemic based on their ante-natal surveillance data with limited data on HIV incidence due to the difficulty in accurately measuring HIV incidence rates. A number of studies conducted among non-pregnant women in parts of east and southern Africa suggest prevalence rates ranging from 14.5% (95% CI 11.2 – 18.4) in east Africa to 38.7% (95% CI 34.2 – 43.3) in Lusaka (Zambia) and 39.5% (95% CI 35.1 – 44.0) in Durban, South Africa [5]. There have been reports of a decline or stabilizing in HIV prevalence among women in southern Africa [6,7]. However, HIV incidence data from large scale clinical trials and cohort studies suggests that the low prevalence masks high HIV incidence rates [8-11]. Risk factor analysis of these cohorts of women from various HIV prevention trials suggest that being under the age of 25 years, having had one sexually transmitted infection (STI) in the past and being unmarried were significantly associated with high risk of HIV seroconversion [12,13]. Rehle *et al.* substantiated these results in the 2013 Human Sciences Research Council (HSRC) household survey which showed that being young and unmarried increased the risk of HIV acquisition among South African women [14].

Factors that increase women's vulnerability to HIV in Africa

The disproportionate impact of the HIV epidemic on women can be attributable to several factors including

* Correspondence: Gita.Ramjee@mrc.ac.za
[1]HIV Prevention Research Unit, South African Medical Research Council, 123 Jan Hofmeyr Road, Westville, Durban 3629, South Africa
[2]London School of Hygiene and Tropical Medicines, Keppel Street, London WC1E, 7HT, UK

biological, social, behavioral, cultural, economic and structural. In SSA a combination of these factors has led to the disparate increase in HIV infection rates among women compared to their male counterparts [15].

Biological risk factors

Women are at a greater physiological risk of contracting HIV than men. This is in part because women have a greater mucosal surface area exposed to pathogens and infectious fluid for longer periods during sexual intercourse and are likely to face increased tissue injury. Young women are at particularly high risk due to cervical ectopy which facilitates greater exposure of target cells to trauma and pathogens in the vagina [16]. It has been well documented that STIs increase the risk of HIV acquisition [17]. For women, the risk is increased due to difficulty in diagnosing STIs which are often asymptomatic in presentation [18], thus making treatment difficult [16]. A study by Ramjee *et al.* [5] determined the prevalence of STIs (such as *Neisseria Gonorrhea, Chlamydia Trachomatis, Syphilis,* and *Trichomonas Vaginalis)* at 4 clinical trials sites namely Durban and Hlabisa (South Africa), Lusaka (Zambia) and Moshi (Tanzania). The study showed that women at the South African sites were 3 times more likely to acquire an STI than participants at the Tanzanian and Zambian sites. Studies on HIV/STI "hot spots" among women in communities in the greater Durban area in the province of KwaZulu-Natal (South Africa) theorize an overlap of prevalence and incidence of these infections, suggesting increased risk of HIV acquisition in STI/HIV "hot spot" areas within these communities [19].

Hormones such as progesterone are reported to be playing a role in a woman's biological vulnerability to HIV infection. Observational evidence suggests that progesterone containing injectable contraception depot medroxyprogesterone acetate (DMPA) may be putting women at higher risk of HIV acquisition [20-23]. There is however some conflicting studies which have not observed this risk [24-26]. Injectable contraception is one of the most widely used contraceptive methods of choice among women in SSA, the use of which is on the rise in certain countries such as Kenya, Madagascar and Malawi [27]. Based on conflicting evidence on the role of DMPA on HIV acquisition, the World Health Organization (WHO) released a statement recommending that women on hormonal injectable progestin contraception should be counseled to use condoms in conjunction with pregnancy prevention methods to prevent HIV acquisition [28].

Studies in Uganda, Rwanda and Zimbabwe have shown that pregnant women are at a higher risk of HIV infection than lactating or other women, possibly due to physiological changes that a woman undergoes during pregnancy [29]. High levels of oestrogen and progesterone either during pregnancy or from exogenous sources could cause changes in the structure of the genital mucosa or cause immunological changes, such as an increase in mucosal lymphoid aggregates or hormone-induced overexpression of co-receptors associated with HIV infection. Increased levels of oestrogen are also associated with cervical ectopy in young women which in turn increases risk to HIV infection [29].

Supporting evidence suggests that women have a window of vulnerability approximately seven to ten days after ovulation in their menstrual cycle in which the potential for viral infectivity in the female reproductive tract is increased. This is due to the suppressing influence of sex hormones on the innate, humoral and cell-mediated immune systems. This takes place in the upper and lower female reproductive tract, and overlaps with the upregulation of co-receptors for HIV uptake and the recruitment of potentially infectable cells [30].

Contextual variability in risk

For women in SSA, probabilities of HIV exposure, acquisition and transmission is influenced by a range of factors such as infectiousness of the male partner according to the stage of the disease, or presence of ulcers in the male partner in the event of unprotected sexual intercourse. At a broader societal level, several factors influence the scale and rate of the epidemic spread such as overall HIV and STI prevalence, sexual practices, marriage and other cultural norms including structural factors not in control of the individual.

The dominant patriarchal culture and society in Africa exacerbates women's inferiority and their disparate health status. Here, the needs and desires of women are not considered significant and often women play no part in sexual decision making, nor are they allowed to express their sexuality [31,32]. There may be violent consequences if a woman were to take the initiative in sex, suggest condom use or refuse sexual advances [31]. In certain cultures men are regarded as the heads of the family, decision-makers and the ones who control resources and finances while women are expected to respect their husbands, accept polygamous relationships and fulfill family and community tasks [33]. Cultural expectations of masculinity encourage men to assume the patriarchal attitude that wives, partners and daughters are the possessions of men, and most husbands expect or demand their conjugal 'rights' [33]. One cultural practice that perpetuates the idea that a woman is her husband's property is "bride payments", where the bride's family receives financial compensation from the potential husband. Due to the issue of bride payment or "lobola" many men in relationships are unable to "pay" for the woman they would like to marry resulting in many men moving from one relationship to another leaving the woman (more likely with his children) to economically fend for herself and the children [34,35]. Women then look for other partners resulting in a complex web of cultural practice and multiple partnerships placing both men and women at high risk of HIV infection.

In countries such as Malawi, Kenya, Zambia, and Botswana, it is widely believed that a widow becomes unclean after her late husband's burial ceremonies. In cleansing rituals, an unprotected sexual act is believed to purify the recipient through the semen entering the woman's body [36]. Community elders identify a man with whom the widow has to have sex; someone who has often had several sexual partners in the process of cleansing others. These practices often put widowed women at greater risk of HIV and other STI infection [36]. The ritual is also practiced in other situations, such as after a birth the mother, regardless of marital status, has unprotected sex with a man believing the act will cleanse the baby and encourage health; after miscarriage; and where a man has acquired a boat for fishing, a woman has sex with the man to cleanse away evil spirits which may capsize the boat [36]. Sexual cleansing is also believed to 'cleanse' people living with HIV; in some African countries it is believed that sex with a virgin can cure the disease [16,36].

The practice of "dry sex" is reportedly high in some southern African countries [36]. This practice involves inserting drying agents into the vagina (herbs, a dry cloth, or even chemicals) to produce the required tight, dry and "hot" vagina. This practice is believed to provide heightened sexual pleasure for the male partner. For women, it causes friction and possible tearing of delicate vaginal mucosal lining, increasing the risk of HIV acquisition. Use of harmful chemicals can cause inflammation and lesions and alter the natural vaginal pH level, potentially increasing women's risk of contracting HIV. However, no studies have confirmed the role of "dry sex" in HIV acquisition [29,36,37]. Deeply entrenched traditional and cultural practices; often interwoven with religious beliefs make change in behaviour very difficult and complex [36].

Virginity testing, (a physical examination of girls and women to determine whether the hymen is unbroken), is now widely regarded as a human rights abuse. Although virginity testing was a common traditional practice among unmarried couples in South Africa and Uganda, it was, until recently, no longer commonplace. However, in an attempt to promote abstinence among girls, this practice has seen resurgence [36]. A concern with this 'forced abstinence' is that girls and unmarried women may engage in risky anal sex to avoid failing virginity tests, placing them at even higher risk of HIV acquisition [36].

In many African countries, young girls are encouraged or forced to marry older men [36,38] which can make young girls vulnerable to HIV infection in several ways. The change from virginity to frequent unprotected sex increases their risk of HIV infection. Even if they were sexually active prior to marriage, marriage usually drastically increases the frequency of unprotected sex [39]. In Malawi, for example, consent to sex is assumed within a marriage and therefore marital rape does not exist [31,36]. Many African countries condone polygamy [38], which means that an adolescent bride is likely to be a second or third wife [39]. Women who marry as adolescents are also more likely to receive less formal education and have less exposure to HIV prevention messages [38,39]. A study in Durban, South Africa, demonstrated that if age of sexual debut was 15 or younger, the women were more likely to be HIV positive compared to women who had their sexual debut at the age of 21 or older (Hazard ratio of 1.97; 95% CI 1.07 to 3.63, $p = 0.029$) [40].

Socioeconomic vulnerabilities

In the last two decades, nearly all SSA countries have faced slowing economic growth which has influenced spending on social services [32]. This has further impoverished African populations, with increases in unemployment rates and the decrease in provision of social services, including education and health services. The deterioration of education, health, and other social services implies a loss of opportunities for HIV prevention [32], particularly in women.

Poverty is another driving force of HIV transmission in women [33]. Evidence from SSA, Asia and Latin America demonstrates that greater national-level income inequality is associated with higher HIV prevalence rates [41,42]. Low economic status has been associated with earlier sexual experience, lower condom use at last sex act, having multiple sex partners, increased chances that the first sex act is non-consensual, and a greater likelihood of having had transactional sex or physically forced sex [15]. Many women resort to transactional sex to sustain their livelihoods and young girls are often coerced into sexual activities with older men to survive [32,33]. Cash transfers among secondary school-aged young women in Malawi showed that such transfers can encourage women to reduce their risky sexual behaviour, and resulted in decreased teenage pregnancy, in addition to lower self-reported sexual activity [33]. In conditions of poverty, HIV risk becomes a low priority among people's daily concerns. Young people growing up in poor conditions have little access to schooling and therefore few prospects for their future. Sex becomes a way to pass time due to a lack of recreational facilities [32].

Transactional sex (sex for money) is common in SSA. Many women engage in sex work which is defined as the provision of sexual services in exchange for money, goods, or other benefits [43]. Globally, female sex workers (FSWs) are at high risk of HIV infection and are 13.5 times more likely to be living with HIV than other women [2]. An estimated fifteen percent of HIV in the general female adult population is attributable to (unsafe) female sex work. The region with the highest attributable fraction is SSA with

98,000 HIV-related deaths [44] compared to an estimated 106,000 deaths worldwide which are a result of female sex work [45]. FSW is an important contributor to HIV transmission and the global HIV burden. Studies from South Africa and Kenya suggest sex workers engage in high risk behavior such as dry sex [46,47] and anal sex (fetching a high price) which further increase their risk.

Behavioral vulnerabilities

It is well documented that behavioral change can lead to a decrease in HIV acquisition [48]. These include use of methods such as abstinence or delaying sexual debut, condoms, safe sex, monogamy, reduction in number of partners, voluntary counseling and testing etc. However abstinence is not an option for many women. A South African household survey showed that 7.8% of women aged 15–24 years had had sexual intercourse by the age of 14 [49]. An association has been shown between early age of sexual debut and ensuing risky sexual behaviors [50], such as having multiple partners and decreased contraceptive and condom use [51,52]. Studies in Africa demonstrated a correlation between having sex at an early age and the HIV incidence [53,54]. It is thought that the delay of sexual debut may have been one of the crucial changes in behavior which led to a decline in HIV infection in Uganda [40,55,56].

Concurrent partnerships are powerful transmitters of HIV in the community [57]. Concurrent sexual partnerships, with two or more partners, are common practices in Africa. Partner reduction and fidelity appear to be the main behavioral changes accountable for the decrease in Kenya's HIV infection rates. This fall in HIV infection rates as a result of partner reduction has also been observed Zimbabwe, Côte d'Ivoire, Malawi and Ethiopia [58].

The vulnerability to HIV infection increases by engaging in unprotected anal sex by 13 fold compared to oral sex [59]. This is primarily due to the fragility of the rectal mucosa [29]. Although it is difficult to ascertain the percentage of women who participate in heterosexual anal sex in Africa, some studies and surveys have shown that between five [60] and twelve per cent [61] of women in the general community in South Africa report engaging in anal sex. However, this practice could be as high as forty per cent in female sex workers [59]. Effective HIV prevention measures exist and have been successfully targeted at key populations in many settings. It is however difficult to attract this high risk population group due to the different settings in which the FSWs conduct their business. Regular surveillance, prevention and treatment of HIV among FSWs would benefit this often neglected vulnerable group and the general population as a whole [2].

Alcohol abuse in much of Africa is characterized by irregular episodes of heavy drinking, frequently in the form of weekend bingeing [29]. These drinking patterns may have independent effects on sexual decision-making, and on condom-negotiation skills and correct condom use. Studies have demonstrated that women with heavy episodic drinking patterns are more prone to use condoms inconsistently and incorrectly, experience sexual violence; and acquire an STI, including HIV [29,62].

Structural vulnerabilities

Many structural vulnerabilities place women at risk including gender inequality and gender based violence (GBV) [63], migration and health seeking related stigma [64]. Gender inequality is created and perpetuated in part by social norms that demand culturally appropriate roles and conduct for men and women [65]. Hierarchical gender roles such as notions of male sexual entitlement, the low social value and power of women, and ideas of manhood linked to the control of women result in lower levels of education among women; few public roles for women; the lack of family, social and legal support for women; and the lack of economic power for women [65,66]. Institutionalized economic inequalities keep money, land, and other resources out of women's reach, causing women to be financially dependent on men, more likely to practice transactional sex, less likely to be able to negotiate safe sex or condom use with a partner, and more at risk of violence [6,16,49,65,67].

Gender norms promote multiple concurrent sexual partners for men while women are expected to be monogamous and unquestioning of their partner's behavior [49,65]. However, recent data from several African studies show that many women are almost as likely as men to bring HIV into the partnership [68]. Sexual negotiation or refusal by a woman may result in suspicions of infidelity and result in intimate partner violence [49], which is often tolerated by these societies [65]. Women's sexual subordination exposes them to elevated reproductive health risks including maternal mortality, unsafe abortion, coerced sex and rape, STIs and HIV [63].

Violence against women is a global problem and a well-recognized risk factor for HIV and other STIs [16,63,69]. In certain countries, over 50% of women report physical assault by an intimate partner, with one third to one half of physically abused women also reporting sexual coercion [65,70]. Abusive men are more likely to have additional sexual partners unknown to their wives [69]. Experiences of sexual violence have also been associated with drug and alcohol use, early sexual debut, having multiple sexual partners, trading sex for money and drugs and less contraceptive use [66]. Women who live in poverty, younger women and uneducated women are especially affected by intimate partner violence [70-72]. A South African study found that 12% of new HIV infections in women were attributable to intimate partner violence [71], while GBV increased the risk of HIV infection by 55% in a Ugandan study [73].

Discrimination is often based on gender, race/ethnicity, sexual orientation, and HIV status [74]. Stigma and fear of status disclosure has been a large factor in individuals seeking HIV testing and subsequent treatment and care [33,75]. Stigma can occur at different levels, including community, interpersonal, legislative and institutional (e.g. workplaces, schools and health facilities) levels [75]. Women often suffer the heaviest burden of HIV stigma and discrimination, as they are often expected to uphold the moral traditions of their societies; being HIV infected is considered evidence that they have failed in this regard [33,74]. HIV positive women experience discrimination, stigma and other human rights violations within families and communities, by legal and social services, in health-care settings, and in their work environment. Health-care settings often refuse to provide information or provide the wrong information on HIV prevention and treatment, sexual and reproductive health, and family planning [33]. HIV positive women have also experienced the denial of services, lack of confidentiality, harsh and judgmental treatment, and lack of informed consent [33]. As a result of stigma, women are often reluctant to seek HIV testing and are not empowered to enact HIV prevention [74].

Migration trends in Africa vary in terms of their spatial, temporal and social characteristics. Many individuals migrate due to better job prospects or are forced to migrate due to political instability, war and famine [32]. Worldwide, mobile populations have higher HIV infection rates than non-mobile populations irrespective of HIV prevalence in the origin or destination location [74]. Mobility per se can encourage high risk sexual behavior and more than often migrants' social networking creates opportunities for sexual networking. Women are becoming more mobile and are migrating for economic survival. However in many cases, lack of education often restricts them to unskilled jobs such as informal trading, commercial sex work and domestic work among others. A study conducted in South Africa among migrant and non-migrant women showed that migrant women were older, more likely to be married and had more than one sexual partner and were less likely to use condoms compared to non-migrant women. Migrant women were 1.6 times more likely to be infected with HIV than non-migrants [76].

Urbanization has also fuelled the rapid spread of HIV. In SSA, urban HIV prevalence is higher than rural populations [32]. Urbanization replaces the traditional village norms for an urban modern culture with fewer restrictions on sexual behaviour and marriage. Additionally, the loss of culture and social networks are related to social problems such as drug abuse, which fosters high-risk behaviour [32]. Political conflicts and war are commonplace in Africa and affects the risk of HIV/AIDS by interrupting normal social and risk networks, increasing poverty and social instability and weakening or destroying medical infrastructure [74]. Military conflict can cause changes in risk behavior, and war or civil strife often cause massive displacements of people [74], interrupt social cohesion and relationships, and encourages promiscuity and commercial sex; forced migration of people from low HIV prevalence areas to areas of high HIV prevalence [32]. Women who are temporarily displaced or in transit as a result of war or violence are more likely to report having received goods or money for sex [62].

HIV prevention strategies targeted at women

Given the magnitude of women's vulnerability to HIV acquisition as described above, it is not surprising that there is a worldwide call to address the high HIV infection rates reported among women in SSA and elsewhere. Biomedical, behavioural and structural interventions have been investigated to reduce women's vulnerability to HIV acquisition but also HIV incidence in general.

Biomedical interventions

Male condoms in general remain the most effective method of HIV prevention. However condom use or negotiation thereof is not always in the woman's hands. Although female condoms are available, the use still requires negotiation. Thus female-initiated prevention methods have been investigated.

Microbicides are products with anti-HIV properties developed in numerous formulations for prevention of HIV. Microbicides were initially developed for vaginal application but are now also tested for rectal application [77]. Over the past decade several microbicides with varying actions such as membrane disruption activity (surfactants), prevention of virus attachment to target cells (polyanions), and buffering agents have been tested with limited success primarily due to lack of specificity against HIV and poor adherence to interventions by women [10,11,78-80]. More recently, products containing anti-retorviral (ARV) agents commonly used in HIV therapeutics were tested. A study of tenofovir based vaginal gel in South Africa showed a 39% (95% CI 6 to 60) reduction in HIV acquisition [81]. The greater the adherence to the product, the better was the efficacy in HIV prevention. Unfortunately the results were not replicated in a larger study conducted in several countries in SSA using the same gel [82]. The main reason for lack of efficacy was poor adherence. Further research is being undertaken to ascertain women's reluctance to use such interventions given the high risk of HIV acquisition in this region. A study with a long-acting vaginal ring with a drug called Dapivirine is currently ongoing (ASPIRE) [83]. Lessons from microbicide trials suggest the need to better understand social, cultural and traditional contexts of women in Africa while developing interventions for HIV prevention.

Success with research among HIV discordant couples showed a decrease in HIV acquisition when a negative partner in a dicordant partnership was provided with oral pre-exposure prophylaxis (PrEP). Partners taking oral tenofovir or tenofovir plus emtricitibine (Truvada) as prophlaxis had a reduced rate of HIV acquisition 67% (95% CI 44 to 81) and 75% (95% CI 55 to 87) respectively [84]. The higher the adherence the greater the efficacy. Unfortunately a study among women in east and southern Africa testing the same drug, Truvada, for HIV prevention did not show any efficacy in preventing HIV due to poor adherence to the study product [85].

Treatment with ARV for prevention (TasP) has been reported to be highly efficacious (96%) among both men and women in a discordant couple relationship where the positive partner was provided ARV treatment to reduce HIV transmission to the negative partner [86]. Thefore it appears that when both sexual partners have the knowledge of their HIV status and are targeted together for HIV prevention the intervention is likely to be aceptable and used.

Behavioral interventions

HIV counseling and testing is recognized as a critical component for all HIV prevention interventions. Testing provides the opportunity to identify people who are HIV positive and in need for treatment and care and can also identify people who are HIV negative and referred for HIV prevention and care. Regular HIV testing will be critical for prevention interventions using PrEP. HIV counseling and testing not only allows women, couples, and families to learn their HIV status and obtain personalized risk reduction counseling and further care appropriate to their status, but can also assist communities in addressing stigma and discrimination associated with HIV/ AIDS [87,88].

Peer education interventions in developing countries have shown a significant increase in HIV knowledge and increased condom use. However, these programs have shown only a moderate improvement of behavioral outcomes, with no significant effect on biological outcomes [89]. Kenyan peer educators were able to increase protected sex among sex workers by providing condoms; facilitating HIV testing, treatment and care facilities and providing STI and HIV education [90]. In South Africa, the Stepping Stones program used participatory learning approaches to build communication skills, knowledge, and risk awareness. The program saw a 33% reduction in Herpes simplex virus-2 (HSV-2) incidence and improved several reported risk behaviors in men, such as transactional sex and intimate partner violence, although no decrease in HIV incidence was noted [91]. In developing countries, many mass media interventions have targeted changing HIV-related knowledge, behaviors and attitudes. At least half of these studies which reported outcomes such as condom use, reduction in risky sexual behavior, awareness of the modes of HIV transmission, HIV risk perception, ability to negotiate condom use and sexual abstinence showed a positive impact on the knowledge of HIV transmission and the decrease of risky sexual behavior [92]. Zambia has implemented several health communication programs focusing on HIV prevention and people who had been exposed to these radio and television programs were more likely to have ever used a condom [93]. In Nigeria, mass-media campaigns via television, radio and printed advertisements to increase the use of family planning, HIV/AIDS services and child survival demonstrated that people were twice as likely to know that HIV risk is reduced by condoms and one and a half times as likely to discuss HIV with their partner if they had high exposure to the program [94].

It is widely known that women who have an early sexual debut participate in risky sexual behavior, such as having multiple partners, higher STI incidence and decreased condom and contraceptive use [51,52]. High level governmental encouragement of the delay of sexual debut could have contributed to the decline in Uganda's HIV infection [55,56].

Concurrent sexual partnerships are recognized as being significantly responsible for the transmission of STIs, particularly heterosexual HIV transmission. Evidence implies that concurrent partnerships can increase the size of an HIV epidemic, the speed at which it infects a population and its persistence within a population [57]. Uganda adopted a "Zero Grazing" campaign in the 1980's, where having concurrent partners was discouraged. This campaign showed a 50% reduction in the number of people reporting casual and multiple partners between 1989 and 1995 [58,95]. It is also believed that partner reduction and fidelity are the main behavioral changes responsible for the decline in Kenya's HIV infection rates. Similar behavior changes have been reported in Cote d'Ivoire, Zimbabwe, Ethiopia and Malawi which may be responsible for their decrease in HIV prevalence [58].

Structural interventions

Structural interventions attempt to change the social norms that worsen HIV vulnerability. The South African IMAGE project sought to decrease gender based HIV vulnerabilities such as sexual violence, women's lack of knowledge about HIV and its transmission and women's economic dependency on men. The study partnered with a local microfinance institution to permit women to participate in microenterprises, while providing them with HIV education and a forum to discuss action against gender-based violence. These women improved their household wellbeing and empowerment, in addition to the significant reduction in gender-based violence [64].

Microfinance programs attempt to ease poverty by offering access to credit, savings or business skills. In

South Africa, a study using an integrated curriculum of gender equity, anti-violence work and HIV/AIDS education together with an existing microfinance program demonstrated higher levels of HIV-related communication by women in addition to a 55% reduction in domestic violence. Women in this study were less likely to have had unprotected sex at their last sex act and more likely to have accessed HIV Counselling and Testing [96]. In Malawi, girls receiving cash transfers had a lower prevalence of HIV and HSV-2 than those who were not because of less sexual activity, delayed sexual debut, having younger and fewer partners and decreased transactional sex [88]. A Tanzanian trial suggested a 25% lower incidence of STIs in both women and men receiving monetary incentives [88]. A Kenyan project provided HIV and safe sex education, small business management training and startup funds to women engaged in sex work. The project showed an increased sense of pride and wellbeing, a decrease in the number of sexual partners and an increase in condom use [97]. In response to the increase in HIV incidence caused by migration, a project in Tanzania distributed and promoted condom use, raised HIV awareness, encouraged reduction in the overall number of sexual partners and encouraged peer-based STI/HIV education among truck drivers. The number of condoms distributed increased by 100 000 and HIV awareness among truck drivers increased [97].

Education reduces risk of HIV infection, boosts self-esteem, and provides alternatives for earning a livelihood [50]. Communities and individuals with greater school education may be at decreased risk of HIV infection due to the adoption of protective lifestyles and behaviour [98]. People with little or no education have limited access to safe-sex information. For example, condom use is associated with higher education levels [32]. Keeping young girls in school has also showed a reduction in their risk of contracting HIV. Studies show that the expansion of primary and secondary schooling for girls in southern Africa will help reduce their vulnerability to HIV [99].

Policy structural factors play a major role in HIV transmission and Uganda is the best example of successful policy changes and the link to decreased HIV transmission. The Ugandan government committed itself to extensive training of trainers, mass media, health education campaigns, countrywide messaging and district mobilization causing changes in sexual behavior, social norms and HIV prevalence [100]. Research in Uganda has demonstrated the connection between a country's government recognition of the importance of HIV and the subsequent development of better government interventions to HIV [97].

Conclusion

Convincing evidence from biological, epidemiological, sociocultural and structural challenges identify women's vulnerability to HIV infection in SSA. The evidence shows that women in SSA are at higher risk of HIV infection compared to their male counterparts. Through gender power dynamics, women are embedded in relationships which increase their risk even more. Other than personal behavior, several other issues such as structural influences are identified which are beyond women's control and are likely to affect women globally. Given the unacceptably high prevalence and incidence rates of HIV in young women in southern Africa, every effort to mitigate this risk is urgently needed with a combination of biomedical, behavioural and structural interventions targeted not only to the women but their sexual partner(s) as well. Recent advances in the HIV prevention field need to be stepped up by implementing appropriate HIV prevention packages taking into consideration the cultural environment, biological, socio-economic and structural risks facing women.

Competing interests

The authors declare that they have no competing interests.

Authors' contributions

Both GR and BD contributed to the drafting of the manuscript. Both authors read and approved the final manuscript.

Acknowledgements

Dr. Duduzile Ndwandwe for her assistance in preparing this manuscript.
Dr. Renee Street for her review of the final manuscript.

References

1. UNAIDS: *Report on the Global AIDS Epidemic.* Geneva, Switzerland: Joint United Nations Program on HIV/AIDS (UNAIDS); 2012.
2. UNAIDS: *Global Report on the Global AIDS epidemic.* Geneva, Switzerland: Joint United Nations Program on HIV/AIDS (UNAIDS); 2013.
3. UNAIDS: *Every minute, a young woman is infected with HIV.* Geneva, Switzerland: Joint United Nations Program on HIV/AIDS (UNAIDS); 2012.
4. UNAIDS: *World AIDS Day Report.* Geneva: UNAIDS; 2012.
5. Ramjee G, *et al*: **The value of site preparedness studies for future implementation of phase 2/IIb/III HIV prevention trials: experience from the HPTN 055 study.** *J Acquir Immune Defic Syndr* 2008, **47**(1):93–100. 10.1097/QAI.0b013e31815c71f7.
6. UNAIDS: *How Africa turned AIDS around.* 2013.
7. Rehle TM, *et al*: **A decline in new HIV infections in South Africa: estimating HIV incidence from three national HIV surveys in 2002, 2005 and 2008.** *PloS One* 2010, **5**(6):e11094.
8. Karim QA, *et al*: **Stabilizing HIV prevalence masks high HIV incidence rates amongst rural and urban women in KwaZulu-Natal, South Africa.** *Int J Epidemiol* 2011, **40**(4):922–930.
9. Ramjee G: *Zero new infections: a myth or reality, in 6th SA AIDS conference.* Durban, South Africa; 2013.
10. Karim SSA, *et al*: **Safety and effectiveness of BufferGel and 0.5% PRO2000 gel for the prevention of HIV infection in women.** *AIDS (London, England)* 2011, **25**(7):957.
11. McCormack S, *et al*: **PRO2000 vaginal gel for prevention of HIV-1 infection (Microbicides Development Programme 301): a phase 3, randomised, double-blind, parallel-group trial.** *Lancet* 2010, **376**(9749):1329–1337.
12. Wand H, Ramjee G: **Assessing and evaluating the combined impact of behavioural and biological risk factors for HIV seroconversion in a cohort of South African women.** *AIDS Care* 2012, **24**(9):1155–1162.
13. Wand H, Whitaker C, Ramjee G: **Geoadditive models to assess spatial variation of HIV infections among women in Local communities of Durban, South Africa.** *Int J Health Geogr* 2011, **10**(1):28.
14. Rehle T, Shisana O: *HSRC National Survey 6th SA AIDS Conference.* Durban; 2013.

15. Mabala R: **From HIV prevention to HIV protection: addressing the vulnerability of girls and young women in urban areas.** *Environ Urban* 2006, **18**(2):407–432.
16. Ackermann L, Klerk GW: **Social factors that make South African women vulnerable to HIV infection.** *Health Care Women Int* 2002, **23**(2):163–172.
17. Kalichman SC, Pellowski J, Turner C: **Prevalence of sexually transmitted co-infections in people living with HIV/AIDS: systematic review with implications for using HIV treatments for prevention.** *Sex Transm Infect* 2011, **87**(3):183–190.
18. Connolly CA, *et al*: **Incidence of sexually transmitted infections among HIV-positive sex workers in KwaZulu-Natal, South Africa.** *Sex Transm Dis* 2002, **29**(11):721–724.
19. Ramjee G, Wand H: **Geographical clustering of high risk sexual behaviors in "Hot-spots" for HIV and sexually transmitted infections in Kwazulu-Natal, South Africa.** *AIDS Behav* 2013, 1–6. DOI: 10.1007/s10461-013-0578-x.
20. Baeten JM, *et al*: **Hormonal contraceptive use, herpes simplex virus infection, and risk of HIV-1 acquisition among Kenyan women.** *Aids* 2007, **21**(13):1771–1777.
21. Ramjee G, Wand H: **Population-level impact of hormonal contraception on incidence of HIV infection and pregnancy in women in Durban, South Africa.** *Bull World Health Organ* 2012, **90**(10):748–755.
22. Heffron R, *et al*: **Use of hormonal contraceptives and risk of HIV-1 transmission: a prospective cohort study.** *Lancet Inf Dis* 2012, **12**(1):19–26.
23. Wand H, Ramjee G: **The effects of injectable hormonal contraceptives on HIV seroconversion and on sexually transmitted infections.** *Aids* 2012, **26**(3):375–380.
24. Kleinschmidt I, *et al*: **Injectable progestin contraceptive use and risk of HIV infection in a South African family planning cohort.** *Contraception* 2007, **75**(6):461–467.
25. Myer L, *et al*: **Prospective study of hormonal contraception and women's risk of HIV infection in South Africa.** *Int J Epidemiol* 2007, **36**(1):166–174.
26. Kiddugavu M, *et al*: **Hormonal contraceptive use and HIV-1 infection in a population-based cohort in Rakai, Uganda.** *Aids* 2003, **17**(2):233–240.
27. Adetunji J: **Rising popularity of injectable contraceptives in sub-Saharan Africa.** *African Popul Stud* 2011, **25**(2):587–604.
28. Organization WH: *Hormonal contraception and HIV: technical statement.* Geneva, Switzerland: World Health Organization; 2012.
29. Chersich MF, Rees HV: **Vulnerability of women in southern Africa to infection with HIV: biological determinants and priority health sector interventions.** *Aids* 2008, **22**:S27–S40.
30. Wira CR, Fahey JV: **A new strategy to understand how HIV infects women: identification of a window of vulnerability during the menstrual cycle.** *AIDS (London, England)* 2008, **22**(15):1909.
31. Duffy L: **Culture and context of HIV prevention in rural Zimbabwe: the influence of gender inequality.** *J Transcult Nurs* 2005, **16**(1):23–31.
32. Buvé A, Bishikwabo-Nsarhaza K, Mutangadura G: **The spread and effect of HIV-1 infection in sub-Saharan Africa.** *Lancet* 2002, **359**(9322):2011–2017.
33. UN: *Women out loud: How women living with HIV will help the world ends AIDS, in United Nations Joint Programme on HIV/AIDS.* Geneva, Switzerland: Joint United Nations Program on HIV/AIDS (UNAIDS); 2012.
34. Mfecane S: **Living with HIV as a man: implications for masculinity.** *Psychol Soc* 2008, **36**:45–59.
35. Montgomery CM, *et al*: **Men's involvement in the South African family: engendering change in the AIDS era.** *Soc Sci Med* 2006, **62**(10):2411–2419.
36. Maleche A, Day E: *Traditional cultural practices and HIV: reconciling culture and human rights.* Working Paper for the Third Meeting of the Technical Advisory Group of the Global Commission on HIV and the Law, 7–9 July 2011. 2011. http://kelinkenya.org/wp-content/uploads/2010/10/TRADITIONAL-CULTURAL-PRACTICESHIV-RECONCILING-CULTURE-AND-HUMAN-RIGHTS.pdf.
37. Hilber AM, *et al*: **Intravaginal practices, vaginal infections and HIV acquisition: systematic review and meta-analysis.** *PLoS One* 2010, **5**(2):e9119.
38. Samuels F, Blake C, Akinrimisi B: *HIV vulnerabilities and the potential for strengthening social protection responses in the context of HIV in Nigeria.* London, UK: The Overseas Development Institute; 2012.
39. Clark S, Bruce J, Dude A: **Protecting young women from HIV/AIDS: the case against child and adolescent marriage.** *International Family Planning Perspectives* 2006, **32**(2):79–88.
40. Wand H, Ramjee G: **The relationship between age of coital debut and HIV seroprevalence among women in Durban, South Africa: a cohort study.** *BMJ Open* 2012, **2**:e000285.
41. Gillespie S, Kadiyala S, Greener R: **Is poverty or wealth driving HIV transmission?** *Aids* 2007, **21**:S5–S16.
42. Piot P, Greener R, Russell S: **Squaring the circle: AIDS, poverty, and human development.** *PLoS Med* 2007, **4**(10):e314.
43. Vandepitte J, *et al*: **Estimates of the number of female sex workers in different regions of the world.** *Sex Transm Infect* 2006, **82**(Suppl 3):iii18–iii25.
44. WHO: *Preventing HIV among sex workers in sub-Saharan Africa: a literature review.* Geneva: WHO; 2011.
45. Pruss-Ustun A, *et al*: **HIV due to female sex work: regional and global estimates.** *PLoS One* 2013, **8**(5):e63476.
46. Schwandt M, *et al*: **Anal and dry sex in commercial sex work, and relation to risk for sexually transmitted infections and HIV in Meru, Kenya.** *Sex Transm Infect* 2006, **82**(5):392–396.
47. Luseno WK, *et al*: **Substance use, sexual risk, and violence: HIV prevention intervention with sex workers in Pretoria.** *AIDS Behav* 2006, **10**(2):131–137.
48. Coates TJ, Richter L, Caceres C: **Behavioural strategies to reduce HIV transmission: how to make them work better.** *Lancet* 2008, **372** (9639):669–684.
49. Pettifor AE, *et al*: **Sexual power and HIV risk, South Africa.** *Emerg Inf Dis* 2004, **10**(11):1996.
50. Glynn JR, *et al*: **Age at menarche, schooling, and sexual debut in northern Malawi.** *PLoS One* 2010, **5**(12):e15334.
51. Greenberg J, Magder L, Aral S: **Age at first coitus a marker for risky sexual behavior in women.** *Sex Transm Dis* 1992, **19**(6):331–334.
52. Manning WD, Longmore MA, Giordano PC: **The relationship context of contraceptive use at first intercourse.** *Family Planning Perspectives* 2000, **32**(3):104–110.
53. Boileau C, *et al*: **Sexual and marital trajectories and HIV infection among ever-married women in rural Malawi.** *Sex Transm Infect* 2009, **85**(Suppl 1):i27–i33.
54. Pettifor AE, *et al*: **Early age of first sex: a risk factor for HIV infection among women in Zimbabwe.** *Aids* 2004, **18**(10):1435–1442.
55. Laga M, *et al*: **To stem HIV in Africa, prevent transmission to young women.** *Aids* 2001, **15**(7):931–934.
56. Asiimwe-Okiror G, *et al*: **Change in sexual behaviour and decline in HIV infection among young pregnant women in urban Uganda.** *Aids* 1997, **11**(14):1757–1763.
57. Mah TL, Halperin DT: **Concurrent sexual partnerships and the HIV epidemics in Africa: evidence to move forward.** *AIDS Behav* 2010, **14**(1):11–16.
58. Potts M, *et al*: **Reassessing HIV prevention.** *Science* 2008, **320**(5877):749.
59. Karim SS, Ramjee G: **Anal sex and HIV transmission in women.** *Am J Public Health* 1998, **88**(8):1265–1266.
60. Lane T, *et al*: **Heterosexual anal intercourse increases risk of HIV infection among young South African men.** *Aids* 2006, **20**(1):123–125.
61. Simbayi LC, *et al*: **Risk factors for HIV-AIDS among youth in Cape Town, South Africa.** *AIDS Behav* 2005, **9**(1):53–61.
62. Scorgie F, *et al*: **Socio-demographic characteristics and behavioral risk factors of female sex workers in sub-saharan Africa: a systematic review.** *AIDS Behav* 2012, **16**(4):920–933.
63. Murphy EM, *et al*: **Was the "ABC" approach (abstinence, being faithful, using condoms) responsible for Uganda's decline in HIV?** *PLoS Med* 2006, **3**(9):e379.
64. Gupta GR, *et al*: **Structural approaches to HIV prevention.** *Lancet* 2008, **372**(9640):764–775.
65. Gupta GR: **How men's power over women fuels the HIV epidemic: It limits women's ability to control sexual interactions.** *Br Med J* 2002, **324**(7331):183.
66. Jewkes RK, Levin JB, Penn-Kekana LA: **Gender inequalities, intimate partner violence and HIV preventive practices: findings of a South African cross-sectional study.** *Soc Sci Med* 2003, **56**(1):125–134.
67. Leclerc-Madlala S: **Age-disparate and intergenerational sex in southern Africa: the dynamics of hypervulnerability.** *Aids* 2008, **22**:S17–S25.
68. Serwadda D, *et al*: **The social dynamics of HIV transmission as reflected through discordant couples in rural Uganda.** *Aids* 1995, **9**(7):745–750.

69. Higgins JA, Hoffman S, Dworkin SL: **Rethinking gender, heterosexual men, and women's vulnerability to HIV/AIDS.** *Am J Public Health* 2010, **100** (3):435–445.
70. Kim J, *et al*: **Exploring the role of economic empowerment in HIV prevention.** *Aids* 2008, **22**:S57–S71.
71. Jewkes RK, *et al*: **Intimate partner violence, relationship power inequity, and incidence of HIV infection in young women in South Africa: a cohort study.** *Lancet* 2010, **376**(9734):41–48.
72. Campbell JC, *et al*: **The intersection of intimate partner violence against women and HIV/AIDS: a review.** *Int J Inj Contr Saf Promot* 2008, **15**(4):221–231.
73. Vyas S, Watts C: **How does economic empowerment affect women's risk of intimate partner violence in low and middle income countries? A systematic review of published evidence.** *J Int Dev* 2009, **21**(5):577–602.
74. Poundstone K, Strathdee S, Celentano D: **The social epidemiology of human immunodeficiency virus/acquired immunodeficiency syndrome.** *Epidemiol Rev* 2004, **26**(1):22–35.
75. Pulerwitz J, *et al*: **Reducing HIV-related stigma: lessons learned from Horizons research and programs.** *Public Health Rep* 2010, **125**(2):272–281.
76. Lurie MN, *et al*: **The impact of migration on HIV-1 transmission in South Africa: a study of migrant and nonmigrant men and their partners.** *Sex Trans Dis* 2003, **30**(2):149–156.
77. McGowan I: **Rectal microbicides: a new focus for HIV prevention.** *Sex Transm Infect* 2008, **84**(6):413–417.
78. Van Damme L, *et al*: **Effectiveness of COL-1492, a nonoxynol-9 vaginal gel, on HIV-1 transmission in female sex workers: a randomised controlled trial.** *Lancet* 2002, **360**(9338):971–977.
79. Skoler-Karpoff S, *et al*: **Efficacy of Carraguard for prevention of HIV infection in women in South Africa: a randomised, double-blind, placebo-controlled trial.** *Lancet* 2008, **372**(9654):1977–1987.
80. Van Damme L, *et al*: **Lack of effectiveness of cellulose sulfate gel for the prevention of vaginal HIV transmission.** *N Engl J Med* 2008, **359**(5):463–472.
81. Abdool Karim Q, *et al*: **Effectiveness and safety of tenofovir gel, an antiretroviral microbicide, for the prevention of HIV infection in women.** *Science* 2010, **329**(5996):1168–1174.
82. Marrazzo J, *et al*: **Pre-exposure prophylaxis for HIV in women: daily oral tenofovir, oral tenofovir/emtricitabine, or vaginal tenofovir gel in the VOICE Study (MTN 003).** In *20th Conference on Retroviruses and Opportunistic infections.* Atlanta, USA: 2013 CROI conference; 2013.
83. *Network, M.T. MTN 020. 09 October 2013.* Available from: http://www.mtnstopshiv.org/studies/3614.
84. Baeten JM, *et al*: **Antiretroviral prophylaxis for HIV prevention in heterosexual men and women.** *N Engl J Med* 2012, **367**(5):399–410.
85. Van Damme L, *et al*: **Preexposure prophylaxis for HIV infection among African women.** *N Engl J Med* 2012, **367**(5):411–422.
86. Cohen MS, *et al*: **Prevention of HIV-1 infection with early antiretroviral therapy.** *N Engl J Med* 2011, **365**(6):493–505.
87. Grabbe KL, *et al*: **Increasing access to HIV counseling and testing through mobile services in Kenya: Strategies, utilization and cost-effectiveness.** *J Acquir Immune Defic Syndr* 2010, **54**(3):317.
88. Padian NS, *et al*: **HIV prevention transformed: the new prevention research agenda.** *Lancet* 2011, **378**(9787):269–278.
89. Medley A, *et al*: **Effectiveness of peer education interventions for HIV prevention in developing countries: a systematic review and meta-analysis.** *AIDS Educ Prev* 2009, **21**(3):181–206.
90. Luchters S, *et al*: **Impact of five years of peer-mediated interventions on sexual behavior and sexually transmitted infections among female sex workers in Mombasa, Kenya.** *BMC public health* 2008, **8**(1):143.
91. Jewkes R, *et al*: **Impact of stepping stones on incidence of HIV and HSV-2 and sexual behaviour in rural South Africa: cluster randomised controlled trial.** *Br Med J* 2008, **337**:a506. doi:10.1136/bmj.a506.
92. Bertrand JT, *et al*: **Systematic review of the effectiveness of mass communication programs to change HIV/AIDS-related behaviors in developing countries.** *Health Educ Res* 2006, **21**(4):567–597.
93. Van Rossem R, Meekers D: **The reach and impact of social marketing and reproductive health communication campaigns in Zambia.** *BMC Public health* 2007, **7**(1):352.
94. Keating J, Meekers D, Adewuyi A: **Assessing effects of a media campaign on HIV/AIDS awareness and prevention in Nigeria: results from the VISION Project.** *BMC Public health* 2006, **6**(1):123.
95. Shelton JD, *et al*: **Partner reduction is crucial for balanced "ABC" approach to HIV prevention.** *Br Med J* 2004, **328**(7444):891.
96. Dworkin SL, Blankenship K: **Microfinance and HIV/AIDS prevention: assessing its promise and limitations.** *AIDS Behav* 2009, **13**(3):462–469.
97. Parker RG, Easton D, Klein CH: **Structural barriers and facilitators in HIV prevention: a review of international research.** *Aids* 2000, **14**:S22–S32.
98. Gregson S, *et al*: **Community group participation: Can it help young women to avoid HIV? An exploratory study of social capital and school education in rural Zimbabwe.** *Soc Sci Med* 2004, **58**(11):2119–2132.
99. Jukes M, Simmons S, Bundy D: **Education and vulnerability: the role of schools in protecting young women and girls from HIV in southern Africa.** *Aids* 2008, **22**:S41–S56.
100. Slutkin G, *et al*: **How Uganda reversed its HIV epidemic.** *AIDS Behav* 2006, **10**(4):351–360.

3

Prevalence of intestinal parasites and associated risk factors among HIV/AIDS patients with pre-ART and on-ART attending dessie hospital ART clinic, Northeast Ethiopia

Assefa Missaye[1], Mulat Dagnew[2*], Abebe Alemu[3] and Agersew Alemu[3]

Abstract

Background: Intestinal parasites are a major concern in most developing countries where HIV/AIDS case are concentrate and almost 80% of AIDS patients die of AIDS-related infections. In the absence of ART, HIV/AIDS patients in developing countries unfortunately continue to suffer from the consequences of opportunistic parasites. But this prevalence has dramatically decreased in countries where antiretroviral agents are widely available. Therefore, the aim of this study was to assess the prevalence of intestinal parasite and risk factor among pre- ART and on ART adult HIV/ AIDS patients attending ART clinic in Dessie hospital.

Methods: A comparative cross-sectional study was conducted among pre-ART and on ART adult HIV/AIDS patients of Dessie Hospital. A total of 272 (136 from each group) study subjects were selected by using systematic random sampling. Stool sample was collected and processed using direct wet mount, formol-ether concentration technique and modified Ziehl-Neelson staining techniques. A structured questionnaire was used to collect data on Sociodemographic & associated risk factors. Data was entered and analyzed by using SPSS 16 software and logistic regressions were applied to assess any association between explanatory factors and outcome variables.

Results: The overall prevalence of IP in pre-ART and on-ART was 39% and 17.6%, respectively with significant decrease of intestinal parasite in the ART era ($p < 0.001$). All *Cryptosporidium* spps infections were found in the pre-ART patients and significantly associated for lower CD4 <200cells/mm^3. Absence of toilet (AOR = 7.57; 95% CI = 1.3,44.22), source of water (AOR = 6.03; 95% CI = 1.14,31.98), living condition (AOR = 13.29, 95% CI = 5.14, 34.35); WHO stage (AOR = 6.06; 95% CI = 2.49,14.74) and ART status (AOR = 7.55; 95% CI = 3.24,17.59) have significant association with prevalence of intestinal parasite.

Conclusion: The overall prevalence of IP was differ by ART status and opportunistic parasite like *cryptosporidium spps* were found in low CD4 counts in ART naive patients. This study identified some environmental and some clinical finding as determinant factor for IP infections. Therefore, public health measures and adherence to ART should be strengthened to improve the quality of life of these patients.

Keywords: Intestinal parasite, ART, CD4

* Correspondence: dagnewmulat@gmail.com
[2]Department of Medical Microbiology, School of Biomedical and Laboratory Sciences, College of Medicine and Health Sciences, University of Gondar, Gondar, Ethiopia
Full list of author information is available at the end of the article

Background

Intestinal parasitic infections which are caused either by protozoa or helminths or both are among the most widespread of human infections worldwide. It is estimated that as much as 60% of the World's population is infected with intestinal parasites which may play a significant role in morbidity due to intestinal infections [1]. The rate of infection is also remarkably high in Sub-Saharan Africa, where the majority of Human Immune Deficiency Virus (HIV) /Acquired Immunodeficiency Syndrome (AIDS) cases are concentrated where factors including poverty and malnutrition could promote transmission of both infections in the region [2].

Like in many other developing countries, intestinal parasites are widely distributed in Ethiopia largely due to the low level of environmental and personal hygiene, contamination of food and drinking water that results from improper disposal of human excreta [3]. Intestinal parasites as a major concern in most developing countries have been pronounced with the co-occurrence of malnutrition and HIV/AIDS. Opportunistic parasitic infections are a common feature in HIV/AIDS infections where almost 80% of AIDS patients die of AIDS-related infections including intestinal parasites rather than of the HIV infection itself which usually occur late in the course of HIV infection when Cluster of Differeation (CD4) + T-cell count has been severely depleted mostly below 200cells/mm3 [4-6].

In the absence of Anti Retroviral Therapy (ART) HIV/AIDS patients in developing countries unfortunately continue to suffer the consequences of opportunistic parasites [7]. Patients enrolling into ART programmes with very low CD4 cell counts have heightened risk of morbidity and mortality before ART [8]. There is evidence that the control of these opportunistic parasitic infections in HIV-positive persons under HAART is also induced by the inhibition of the aspartylprotease of the parasites and by the reconstitution of the immune system of the patient [9,10]. However, patients in resource limited settings typically start ART programmes with advanced symptomatic disease and very low blood CD4 cell counts which predisposes them to high rates of both clinical and subclinical opportunistic infections [8]. Therefore, this study was aimed to assess the prevalence of intestinal parasites and associated risk factors in both pre-ART and ART patients in Dessie hospital.

Materials and methods

Study design, period and area

A comparative cross-sectional study was conducted from February 1 to April 30, 2012. The study was carried out in Dessie Hospital (DH) ART clinic, South Wollo zone of Amhara regional state, Northeast Ethiopia. Dessie Hospital is found in Dessie town with a distance of 400 km from the capital city of the county, Addis Ababa. According to the 2007 population and housing census, the town had total population of 151,094 and among these, 72,891 was males and 78,203 were females [11]. Dessie Hospital was founded in 1962 and has 17 departments with 300 beds. The Hospital is giving service for 14,114 pre-ART and 10,484 on-ART HIV/AIDS patients.

Sample size and sampling techniques

Epidemiological Information (EpiInfo) soft ware was used for sample size determination and it gave a sample size of 136 for pre-ART and 136 for on-ART with total sample size of 272 by taking proportion from previous study: Proportion of pre-ART (p1) = 43.5%, Proportion of on-ART (p2) = 24.5%, Odds =2 [12] for pre-ART and on-ART respectively, Marginal error (w) = 5%.

A systematic random sampling technique was used by considering Dessie hospital ART clinic on average gave ART service for 25 pre-ART and 75 for ART adults per day. Since the sample collection period for this study was for two months, the total amount of adult pre-ART and on-ART HIV/AIDS patients that came to the hospital for service was 1500 (N1) and 4500 (N2) respectively and to determine K, the following formula was used, K1 (for pre-ART) = N1/n1 = 1500/136 = 11, so every 11th pre-ART adult HIV/AIDS patients that came to the ART clinic from January to March was included in the sample until the required sample was achieved. Similarly K2(for on-ART) = N2/n2 = 4500/136 = 33 for on-ART adult HIV/AIDS patients, so every 33th on-ART adult HIV/AIDS patients came to the ART clinic from February to March was included in the sample until the required sample was achieved.

Operational definitions

Pre-ART patients: The person who were found HIV positive but not eligible for ART.

ART patients-The person who were found HIV positive, eligible and started ART already.

Good living condition-low degree of crowding, tape water supply, proper disposal of excreta and cemented and finished type of floor.

Data collection and processing

A pre-tested structured questionnaire was utilized to collect socio-demographic characteristics, clinical information and other risk factors. The questionnaires were pretested and validated before two weeks in the study time in Selam private Hospital in Dessie on 20 HIV positive patients. A single fresh stool was collected with a labelled stool cup from 272 study participants following standard procedures by laboratory technologist who worked at the ART clinic. A direct saline and iodine wet mount of each sample was used to detect intestinal parasites microscopically. The wet mounts were examined under light microscope at 100 and 400× magnifications [13].

Formol ether concentration method

A portion of each fresh stool sample was taken and processed. Briefly, 1 g of stool was placed in a clear 15 ml conical centrifuge tube containing 7 ml formalin saline by using applicator stick. The resulting suspension was filtered through a sieve into another conical tube. After adding 3 ml of diethyl ether to the formalin solution, the content was centrifuged at 3200 rpm form 3 minutes. The supernatant was poured away and the tube was replaced in its track. Finally, smear was prepared from the sediment and observed under light microscope with a magnification of 100× and 400× [13].

Modified ziehl neelsen staining method

A small portion of the fresh stool sample was processed for detection of opportunistic parasites using the Ziehl Neelsen method. Thin smear was prepared directly from sediment of concentrated stool and allowed to air dry. The slides were then fixed with methanol for 5 minutes and stained with carbol fuchsine for 30 minutes. After washing the slides in tap water, they were decolorized with acid alcohol for 1–3 minutes and stained in methylene blue for 1 minute. The slides were then washed in tap water and observed under light microscope with a magnification of 1000X (12).

Quality control and data analysis

Data collectors were trained and the questioners were pretested before the study time. After data collection process, the data were checked for completeness and any incomplete or misfiled questionnaires filed again. Then the result of laboratory examination was recorded on well prepared format carefully and finally attached with the questionnaire. Data were double entered and analyzed by using SPSS-16 database software programme. Descriptive statistics were used to give a clear picture of background variables like age, sex and other variables in well-structured questionnaire. The frequency distribution of both dependent and independent variables were worked out and the association between the independent and dependent variables were measured and tested using OR and 95% CI. The relative contribution of each selected variables to the outcome of interest were assessed using logistic regression.

Ethical consideration

Ethical clearance was obtained from University of Gondar College of Medicine and Health Sciences School of Biomedical and Laboratory Sciences ethical clearance committee. Permission to conduct the study was also obtained from Dessie Hospital ART clinic. Additionally, after explaining the importance, purpose and procedure of the study briefly a written consent was obtained from study participants. Anyone not willing to take part in the study had full right to do so and confidentiality of the study participants was also maintained. Any study participant who was positive for intestinal parasite was referred to physicians for treatment.

Results

Socio-demographic characteristics of the respondents

A total of 272 study participants were included for the analysis of this study. Out of these, 136 were pre-ART (group 1) and 136 were on-ART (group 2). Comparatively, in the Pre-ART and on-ART groups the distribution by sex revealed a predominance of female cases that was 82 (60%) and 78 (57.4%), respectively. The majority of pre-ART (67%) and on-ART (55%) study participants were in the age range of 18–35 years with median age of 32 years (range 18–65 years) and 35 years range (18–63 years); respectively. Majority of pre-ART and on-ART study participants 106 (78%) and 113 (83%) were urban residence; respectively. The assessment of educational status of HIV positives involved in the survey showed 42 (30.9%) of group 1 and 44 (32.4%) of group 2 were able to read and write. Moreover, 44.9% and 46.3% of group 1 and group 2 had <500 birr monthly income, respectively (Table 1).

Prevalence of intestinal parasite in pre-ART and on-ART adult HIV/AIDS patients

A total of 272 stool samples from both groups were examined for intestinal parasitic infections. The overall prevalence of IP in pre-ART was 39% and from these the prevalence of protozoan, helminthic and both protozoan and helminths were 31%, 7.4% and 0.7%; respectively. The prevalence of opportunistic intestinal parasites were 2.2% and from these 1.5% for *Cryptosporidium* spps followed by *I. belli* 0.7%. The most prevalent protozoan parasites and helminths in ART naïve patients were trophozoite of *E.histolytica/dispar* and *A. lumbricoides* with respective prevalence of 19.1% and 2.9% (Table 2).

The overall prevalence of IP among on-ART was 17.6% and from these the prevalence of protozoan, helminthic was 12.5% and 5.1%, respectively. But none of the ART patients were indentified with opportunistic parasites and mixed infection (both protozoan and helminthic infection). The most prevalent protozoan parasites and helminths among ART patients were trophozoite of *E.histolytica/dispar* and *A.lumbricoides* with respective prevalence of 5.1% and 2.2%. The overall prevalence of IP in the pre-ART (39%) was higher when compared to ART groups (17.5%) indicating statistically significant decrease of intestinal parasite in ART patients ($p < 0.001$) (Table 2).

Table 1 Associations of sociodemographic factors of adult HIV patients with prevalence of intestinal parasite by ART status using binary logistic regression in Dessie Hospital ART clinic, Feb.-March 2012 (N = 272)

VARIABLES	Intestinal parasite prevalence						COR (95% CI)
	Pre-ART n = 136		On-ART n = 136		Total N = 272		
	Positive n (%)	Negative n (%)	Positive n (%)	Negative n (%)	Positive n (%)	negative n (%)	
Age groups							
18-35 yrs	34(37.4)	57(62.6)	15(20)	60(80)	49(30)	117(70)	1. 26(0. 25, 6.4)
36-53 yrs	17(40.5)	25(59.5)	9(16.1)	47(83.9)	26(26.5)	72(73.5)	1.08(0.21, 5.7)
54-65 yrs	2(66.7)	1(33.3)	0(0)	5(0)	2(25)	6(75)	1*
Sex							
Male	20(37)	34(63)	12(20.7)	46(79.3)	32(28.6)	80(71.4)	1*
Female	33(40.2)	49(59.8)	12(15.4)	66(84.6)	45(28)	115(72)	0.98(0.57, 1.7)
Residence							
Urban	41(38.7)	65(61.3)	14(12.4)	99(87.6)	55(25)	164(75)	1*
Rural	12(40)	18(60)	10(43.5)	13(56.5)	22(41.5)	31(58.5)	2.12(1.13,4.0)**
Marital status							
Single	22(42.3)	30(57.7)	4(9.3)	39(90.7)	26(27.4)	69(72.6)	0.93(0.53,1.62)
Married	31(36.9)	53(63.1)	20(21.5)	73(78.5)	51(29)	126(71)	1*
Educational Status							
Illiterate	1(33.3)	2(66.7)	2(16.7)	10(83.3)	3(20)	12(80)	1.44(.28, 7.5)
Read and write	19(45.2)	23(54.8)	6(13.6)	38(86.4)	25(29.1)	61(70.9)	2.36(.74,7.51)
Primary education	16(37.2)	27(62.8)	10(29.4)	24(70.6)	26(33.8)	51(66.2)	2.93(.92, 9.37)
Secondary education	13(38.2)	21(61.8)	6(18.2)	27(81.8)	19(28.4)	48(71.6)	2.28(.69,7.46)
College and above	4(28.6)	10(71.4)	0(0)	13(100)	4(14.8)	23(85.2)	1*
Occupation							
Gov't employer	13(38.2)	21(61.8)	6(19.4)	25(80.6)	19(29.2)	46(70.8)	1*
Merchant	8(42.1)	11(57.9)	0(0)	9(100)	8(28.6)	20(71.4)	.97(0.36,2.58)
Farmer	10(58.8)	7(41.2)	9(42.9)	12(57.1)	19(50)	19(50)	2.42(1.06,5.56)**
Student	1(33.3)	2(66.7)	0(0)	2(100)	1(20)	4(80)	.61(0.06,5.78)
Daily laborers	11(45.8)	13(54.2)	3(12)	22(88)	14(28.6)	34(71.4)	.97(0.43, 2.19)
House wife	4(36.4)	7(63.6)	2(10.5)	17(89.5)	6(20)	24(80)	.61(.21,1.72)
Others	6(21.4)	22(78.6)	4(13.8)	25(86.2)	10(17.5)	47(82.5)	.52(.22,1.2)
Income							
<500 birr	25(41)	36(59)	7(11.1)	56(88.9)	32(25.8)	92(74.5)	.93(.43-2.02)
500-1000 birr	18(35.3)	33(64.7)	15(28.3)	38(71.7)	33(31.7)	71(68.3)	1.24(.57, 2.7)
>1000 birr	10(41.7)	14(58.3)	2(10)	18(90)	12(27.3)	32(72.7)	1*

Association of intestinal parasite with CD4 among pre-ART and on-ART adult HIV/AIDS patients

The study participants who were pre-ART consisted of 51 (37.5%) with CD4 count > 500 cells/mm^3, 56 (41.2%) with CD4 count 200–500 cells/mm^3 and 29 (21.3) patients with CD4 count < 200 cells/mm^3. All the three opportunistic parasites were found in ART naive patients <200 cells/mm^3 CD4 T-cell counts and from these all *Cryptosporidium spps* infections were significantly associated with < 200 cells/mm^3 CD4 T-cell counts (p = 0.024).

The study participants who were on-ART consisted of 47 patients (34.6%) with CD4 count > 500 cells/mm^3, 72 patients (52.9%) with CD4 count 200–500 cells/mm^3 and 17 patients (12.5%) with CD4 count < 200 cells/mm^3. Among the 17 on-ART patients with CD4 count < 200 cells /μl, parasites were identified in 9 (52.9%) patients

Table 2 Prevalence of intestinal parasites in HIV positive patients with regard to their ART status in Dessie referral Hospital ART clinic, February1 -March 30, 2012(N = 272)

Parasite identified	ART status		X^2	-value
	Pre-ART No (%)	On-ART No (%)		
Tro.*E.histolytica/dispar*	26(19.1)	7(5.1)	12.450	<0.00001
Tro.*G.lamblia*	13(9.6)	6(4.4)	2.773	0.096
Cyst of *E.histolytica*	5(3.7)	5(3.7)	0	Nd
Cyst of *G.lamblia*	1(0.7)	0(0)	1.004	0.50
I.belli	1(0.7)	0(0)	1.004	0.50
Cryptosporidium spps	2(1.5)	0(0)	2.015	0.49
A.lumbricoides	4(2.9)	3(2.2)	0.147	1.0
T.tricuria	1(0.7)	1(0.7)	0	1.0
E.vermicularis	0(0)	1(0.7)	1.004	0.50
S.stercolaris	1(0.7)	1(0.7)	0	1.0
Taenia spps	3(2.2)	1(0.7)	1.015	0.62
H.nana	2(1.5)	0(0)	2.015	0.49
S.mansoni	1(0.7)	0(0)	1.004	0.5
protozoan	42(31)	17(12.5)	16.435	0.001
Helminths	10(7.4)	7(5.1)		
protozoa + helminths	1(0.7)	0(0)		
Total	53(39)	24(17.6)	15.235	0.00001

(X^2) = Pearson chi-square test, nd = not determined.

which was statistically significant associated with < 200 cells/mm^3 CD4 counts (p = 0.0001) (Table 3).

Associated factors for intestinal parasite among adult HIV/AIDS patients attending ART clinic

Sociodemographic variables in relation to IP prevalence were analyzed by using binary logistic regression model. Place of residence and occupational categories were identified as the major socio-demographic determinants of intestinal parasite among adult HIV/AIDS patients by binary logistic regression. Being rural residence were almost 2 times more likely to had intestinal parasite than those of urban residence (COR = 2.12; 95% CI: 1.13, 3.96) and farmers by occupational categories were almost 2 times more likely to harbour intestinal parasite than government employed (COR = 2.42; 95% CI:1.06,5.56,). However, regarding other socio-demographic characteristics like sex, age group, educational status, monthly income did not show any association with parasite positivity (Table 1).

From the selected environmental and clinical variables as determinant factors for intestinal parasite infection absence of toilet, using river/unprotected water for drinking, having indiscriminate waste disposal system, having contact with animal feaces, having poor living condition, having <200 CD4 counts, being WHO stage III and being Pre-ART were significantly associated with intestinal parasitic infection among adult HIV/AIDS patients in the binary logistic regression with corresponding crude odds ratio of [COR = 6.320; 95% CI: 1.89; 21.191], [COR = 14.2; 95% CI: 3.9, 51.1], [COR = 7.3; 95% CI: 4.04, 13.31], [COR = 3.6; 95% CI: 1.27, 9.92)], [COR = 8.3; 95% CI: 4.52-15.23], [COR = 4.15,95% CI: 1.98,8.72], [COR = 8.4; 95% CI: 3.99, 17.7] and [COR = 2.98; 95% CI: 1.70, 5.22] respectively (Table 4).

Multivariate analysis was adjusted for potential confounding factors such as residence, living condition, absence of toilet, ART status, WHO stage, and CD4. Adult HIV/AIDS patients who do not have toilet in their home were almost 8 times (AOR = 7.57; 95% CI = 1.3, 44.22) more likely to have intestinal parasite than those who have toilet (Table 4). Adult HIV/AIDS patients whose source of water were river/unprotected are almost 6 times (AOR = 6.03; 95% CI: 1.14, 31.97) more likely to be infected for intestinal parasite than those whose source of water is tape water. Concerning living condition those HIV/AIDS patients who had poor living condition are 13 times (AOR = 13.29; 95% CI: 5.14, 34.35) more likely to have parasite than those who have good living condition. Regarding WHO stage those Stage III (AOR =6.06; 95% CI: 2.49, 14.74) patients are 6 times more likely to IP than stage I. With respect to ART status pre-ART patients are 8 times (AOR = 7.55; 95% CI: 3.24, 17.59) more likely to intestinal parasite (Table 4).

Discussion

This study showed the prevalence of common and opportunistic intestinal parasite among adult HIV/AIDS patients with pre-ART and on-ART in Dessie referral Hospital ART clinic with total prevalence of 39% and 17.6% in pre-ART and on-ART patients; respectively.

The prevalence of intestinal parasite among pre-ART patients was (39%) in this study in line with that of Cameroon study (40.5%), Gondar (43.5%) [12,14]. However; lower in studies Brazil (63.9%), in selected ART centers of Adama, Afar and Dire-Dawa (52%), Arbaminch Chencha and Gideo (45%), in different parts of Ethiopia (57.2%) ([15-17], unpublished data). This low prevalence in this study might be due to geographic difference in sample size (more than one study area for most reports), considering those patients with, time gap where those studies were done averagely four years ago but nowadays there is a better awareness of the patients about intestinal parasite infection and their cause. They may be diagnosed for parasites by direct wet mount and treated as well.

The prevalence of IP among on-ART patients was 17.6% in this study which was lower than reported in Brazil (24%), Congo (24.6%), Nigeria (30%), in selected ART centers of Adama, Afar and Dire-Dawa (48%), different parts of Ethiopia (42.8%) and Gondar (24.3%) [12,15-19] but it was higher than that of Cameroon (8.5%) [14]. These might be due better follow-up through laboratory

Table 3 Prevalence of intestinal parasite among pre-ART individuals (n = 53) and on-ART HIV positive individuals (n = 24) in relation to their CD4 counts in Dessie referral Hospital ART clinic, 2012

Parasite identified	Pre-ART				On-ART			
	CD4 category			p-value	CD4 category			p-value
	>500 Cell/mm^3 no (%)	200-500 Cell/mm^3 no (%)	<200 Cell/mm^3 no (%)		>500 cell/mm^3 no (%)	200-500 cell/mm^3 no (%)	<200 cell/mm^3 no (%)	
Tro.*E.histolytica/dispar*	7(26.9)	9(34.6)	10(38.5)	.057*	2(28.6)	2(28.6)	3(42.9)	.042**
Tro.*G.lamblia*	2(15.4)	4(30.8)	7(53.8)	.009*	0(0)	0(0)	6(100)	<.001
Cyst *G.lamblia*	1(100)	0(0)	0(0)	.432	0(0)	0(0)	0(0)	Nd
Cyst*E.histolytica/dispar*	5(100)	0(0)	0(0)	.013	4(80)	1(20)	0(0)	.090**
I.belli	0(0)	0(0)	1(100)	.156**	0(0)	0(0)	0(0)	Nd
Cryptosporidium spps	0(0)	0(0)	2(100)	.024**	0(0)	0(0)	0(0)	Nd
A.lumbricoides	1(25)	3(75)	0(0)	.334**	1(33.3)	2(67.7)	0(0)	.78**
T.tricuria	1(100)	0(0)	0(0)		3(100)	0(0)	0(0)	.39**
E.vermicularis	0(0)	0(0)	0(0)	Nd	0(0)	0(0)	1(100)	.03**
S.stercolaris	0(0)	1(100)	0(0)	.487**	0(0)	1(100)	0(0)	.64**
Teania spps	1(33.3)	1(33.3)	1(33.3)	.875**	0(0)	1(100)	0(0)	.64**
H.nana	0(0)	2(100)	0(0)	.235**	0(0)	0(0)	0(0)	Nd
S.mansoni	0(0)	1(100)	0(0)	.487**	0(0)	0(0)	0(0)	Nd
Protozoan	14(27.5)	11(19.6)	17(58.6)	.014*	6(12.8)	3(4.2)	8(47.1)	.001*
Helminths	3(5.9)	6(10.7)	1(3.4)		2(4.3)	4(5.6)	1(5.9)	
protozoa + helminths	0(0)	1(1.8)	0(0)		0(0)	0(0)	0(0)	
Total	17(33.3)	18(32.1)	18(62.1)	.016*	8(17)	7(9.7)	9(52.9)	.00001*

tests and better awareness of the patients themselves in adopting prevention and treatment measures against intestinal parasites. Antihelminthics may be given for ART patients for deworming purpose.

This study revealed that statistically significant reduction of intestinal parasite in the ART era ($p < 0.001$).This finding was in line with previous studies done in Brazil and in different parts of Ethiopia where those studies indicated significant decrease intestinal parasite in the ART era [15-17]. These might be due to the use of HAART with improvement in immunologic conditions of the patients and better response to infections including parasitic ones or even with a direct action on certain enteroparasites, better clinical handling of the patients with constant updating of protocols for treatment and prophylaxis besides their better follow-up through laboratory tests.

This study showed statistical significant difference of *E.histolytica/dispar* between pre-ART and on-ART groups. This is an indication that ART also contributes to the reduction of some non-OIPs even though no evidence that support whether it is the effect of ART or not. However; for other species specific intestinal parasite detected and identified in this study there was no statistically significant difference between the groups and this result was in agreement with study done in Gondar where authors report no statistically significant difference of species specific intestinal parasite between the two groups [12].

The prevalence of *cryptosporidium spps* (1.5%) in pre-ART patients in this study is much lower than Brazil (8.1%), Nepal (31.4%), selected ART centers of Adama, Afar and Dire-Dawa (8%), Nekemet (25%) and that of Gondar (8.7%) [12,15,16,20,21]. The prevalence of *I.belli* (0.7%) in the pre-ART groups in this study is lower than in Brazil (4.8%), Nepal (2.9%), selected ART centers of Adama, Afar and Dire-Dawa (5%) and Nekemet (11.7%) [15,16,20,22]. The existence of such variation may be explained by the difference in geographic location, general hygiene of the population as reported from elsewhere and moreover study participants were recruited without considering their diarrhoea.

This study indicated that all of *cryptosporidium spps* infections among pre-ART groups were found significantly associated with lower <200 cells/mm^3 CD4 count when compared to the ART experienced patients without this parasite infection in any of CD4 category. This may be due to the fact that opportunistic parasites are known to resolve spontaneously with immune restoration among HIV/AIDS patients on ART [9,10]. The association of these parasite for lower 200 cells/mm^3 CD4 count was in line with that of Varasani (97.8%), India (83%), in selected ART centers of

Table 4 Associations of selected environmental and clinical findings of adult HIV patients with prevalence of intestinal parasite by ART status using binary and multiple logistic regression in Dessie Hospital ART clinic, Feb-March.2012 (N = 272)

	Intestinal parasite prevalence							
VARIABLES	Pre-ART		On-ART		Total			
	n = 136		n = 136		N = 272			
	Positive n (%)	Negative n (%)	Positive n (%)	Negative n (%)	Positive n (%)	negative n (%)	COR (95% CI)	AOR (95% CI)
Presence of toilet								
Yes	49(37.7)	81(62.3)	19(15)	110(85)	68(26)	191(74)	1*	1*
No	4(66.7)	2(33.7)	5(71.4)	2(28.6)	9(69.2)	4(30.8)	6.3(1.9,21.2)**	7.6(1.3,44.2)**
Source of water								
Tape water	45(35.2)	83(64.8)	18(14)	109(86)	63(25)	192(75)	1*	1*
River/unprotected	8(100)	0(0)	6(66.7)	3(33.3)	14(82.4)	3(17.6)	14.2(3.9651.1)**	6.03(1.2, 31.9)**
Waste disposal								
Indiscriminate	26(74.3)	9(25.7)	18(46.2)	21(53.8)	44(59.5)	30(40.5)1	7.3(4.0-13.3)**	
Collected	27(26.7)	74(73.3)	6(6.2)	91(93.8)	33(17)	65(83)	1*	
Presence of animal								
Yes	10(45.5)	12(54.5)	7(35)	13(65)	17(40.5)	25(59.5)	1.93(.97-3.81)	
No	43(37.7)	71(62.2)	17(14.5)	99(85.3)	60(26)	170(74)	1*	
Contact with animal feaces								
Yes	5(50)	5(50)	4(66.7)	2(33.3)	9(56.2)	7(43.8)	3.56(1.3-9.9)**	
No	48(38.1)	78(61.9)	20(15)	110(85)	68(27)	188(73)	1*	
Living condition								
Poor	26(78.8)	7(21.2)	18(47.4)	20(52.6)	44(62)	27(38)	8.3(4.5,15.2)**	13.3(5.14,34.4)**
Good	27(26.2)	76(73.8)	6(6.1)	92(93.9)	33(16)	168(84)	1*	1*
CD4 categorized								
<200cell/mm^3	18(62.1)	11(37.9)	9(52.9)	8(47.1)	27(58.7)	19(41.3)	4.15(1.98-8.72)**	
200-500cell/mm^3	18(32.1)	38(67.9)	7(9.7)	65(90.3)	25(20)	103(80)	.71(.38-1.33)	
>500cell/mm^3	17(33.3)	34(66.7)	8(17)	39(83)	25(25.5)	73(74.5)	1*	
WHO stage								
Stage I	24(30)	56(70)	5(6.7)	70(93.3)	29(19)	126(81)	1*	1*
Stage II	13(41.9)	18(58.1)	3(7.7)	36(92.3)	16(22.9)	54(77.1)	1.29(.67-2.56)	1.31(.56, 3.06)
Stage III	15(62.5)	9(37.5)	14(70)	6(30)	29(65.9)	15(34.1)	8.4(3.99-17.65)**	6.1(2.49,14.74)**
Stage IV	1(100)	0(0)	2(100)	0(0)	3(100)	0(0)	Nd	Nd
ART status								
Pre-ART	53(39)	83(61)	53(39)	83(61)	77(28)	195(72)	2.98(1.7,5.2)**	7.55(3.24,17.6)**
On-ART	24(17.6)	112(82.4)	24(17.6)	112(82.4)			1*	

*Reference category, ** significant association.

Adama, Afar and Dire-Dawa (62.5%), in different part of Ethiopia (76.9%) and Hawassa (72%) [16,17,21,23,24].

This study showed that 69.2% of parasite positive HIV/AIDS patients did not have toilet in their home and they were almost 8 times more likely (AOR = 7.566, 95% CI = 1.3- 44.22) to had parasitic infection than those who had toilet in their home. This finding was supported by study done in Nigeria which showed 50% parasite positive patients did not have toilet in their home and also by another study done in Malaysia which showed indiscriminate defecation was significantly associated with parasite positivity with the odds of (OR = 5.01; 95% CI = 3.30–7.62). The higher AOR of this study when compared to Malaysian might be due difference in study population since this study consider HIV/AIDS patients who are immune suppressed but study in Malaysia consider total population [19,25].

Using river water as predictor of IP infection by indicating 82.4% of parasite positive HIV/AIDS were using river water and they were 6 times (AOR = 6.03; 95% CI =1.14, 31.97) more likely to harbour IP than those using tape water. This finding was also supported by study done in Nigeria where 54.6% of parasite infected HIV patients were using river/unprotected water for drinking purpose and by other previous study done in Malaysia which showed that those community residence using river water/untreated water were almost 2 times to had IP infection than those using tape or treated water with the odds ratio of (OR = 2.08; 95% CI = 1.36–3.21). The relatively higher OR of the present study when compared to Malaysian might be due to difference in study population since this study consider HIV/AIDS patients who are immune suppressed but study in Malaysia consider total population [19,25].

This study revealed that poor living condition as one of determinant factor for intestinal parasitic infections by indicating that 62% of parasite positive patients had poor living condition and 13 times more likely (AOR =13.29; 95% CI = 5.14, 34.35) to infected with IP than those with good living condition. The association between poor living condition and intestinal parasite infection was also indicated by previous studies in selected ART centers of Adama, Afar and Dire-Dawa (87.5%) and in different part of Ethiopia (87.6%) of parasite positives were in poor living condition [16,17].

The present finding revealed that being WHO stage III as one of predictor of intestinal parasite infection where stage III patients were 6 times (AOR = 6.06, 95% CI =2.49, 14.74) more likely to have IP than stage I patients and there was study in Nekemet supporting the finding of this study by indicating that the prevalence OIP increased with increasing WHO stage [22].

Considering ART as protective factor those pre-ART patients were almost 8 times (AOR = 7.55; 95% CI =3.24-17.59) more likely to harbour IP than ART experienced patients and this finding was in line with that of Brazil where they indicated those pre-ART patients were almost 6 times more likely to had any intestinal parasite infection than those on-ART patients [15].

In this study, we have done only normal saline, iodine, formol-ether concentration and modified Ziehl-Neelsen staining method for detection of common and opportunistic intestinal parasites. We have not used water-ether sedimentation method for *Microsporidia and* other methods like Molecular techniques and immuno flouscent techniques sensitive for parasites. In addition to this, patients may be diagnosed for parasites and treated as well before. Antihelminthics may be given for deworming purpose. Because of this fact prevalence of intestinal parasites were under estimated in this study.

Conclusion

The prevalence of intestinal parasites found to be higher in ART naive than attending ART patients. High proportions of intestinal parasites were associated with lower CD4 counts in both pre-ART and on-ART patients. Infections with opportunistic intestinal parasite were associated with lower CD4 counts in ART naïve patients only. Increasing the immune status of HIV infected patients with anti-retroviral therapy may help to reduce acquisition of parasites. Using river/unprotected, absence of toilet in the home, poor living condition, being WHO stage III and being pre-ART significantly increased the prevalence of intestinal parasite in the study area. Public health measures should continue to emphasize the importance of environmental and personal hygiene as well as provide and monitor the quality of drinking water aiming to obtain a better quality of life for those patients. Stool examination should be routinely performed in the follow-up of patients with HIV/AIDS attending ART clinic in order to optimize treatment of institution and other preventive measures. Moreover large scale longitudinal study is needed to determine the effect of ART for both opportunistic and non-opportunistic parasite.

Competing interests

The authors declare that they have no competing interests.

Authors' contributions

AM was the primary researcher, conceived the study, designed, participated in data collection, conducted data analysis, drafted and finalized the manuscript for publication. AA, MD and AA assisted in data collection and reviewed the initial and final drafts of the manuscript. AM, MD, AA and AA interpreted the results, and reviewed the initial and final drafts of the manuscript. All authors read and approved the final manuscript.

Acknowledgements

We acknowledge University of Gondar for funding this study. We are greatly appreciate Dessie Hospital Laboratory for cooperation during the study. We are also grateful to the HIV AIDS patients who participated in this study.

Author details

[1]Dessie regional laboratory, Amhara regional state, Northeast Ethiopia. [2]Department of Medical Microbiology, School of Biomedical and Laboratory Sciences, College of Medicine and Health Sciences, University of Gondar, Gondar, Ethiopia. [3]Department of Medical Parasitology, School of Biomedical and Laboratory Sciences, College of Medicine and Health Sciences, University of Gondar, Gondar, Ethiopia.

References

1. World Health Organization: **Prevention and control of intestinal parasitic infections.** *WHO Technical Report* 1987, **749:**1–86.
2. UNAIDS/WHO: *HIV Epidemic Update.* Geneva: UNAIDS; 2002.
3. Kumie A, Ali A: **An overview of environmental health status in Ethiopia with particular emphasis to its organization, drinking water and sanitation: a literature survey.** *Ethiop J Health Dev* 2005, **19:**89–103.
4. Kam KM: **Gut parasites in general practice in Hong Kong.** *J Trop Med Hyg* 1994, **97:**117–120.
5. Kelly P: **Diarrhoea and AIDS: recent developments in the African settings.** *African Health* 1998, **1:**16–18.

6. Shah UV, Purohit BC, Chandralekha D, Mapara MH: **Co- infection with *cryptosporidium, isospora* and *S. stercoralis* in a patient with AIDS- a case report.** *Ind J Med Micr* 2005, **21**:137–138.
7. Maggi P, Larocca A, Quarto M, Serio G, Brandonisio O, Angarano G: **Effect of antiretroviral therapy on cryptosporidiosis and microsporidiosis in patients infected with human immunodeficiency virus type 1.** *Eur J Clin Microbiol Infect Dis* 2000, **19**:213–217.
8. Lawn SD, Myer L, Orrell C, Bekker LG, Wood R: **Early mortality among adults accessing a community-based antiretroviral service in South Africa: implications for programme design.** *AIDS* 2005, **19**:2141–2148.
9. Alfonso Y, Monzote L: **HIV protease inhibitors: effect on the opportunistic protozoan parasites.** *Open Med Chem J* 2011, **5**:40–50.
10. Willemot P, Klein MB: **Prevention of HIV-associated opportunistic infections and diseases in the age of highly active antiretroviral therapy.** *Expert Rev Anti Infect Ther* 2004, **2**:521–532.
11. *FDRE, Census Commission. Summary and statistical report of the 2007 population and housing census. Dec. 2008. Addis Ababa.* http://www.csa.et.gov/pdf (accessed on March 10, 2011).
12. Telele NF, Damte DG, Selassie S: **Intestinal parasitic infections among HIV seropositives and seronegatives adult patients presented with diarrhea in Gondar, North west Ethiopia.** *Revi Ant Infec Dis* 2010, **3**:7–8.
13. Cheesbrough M: *Medical laboratory manual for tropical countries*, Volume 1. 2nd edition. Cambridge press; 1992:208–210.
14. Sarfati C, Bourgeois A, Menotti J, Liegeois F, Moyou-Somo R, Delaporte E, Derouin F, Ngole EM, Molina JM: **Prevalence of intestinal parasites including microsporidia in human immunodeficiency virus–infected adults in Cameroon: a cross-sectional study.** *AmJTrop Med Hyg* 2006, **74**(Suppl 1):162–164.
15. Rodrigues Bachur TP, Vale JM, Branco Coêlho IC, de Sales Queiroz TR, Souza Chaves BC: **Enteric parasitic infections in HIV/AIDS patients before and after the highly active antiretroviral therapy in Brazil.** *Bra J Infe Dis* 2008, **12**(Suppl 2):115–122.
16. Adamu H, Petros B: **Intestinal protozoan infections among HIV positive persons with and without antiretroviral treatment (ART) in selected ART centers in adama, afar and dire-dawa, Ethiopia.** *Ethiop J Health Dev* 2009, **23**(Suppl 2):133–140.
17. Adamu H: *The prevalence of intestinal parasites and molecular characterization of cryptosporidium species in Ethiopia*, Dissertation paper. Addis Ababa, Ethiopia; 2010.
18. Wumba R, Longo-Mbenza B, Mandina M, Odio Wobin T, Biligui S, Sala J, Breton J, Breton J, Thellier M: **Intestinal parasites infections in hospitalized AIDS patients in Kinshasa.** *DemRCP* 2010, **17**:321–328.
19. Wokem GN, Chukwu C, Nwachukwu BC: **Prevalence of intestinal parasites seen in HIV sero-positive subjects in Port Harcourt, Nigeria.** *Niger J Parasitol* 2008, **29**(Suppl 2):115–120.
20. Sucilathangam G, Velvizhi G, Palaniappan TT: **The prevalence of coccidian parasites in and around tirunelveli in HIV positive individuals and its correlation with the CD4 count.** *J Clin Diagn Res* 2011, **5**(Suppl 6):1182–1186.
21. Assefa S, Erko B, Medhin G, Assefa Z, Shimelis T: **Intestinal parasitic infections in relation to HIV/AIDS status, diarrhea and CD4 T-cell count.** *BMC Infect Dis* 2009, **9**:1551–1556.
22. Dufera M, Petros B, Endeshaw T, Mohammed H, Kassu A: **Opportunistic intestinal protozoan parasites among HIV positive patients on antiretroviral therapy at Nekemte hospital, West Ethiopia.** *Ethiop J Health Biomed Sci* 2008, **1**(Suppl 1):11–17.
23. Tuli L, Gulati KA, Sundar S, Mohapatra TM: **Correlation between CD4 counts of HIV patients and enteric protozoan in different seasons – An experience of a tertiary care hospital in Varanasi (India).** *BMCG* 2008, **8**(Suppl 36):1–6.
24. Basnet A, Sherchan JB, Rijal B, Sharma S, Khadga P: **Detection of coccidian parasites and their clinical manifestation, treatment and prophylaxis in HIV infected patients in Tribhuvan University teaching hospital.** *Scientific world* 2010, **8**(Suppl 8):51–55.
25. Ngui RS, Ishak S, Chow Sek Chuen CS, Rohela Mahmud R, Lim YAL: **Prevalence and risk factors of intestinal parasitism in rural and remote west Malaysia.** *Plosntds.org* 2011, **5**(Suppl 3):1–7.

4

Virologic and immunologic outcome of HAART in Human Immunodeficiency Virus (HIV)-1 infected patients with and without tuberculosis (TB) and latent TB infection (LTBI) in Addis Ababa, Ethiopia

Desta Kassa[1,2*], Gebremedhin Gebremichael[1], Yodit Alemayehu[1], Dawit Wolday[3], Tsehaynesh Messele[1] and Debbie van Baarle[2]

Abstract

Background: HIV/TB coinfection remains a major challenge even after the initiation of HAART. Little is known about *Mycobacterium tuberculosis (Mtb)* specific immune restoration in relation to immunologic and virologic outcomes after long-term HAART during co-infections with latent and active TB.

Methods: A total of 232 adults, including 59 HIV patients with clinical TB (HIV + TB+), 125 HIV patients without clinical TB (HIV + TB-), 13 HIV negative active TB patients (HIV-TB+), and 10 HIV negative Tuberculin Skin TST positive (HIV-TST+), and 25 HIV-TST- individuals were recruited. HAART was initiated in 113 HIV + patients (28 TB + and 85 TB-), and anti-TB treatment for all TB cases. CD4+ T-cell count, HIV RNA load, and IFN-γ responses to ESAT-6/CFP-10 were measured at baseline, 6 months (M6), 18 months (M18) and 24 months (M24) after HAART initiation.

Results: The majority of HIV + TB- (70%, 81%, 84%) as well as HIV + TB + patients (60%, 77%, 80%) had virologic success (HIV RNA < 50 copies/ml) by M6, M18 and M24, respectively. HAART also significantly increased CD4+ T-cell counts at 2 years in HIV + TB + (from 110.3 to 289.9 cells/μl), HIV + TB- patients (197.8 to 332.3 cells/μl), HIV + TST- (199 to 347 cells/μl) and HIV + TST + individuals (195 to 319 cells/μl). Overall, there was no significant difference in the percentage of patients that achieved virologic success and in total CD4+ counts increased between HIV patients with and without TB or LTBI. The *Mtb* specific IFN-γ response at baseline was significantly lower in HIV + TB + (3.6 pg/ml) compared to HIV-TB + patients (34.4 pg/ml) and HIV + TST + (46.3 pg/ml) individuals; and in HIV-TB + patients compared to HIV-TST + individuals (491.2 pg/ml). By M18 on HAART, the IFN-γ response remained impaired in HIV + TB + patients (18.1 pg/ml) while it normalized in HIV + TST + individuals (from 46.3 to 414.2 pg/ml).

Conclusions: Our data show that clinical and latent TB infections do not influence virologic and immunologic outcomes of ART in HIV patients. Despite this, HAART was unable to restore optimal TB responsiveness as measured by *Mtb* specific IFN-γ response in HIV/TB patients. Improvement of *Mtb*-specific immune restoration should be the focus of future therapeutic strategies.

Keywords: HIV, Tuberculosis, HAART

* Correspondence: dkassa2003@gmail.com
[1]Infectious and non-infectious diseases research directorate, Ethiopian Health and Nutrition Research Institute (EHNRI), P.O. Box 1242, Addis Ababa, Ethiopia
[2]Department of Internal Medicine and Infectious Diseases and Department of Immunology, University Medical Center Utrecht, Utrecht, The Netherlands
Full list of author information is available at the end of the article

Background

Human immunodeficiency virus/Acquired immunodeficiency syndrome (HIV/AIDS) associated morbidity and mortality has reduced substantially since the introduction of Highly Active Antiretroviral Therapy (HAART) in the mid 90's [1,2]. Access to Antiretroviral Therapy (ART) in low and middle income countries has been expanded following the launche of "3 by 5" global initiative [3], though only 54% of those eligible for ART were on treatment by 2011 [2]. In Ethiopia, where free ART was started in 2005, >250,000 (~79%) of the adults requiring ART were actually treated [4].

The primary goal of HAART is to suppress HIV-1 RNA lower than the detection level (LDL) of the assay within 3 to 6 months on treatment and restore immunologic function, to reduce morbidity and mortality, to reduce vertical transmission, and improve quality of life [5]. However, there are still un-resolved problems including early mortality [6], incomplete responses [7], variations in HAART outcomes [8], lack of universal consensus to define treatment failures and time to start ART [9], drug resistance [10] and lost to follow-ups [7].

While HIV RNA testing is the golden standard to monitor patients on ART [8], due to costs and technical demands of the HIV RNA test, CD4+ T cell measurements are recommended for resource poor settings [11]. Immunologic parameters, however, have lower performance to identify virologic failures which could lead to premature change or to continuous use of failed regimens reviewed in [12]. This leads to higher morbidity and mortality rates and more complex resistance in settings where virologic tests are not available [13]. Therefore, accurate diagnosis of treatment failure is necessary in settings where free ART service is accelerating and patient monitoring is exclusively dependent on clinical and CD4+ T cell measurements like in Ethiopia.

Furthermore, despite that HAART has significantly reduced morbidity and mortality in HIV/TB patients [14], studies showed defects of immune response in HIV/TB patients on HAART including suboptimal restoration of CD4+ T cells in number, phenotype and function [15,16], and incomplete TB specific immune restoration [17]. Higher TB incidence in individuals on continuous HAART as compared to the HIV negative local population, which could be due to incomplete immune restoration specific to TB, was also reported [18]. However, data regarding the magnitude of immune restoration specific to *Mtb* in relation to CD4+ and virologic responses to long-term HAART in patients with TB and LTBI is limited.

Overall, although extensive studies aiming to evaluate ART outcomes have been performed, the studies are predominantly from developed countries, and they are different in study design, ex-/inclusion criteria, ethnicity, ART experience, ARV regimen, duration, and definitions, which makes it difficult to generalize HAART outcomes in different countries [19]. Especially in Ethiopia, like in many HIV/TB endemic settings, little data is available [20,21] regarding HAART outcome in patients with and without active TB and LTBI.

In summary, these studies strongly support the need of recent data from well defined longitudinal cohort studies on HAART, which is crucial to provide answers and insights to the HAART related challenges and develop and update national ART guidelines [19,22].

The aim of this observational cohort study which comprised three clinical groups including HIV + TB+, HIV + TB-, and HIV-TB + patients, and two control groups including HIV-TST+, and HIV-TST- individuals , was to evaluate the long-term outcome of HAART by comprehensively measuring key parameters including mortality, virologic and immunologic responses, and *Mtb* specific immune restoration by measuring IFN-γ production in response to Early Secretory Antigenic Target-6/Culture Filtrate Protein-10 (ESAT-6/CFP-10).

Results

Characteristics of the study population at enrolment

Demographic, clinical and laboratory data of the study populations at baseline are shown in Table 1. A total of 232 participants were included. Thirteen HIV-TB+, 59 HIV + TB+, 125 HIV + TB- (of whom 43 were HIV + TST+, and 82 HIV + TST-), 10 HIV-TST+, and 25 Controls (HIV-TST-) were enrolled. HIV + TB + patients had lower numbers of CD4+ T cells ($p = 0.003$), total Lymphocyte count (TLC) ($p = 0.001$), Hemoglobin (Hgb) (g/dl) ($p = 0.02$), Body Mass Index (BMI) (Kg/m^2) ($p = 0.002$), CD4% ($p = 0.006$), but higher HIV RNA levels ($p = 0.02$) than HIV + TB- patients. There was no significant difference in CD4+, TLC, Hgb, BMI, CD4% and HIV RNA tests between HIV + TST- and HIV + TST + individuals (data not shown). Of special interest, 10 (6.3%) of the ART naïve HIV patients had HIV RNA < 50 copies/ml (LDL) at enrolment. The mean CD4+ T cell count of these subjects was 476.1 (SD ± 260.7 cells/μl).

At enrolment, more than 50% of the HIV + TB + patients had advanced diseases stages (anemic, malnourished, WHO stages 3 plus 4, and immunosuppressed) while only 15-36% of the HIV + TB- patients had these advanced disease stages. There was also a higher percentage of chronic hepatitis B virus coinfection in the HIV + TB + patients, (19.3%), followed by the HIV + TB-, (7.2%), and healthy controls (4.2%) (Table 1).

Outcome of HAART

ART initiation, mortality and follow-up status

A total of 113 (61.4%) HIV patients including 28 HIV + TB + and 85 HIV + TB- [of whom 31 were HIV + TST +

Table 1 Baseline characteristics of the study populations (n = 232)

	HIV + TB+ (n = 59)	HIV + TB- (n = 125)	HIV-TB+ (n = 13)	HIV-TST+ (n = 10)	HIV-TST (n = 25)
Demographic data					
Age, years	33.1 ± 8.7	33.2 ± 7.3	28.5 ± 9.5 [b]	26.6 ± 7.4,	24.6 ± 6.6
Female, n (%)	28 (47.5)	83 (66.4)	6 (46.2)	6 (60)	16 (64)
Clinical data					
CHBV coinfection, n (%)	11/57 (19.3)	8/112 (7.2)	3 (15)	2 (20)	1 (4)
WHO stage, n (%)					
I + II	3/50 (6)	80 (64)			
III + IV	47/50 (94)	45 (36)	NA	NA	NA
BMI, kg/m2	18.9 ± 3.1[a]	21.3 ± 3.5	18.9 ± 2.8	21.4 ± 2.5	21.4 ± 2.0
BMI < 18.50 kg/m^2, n (%)	29 (49.2)	18/124 (14.6)	6 (46)	8 (80)	24 (96)
Laboratory data					
Hgb, g/dl	12.2 ± 3.7 [a]	13.2 ± 2.5	13.5 ± 2.5 [b]	16.4 ±1.8 [c]	18.0 ± 2.1
Hgb < 12 g/dl (anemic), n (%)	23/43 (53.5)	29/107 (27.1)	2 (23)	0	0
CD4+ count/μl	173.7 ± 180.8 [a]	279.2 ± 212.4	478.1 ± 253 [b]	787.3 ± 274	754.8 ± 241
CD4+ category, n (%)					
< 100	27 (48.2)	26 (22.2)	1 (1.7)	0	0
100 -200	12 (21.4)	26 (22.2)	6 (10.0)	0	0
> = 201	17 (30.3)	65 (55.6)	53 (88.3)	10 (100)	25 (100)
TLC	1175 ± 754 [a]	1626 ± 750	1485 ± 895 [b]	1975 ± 1483	1.668 ± 559
HIV RNA (log10copies/ml)	4.5 ± 0.8 [a]	4.1 ± 0.9	NA	NA	NA
HIV RNA category, n (%)					
LDL	1 (2.2)	9 (8.0)			
<= 100000	14 (30.4)	97 (85.8)			
>100000	32 (69.6)	16 (14.2)	NA	NA	NA

Data are means ± standard deviations (SD) unless stated; *n (%)* Number of patients, **CHBV** chronic Hepatitis B Virus, defined as the presence of hepatitis surface antigen (HBsAg) in the plasma, **BMI** Body mass index, **Hgb** Hemoglobin, **TLC** total lymphocyte, **HIV RNA** plasma viral load, **LDL** lower than detection limit (HIV RNA < 50 copies/ml), **WHO** World Health Organization, **NA**: not applicable.
[a] Comparing HIV + TB + and HIV + TB-; *P < 0.05.*
[b] Comparing HIV + TB + and HIV-TB+; *P < 0.05.*
[c] Comparing HIV-TST + and HIV-TST- ; *P < 0.05.*

and 54 were HIV + TST-], initiated ART and were followed for a median of 23.9 (IQR 22.5-24.4) months. The majority (78%) of the HIV + TB- patients received D4T + 3TC + NVP HAART regimens. At ART initiation, HIV + TB + patients had lower mean CD4+ T cells (*p = 0.005*), CD4% (*p = 0.03*), TLC (p = 008), and BMI (*p < 0.0001*) than HIV + TB- patients (Table 2).

At 2 years, 18 (9.8%) patients died of which 63% within the first 24 weeks. The risk factors for early mortality in the HIV patients with and without TB were advanced disease stages including baseline CD4+ count <100 cells/μl (OR: 5.7, 95% CI 1.8 – 17.2, *p = 0.03*), WHO-stages III plus IV (OR: 4.8 95% CI 1.3-17.5, *p = 0.01*), and BMI < 18.5 kg/m2 (OR: 1.2 95% CI 0.37-3.8, *p = 0.77*) (data not shown).

Overall, at M6, M18 and M24 of follow-up time, 21/59 (35.6%), 21/51 (41.2%) and 23/41 (56.1) of the HIV + TB + patients; and 27/125 (21.6%), 36/120 (30%) and 43/115 (37.4%) of the HIV + TB- patients, respectively, were lost to follow-up (more than 60 days late for a scheduled date of clinic visit).

Virologic outcomes

We measured virologic outcomes by determining the HIV RNA level as well as the proportion of patients with virologic success. In both HIV + TB + and HIV + TB- patients, the mean HIV RNA level significantly declined after HAART (p < 0.05 and p < 0.001, respectively) (Figure 1A). There was no significant difference in mean HIV RNA decline between patients with and without TB or LTBI (Figure 1A & B).

By M24 on HAART, the majority of the individuals (>80%) achieved virologic success (HIV RNA < 50 copies/ml). There was no significant difference in the

Table 2 Therapeutic, clinical and immunovirologic characteristic of the study participants at ART initiation (n = 113)

	HIV + TB+	HIV + TB-	*p value*
No of patients initiated ART	28	85	
Demographic			
Female, n (%)	14 (50)	56 (65.7)	
Age, years	34.1 ± 8.3	34.4 ± 7.7	
Treatment			
Mean follow-up days before ART initiation	78.7	37.7	
Mean delay in commencing HAART following TB treatment, days	100		
HAART regimen at ART initiation, n (%)			
D4T/3TC/NVP	4 (15)	66 (78)	
D4T/3TC/EVZ	11(41)	2 (2)	
AZT/3TC/NVP	7(26)	12 (14)	
AZT/3TC/EVZ	5 (16)	4 (5)	
Others		1 (1)	
Cortimoxzole treatment, n (%)	15 (83.3%)	58 (59.2%)	
BMI and Laboratory values at ART initiation			
BMI (kg/m^2)	18.1 ± 2.5	21.3 ± 3.7	0.0001
CD4+ (cells/µl)	110.3 ± 71.3	197.8 ± 153.2	0.005
CD4%	10.1 ± 5.3	14.6 ± 9.9	0.033
TLC (cells/µl)	1078 ± 512	1521 ± 692	0.007
Hgb (g/dl)	13.4 ± 3.4	13.0 ± 2.5	0.68
HIV RNA (log$_{10}$copies/ml)	4.3 ± 0.9	4.3 ± 0.9	0.73
Follow-up outcomes			
Deaths, n (%)	8/59 (13.6)	10/125 (8.0%)	

Data in mean ± standard deviation (SD) unless stated; *n* number of patients, D4T Stavudine, 3TC lamividine, NVP Nevirapine, EVZ Efavirenz, AZT Zidovudin, BMI Body mass index, Hgb Hemoglobin, TLC total lymphocyte count; M6, M18 and M24 = 6, 18 and 24 months after HAART initiation.

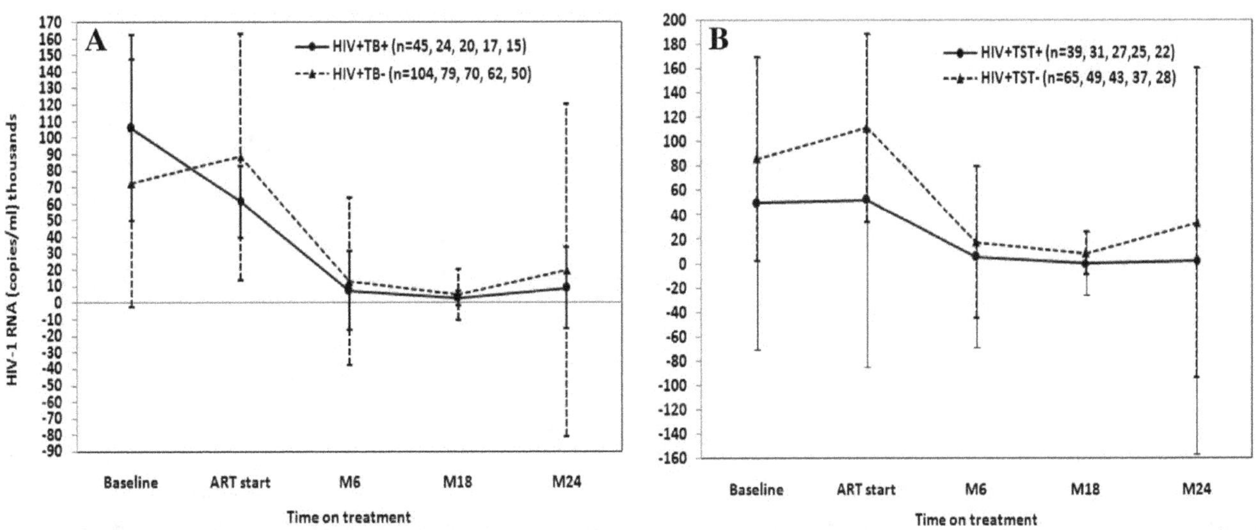

Figure 1 Changes in HIV RNA level (copies/ml) over time after the start of HAART. HIV RNA was measured at baseline, at ART start and at six month (M6), M18 and M24 of HAART in HIV patients with TB (HIV + TB+) (continuous line) and without TB (HIV + TB-) (dotted line) **(A)**, and HIV + TB- patients sub-grouped as those with TST positive (HIV + TST+) (continuous line) and TST negative (HIV + TST-) (dotted line) **(B)**. Values are shown as mean and standard deviation. n = number of participants per visit.

proportion of patients achieving virologic success between individuals with and without TB or LTBI (Figure 2A & B). Moreover, whereas 28 (85%) of the patients on HAART maintained HIV RNA < 50 copies/ml at M6, M18 and M24 (ever suppressed), 5 (15%) never reached HIV RNA < 50 copies/ml (never suppressed).

At M6, 13 (19%) HIV + TB- patients had virologic failure (HIV RNA >5000 copies/ml), for which baseline BMI < 18.5 kg/m^2, CD4+ count < 100 cells/μl, and WHO stages 3 and 4 [OR: 3.8, 2.3, 4.9; $p = 0.05$, 0.32, 0.02, respectively] were risk factors. Other factors like sex (OR: 0.51) age (OR: 0.41), Hgb (OR: 0.19), and HIV RNA (OR: 0.89) were not associated with the risk of virologic failures (Table 3).

Immunologic responses

Quantitative restoration of CD4+ cells is one of the principal evidences for immune recovery during HAART. There was a significant increase in CD4+ T cell count at M6, M18 and M24 of HAART in both the HIV + TB- ($P < 0.001$ for all) as well as the HIV + TB + patients (p = 0.02, 0.001, 0.001, respectively); and in the HIV + TST + ($p = 0.03$, 003, 0.04, respectively) as well as in the HIV + TST- ($P < 0.001$ for all) (Figure 3A & B).

There was no significant difference in the total CD4+ T cells reached by M6, M18 and M24 in HIV + TB + vs. HIV + TB- ($p = 0.37$, 0.63 and 0.56, respectively) and in HIV + TST + vs. HIV + TST- (*p = 0.77, 0.62, and 0.74,* respectively) (Figure 3A & B). Interestingly, although the study population was small, HIV/TB patients coinfected with HBV (n = 9) showed the least increase in CD4+ T cells (Figure 3A).

There was an overall increase in CD4+ count over the two years with an average increase of 6.7 cells/μl per month in the HIV + TB- patients, and 5.9 cells/μl per month in the HIV + TB+. CD4+ increase was highest in the first six months. Despite lower CD4+ T cell count at ART initiation in HIV + TB + patients (110 CD4+ cell/μl) than HIV + TB- patients (198 CD4+ cell/μl) (p = 0.001), there was no significant difference in the net increase of CD4+ T cells per month as well as in the total CD4+ cells achieved at each time point between the patients with and without TB.

Overall, at two years on HAART, the total CD4+ cells in all clinical groups was still lower by more than two fold compared to healthy controls (HIV-TST-) (771 CD4+ cells/μl) (Figure 3A and B). Moreover, the proportion of patients that attained the critical CD4+ count of ≥ 200 cells/μl by two years on ART was 19 (68%) for HIV + TB-, and 8 (73%) for the HIV + TB+. Six (21%) of the HIV + TB- but none of the HIV + TB + patients had CD4+ count >500 cells/μl (super responders).

At M6, M18 and M24 of HAART, 45%, 30%, 42% of the HIV + TB- and 54%, 43%, and 30% of the HIV + TB + patients, respectively, were diagnosed with immunologic failure (an increase of less than 50 cells/ μl by M6, and less than 100 cells/ μl by M18 and M24 of HAART). The risk factors for immunologic failure at M6 of HAART for the HIV + TB- patients were WHO stages 3 + 4 [OR: 4.3, p = 0.01], and CD4+ < 100 cells/μl) [OR: 5.6, p = 0.008] at baseline (Table 3).

As shown in Figure 4, for the HIV + TB- patients on ART, the CD4+ increase was steeper in women, in patients with older age, patients with baseline HIV RNA < 10000

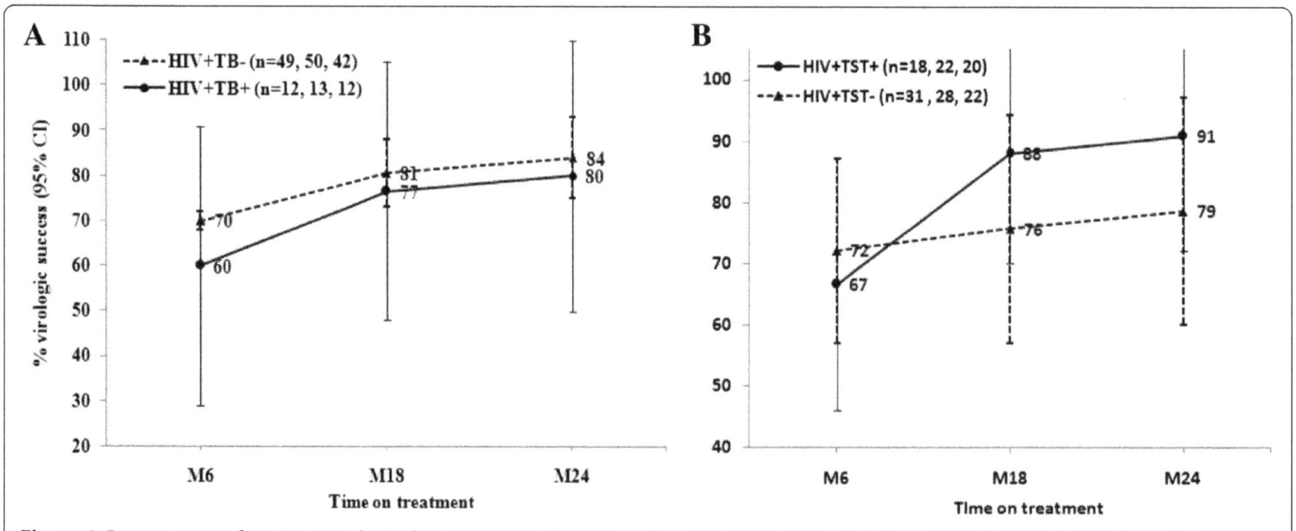

Figure 2 Percentages of patients with virologic success (plasma HIV RNA < 50 copies/ml) with 95% confidence interval (95% CI) overtime on HAART. HIV RNA was measured at six month (M6), M18 and M24 of treatment in HIV patients with TB (HIV + TB+) (continuous line) and without TB (HIV + TB- (dotted line) **(A)**, and HIV + TB- patients sub-grouped as those with TST positive (HIV + TST+) (continuous line) and TST negative (HIV + TST-) (dotted line) **(B)**. Percentage of patients with virologic success per follow up visit are shown on the line graphs; n = number of participants per visit.

Table 3 Logistic regression analysis showing odds ratio for factors associated with the risk of immunologic and virologic failures of the HIV patients with no TB (HIV + TB-) at six months of ART

	Risk of immunologic failure (an increase of CD4+ < 50 cells/μl) at 6 months (n = 56)			Risk of virologic failure (HIV RNA > 5000 cells/μl) at 6 months (n = 69)		
	OR	95% CI	P value	OR	95% CI	P value
Sex						
Male	1			1		
Female	0.62	1.0-1.9	0.40	0.51	0.12-2.1	0.93
Age (years)						
36-60	1			1		
16–35	0.65	0.21-2.0	0.44	0.41	0.10- 1.7	0.21
BMI						
<18.50	1			1		
> = 18.50	0.90	0.25- 3.29	0.87	3.75	1.0-14.4	0.05
Hgb						
< 12	1			1		
> = 12	0.38	0.08-1.7	0.21	0.19	0.02-1.6	0.13
CD4+ count/μl						
> = 100	1			1		
<100	5.6	1.6-20.1	0.008	2.3	0.45- 11.2	0.32
> = 200	1			1		
>200	0.22	0.07-0.73	0.01	0.89	0.24-3.2	0.85
HIV RNA copies/ml						
> = 100000	1			1		
<100000	1.2	0.3- 5.3	0.82	0.38	0.04- 3.3	0.4
WHO stages						
I + II	1			1		
III + IV	4.3	1.4-13.4	0.01	4.9	1.2-19.9	0.02
TB coinfection						
No	1			1		
Yes	1.4	0.4-1.8	0.5	0.23	0.03-1.9	0.17

OR Odds ratio, 95% CI 95% confidence Interval; n = total number of participants who have CD4+ count and plasma HIV RNA measurement at 6 month of HAART.

copies/ml, and CD4+ count > 200 cells/μl with the difference becoming larger over time. More interestingly, the total CD4+ T cell count achieved in the HIV + TB- patients started ART at CD4+ > 200, was two fold higher than those started ART at < 200 cells/μl (495.0 vs. 243.2 cells/μl, respectively, (*P = 0.007*). This indicated that advanced pre-treatment immunodeficiency is the most important factor for diminished restoration of CD4 cell counts after HAART.

Mtb antigen specific IFN-γ response before and after HAART

Although quantitative measurement of CD4+ counts and HIV RNA level provides a general insight in immune recovery, measuring qualitative restoration of TB specific immune responses will provide insight whether antigen specific immune responses are also restored. Therefore, we measured *Mtb* antigen (ESAT-6/CFP-10) specific IFN-γ responses during HAART (Figure 5). Compared to IFN-γ response in LTBI individuals (HIV-TST+) (491.2 pg/ml) at baseline, there was significantly lower IFN-γ production in HIV + TB + (3.6 pg/ml) (*p = 0.004*), in HIV-TB + (34.4 pg/ml) (*p = 0.004*), and in HIV + TST + (46.3 pg/ml) patients (*p = 0.002*). Moreover, IFN-γ production at baseline was significantly lower in HIV + TB + compared to HIV-TB + (*p = 0.02*) and HIV + TST + (*p = 0.04*) patients, and in HIV + TST + compared to HIV-TB + (*p = 0.004*).

In the HIV + TST + individuals, following initiation of HAART, although the level of IFN-γ did not change by M6 (44.3 pg/ml), it increased sharply after that and normalized by M18 of treatment (414.2 pg/ml) (*p = 0.007*) and reached similar level as HIV-TST +

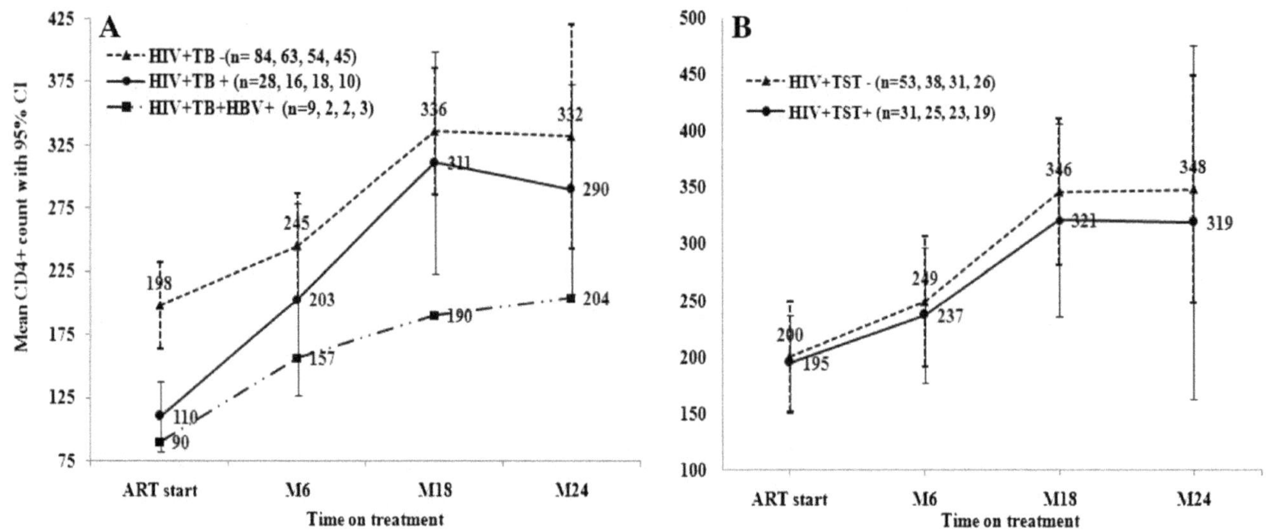

Figure 3 Mean CD4+ count increase (cells/μl) with 95% Confidence interval (95% CI) over time after the start of HAART. CD4+ T cell count was measured at ART start, six month (M6), M18, and M24 of HAART in HIV patients with TB (HIV + TB+) (continuous line), with no TB (HIV + TB-) (dotted line), and HIV patients with TB and HBV (HIV + TB + HBV) (dash line) **(A)**, and HIV + TB- patients sub-grouped as those with TST positive (HIV + TST+) (continuous line) and those TST negative (HIV + TST-) (dash line) **(B)**. Number of CD4+ T cell counts per follow-up visit are shown on the line graphs; n = number of participants per visit.

individuals (491.2 pg/ml) ($p > 0.05$). In contrast, there was no significant increase in *Mtb* specific immunity for the HIV patients with TB (HIV + TB+) on TB treatment and on HAART by M6 (31.7 pg/ml) as well as by M18 (18.1 pg/ml) of treatment. For the HIV negative TB patients (HIV-TB+) on TB treatment, mean IFN-γ production significantly increased by M6 (181 pg/ml) ($p = 0.005$)

To see whether the poor *Mtb*-specific recovery is due to lower CD4 recovery, we correlated the increase in CD4+ cell count in the HIV + TB + patients after HAART with IFN-γ production upon stimulation with ESAT-6/

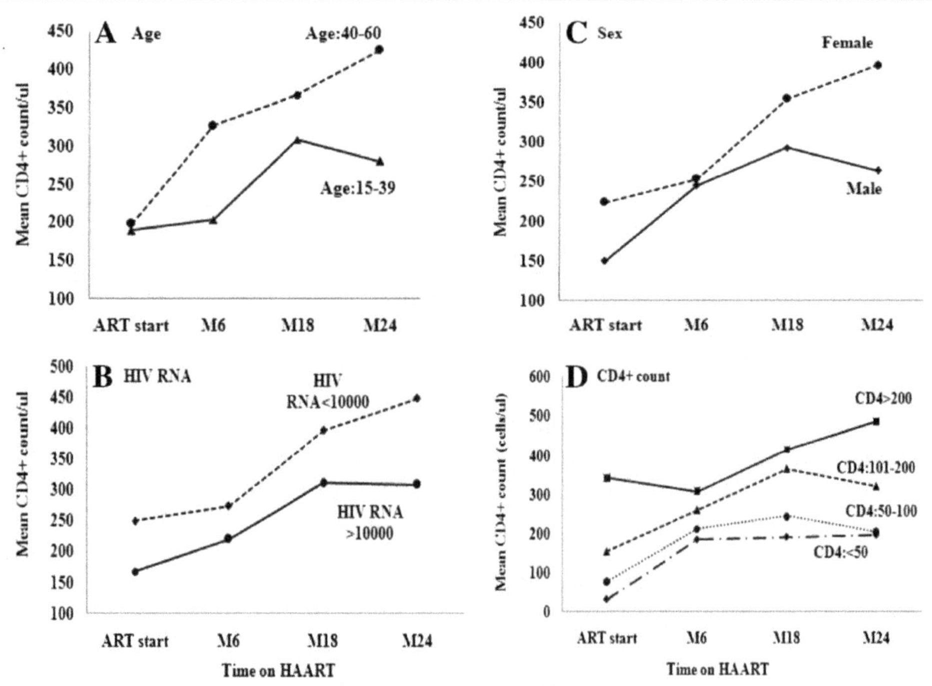

Figure 4 Mean CD4+ count increase (cells/μl) over time after the start of HAART in HIV patients with no TB (HIV + TB-) according to the baseline category of (A) Age, (B) HIV RNA (copies/ml), (C) Sex, and (D) CD4+ count (cells/μl).

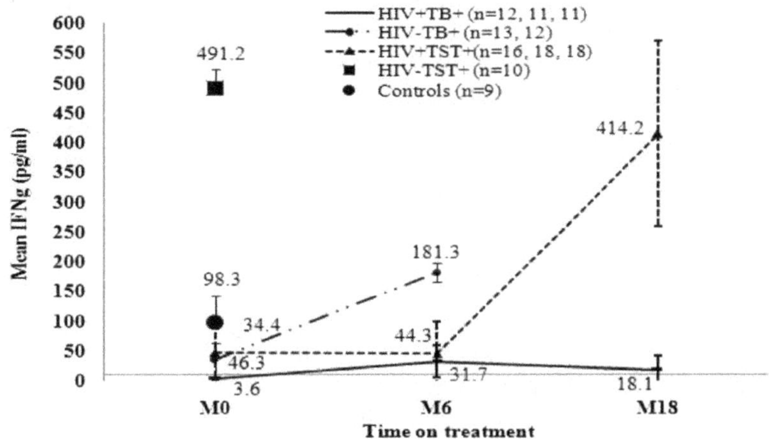

Figure 5 Restoration of *Mtb* specific IFN-γ (pg/ml) response overtime after the start of HAART and TB treatment. Level of IFN-γ (pg/ml) was measured at baseline (M0), and at six (M6) and M18 of treatment in 7th day culture supernatants of whole blood stimulated with *Mtb* specific (ESAT-6/CFP-10) antigen. **HIV + TB+**: HIV patients with TB (continuous line); **HIV-TB**: HIV negative TB patients (long-dash line); **HIV + TST+**: HIV positive tuberculin skin test (TST) positive patients (dot line); **HIV-TST+**: HIV negative TST positive individuals (square dot); and Controls (HIV-TST-) (circle dot). Mean of IFN-γ (pg/ml) with standard deviation per follow-up visit are shown on the line graph; n = number of participants per visit shown on the legend.

CFP-10 (immune function specific to TB). No significant correlation between CD4+ T cell count recovery and IFN-γ production was found *(r = 0.19, p = 0.40, n = 22)*. In contrast, however, there was a strong positive correlation between the recovery of CD4+ cells and IFN-γ production in the HIV negative active TB patients (HIV-TB+) following TB treatment for six months *(r = 0.71, p = 0.0007, n = 19)* (Figure 6).

Discussions

In this study, we determined the long-term outcome of HAART in HIV patients with and without TB and LTBI by comprehensively measuring HIV RNA suppression, CD4+ T-cell recovery, and immune reconstitution specific to *Mtb*.

The goal of ART is to suppress HIV-1 RNA below the detection limit of the assay within 12–24 weeks [5], or to less than 0·5-0·75 log copies/ml by 4 weeks [23]. In this study, 84% of the non-TB patients on HAART had HIV RNA <50 copies/ml at 24 months on ART. This is comparable to most studies from Africa [24,25], Europe [15,26], and United States [27].

Nevertheless, 19% of the non-TB patients in this study were virologic failures (HIV RNA > 5000 copies/ml) at 6 months of ART. Reports from Cameroon [28] and Brazil [29] also showed virologic failure (HIV RNA > 400 copies/ml) in 13% and 28% of patients at 6 months on ART. As reported by Tuboi SH *et al.* [29], malnutrition and advanced WHO stages were risk factors for virologic failure in this study, which strongly indicate the

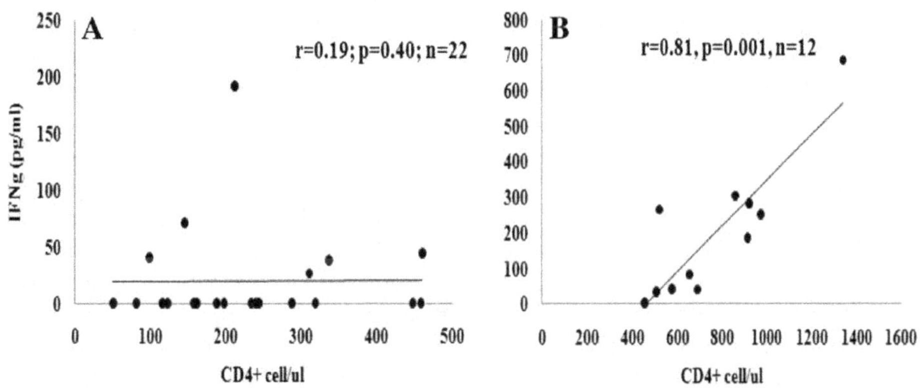

Figure 6 Spearman correlation between IFN-γ production and absolute CD4+ count recovery after the start of HAART and TB treatment. (A) HIV positive patients with active TB (HIV + TB+) at 6th and 18th months of HAART and TB treatment, and **(B)** HIV negative TB patients (HIV-TB+) at six months of TB treatment. IFN-γ secretion was measured in 7th day culture supernatants of whole blood stimulated with *Mtb* specific antigen (ESAT-6/CFP-10). r = correlation coefficient.

need of earlier identification of eligible patients and earlier initiation of HAART for better treatment outcome.

Interestingly, comparable to other reports [15,30], also 80% of the HIV patients with TB in this study had HIV RNA < 50 copies/ml at 24 months on HAART, which is similar to viral suppression in patients without TB (Figures 1 & 2) and has been reported recently in another study [31]. In contrast, others have reported a high hazard ratio for virologic failure in patients with TB on ART [32].

Since many patients in Sub-Saharan Africa present to the health facilities with advanced disease stages and low CD4 cell counts [24], they may have limited advantage for CD4+ recovery after ART [17]. However, despite the overall lower baseline CD4+ count of the healthy Ethiopians [33], and the lower CD4+ count at ART start (197 cells/ μl) in HIV patients without TB in this study, the increase in CD4+ cells after two years on ART (332 cells/μl) was comparable with a recent report from Ethiopia [34], and other reports from Africa [24], in low-income countries (Africa, Latin America and Asia) [35], and the United States [27,36]. The mean CD4+ increase by 24 month on ART in this study (6.7 cells/μl/month) was also comparable to a report from South Africa [37].

However, 45% of the non-TB patients in this study had immunologic failure (an increase of <50 CD4+ cells/μl) at 6 months, while 32% failed to restore CD4+ T cell count to ≥ 200 cells/μl by 2 years on ART, which is similar to a study from Nigeria [38]. Similar to Lifson *et al.* [36], advance WHO stages and lower CD4+ count at baseline were risk factors for immunologic failure, which strongly suggests the need for earlier identification of eligible patients and initiation of HAART.

Furthermore, since more than 50% of the HIV/TB patients in Sub-Saharan Africa presented to the health facilities at advanced disease stages and start ART at CD4+ counts of 100–150 cells/μl [16,24] the benefit of patients on ART could be limited [28,39]. More than 50% of the HIV/TB patients in our cohort had advanced disease stage at enrolment and the CD4+ count at ART initiation was 110 cells/μl (Table 2). Interestingly, however, we observed no difference in the CD4+ cell increase over time on HAART in patients with and without TB as reported by Lawn SD *et al.* [40] and Dronda F *et al.* [31]. In contrast, others reported reduced CD4+ recovery after ART in patients with TB [15,41,42]. Interestingly, although the study sample was small, we did observe reduced CD4+ recovery in HIV/TB patients co-infected with HBV (Figure 3A) as reported by Pe' rez-Molina JA *et al.* [43].

Overall, the total CD4+ count achieved by 2 years on HAART in patients with TB (290 cells/μl) and without TB (332 cells/μl) in this study was comparable to findings from African and other developed countries, although it was still lower compared to the healthy Ethiopian populations (754.8 cells/μl). This poses the question whether immune function is restored after 2 year of HAART. Therefore, the *Mtb* specific immune restoration after 18 month on HAART was investigated.

It has been estimated that, if HAART is accessible to all patients with CD4+ < 200 cells/μl and would restore optimal immune responses specific to *Mtb*, the cumulative incidence of TB would decrease by 22% over 20 years [44]. However, if immune restoration to *Mtb* is incomplete, there would be a substantial number of patients on HAART which are continuously at high risk for TB. In this study we measured the level of IFN-γ, a cytokine which plays a key role in the control of *Mtb* infection [45] in response to *Mtb* specific antigen (ESAT-6/CFP-10) [46].

We observed lower IFN-γ secretion in HIV negative TB patients compared to LTBI individuals at baseline as reported by Hanna LE *et al.* [47]. Coinfection with HIV severely decreased the secretion of IFN-γ in both groups. Furthermore, in support to previous reports [41,42,48], IFN-γ production after 18 month of HAART was not restored in HIV patients with TB while it was normalized in those with LTBI. Among the possible factors contributing to the impaired IFN-γ response in the HIV/TB patients are exhaustion of immune system [47] defined as a reduced proliferation of immune cells and impaired cytokine production due to infection with HIV [49] and *Mtb* [50] , and depletion of *Mtb* specific CD4+ cells due to direct infection with HIV [15]. Our observation that there was no correlation between CD4+ count recovery after HAART and level of IFN-γ production in the HIV + TB + patients, unlike to that of HIV-TB + patients where there was a strong correlation between CD4+ T cell recovery and IFN-γ production following TB treatment (Figure 5), suggests that other factors may play a role in the impaired functional recovery of *Mtb* specific immune responses in the HIV + TB + patients. Among the strategies proposed to boost immune restoration specific to TB after HAART are early initiation of HAART and isoniazid prophylaxis, and adjunctives such as BCG vaccination or co-administration of IL-2 [48,51].

Overall, addressing the long-term outcome of HAART by comprehensively measuring the key parameters of ART responses in a well defined cohort of patients with and without active TB and LTBI is the major strength of this study. The study addressed immune responses after HAART not only by measuring the absolute CD4+ cell recovery as a proxy for immune restoration but also by measuring IFN-γ response specific to *Mtb.* However, the fact that there is no golden standard definition of LTBI could be counted as limitations of the study

Conclusions

In this observational cohort study, we showed sustained outcomes of long-term HAART in HIV patients with and without TB and LTBI as evidenced by clinical, immunologic and virologic data. Advanced pre-ART disease stages were the risk factors for diminished CD4+ and virologic responses to HAART and high mortality, which strongly indicated the need of early identification of eligible patients and early access to care and treatment. *Mtb* specific immune reconstitution in HIV/TB patients remained impaired after 18 months on HAART, which suggested the need of strong prevention, earlier diagnosis, and treatment of TB, as well as earlier initiation of HAART. Factors contributing to impaired *Mtb* specific immune restoration in HIV/TB patients after HAART need to be investigated in order to develop intervention methods which could boost the immune response. In addition, we should do further study on the immunological mechanisms associated with HIV/TB coinfection.

Materials and methods

Study populations and settings

This observational cohort study was performed from April 2007-February 2011 at St Peter Specialized Referral TB Hospital, Akaki and Kality Health centers in Addis Ababa, Ethiopia. Adults of both sexes who were naïve to ART and TB treatment were enrolled after informed and written consent was sought.

Diagnosis of active tuberculosis (TB) was based on both clinical and bacteriological evidences. At least two sputum smears stained by the Ziehil-Neelsen direct method were required to be microscopy positive for Acid Fast Bacilli (AFB) [52]. Except for TB patients, Mantoux Tuberculin Skin Testing (TST) for tuberculin was done for all participants. A diameter of skin induration with ≥ 10 mm in HIV un-infected, and ≥ 5 mm in HIV-infected individuals was graded as TST positive (TST+), and was considered as a LTBI [52].

The study participants were enrolled in 5 clinical groups: HIV patients with TB (HIV + TB+), and without TB (HIV + TB-) [sub-grouped further as Tuberculin Skin Test (TST) positive (HIV + TST+) and TST negative HIV + TST-], HIV negative TB cases (HIV-TB+), HIV-TST+, and controls (HIV-TST-). After enrolment, the HIV + TB+, HIV + TB-, and HIV-TB + groups were scheduled for follow-up (FU) clinic visits at sixth month (M6), M18 and M24.

At enrolment and during FU visit, each participant was interviewed using a standard questionnaire and detailed clinical, anthropometric and demographic data were recorded by a clinician or a nurse. A total of 20 ml heparinized venous blood was collected and transported immediately to the National HIV Referral Laboratory (NHL), at EHNRI. HAART was prescribed for eligible HIV patients and anti-TB treatment for all the TB cases free of charge as per the national guidelines. Antibiotic prophylaxis was also prescribed by the physician at enrolment or during the clinic follow-up visits [52].

Laboratory tests

Laboratory examinations of blood were performed by automated machines following the manufacturer's protocol. Hematological values were determined using Cell Dyn (Abbott laboratories, Abott Par IC Jl 60064, USA); CD4+ T cell counts were determined using Becton Dickinson (BD) FACSCalibur (Becton Dickinson, San Jose, USA); and Plasma HIV-1 RNA load was measured using the NucliSens EasyQ NASBA diagnostic 2007/1 (Organon, Teknika) which has a detection range of 50–3,000,000 copies/ml. The level of IFN-γ (pg/ml) in the 7th day whole blood culture supernatant stimulated with *Mtb* specific antigen (ESAT-6/CFP-10) was measured by xMAP multiplex technology (Luminex, Austin TX, USA), using Biosource reagents (Biosource, Camarillo, USA), and analyzed with the STarStation v2.0 software (Applied Cytometry Systems, United Kingdom) as described previously [53].

Definitions

Based on data from different studies [54,55], the national [56] and international [11] guidelines, and considering the small sample size in this study, we choose the following cut-off values to define HAART outcomes. *Body mass index (BMI)* (kg/m^2) was categorized as malnutrition (BMI <18.50) and normal (18.50 ≥ BMI ≤ 24.99), and anemia was defined as hemoglobin (Hgb) <12 g/dl [57]; *virologic success* was defined as achieving a viral suppression (HIV RNA < 50 copies/ml, or lower than the detection level (LDL) of the assay) after HAART, and *virologic failure* as a single HIV RNA >5000 copies/ml after a minimum of 6 months on HAART [11]. *Immunologic success* was defined as an increase of ≥ 50 CD4+ cells/μl at M6 and ≥100 cells/μl at M18 and M24 from that at ART initiation; *immunologic failure* as a failure to increase ≥ 50 cells/μl at M6, or ≥100 cells/μl at M18 and M24; and *super-responders* as patients able to achieve CD4+ count of >500 cells/μl after 2 years of HAART.

Statistical analysis

Data entered using Microsoft Access (DBse XI) was double-checked for discrepancies. All data analysis was done using Intercooled STATA version 11.0 (College Station, Texas, USA). Descriptive analyses including counts and frequencies for categorical variables, and mean (standard deviation, SD) or median (interquartile range, IQR) for continuous variables were computed. Results were compared using chi-square test and Fisher's exact test for categorical variables and non-parametric tests (Wilcoxon signed rank test and Mann–Whitney U test) for continuous variables. Fixed (sex, groups) and time-updated variables (age, CD4+ count, HIV RNA, BMI, Hgb, TLC, co-infections) were included in the logistic regression analysis to identify risk factors for failed immunologic and virologic responses to HAART. A p-value of < 0.05 was considered as statistical significant.

Competing interests

The authors declare that they have no competing interests.

Authors' contributions

DK was a lead author on planning, implementation of the study, data analysis, and writing of the draft, interim and final version of the manuscript; GG and YA participated in different laboratory tests; AA participated in counseling the study participants, filling study questionnaires and sample collection; DW, TE and DB – participated in providing advice and help during data analysis and also offered inputs and recommendations during the draft, interim and final version of the manuscript. All authors have seen and approved the final manuscript.

Acknowledgements

This work, which is part of an ongoing longitudinal study entitled "Biomarkers of protective immunity against tuberculosis in the context of Human Immunodeficiency Virus/Acquired immunodeficiency Syndrome (HIV/AIDS) in Africa" [58], was supported by the Bill & Melinda Gates Foundation through the Grand Challenges in Global Health Initiative, grant no. 37772.
This work has been presented in part to the "Australian HIV/AIDS conference 2012" Melbourne, Australia, October 17–19, 2012 (poster number 311).
We would like to thank all patients participating in this cohort study, all the study nurses involved, and the data clerk.

Author details

[1]Infectious and non-infectious diseases research directorate, Ethiopian Health and Nutrition Research Institute (EHNRI), P.O. Box 1242, Addis Ababa, Ethiopia. [2]Department of Internal Medicine and Infectious Diseases and Department of Immunology, University Medical Center Utrecht, Utrecht, The Netherlands. [3]Medical Biotech Laboratory, Addis Ababa, Ethiopia.

References

1. Palella FJ, Delaney KM, Moorman AC: **Declining morbidity and mortality among patients with advanced human immunodeficiency virus infection.** *N Engl J Med* 1998, **38:**853–860.
2. Joint United Nations Programme on HIV/AIDS (UNAIDS): *Report on the global AIDS epidemic, 2012, "UNAIDS / JC2417E".* http://www.unaids.org/en/media/unaids/contentassets/documents/epidemiology/2012/gr2012/20121120_UNAIDS_Global_Report_2012_en.pdf.
3. World Health Organization (WHO): *Treating 3 million by 2005: making it happen. The WHO strategy. Geneva, World Health Organization, 2003.* http://www.who.int/3by5/publications/documents/isbn9241591129.
4. Federal HIV/AIDS Prevention and Control Office (FHAPCO): *Multi-sectoral HIV/AIDS response monitoring and evaluation: Annual report*; 2011. http://www.HAPCO.gov.et or http://www.etharc.org.
5. Volberding PA, Deeks SG: **Antiretroviral therapy and management of HIV infection.** *Lancet* 2010, **376:**49–62.
6. Collazos J, Asensi V, Carton JA: **CD4 Responses in the Setting or Suboptimal Virological Responses to Antiretroviral Therapy: Features, Outcomes, and Associated Factors.** *AIDS Res Hum Retroviruses* 2009, **25**(7):647–655.
7. Menéndez-Arias L: **Molecular basis of human immunodeficiency virus drug resistance: an update.** *Antiviral Res* 2010, **85**(1):210–31.
8. Nicastri E, Chiesi A, Angeletti C, Sarmati L, Palmisano L, Geraci A, *et al*: **Italian Antiretroviral Treatment Group (IATG): clinical outcome after 4 years follow-up of HIV-seropositive subjects with incomplete virologic or immunologic response to HAART.** *J Med Virol* 2005, **76:**153–60.
9. Carpenter CC, Cooper DA, Fischl MA, Gatell JM, Gazzard BG, Hammer SM, *et al*: **Antiretroviral therapy in adults: updated recommendations of the International AIDS Society-USA Panel.** *JAMA* 2000, **283**(3):381–390.
10. Jevtovic D, Salemovic D, Ranin J, Pešic'I, Žerjav S, Djurkovic'-Djakovic O: **The dissociation between virological and immunological responses with HAART.** *Biomed Pharmacother* 2005, **59:**446–451.
11. WHO: *Antiretroviral therapy for HIV infection in adults and adolescents: recommendations for a public health approach*; 2010. Revision. http://whqlibdoc.who.int/publications/2010/9789241599764_eng.pdf.
12. Misgena DK: **The pattern of immunologic and virologic responses to Highly Active Antiretroviral Treatment (HAART): Does success bring further challenges?** *Ethiop. J. Health Dev* 2011, **25**(1):61–70.
13. Gupta RK, Hill A, Sawyer AW, Cozzi-Lepri A, Wyl V, Yerly S, *et al*: **Virological monitoring and resistance to first-line highly active antiretroviral therapy in adults infected with HIV-1 treated under WHO guidelines: a systematic review and meta-analysis.** *Lancet Infect Dis* 2009, **9:**409–417.
14. Egger S, Petoumenos K, Kamarulzaman A, Hoy J, Sungkanuparph S, Chuah J, Falster K, *et al*: **Long-Term patterns in CD4 response are determined by an interaction between baseline CD4 cell count, viral load, and time: The Asia Pacific HIV observational database (APHOD).** *J Acquir Immune Defic Syndr* 2009, **50:**513–520.
15. Cingolani A, Cozzi Lepri A, Castagna A, Goletti D, De Luca A, Scarpellini P, Fanti I, Antinori A, *et al*: **Impaired CD4 T-Cell Count Response to Combined Antiretroviral Therapy in Antiretroviral-Naive HIV-Infected Patients Presenting With Tuberculosis as AIDS-Defining Condition.** *Clin Infect Dis* 2011, **54:**853–61.
16. Lawn SD, Kranzer K, Wood R: **Antiretroviral therapy for control of the HIV-associated tuberculosis epidemic in resource-limited settings.** *Clin Chest Med* 2009, **30:**685–99.
17. Lederman HM, Williams PL, Wu JW, Evans TG, Cohn SE, McCutchan JA, *et al*: **Incomplete immune reconstitution after initiation of highly active antiretroviral therapy in human immunodeficiency virus-infected patients with severe CD4+ cell depletion.** *J Infect Dis* 2003, **188:**1794–1803.
18. Gupta A, Wood R, Kaplan R, Bekker L-G, Lawn SD: **Tuberculosis Incidence Rates during 8 Years of Follow-Up of an Antiretroviral Treatment Cohort in South Africa: Comparison with Rates in the Community.** *PLoS One* 2012, **7**(3):e34156.
19. Marimoutou C, Chêne G, Mercié P, Neau D, Farbos S, Morlat P, Ceccaldi J, *et al*: **Prognostic factors of combined viral load and CD4+ cell count responses under triple antiretroviral therapy, Aquitaine cohort, 1996–1998.** *J Acquir Immune Defic Syndr* 2001, **27:**161–167.
20. Horst R, Collin SM, Ritmeijer K, Bogale A, Davidson Rt N: **Concordant HIV Infection and Visceral Leishmaniasis in Ethiopia: The Influence of Antiretroviral Treatment and Other Factors on Outcome.** *Clin Infect Dis* 2008, **46**(11):1702–1709.
21. Huruy K, Kassu A, Mulu A, Wondie Y: **Immune restoration disease and changes in CD4+ T-cell count in HIV- infected patients during highly active antiretroviral therapy at Zewditu memorial hospital, Addis Ababa, Ethiopia.** *AIDS Res Ther* 2010, **7:**46.
22. Sabin CA: **Cohort studies: to what extent can they inform treatment guidelines?** *Curr Opin Infect Dis* 2010, **23**(1):15–20.
23. US Health and Human Services (UHHS): *Guidelines for the use of antiretroviral agents in HIV-infected adults and adolescents.* Washington, DC: DHHS; 2001.
24. Hammond R, Harry TC: **Efficacy of antiretroviral therapy in Africa: effect on immunological and virological outcome measures – a meta-analysis.** *Int J STD AIDS* 2008, **19:**291–296.
25. Bussmann H, Wester CW, Ndwapi N, Grundmann N, Gaolathe T, Puvimanasinghe J, *et al*: **Five-year outcomes of initial patients treated in Botswana's National Antiretroviral Treatment Program.** *AIDS* 2008, **22:**2303–2311.
26. Geretti AM, Harrison L, Green H, Sabin C, Hill T, Fearnhill E, *et al*: **Effect of HIV-1 subtype on virologic and immunologic response to starting highly active antiretroviral therapy.** *Clin Infect Dis* 2009, **48**(9):1296–305.
27. Marconi VC, Grandits GA, Weintrob AC, Chun H, Landrum ML, Ganesan A, Infectious Disease Clinical Research Program HIV Working Group (IDCRP), *et al*: **Outcomes of highly active antiretroviral therapy in the context of universal access to healthcare: the U.S. Military HIV Natural History Study.** *AIDS Res Ther* 2010, **7:**14.

28. Rougemont M, Stoll BE, Elia N, Ngang P: **Antiretroviral treatment adherence and its determinants in Sub-Saharan Africa: a prospective study at Yaounde Central Hospital, Cameroon.** *AIDS Res Ther* 2009, **6**:21.
29. Tuboi SH, Harrison LH, Sprinz E, Albernaz RK, Schechter M: **Predictors of virologic failure in HIV-1-infected patients starting highly active antiretroviral therapy in Porto Alegre, Brazil.** *J Acquir Immune Defic Syndr* 2005, **40**:324–8.
30. Zanoni BC, Phungula T, Zanoni HM, France H, Feeney ME: **Impact of tuberculosis cotreatment on viral suppression rates among HIV-positive children initiating HAART.** *AIDS* 2011, **25**:49–55.
31. Dronda F, Sobrino P, Hernández-Novoa B, Caro-Murillo AM, Montero M, Iribarren JA, *et al*: **Response to HAART in treatment-naive HIV-infected patients with a prior diagnosis of tuberculosis or other opportunistic infections.** *Curr HIV Res* 2011, **9**:229–36.
32. Lartey M, Sagoe KW, Yang H, Kenu E, Xexemeku F, Oliver-Commey J, *et al*: **Viral decay rates are similar in HIV-infected patients with and without TB coinfection during treatment with an Efavirenz-based regimen.** *Clin Infect Dis* 2011, **52**(4):547–50.
33. Mekonnen Y, Geskus RB, Hendriks JC, Messele T, Borghans J, Miedema F, *et al*: **Low CD4 T cell counts before HIV-1 seroconversion do not affect disease progression in Ethiopian factory workers.** *J Infect Dis* 2005, **192**(5):739–748.
34. Assefa Y, Kiflie A, Tekle B, Mariam DH, Laga M, Van Damme W: **Effectiveness and acceptability of delivery of antiretroviral treatment in health centres by health officers and nurses in Ethiopia.** *J Health Serv Res Policy* 2012, **17**(1):24–9.
35. Nash D, Katyal M, Brinkhof MW, Keiser O, May M, Hughes R, Dabis F, *et al*: **Long-term immunologic response to antiretroviral therapy in low-income countries: a collaborative analysis of prospective studies.** *AIDS* 2008, **22**:2291–2302.
36. Lifson AR, Krantz EM, Eberly LE, Matthew Dolan J, Marconi VC, Weintrob AC: **Long-term CD4+ lymphocyte response following HAART initiation in a U. S. Military prospective Cohort.** *AIDS Res Ther* 2011, **8**(1):2.
37. Julg B, Poole D, Ghebremichael M, Castilla C, Altfeld M, Sunpath H, *et al*: **Factors Predicting Discordant Virological and Immunological Responses to Antiretroviral Therapy in HIV-1 Clade C Infected Zulu/Xhosa in South Africa.** *PLoS One* 2012, **7**(2):e31161.
38. Rawizza HE, Chaplin B, Meloni ST, Eisen G, Rao T, Sankalé JL, *et al*: **Immunologic Criteria Are Poor Predictors of Virologic Outcome: Implications for HIV Treatment Monitoring in Resource-Limited Settings.** *Clin Infect Dis* 2011, **53**(12):1283–90.
39. Sanne IM, Westreich D, Macphail AP, Rubel D, Majuba P, Van Rie A: **Long term outcomes of antiretroviral therapy in a large HIV/AIDS care clinic in urban South Africa: a prospective cohort study.** *J Int AIDS Soc* 2009, **12**:38.
40. Lawn SD, Myer L, Bekker LG, Wood R: **Burden of tuberculosis in an antiretroviral treatment programme in sub-Saharan Africa: impact on treatment outcomes and implications for tuberculosis control.** *AIDS* 2006, **20**:1605–12.
41. Elsherbiny D, Ren Y, McIlleron H, Maartens G, Simonsson US: **Population pharmacokinetics of lopinavir in combination with rifampicinbased antitubercular treatment in HIV-infected South African children.** *Eur J Clin Pharmacol* 2010, **66**:1017–23.
42. Lazaro E, Coureau G, Guedj J, Blanco P, Pellegrin I, Commenges D, *et al*: **Change in T-lymphocyte count after initiation of highly active antiretroviral therapy in HIV-infected patients with history of Mycobacterium avium complex infection.** *Antivir Ther* 2006, **11**(3):343–50.
43. Pe' rez-Molina JA, Dı'az-Mene'ndez M, Plana MN, Zamora J, Lo'pez-Ve'lez R and and Moreno S: **Very late initiation of HAART impairs treatment response at 48 and 96 weeks: results from a meta-analysis of randomized clinical trials.** *J Antimicrob Chemother* 2012, **67**:312–321.
44. Williams BG, Dye C: **Antiretroviral therapy for TB control in the era of HIV/AIDS.** *Science* 2003, **301**:1535–37.
45. Flynn J: **Immunology of tuberculosis and implications in vaccine development.** *Tuberculosis* 2004, **4**:93–101.
46. Pollock JM, Andersen P: **The potential of the ESAT-6 antigen secreted by virulent mycobacteria for specific diagnosis of tuberculosis.** *J Infect Dis* 1997, **175**(5):1251–4.
47. Hanna LE, Nayak K, Subramanyam S: **Incomplete immunological recovery following anti-tuberculosis treatment in HIV-infected individuals with active tuberculosis.** *Indian J Med Res* 2009, **129**(5):548–54.
48. Lawn SD, Bekkera L-G, Wood R: **How effectively does HAART restore immune responses to *Mycobacterium tuberculosis*? Implications for tuberculosis control.** *AIDS* 2005, **19**:1113–1124.
49. Wherry EJ: **T cell exhaustion.** *Nat Immunol* 2011, **12**:492e9.
50. Wang X, Cao Z, Jiang J, Niu H, Dong M, Tong A, *et al*: **Association of mycobacterial antigen-specific CD4+ memory T cell subsets with outcome of pulmonary tuberculosis.** *J Infect* 2010, **60**:133e9.
51. Marchetti G, Franzetti F, Gori A: **Partial immune reconstitution following highly active antiretroviral therapy: can adjuvant interleukin-2 fill the gap?** *J Antimicrob Chemother* 2005, **55**:401–409.
52. Federal Ministry of Health (FMOH): *Manual of Tuberculosis, Leprosy and TB/HIV prevention and control programme.* 3rd edition. Addis Ababa, Ethiopia; 2005. http://www.moh.gov.et/English/Resources/Documents/FMOH_Guidelines forTBL_TB_HIV.pdf.
53. Fulton RJ, McDade RL, Smith PL, Kienker LJ, Kettman JR Jr: **Advanced multiplexed analysis with the FlowMetrix system.** *Clin Chem* 1997, **43**(9):1749–1756.
54. Hammer SM, Eron JJ Jr, Reiss P, Schooley RT, Thompson MA, Walmsley S, Cahn P, Fischl MA, Gatell JM, Hirsch MS, Jacobsen DM, Montaner JS, Richman DD, Yeni PG, Volberding PA: **International AIDS Society-USA. Antiretroviral treatment of adult HIV infection: 2008 recommendations of the International AIDS Society-USA panel.** *JAMA* 2008, **6;300**(5):555–570.
55. Murphya RA, Sunpathb H, Luc Z, Chelinb N, Losinac E, Gordond M, *et al*: **Outcomes after virologic failure of first-line ART in South Africa.** *AIDS* 2010, **24**:1007–1012.
56. Federal Ministry of Health (FMOH)-Federal HIV/AIDS Prevention and Control Office (HAPCO) (FMOH/FHAPCO): *Single Point HIV Prevalence Estimate, Addis Ababa, June 2007.* http://www.etharc.org/aidsineth/publications/singlepointprev_2007.pdf.
57. Blanc B, Finch CA, Hallberg L: **Nutritional anaemias. Report of a WHO Scientific Group.** *WHO Tech Rep Ser* 1968, **405**:1–40.
58. Kaufmann SHE, Parida SK: **Tuberculosis in Africa: Learning from Pathogenesis for Biomarker Identification.** *Cell Host Microbe* 2008, **4**(3):219–228.

5

Population specific reference ranges of CD3, CD4 and CD8 lymphocyte subsets among healthy Kenyans

Erick M Bosire[1*], Anthony K Nyamache[2], Michael M Gicheru[1], Samoel A Khamadi[3], Raphael W Lihana[3] and Vincent Okoth[3]

Abstract

Background: The enumeration of absolute CD4 counts is of primary importance for many medical conditions especially HIV infection where therapeutic initiation depends on the count. These ranges tend to vary across populations. However, these ranges have not been comprehensively established in the Kenyan population. Therefore, this study aimed at establishing the reference ranges for the CD4 and CD8 T-lymphocytes in normal healthy individuals in Kenya.

Methods: A total of 315 individuals of the ages between 16 and 60 years old, in 5 different regions of the country, were recruited into the study. They were screened for diseases that potentially cause lymphocyte homeostasis perturbation. CD4/CD8 Counts were performed by use of a FACSCalibur flow cytometer (Becton-Dickinson, NJ) equipped with automated acquisition and analysis software. Results were analysed according to age, sex and region.

Results: Results were presented as means and ranges (in parenthesis) generated non parametrically as 2.5 and 97.5 percentiles as follows; In general population; CD3 1655 (614-2685 cells/μL), CD4 920 (343-1493 cells/μL), and CD8 646 (187-1139 cells/μL), while according to sex, females; CD3 1787 (697-2841 cells/μL), CD4 1010 (422-1572 cells/μL), CD8 659 (187-1180 cells/μL); males; CD3 1610 (581-2641 cells/μL), CD4 889(320-1459 cells/μL) and CD8 644 (185-1140 cells/μL). The general reference ranges for CD4/CD8 ratios were as follows; general population 1.57(0.50-2.74), males 1.51(0.49-2.64) and females 1.69(0.55-2.95).

Conclusion: The lymphocyte reference ranges for the Kenyan population are fairly comparable to those established in other African populations. The ranges also differ appreciably from those established in Germany, Italy and Switzerland. Furthermore, the study reported significant differences in the ranges of different population clusters within Kenya, as well us between males and females.

Keywords: CD4/CD8 count, Lymphocyte subsets, HIV-1, Flow cytometry, Reference ranges

Introduction

Lymphocytes co-ordinate the immune system's response and play a central role in cell mediated immunity [1]. Lymphocyte subset may include; Helper T cells (CD4 T-cells), Cytotoxic T cells (CTLs or CD8 T-cells), Memory T cells and Regulatory T cells (Treg cells). Upon encounter with antigens, CD4 T cells become activated and proliferate rapidly secreting cytokines that sends signals and maintain active immune response. On the other hand, the CD8 T-cells destroy virally infected cells and tumor cells, and remain inactivated when there is no foreign antigen. In human immunodeficiency virus-1 (HIV-1) infected individuals, lymphocytes (specifically CD4 T-cells) are the viral prime targets. Therefore in these individuals, a CD4 count provides a picture of immune system competence, with higher CD4 counts typically signifying healthier immune systems [1,2]. In such application, flow cytometry is used to provide absolute counts, percentages and or ratios of these lymphocyte subsets. Besides HIV management, flow cytometric analysis of peripheral blood lymphocyte

* Correspondence: bosireerick@yahoo.com
[1]Department of Zoological Science, Kenyatta University, P.O. Box 43844-0100, Nairobi, Kenya

phenotypes has proven a useful aid in managing a wide range of medical conditions, including autoimmunity, immunodeficiency, infection, malignancy and transplantation [3-5]. Essential to the effective application of this approach is availability of accurate reference values against which results can be meaningfully compared.

Reference ranges that are currently used in Kenya are derived from data obtained from Caucasians who are not African Kenyans. In addition, these ranges do not include age and sex which are very important factors that influence lymphocyte counts [6]. Furthermore, several factors have been associated with these differences in lymphocyte counts. These may include; demographic and genetic factors, current exposure to infectious diseases and behavioral factors on CD3, CD4 and CD8 in HIV-negative populations [1,2,6]. Averagely, healthy African and Asian populations have been shown to have lower CD4 lymphocyte counts than their western European and Caucasian counterparts [2,7,8]. In addition, women tend to have higher CD4 levels than men with comparable demographic and behavioral patterns [8,9]. However, there is still limited data from specific countries to confirm these differences.

The pattern of lymphocyte generation has been shown to affect the levels of circulating lymphocytes in males, females and individuals of different ages. The pattern of T lymphocyte generation in aging has been associated with dynamic changes in thymic and extrathymic functions along with sequential developmental steps from cells to mature cells [10]. Increased absolute numbers of peripheral blood CD4 cells in females compared to males have been reported [11]. This is perhaps due to androgens which accelerate thymocytes apoptosis and subsequently influence T cell repertoire with males tending to have less CD4 cells than females [12,13]. Sex and age related variations in the lymphocyte subsets contribute to age and sex related diseases including autoimmune disorders in females and leukemia or lymphoma in males and elderly patients [14,15]. Other factors which have received little attention but also affect the normal lymphocyte levels include; dietary patterns, body mass index and smoking habits [16-18]. The influence of these many factors point out to the fact that the reference ranges of one population might not be accurately used as a reference range for another. This might give an inaccurate interpretation of the immune status of the individuals.

Several efforts to establish reference ranges have indicated differences in lymphocyte levels between African and Western populations [2,3,9,19]. In one community in Kenya, general clinical ranges have been shown to significantly differ from the ranges from other parts of the continent [20]. These ranges are also appreciably different from those reported in a neighboring country [21]. The two studies in Kenya had indicated a possibility of having remarkably different ranges of lymphocyte subsets within the Kenyan population [20,22]. This necessitates the need for a comprehensive reference range establishment using subjects from different regions of the country. In this study we report comprehensive reference ranges for CD3, CD4 and CD8 cutting across representative regions of the country. The study provides ranges specific for males, females and for different ages.

Materials and methods

Study subjects and samples

A total of 315 adults (222 men and 85 female) were recruited into the study after giving consent. This study was ethically approved by Kenya National ethical Review committee before execution. The individuals who were included in the study were healthy adults between 16 and 55 (categorized as 16-19, 21-30 and 31-55) years of age presenting for routine blood donation at the regional centers. These regional blood transfusion centers included; Mombasa, Nakuru, Kisumu, Embu, and Nairobi. A structured questionnaire was used to collect information on the history and general health status of the donors (See Additional file 1). Donors who confirmed to have a history of conditions that cause immune perturbations were excluded from the study. Further, the samples were screened for HIV, Hepatitis B virus (HBV), Hepatitis C virus (HCV), malaria, and syphilis after blood collection, and samples that tested positive were excluded from the study. Blood samples were collected by venipuncture into EDTA vacutainer tubes and analyzed immediately after collection.

Screening for malaria, syphilis, HIV, HCV and HBV

Enzyme linked immunoassays were used in screening for these conditions. Commercially available kits containing purified antigens were used. The kits included: ICE* Syphilis, Murex anti-HCV (version 4.0), Hepanostika HBsAg Ultra kit, Murex HIV-1.2.0 (Abbot) and malaria antigen detection kit (Creative diagnostics).

Sample collection and analysis

The lymphocyte subsets were analyzed on a FACSCalibur flow cytometer (Becton Dickinson Immunocytometry Systems, San Jose, California) with three monoclonal antibodies (BD Tritest CD4-FITC/CD8-PE/CD3-PerCP reagent) according to the manufacturer's instructions. The FACSCaliber was calibrated and reconfirmed daily using the BD Calibrite beads and BD-FACSComp software, version 2.0 for setting the photomultiplier tube voltages, setting the fluorescence compensation and checking instrument sensitivity before use. A control sample of commercially available whole blood was run daily to optimize the instrument settings. The CD45 versus the side scatter (SSC) dot plot was visually inspected

Table 1 The means and medians of the lymphocyte subsets in the study population

T lymphocyte subset							
	CD3		CD4		CD8		Ratios
	Absolute count*	%×	Absolute count*	%×	Absolute count*	%×	CD4/CD8
Mean	1655	67	920	37	646	26	1.57
Median	1580	67	884	37	559	25	1.47
Ranges	614-2685	50-78	343-1493	24-48	187-1139	13-36	0.50-2.74

*Expressed as cells/μL of blood.
×Expressed as a percentage of total lymphocytes.

to make sure they appear as a bright compact cluster, with low SSC. Analysis did not proceed if populations were diffuse and if there was little or no separation between clusters [15].

Data analysis

Non parametric reference range determination was employed by estimating the 2.5 and 97.5 percentile [23]. The significance of differences between the mean absolute counts and percentages of the Lymphocyte subsets were estimated using the Analysis of Variance (ANOVA) and T-test. Multiple comparisons were done using Tukey's test. Correlation analysis was applied in determining the relationship between lymphocyte subset levels and age.

Results

Among the 315 individuals between the ages 16-60 years, 61.7% (222) were men and 38.4% (85) were female. Their blood samples were analyzed for CD3, CD4 and CD8 lymphocyte subset for establishment of reference ranges. These reference ranges were also compared across the sampled geographical regions, by age as well as sex.

General distribution of the T-lymphocytes for the study population

The CD3, CD4 and CD8 counts and ranges for the general study population were determined. The means, median, percentages and ranges of these lymphocytes, as well as the CD4/CD8 ratios were determined (Table 1).

Lymphocyte subsets in the different Kenyan regions

Mean absolute counts of the different regions were compared using ANOVA. Significantly different means were further subjected to Tukey's test to show differences between each of the regions. The difference in the mean CD3 of Nairobi and Rift valley regions was minimal compared to the difference in the CD3 mean of the Lake Victoria basin region. The Lake Victoria region had the lowest CD3 mean compared to all other regions. These differences in the CD3 absolute count means were

Table 2 Means, medians and ranges of the lymphocyte subsets for the different geographical regions in Kenya

Region	Lymphocyte subset						
		CD3 count	CD3%	CD4 count	CD4%	CD8 count	CD8%
Nairobi	Mean ± SD	1841 ± 486c	69 ± 6a	1046 ± 283c	39 ± 6a	717 ± 260c	26 ± 5c
	Median	1824	69	1007	39	691	26
	Range	908-2661	55-79	517-1506	27-48	266-1165	16-35
Eastern	Mean ± SD	1728 ± 642b	64 ± 7a	949 ± 209b	37 ± 7b	650 ± 329ab	24 ± 6ab
	Median	1617	64	959	37	529	22
	Range	813-2512	47-77	512-1320	21-50	213-1083	11-34
Rift valley	Mean ± SD	1876 ± 883d	67 ± 8b	1029 ± 559ab	37 ± 7c	752 ± 421d	27 ± 8b
	Median	1666	68	902	36	640	26
	Range	660-3074	50-80	345-1703	23-47	217-1315	13-39
Lake Victoria	Mean ± SD	1195 ± 449abcd	66 ± 7c	690 ± 263abc	38 ± 6d	454 ± 231acd	25 ± 7d
	Median	1137	67	630	38	401	24
	Range	471-1886	50-77	275-1081	26-47	135-791	12-36
Coast	Mean ± SD	1617 ± 574a	66 ± 7d	881 ± 333a	36 ± 7a	675 ± 289a	28 ± 6a
	Median	1502	67	854	36	602	28
	Range	572-2708	51-77	281-1540	22-47	210-1179	16-37

The absolute counts of CD4, CD3 and CD8 are presented as cells/μL of blood.
Means followed by the same letters within a column are not significantly different from each other according to Tukey's test.

significant. General reference ranges were also determined as mentioned earlier ($P < 0.05$; Table 2).

T-lymphocyte subset for males and females

Females had a significantly higher CD3 mean absolute counts ($P < 0.05$) compared to men. There were significant differences in CD4 counts for males and females. However, there were no significant differences in the mean CD8 absolute counts. T lymphocyte subset reference ranges for males and females separately were also determined at 2.5 and 97.5 percentiles (Table 3).

Table 3 Means, medians and ranges of the lymphocyte subsets for males and females

Lymphocyte subset	Sex		p-value
	Female	Male	
CD3 Absolute count*			
N	85	222	
Mean	1787	1610	0.039
Median	1701	1529	0.016
Ranges	697-2841	581-2641	
CD3% ×			
Mean	68	66	0.026
Median	69	66	0.024
Ranges	54-78	49-78	
CD8 Absolute count*			
Mean	659	644	0.743
Median	568	558	0.696
Ranges	187-1180	185-1140	
CD8%×			
Mean	25	26	0.133
Median	25	25	0.256
Ranges	14-34	13-37	
CD4 Absolute count*			
Mean	1010	889	0.011
Median	991	855	0.001
Ranges	422-1572	320-1459	
CD4%×			
Mean	40	37	0.001
Median	39	36	0.001
Ranges	23-53	24-46	
CD4/CD8 ratio			
Mean	1.69	1.51	<0.001
Median	1.62	1.44	0.030
Ranges	0.55-2.95	0.49-2.64	

*Expressed as cells/μL of blood.
×Expressed as a percentage of total lymphocytes.

T-lymphocyte subset for the different age groups

The means and medians of the lymphocyte subsets were also determined for the different age groups. There were no significant differences in the mean absolute counts in the age groups that were considered in this study (Table 4).

Comparison of the ranges of the current study with those established by other studies

The reference ranges established in this study showed variations with the ones used in MultiSET (BD FACScaliber) as well as other studies in different populations. The studies compared below included normal (HIV negative)

Table 4 The lymphocyte subset levels in the different age groups

Subset	Age group			
	16-19	20-30	31-55	P value
CD3 Absolute count*				
N	55	196	62	
Mean	1603	1641	1742	0.745
Median	1519	1611	1622	0.595
CD3%×				
N	55	196	62	
Mean	65	67	67	0.180
Median	65	67	67	0.261
CD8 Absolute count*				
N	52	181	61	
Mean	611	641	693	0.870
Median	526	564	636	0.498
CD8%×				
N	52	181	61	
Mean	24	26	27	0.138
Median	23	25	26.	0.090
CD4 Absolute count*				
N	55	196	62	
Mean	912	898	997	0.139
Median	915	882	988	0.254
CD4%×				
N	55	196	62	
Mean	38	37	38	0.222
Median	36	37	37	0.184
CD4/CD8 ratio				
Mean	1.70	1.54	1.54	<0.001
Median	1.63	1.45	1.51	0.135

*Expressed as cells/μL of blood.
×Expressed as a percentage of total lymphocytes.
ANOVA was used to test the differences in means of the lymphocytes in the age groups.

populations in their study populations. Most of the studies were regional, that is, having been conducted in specific countries or in some specific regions within the countries (Table 5).

Discussion

The reference values of the main circulating lymphocyte subsets have been established by many studies throughout the world and have shown some variability according to geographical locations and methodology. Results in Table 5 show comparative values of CD3, CD4 and CD8 subsets levels from other countries, showing variations based on geographical region and platform methods used.

In this study, the mean CD3 count was found to be generally higher compared to those reported in Sweden (1075) but lower in CD3% mean [3]. In comparison with other African countries the lymphocyte counts and percentages were found to be fairly comparable in some cases but in others slightly different. In addition, Kenya like many African countries (Tanzania, Ghana, Senegal and Ethiopia) had lower lymphocyte subset levels compared to those reported in Sweden [3,25,26].

Considering the two important lymphocyte subsets CD4 and CD8, there were striking variations with the other reported ranges within and outside Africa. The mean CD8 value for this study was similar to those obtained in other African countries but slightly higher than those reported in Tanzania and Senegal [8,25]. The CD4 absolute counts were significantly higher than those reported in Ethiopia and Senegal [17] but lower compared to those reported in Kampala Uganda [21]; Table 5. However, the ranges cannot be conclusively compared since the studies differ in experimental set up. For example the study in Uganda included patients who visited an AIDS information center in Kampala, whereas our study was among blood donors across the country. In comparison to other countries outside Africa, the CD4 absolute counts were higher compared to Asian populations [27]. It can be speculated that, these differences in the lymphocyte counts are due to the many factors already mentioned, including genetic predisposition [1-3]. Many of these factors including the genetic influence have not been comprehensively confirmed.

In this study, females had higher absolute counts for CD3 and CD4 lymphocytes compared to males. This was probably due to biological factors (Table 4). It has been speculated that gender and age-related variations within the immune system parameters may contribute to the pathogenesis of several gender and age-related diseases such as autoimmune disorders in female patients [17,19,24]. Further, it has been shown that there are gender differences in the generation of CD8 cells during HIV-1 infection, due to increased immune activation compared to men [28]. However, a comparison of mean CD8 absolute counts between males and females, revealed no significant differences. These findings were consistent with previous studies [2,3,19,24].

The study also compared the differences in absolutes counts across regions. There were significant differences across regions with Lake Victoria region, consistently recording lower lymphocyte counts compared to other regions. The CD8 absolute count of Nairobi were appreciably similar with ones reported by Embree [19] in their controls of a study carried out in Nairobi. These observations show that, there is need to understand the impact of genetic makeup and altitude on the levels of T lymphocytes. The CD4 median absolute counts for the Rift valley (810 cells/μL) were similar to the ones reported in one of the studies in Kericho which is located within the valley ([20] Table 2).

Analysis of the lymphocyte subsets in the different age groups revealed no significant differences. A more comprehensive study design might be required to give a clear picture of the lymphocyte changes with advancing age. It is however well known that the pattern of T lymphocyte generation with age originates from dynamic changes in thymic as well as extrathymic functions, along with

Table 5 Comparison of the reference ranges developed in this study with reference ranges of other populations

Subset	Kenya	MultiSET	Tanzania	Ghana	Italy	Germany	Switzerland
CD3*	613.9048-2685.439	690-2540	NA	NA	600-2460	780-2240	540-1790
CD3%×	50.3433-78.0606	55-84	NA	NA	NA	NA	NA
CD4*	343.5796-1493.167	410-1590	312.2-1367.6	265-1932	490-1670	490-1640	310-1140
CD4%×	23.7048-48.2465	31-60	NA	NA	NA	NA	NA
CD8*	187.1348-1139.389	190-1140	168.2-996.8	162-1590	220-1110	170-880	140-820
CD8%×	13.3894-36.3925	13-41	NA	NA	NA	NA	NA
CD4/CD8 ratio	0.5002-2.7434	NA	1.1-2.5	0.58-4.59	NA	0.9-5.0	1.0-5.0

NA Not available.
*Expressed as cells/μL of blood.
×Expressed as a percentage of total lymphocytes.
Kenya-Current study, MultiSET-BD Biosciences, Tanzania [19], Ghana [2], Italy [24], Germany [25], Switzerland [3].

sequential developmental steps from stem cell to ultimately mature cells [29].

Conclusion

Our study has established ranges and reveals that lymphocyte subsets among the Kenyan population are different from those of other populations in the other populations such as Germany, Italy and Switzerland. However, the ranges are fairly comparable to those reported in some African countries. The ranges are also slightly different from those that are being used currently. This study has established reference ranges for the lymphocyte subsets among healthy Kenyan individuals of the ages between 16-60 years using FACSCalibur flow cytometer (Becton Dickinson Immunocytometry Systems, San Jose, California). The study has further shown the possibility of having varied lymphocyte levels among Kenyan subpopulations, due to many unconfirmed factors. Therefore, the current ranges should be more comprehensively determined and further revised, in order to have accurate comparisons during flow cytometry.

Abbreviations

HIV: Human immunodefieciency virus; CTL: Cytotoxic T lymphocytes; SSC: Side scatter; ANOVA: Analysis of variance.

Competing interests

The authors declare that they have no competing interests.

Authors' contributions

EB designed the study, collected samples, analysed them and drafted the manuscript. MMG helped in data analysis and interpretation and reviewed the manuscript. SAK conceptualized the idea, helped in designing experiment, analysis of the samples, interpretation of data and review of the manuscript. AKN helped in drafting and critically revising the manuscript. RL helped in critically reviewing the manuscript. VO helped in critical review of the paper. All authors read and approved the final manuscript.

Acknowledgements

The authors wish to thank individuals who participated in the study, the staff of all the Regional Blood Transfusion centers for their participation and the Department of Zoological Sciences, Kenyatta University for financial support.

Author details

[1]Department of Zoological Science, Kenyatta University, P.O. Box 43844-0100, Nairobi, Kenya. [2]Department of Plant and Microbial Sciences, Kenyatta University, P. O. Box 43844-0100, Nairobi, Kenya. [3]Kenya Medical Research Institute, Centre for Viral Research, P.O Box 54840-00200, Nairobi, Kenya.

References

1. Ahmadi K, Hall M, Norman P, Vaughan R, Snieder H, Spector T, Lanchbury J: **Genetic determinism in the relationship between human CD4 and CD8 T lymphocyte populations.** *Genes Immunol* 2001, **2:**38–387.
2. Ampofo W, Torpey K, Mukadi Y, Koram K, Nolan K, Amenyah R, Kaitoo E, Antwi P, Ofori-adjei D, Lamptey P: **Normal CD4T lymphocyte levels in HIV seronegative individuals in the Manya/Yilo Krobo communities in the Eastern Region of Ghana.** *Viral Immunol* 2006, **19:**260–266.
3. Bisset L, Lung T, Kaelin M, Ludwig E, Dubs R: **Reference values for peripheral blood lymphocyte phenotypes applicable to the healthy adult population in Switzerland.** *Eur J Haematol* 2004, **72:**203–212.
4. Illoh O: **Current applications of flow cytometry in the diagnosis of primary immunodeficiency diseases.** *Arch Pathol Lab Med* 2004, **128:**23–31.
5. Davis W, Hamilton M: **Uses of flow cytometry to characterize immunodeficiency syndromes in Camelids.** *Small Ruminant Res* 2006, **61**(2):187–193.
6. Ullrich K, Koenigsmann M, Mohren M, Franke A: **Lymphocyte subsets' reference ranges in an age-and gender-balanced population of 100 healthy adults—a monocentric German study.** *Clin Immunol* 2005, **116:**192–197.
7. Howard R, Fasano C, Frey L, Miller C: **Reference intervals of CD3, CD4, CD8, CD4/CD8, and absolute CD4 values in Asian and non-Asian populations.** *Cytometry* 1996, **26:**231–232.
8. Mandy F, Nicholson J, McDougal J: **Revised guidelines for performing single-platform absolute CD4+ T-Cell determinations with CD45 gating for persons infected with human immunodeficiency virus.** *MMWR* 2003, **52:**1–13.
9. Klose N, Coulibaly B, Tebit D, Nauwelaers F, Spengler H, Kynast-Wolf G, Kouyaté B, Kräusslich H, Böhler T: **Immunohematological reference values for healthy adults in Burkina Faso.** *Clin Vaccine Immunol* 2007, **14:**782–784.
10. Lahita R: **Sex hormones and systemic lupus erythematosus.** *Rheum Dis Clin North Am* 2000, **26:**951–968.
11. Vajpayee M, Kaushik S, Sreenivas V, Wig N, Seth P: **CDC staging based on absolute CD4 count and CD4 percentage in an HIV-1-infected Indian population: treatment implications.** *Clin Exp Immunol* 2005, **141:**485–490.
12. Kalayjian R, Landay A, Pollard R, Taub D, Gross B, Francis I, Sevin A, Pu M, Spritzler J, Chernoff M, Namkung A, Fox L, Martinez A, Waterman K, Fiscus S, Sha B, Johnson D, Slater S, Rousseau F, Lederman M: **Age related immune dysfunction in health and in human immunodefieciency virus (HIV) disease: association of age and HIV infection with naive CD8 cell depletion, reduced expression of CD28 on CD8 cells and reduced thymic volumes.** *J Infect Dis* 2003, **187:**1924–1933.
13. Olsen N, Kovacs W: **Effects of androgens on T and B lymphocyte development.** *Immunol Res* 2001, **23:**281–288.
14. Clerici M, Butto S, Lukwiya M: **Immune activation in Africa is environmentally-driven and is associated with upregulation of CCR5: Italian–Ugandan AIDS project.** *AIDS* 2000, **14:**2083–2092.
15. Menard D, Joelle M, Bem M, Kassa E, Gresenguet G, Talarmin A: **Immunohematological reference ranges for adults from the central African republic.** *Clin Diagn Lab Immunol* 2003, **10:**443–445.
16. Schaberge T, Theilacker C, Nitschke O, Lode H: **Lymphocyte subsets in peripheral blood and smoking habits.** *Lung* 1997, **175:**387–394.
17. Mair C, Hawes S, Agne H, Sow P, N'dove I, Manhart L, Fu P, Gottlieb G, Kiviat N: **Factors associated with CD4 lymphocyte counts in HIV-negative Senegalese individuals.** *Clin Exp Immunol* 2007, **151:**432–440.
18. Feldman G, Minkoff H, Schneider F: **Association of cigarette smoking with HIV prognosis among women in the HAART era: a report from the women's interagency HIV study.** *Am J Pub Health* 2006, **96:**1060–1065.
19. Ngowi B, Mfinanga S, Bruun J, Morkve O: **Immunohaematological reference values in human immunodeficiency virus-negative adolescent and adults in rural northern Tanzania.** *BMC Infect Dis* 2009, **9:**1–7.
20. Kibaya R, Bautista C, Sawe F, Schaffer D, Sateren W, Scott P, Michael N, Robb M, Birx D, Souza M: **Reference ranges for the clinical laboratory derived from a rural population in Kericho Kenya.** *PloS ONE* 2008, 3(10):e3327. Doi:10.1371/journal.pone.0003327.
21. Tugume S, Piwowar E, Lutalo T, Mugyenyi P, Grant R, Mangeni F, Pattishall K, Katongole-Mbidde E: **Hematological reference ranges among healthy Ugandans.** *Clin Diagn Lab Immunol* 1995, **2:**233–235.
22. Embree J, Bwayo J, Nagelkerke N, Njenga S, Nyange P, Ndinya-Achola J, Pamba H, Plummer F: **Lymphocyte subsets in human immunodeficiency virus type 1-infected and uninfected children in Nairobi.** *Pediatr Infect Dis J* 2001, **20:**397–403.
23. NCCLS: *How to define and determine reference intervals in the clinical laboratory; approved guideline*, Volume 20. 2nd edition. Wayne, PA: National Committee for Clinical Laboratory Standards; 2000:13. C28-A2.
24. Santagostino A, Garbaccio G, Pistorio A, Bolis V, Camisasca G, Pagliaro P, Girotto M: **An Italian national multicenter study for the definition of**

reference ranges for normal values of peripheral blood lymphocyte subsets in healthy adults. *Haematologica* 1999, **84:**499–504.

25. Koetz K, Bryl E, Spickschen K, O'Fallon W, Goronzy J, Weyand C: **T-cell homeostasis in patients with rheumatoid arthritis.** *Proc Natl Acad Sci USA* 2000, **97:**9203–9208.
26. Nicholson J, Stein D, Mui T, Mack R, Hubbard M, Denny T: **Evaluation of a method for counting absolute numbers of cells with a flow cytometer.** *Clin Diagn Lab Immunol* 1997, **4:**309–313.
27. Chng W, Guat B, Tan S, Kuperan P: **Establishment of adult peripheral blood lymphocyte subset reference range for an Asian population by single-platform flow cytometry: influence of age, sex, and race and comparison with other published studies.** *Clin Diagn Lab Immunol* 2004, **11:**168–173.
28. Meier A, Chang J, Chan E, Pollard R, Sidhu H, Kulkarni S, Wen T, Lindsay R, Orellana L, Mildvan D, Bazner S, Streeck H, Alter G, Lifson J, Carrington M, Bosch R, Robbins G, Altfeld M: **Sex differences in the Toll-like receptor-mediated response of plasmocytoid dendritic cells to HIV-1.** *Nat Med* 2009, **15:**955–959.
29. Globerson A: **Thymocytopoiesis in aging: the bone marrow–thymus axis.** *Arch Gerontol Geriatr* 1997, **24:**141–155.

Predicted HIV-1 coreceptor usage among Kenya patients shows a high tendency for subtype d to be cxcr4 tropic

Veronica Wambui[1], Michael Kiptoo[2], Joyceline Kinyua[2], Irene Odera[2], Edward Muge[1], Peter Muiruri[3], Raphael Lihana[2], Peter Kinyanjui[1] and Elijah M Songok[1,2*]

Abstract

Background: CCR5 antagonists have clinically been approved for prevention or treatment of HIV/AIDS. Countries in Sub-Saharan Africa with the highest burden of HIV/AIDS are due to adopt these regimens. However, HIV-1 can also use CXCR4 as a co-receptor. There is hence an urgent need to map out cellular tropism of a country's circulating HIV strains to guide the impending use of CCR5 antagonists.

Objectives: To determine HIV-1 coreceptor usage among patients attending a comprehensive care centre in Nairobi, Kenya.

Methods: Blood samples were obtained from HIV infected patients attending the comprehensive care centre, Kenyatta National Hospital in years 2008 and 2009. The samples were separated into plasma and peripheral blood mononuclear cells (PBMCs). Proviral DNA was extracted from PBMCs and Polymerase Chain reaction (PCR) done to amplify the HIV *env* fragment spanning the C2-V3 region. The resultant fragment was directly sequenced on an automated sequencer (ABI, 3100). Co-receptor prediction of the *env* sequences was done using Geno2pheno [co-receptor], and phylogenetic relationships determined using CLUSTALW and Neighbor Joining method.

Results: A total of 67 samples (46 treatment experienced and 21 treatment naive) were successfully amplified and sequenced. Forty nine (73%) sequences showed a prediction for R5 tropism while 18(27%) were X4 tropic. Phylogenetic analysis showed that 46(69%) were subtype A, 11(16%) subtype C, and 10(15%) subtype D. No statistical significant associations were observed between cell tropism and CD4+ status, patient gender, age, or treatment option. There was a tendency for more X4 tropic strains being in the treatment experienced group than the naive group: Of 46 treatment experiencing participants, 14(30%) harboured X4, compared with 4(19%) of 21 of the treatment-naïve participants, the association is however not statistically significant ($p = 0.31$). However, a strong association was observed between subtype D and CXCR4 co- receptor usage ($p = 0.015$) with 6(60%) of the 10 subtype D being X4 tropic and 4(40%) R5 tropic.

Conclusion: HIV-1 R5 tropic strains were the most prevalent in the study population and HIV infected patients in Kenya may benefit from CCR5 antagonists. However, there is need for caution where subtype D infection is suspected or where antiretroviral salvage therapy is indicated.

Keywords: Co-receptor usage, HIV-1, Sub-type D

* Correspondence: Esongok@kemri.org
[1]Department of Biochemistry, University of Nairobi, Nairobi 30197-00100, Kenya
[2]Centre for Virus Research, Kenya Medical Research Institute, Nairobi 54848-00200, Kenya
Full list of author information is available at the end of the article

Background

Human immunodeficiency virus (HIV) is the causes of acquired immunodeficiency syndrome (AIDS) [1]. Human immunodeficiency virus has currently surpassed malaria as a leading cause of adult infectious disease mortality worldwide [2]. The Kenya AIDS indicator survey (KAIS), reported by the National AIDS/STIS Control Programme (NASCOP) found that 7.1% of adults (aged 15-64 years) in Kenya were infected with HIV by end of 2007 [3]. HIV is dependent on a host cell for its replication, and requires binding to receptors on the cell surface in order to gain entry. The first receptor is CD4, which is the main receptor and is always the same for each virus particle. There are other two receptors CCR5 and CXCR4 that serve as co-receptors [4]. The co-receptors are used by HIV to infect specific cell types; this phenomenon is referred to as HIV tropism. Non-syncitia-inducing (NSI) strains use the betachemokine receptor, CCR5, for entry and thus able to replicate in macrophages and CD4 positive T-cells. Syncitia inducing (SI) strains replicate in CD4 positive T-cells and use the alpha chemokine receptor, CXCR4 [5]. The preferred phenotypic designations are R5 for the non-syncytium inducing CCR5 using HIV and X4 for the syncytium inducing CXCR4 using HIV [6]. R5 isolates are present early after seroconversion indicating their role in initiation of HIV-1 infection. The eventual use of CXCR4 by X4 isolates of HIV-1 which infect primary T cells and T cell lines closely correspond to the onset of AIDs, although R5 isolates do persist throughout the entire course of infection [6-8]. HIV-1 co-receptor usage has been reported to be fairly stable after HAART therapy [9]. Some ART drugs can lead to suppression of CXCR4 strains of HIV [10]. Of the five HIV-1 gp120 hypervariable domains, V3 has been a target of interest for entry-based inhibitors because of its critical role in defining the specificity of HIV-1 envelope interaction with cellular co-receptor molecules, usually, CCR5 or CXCR4, to facilitate entry into target cells. It encodes the key determinants of viral co receptor usage [11]. Recombinant virus phenotypic entry assays are considered as the gold standard method for determining co-receptor usage [12]. However, their routine use is hampered by technical and cost limitations. Of late the *in silico* approaches are gaining popularity given the simplicity of this strategy and the fact that *env* sequences are increasingly becoming available globally. These include among others, Geno2pheno [co-receptor] which predicts whether the corresponding virus is capable of using CXCR4 or CCR5 as a co receptor [13,14].

By the end of 2007, only 177,000 (40%) of the estimated 470,000 people in need of ART were receiving treatment in Kenya [15]. In Kenya, the first line regimen consists of two nucleoside reverse transcriptase inhibitors (NRTIs) and a non-nucleoside reverse transcriptase inhibitor (NNRTI)/Ritonavir boosted protein inhibitor (PI/r). While the recommended second line regimen consists a fixed drug combination of Didanosine (ddI)/Tenofvir (TDF), Abacavir (ABC) and Lopinavir/ritonavir (LPV/r) [16].

With the introduction of the CCR antagonists for HIV therapy, there is a need to map out the cellular tropism of circulating HIV-1 strains in Kenya. The HIV-1 subtype diversity in Kenya may have an influence on how the CCR5 antagonists are used in Kenya following studies done in Uganda that have demonstrated a high tendency for subtype D to be CXCR4 [17,18]. We therefore carried out a preliminary analysis to determine co-receptor usage in HIV-infected patients attending an outpatient clinic at a tertiary hospital in Nairobi, Kenya. Furthermore, we aimed to evaluate if a correlation exists between HIV-1 tropism, HIV-1 subtypes, and current antiretroviral treatment strategies in Kenya.

Methods

Study population

This was a cross sectional study. The population consisting of antiretroviral therapy experienced patients and treatment naive patients were recruited from the Comprehensive.

Care Centre, Kenyatta National Hospital in 2008 and 2009. The fixed dose combinations for the treatment group were: Zidovudine (AZT)/Stavudine (d4T) + Lamivudine (3TC) + Nevirapine (NVP)/Efavirenz (EFV) and Teno fovir Disoproxil Fumarate (TDF)/Abacavir (ABC) + 3TC/ Didanosine (ddI) + Liponavir/Ritonavir (LPV/r*). The blood from all the subjects was collected for CD4+ count detec tion and the peripheral blood mononuclear cells (PBMCs) for isolating HIV-1 strains. All subjects signed informed consent forms before blood collection. This study was approved by the Kenya medical Research Institute Scientific Steering Committee and Ethical Review Board (Ref. KEMRI SSC No. 1252).

CD + T cell counts and PBMC extraction

CD4+ T cell counts of peripheral blood were determined using FACSCOUNT (Becton-Dickinson, Beiersdorf, Germany). Peripheral blood mononuclear cells were extracted from whole blood by density gradient centrifugation and stored at −30°C.

Extraction and amplification of proviral HIV DNA

Samples were archived, thawed and proviral DNA extracted using Gibco BRL攵 kit as per Manufacturers instructions. A part of the HIV-1 group M env gene covering the C2V3 region (corresponding to 6975–7520 nt in HIV-1 HXB2) was amplified by nested polymerase chain reaction (PCR) with primers M5(5'-CCCCTATTCCTTTTCCCCTTCTT

TTAAAA-3') and M10(5'- CCAATTCCCATACATTATT GTGCCCCAGC TGG-3') in the first round and M3(5'-GTCAGCAA CAGTACAATGACACATGG-3') and M8 (5'- TCCTTCCATGGGAGGGGACTACATTGC-3') in the second round according to manufacturers instructions. Amplification was done with one cycle of 10 min at 95°C, 35 cycles of 30s at 95°C, 30s at 55°C and 1 min at 72°C followed by a final extension of 10 min at 72°C. PCR amplification was confirmed by visualization with ethidium bromide staining of the gel.

Sequencing and subtyping of the C2V3 env region

The resultant 550 bp fragment was sequenced using an automated ABI 3100 sequencer. Sample nucleotide sequences were aligned with HIV-1 subtype/circulating recombinant form (CRF) reference sequences from the Los Almos database using CLUSTAL W with minor manual adjustments. A phylogenetic tree was constructed by the neighbour joining method and its reliability was estimated by 1000 bootstrap replications. The profile of the tree was visualized with Tree View PPC version 1.6.5. To improve the accuracy of subtyping, we used the NCBI Viral Genotyping tools (http://www.ncbi.nlm.nih.gov/projects/genotyping/formpage.cgi) and REGA subtyping tools v2.0 (http://www.bioafrica.net/rega-genotype/html/subtypinghiv.html). The C2-V3 region nucleotide sequences (550 bp) were translated into the corresponding 35 amino acids using Genetic Information Processing Software (Genetyx-Win) version 4.0 (Genetyx, Tokyo, Japan). Sequences with premature stop codons were excluded from further analyses.

Co-receptor usage prediction

Geno2pheno [co-receptor] tool (with a false positive rate of 10%) was used to predict HIV-1 co receptor usage. (http://coreceptor.bioinf.mpi-inf.mpg.de/) was used. Geno2pheno is available at http://co receptor.bioinf.mpi-inf.mpg.de/cgi-bin/co receptor.pl (September 2010). Subtype D genotypic algorithm based on 11/25 and a net charge rules was further used to predict tropism of the sub-type D sequences. One of the following criteria was required for predicting subtype D CXCR4 co-receptor usage: (i) R/K at position 11 of V3; (ii) R at position 25 of V3 and a net charge of ≥ +5; (iii) a net charge of ≥ +6 [14].

Statistical analysis

Correlations of HIV-1 subtype, ART regimen, gender, CD4 count and viral tropism were performed by Chi square test using SPSS v.16 software (IBM Company, New York). P values less than 0.05 were considered statistically significant.

Results

Clinical and general characterization of study population

A total of 67 samples were successfully amplified and sequenced. Of these, 46 individuals were from the ART experienced group while 21 individuals were from the treatment naive group. The mean age of the study population was 39(16–65 years), 23(34%) were male and 44 (66%) were female. The mean CD4 count of the treatment experienced group was 249 cells/mm^3 of whole blood and 375 cells/mm^3 of whole blood for the treatment naive group. Twenty two (48%) of the treatment experiencing group were on AZT/d4T + 3TC + NVP/EFV fixed dose combination while 24(52%) were on TDF/ABC + 3TC/ddI + LPV/r* fixed dose combination.

HIV-1 subtypes

Of the total 67 samples successfully amplified and sequenced, 46(69%) were subtype A 11(16%) subtype C and 10(15%) subtype D (Figure 1).

Predicted co-receptor usage

Of the 67 samples successfully amplified, sequenced and their C2-V3 region 550 bp fragment translated to corresponding 35 amino acids, 49(73%) were predicted to be R5-tropic stains while 18(27%) were predicted to be X4-tropic strains using geno2pheno [co-receptor] bioinformatics tool. There was no discrepancy in tropism prediction for subtype D sequences using Geno2Pheno [co-receptor] and subtype D genotypic algorithm (Table 1). There was a tendency of a higher number of X4 tropic viruses being in the treatment experienced group than the naive group: Of 46 treatment experiencing participants, 14(30%) harboured X4, compared with 4(19%) of 21 of the treatment-naïve participants, the association is however not statistically significant ($p = 0.31$). A strong association was however observed between subtype D and CXCR4 co-receptor usage ($p = 0.015$) (Table 2). There was no association between co-receptor usage and CD4 count, gender and age of the study participants ($p = 0.26$), ($p = 0.97$) and ($p = 0.22$) respectively (Table 2).

Discussion

Despite the impending introduction of CCR5 antagonists as a treatment of option of HIV in Sub-Saharan countries, little is known about HIV co-receptor usage prevalent among infected populations. Our data demonstrates a high prevalence of R5-using strains among patients attending Kenyatta National Hospital HIV/AIDS comprehensive care clinic in Nairobi. This finding is in line with our earlier evaluation of HIV-1 *coreceptor usage* among a sexually transmitted infection clinic attendees and HIV-1 infected infants at a children's home [19,20]. Our data hence confirms the predominance of R5 strains in HIV infected populations in the country.

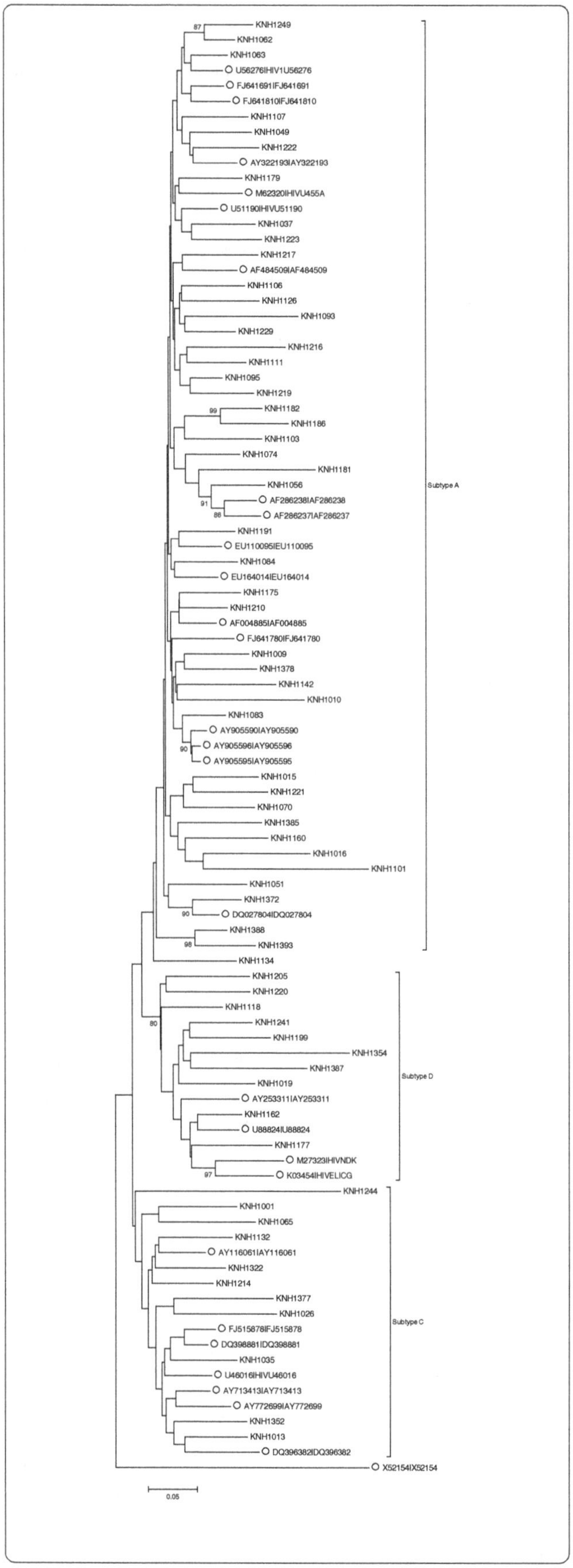

Figure 1 Phylogenetic tree of HIV-1 env-C2V3 region. C2V3 region sequences of the study population were aligned and compared with reference sequences obtained from the Los Alamos HIV database. Phylogenetic relationships were constructed by neighbor-joining method and rooted with X52154. The bootstrap values (of 1000 replicates) above 70% are indicated next to the node. Brackets on the right indicate the subtype clusters while the labelled branches indicate the reference sequences.

Though subtype D constituted only fifteen per cent of the study population, they represented the subtype with highest prevalence of X4 tropic strains. Our observation is in agreement with two other studies done in Uganda. One study aimed to determine whether differences exist in co-receptor use in patients infected with subtypes A & D in a rural Ugandan cohort found the probability of having an X4 virus being higher in subtype D infections than subtype A infections [17]. The second study was conducted among HIV-infected Ugandan infants where tropism assay and phylogenetic methods revealed X4 tropism and subtype D association [18]. Although HIV-1 co-receptor usage and HIV-1 subtype relationship has been well studied in Uganda, less is known about Kenya. Our data therefore confirms the strong relationship between HIV-1 subtype D and X4 infections in Kenya.

HIV-1 subtype D infection is associated with rapid loss of CD4 cells and faster disease progression than any other subtype [21]. Similarly, HIV-1 X4-tropic strains have been confirmed to be associated with faster disease progression compared to HIV-1 R5-tropic strains. Therefore, co-receptor usage could be one explanation for the fast disease progression HIV subtype D strains. In a study aiming to compare the rate of disease progression based on rate of CD4 decline prior to ART, and the initial and subsequent virological response to ART in an ethnically diverse population in south London infected with diverse subtypes, Eastbrook et al. found subtype D to be associated with both a statistically significant four-fold faster rate of CD4 decline and a higher rate of virological rebound on ART compared with subtype A, B, or C. In Uganda, HIV patients infected with subtype D have been shown to have a more severe dementia as compared with those infected with other subtypes [22]. In a follow-up of HIV seropositive women in Daresalam, individuals infected with subtype D experienced the most rapid progression to death. The above associations confirm our findings of subtype D with a higher prevalence of X4 tropic strains.

As use of antiretroviral treatment is now a common feature in HIV/AIDS management, our study also aimed to evaluate if a correlation exists between HIV-1 tropism and currently used therapeutic regimens. The results showed a higher CXCR4 utilization among antiretroviral therapy group than in the treatment naive population,

Table 1 Subtype D sequences tropism prediction by Geno2pheno tool and subtype D genotypic algorithm

Patient ID	Subtype D genotypic algorithm				Geno2Pheno tool
	Amino acid at position 11	Amino acid at position 25	Net charge	Strain	
KNH1220	G	K	6	X4	X4
KNH1118	S	D	4	R5	R5
KNH1019	R	N	9	X4	X4
KNH1177	R	K	6	X4	X4
KNH1162	S	K	6	X4	X4
KNH1387	G	N	5	R5	R5
KNH1354	K	K	4	X4	X4
KNH1076	S	R	11	X4	X4
KNH1109	S	D	5	R5	R5
KNH1241	S	T	5	R5	R5

though the difference was not statistically significant. Some groups in developed countries [23] have found a significantly higher prevalence of X4 viruses among anti-retroviral treatment groups. We caution however that our methodology did not take into effect the presence of dual or mixed CCR5/CXR4 viral strains which have been found to be prevalent in other antiretroviral experienced populations. The mechanism responsible for the emergence of CXCR4- using viruses on antiretroviral treatment groups remains unclear. Several hypotheses have been forwarded. Either, partially suppressive therapy may lead to an increase in HIV-specific T cell responses [24]. Because X4-tropic variants may be more susceptible to cytotoxic T cell responses than R5-tropic viruses, increases in HIV-specific T cell responses during partial treatment-mediated viral suppression might select against X4-tropic viruses [25], or antiretroviral therapy may reduce CCR5 expression on T cells, presumably as a consequence of reductions in T cell activation [26,27], potentially selecting for X4-tropic viruses [28]. Lastly, certain antiretroviral drugs may preferentially select for one virus population, either because of enhanced activity against X4 viruses as has been suggested for enfuvirtide [29] or because of suboptimal drug metabolism in the

Table 2 HIV-1 co-receptor usage and its associated influence factors

	R5 co-receptor usage	X4 co-receptor usage		
CD4 + T count (cells/mm^3)				
CD4 < 200	18 (66.7%)	9 (33.3%)	p = 0.26	
200 = CD4 < 350	15 (93.8%)	19 (6.2%)		
350 = CD4 < 500	11 (73.3%)	4 (26.7%)		
CD4 > =500	5 (55.6%)	4 (44.4%)		
Gender				
Female	32 (72.7%)	12 (27.3%)	p = 0.97	
Male	17 (73.9%)	6 (26.1%)		
Age				
16-25 years	2 (50.0%)	2 (50.0%)	p = 0.22	
26-35 years	15 (83.3%)	3 (16.7%)		
36-45 years	20 (66.7%)	10 (33.3%)		
> 46 years	12 (80.0%)	3 (20.0%)		
Therapeutic regimen				
AZT/d4T + 3TC + NVP/EFV	13 (59.1%)	9 (40.9%)	p = 0.31	
TDF/ABC + 3TC + DDI/LPV/r*	19 (79.2%)	5 (20.8%)		
Treatment Naïve	17 (81%)	4 (19%)		
HIV-1 Subtype				
A	36 (78.3%)	10 (21.7%)	p = 0.261	p = 0.04
C	9 (81.8%)	2 (18.2%)	p = 0.504	
D	4 (40%)	6 (60%)	p = 0.015	

cellular reservoirs for X4 viruses as has been suggested for zidovudine [30].

Our study has two potential shortcomings. First, the small sample size for subtype D and subtype C could have led to the cellular tropism not being well documented for these subtypes, though subtype A has been reported to be the predominant subtype in Kenya. Second, we did not confirm the V3 prediction done by genotypic algorithm by phenotypic assay. Genotypic algorithms have been reported to lack sensitivity for predicting CXCR4 usage [31]. There is therefore need to improve their sensitivity. The genotype-based co-receptor predictors should therefore not be used alone in a clinical setting and even if they approached the sensitivity of phenotypic assays, they would need validation to be used as a wide spread clinical tool.

In conclusion, we infer that HIV-1 R5 tropic strains were more prevalent in the study population suggesting the potential benefit of CCR5 antagonists as a therapeutic option in Kenya. However the observed higher prevalence of X4 strains among subtype D, may call for caution in administration of CCR5 antagonists to patients where subtype D infection is suspected and or where salvage antiretroviral therapy is indicated.

Genebank accession numbers

The sequences from this study has been deposited at the Los Alamos HIV database under accession numbers JN 593245-JN593311.

Competing interests

The authors declare that they have no competing interests.

Authors' contributions

ES and VW conceived the experiment. VW and IO performed the laboratory procedures while PM helped with patient recruitment and clinical follow-up. ES, MK, VW, RL and JK performed bioinformatics and data analysis. VW and ES drafted the manuscript while EM and PK provided scientific guidance. All authors read and approved the final manuscript.

Acknowledgements

We are grateful to the Comprehensive care Centre, Kenyatta National Hospital, for assistance with patient recruitment. We are thankful to Dr. Lyle Mackinnon of University of Manitoba for the critical review of this manuscript. This study was partially funded by Kenya Medical Research Institute.

Author details

[1]Department of Biochemistry, University of Nairobi, Nairobi 30197-00100, Kenya. [2]Centre for Virus Research, Kenya Medical Research Institute, Nairobi 54848-00200, Kenya. [3]Comprehensive Care Centre, Kenyatta National Hospital, Nairobi 2146-00202, Kenya.

References

1. Weiss RA: **How does HIV cause AIDS?** *Science* 2003, **260**(5112):1273–1279.
2. Nelson Michael L: **Host genetic influences on HIV-1 pathogenesis.** *Curr Opin Immunol* 1999, **11**:466–474.
3. National AIDS and STI Control Programme: *Kenya AIDS Indicator Survey 2007.* Nairobi, Kenya: Preliminary Report. Ministry of Health; 2008.
4. Berger E, Murphy P, Farber J: **Chemokine receptors as HIV-1 coreceptors.** *Annu Rev Immunol* 1999, **17**:657–700.
5. Coakley E, Petropoulos CJ, Whitcomb JM: **Assessing chemokine co-receptor usage in HIV.** *Curr Opin Infect Dis* 2005, **18**(1):9–15.
6. Berger EA: **HIV entry and tropism: the chemokine receptor connection.** *AIDS* 1997, **11**:S3–S16.
7. Moore JP, Trkola A, Dragic T: **Co-receptors for HIV-1 entry.** *Curr Opin Immunol* 1997, **9**:551–562.
8. Berger EA, Doms RA, Fenyo EM, Korber BTM, Littman DR, Moore JP, Sattentau QJ, Schuitemaker H, Sodroski J, Weiss RA: **A new classification for HIV-1.** *Nature* 1998, **391**:240.
9. Lehmann C, Daumer M, Boussaad I, Sing T, Beerenwinkel N, Lengauer T, Schmeisser N, Wyen C, Fatkenheuer G, Kaiser R: **Stable co-receptor usage of HIV in patients with ongoing treatment failure on HAART.** *J Clin Virol* 2006, **37**(4):300–304.
10. Philpott S, Weiser B, Anastos K, Kitchen CM, Robinson E, Meyer WA, Sacks HS, Brunner C, Burger H: **Preferential suppression of CXCR4-specific strains of HIV by antiviral therapy.** *J Clin Invest* 2001, **107**(4):431–438.
11. Hwang SS, Boyle TJ, Lyerly HK, Cullen BR: **Identification of the envelope V3 loop as the primary determinant of cell tropism in HIV-1.** *Science* 1991, **253**:71–74.
12. Whitcomb J, Huang W, Fransen S: **Development and characterization of a novel single-cycle recombinant-virus assay to determine HIV-1 coreceptor tropism.** *Antimicrob Agents Chemother* 2007, **51**:566–575.
13. Sing T, Low AJ, Beerenwinkel N, Sander O, Cheung PK, Domingues FS, Buch J, Daumer M, Kaiser R, Lengauer T, Harrigan PR: **Predicting HIV-coreceptor usage based on genetic and clinical covariates.** *Antivir Ther* 2007, **12**:1097–1106.
14. Raymond S, Delobel P, Chaix ML, Cazabat M, Encinas S, Bruel P, Sandres-Saune K, Marchou B, Massip P, Izopet J: **Genotypic prediction of HIV-1 subtype D tropism.** *Retrovirology* 2011, **8**:56.
15. UNAIDS/WHO: *Epidemiological Fact Sheets on HIV and AIDS-Kenya.* 2008. www.who.int/hiv/pub/epidemiology/pubfacts/en/.
16. Ministry Of Health: *Guidelines for Antiretroviral Therapy Drug Therapy in Kenya.* Thirdth edition. Nairobi, Kenya: Ministry Of Health.
17. Kaleebu P, Nankya IL, Yirrell LD, Shafer LA, Shafer LA, Kyosiimire-Lugemwa, Lule BD, Morgan D, Beddows S, Weber J, Whitworth JAG: **Relation between chemokine receptor use, disease stage, and HIV-1 subtypes A and D results from a rural ugandan cohort.** *J Acquir Immune Defic Syndr* 2007, **45**:28–33.
18. Church DJ, Huang W, Mwatha A, Toma J, Stawiski E, Donnell D, Guay AL, Mmiro F, Musoke P, Jackson BJ, Parkin N, Eshleman HS: **HIV-1 tropism and survival in vertically infected Ugandan infants.** *J Infect Dis* 2008, **197**(10):1382–1388.
19. Lihana RW, Khamadi SA, Lwembe RM, Kinyua JG, Muriuki JK, Lagat NJ, Okoth FA, Makokha PE, Songok EM: **HIV-1 subtype and viral tropism determination for evaluating antiretroviral therapy options: an analysis of archived Kenyan blood samples.** *BMC Infect Dis* 2009, **9**:215.
20. Lwembe R, Lihana RW, Ochieng' W, Panikulam A, Mongoina CO, Palakudy T, De Koning H, Ishizaki A, Kageyama S, Musoke R, Owens M, Songok EM, Okoth FA, Ichimura A: **Changes in the HIV type 1 envelope gene from non-subtype B type-1 infected children in Kenya.** *AIDS Res Hum Retroviruses* 2009, **25**(2):141–148.
21. Baeten JM, Chohan B, Lavreys I, Chohan V, McClelland RS, Certain I, Mandaliya K, Jaoko W, Overbaugh J: **HIV-1 sub-type D infection is associated with faster disease progression than sub-type A in spite of similar plasma HIV-1 loads.** *J Infect Dis* 2007, **195**(8):1177–1180.
22. Sacktor N, Nakasuija N, Slolasky R, Rezapour M, Robertson K, Musisi S, Katabira E, Ronald A, Clifford D, Laeyendecker O, Quinn T: **HIV subtype D is associated with dementia compared with subtype A, in immunosuppressed individuals at risk of cognitive impairment in Kampala, Uganda.** *Clin Infect Dis* 2009, **49**:780–786.
23. Hunt PW, Harrigan PR, Huang W, Bates M, Williamson DW, McCune JM, Price RW, Spudich SS, Lampiris R, Hoh T, Leigler JN, Deeks SG: **Prevalence of CXCR4 tropism among antiretroviral treated HIV-infected patients with detectable viremia.** *J Infect Dis* 2006, **194**(7):926–930.
24. Deeks SG, Martin JN, Sinclair E: **Strong cell-mediated immune responses are associated with the maintenance of low-level viremia in antiretroviral-treated individuals with drug-resistant human immunodeficiency virus type 1.** *J Infect Dis* 2004, **189**:312–321.

25. Harouse JM, Buckner C, Gettie A: **CD8+ T cell-mediated CXC chemokine receptor 4-simian/human immunodeficiency virus suppression in dually infected rhesus macaques.** *Proc Natl Acad Sci USA* 2003, **100:**10977–10982.
26. Andersson J, Fehniger TE, Patterson BK: **Early reduction of immune activation in lymphoid tissue following highly active HIV therapy.** *AIDS* 1998, **12:**123–129.
27. Giovannetti A, Ensoli F, Mazzetta F: **CCR5 and CXCR4 chemokine receptor expression and beta-chemokine production during early T cell repopulation induced by highly active anti-retroviral therapy.** *Clin Exp Immunol* 1999, **118:**87–94.
28. Brumme ZL, Goodrich J, Mayer HB: **Molecular and clinical epidemiology of CXCR4-using HIV-1 in a large population of antiretroviral- naive individuals.** *J Infect Dis* 2005, **192:**466–474.
29. Yuan W, Craig S, Si Z, Farzan M, Sodroski J: **CD4-induced T-20 binding to human immunodeficiency virus type 1 gp120 blocks interaction with the CXCR4 coreceptor.** *J Virol* 2004, **78:**5448–5457.
30. Boucher CA, Lange JM, Miedema FF: **HIV-1 biological phenotype and the development of zidovudine resistance in relation to disease progression in asymptomatic individuals during treatment.** *AIDS* 1992, **6:**1259–1264.
31. Low AJ, Dong W, Chan D, Sing T, Ronald S, Jensen M, Pillai S, Good B, Harrigan PR: **Current V3 genotyping algorithms are inadequate for predicting X4 co-receptor usage in clinical isolates.** *AIDS* 2007, **21**(14):17–24.

7

Viral and cellular factors underlying neuropathogenesis in HIV associated neurocognitive disorders (HAND)

Vasudev R Rao†, Arthur P Ruiz† and Vinayaka R Prasad*

Abstract

As the HIV-1 epidemic enters its fourth decade, HIV-1 associated neurological disorders (HAND) continue to be a major concern in the infected population, despite the widespread use of anti-retroviral therapy. Advancing age and increased life expectancy of the HIV-1 infected population have been shown to increase the risk of cognitive dysfunction. Over the past 10 years, there has been a significant progress in our understanding of the mechanisms and the risk factors involved in the development of HAND. Key events that lead up to neuronal damage in HIV-1 infected individuals can be categorized based on the interaction of HIV-1 with the various cell types, including but not limited to macrophages, brain endothelial cells, microglia, astrocytes and the neurons. This review attempts to decipher these interactions, beginning with HIV-1 infection of macrophages and ultimately resulting in the release of neurotoxic viral and host products. These include: interaction with endothelial cells, resulting in the impairment of the blood brain barrier; interaction with the astrocytes, leading to metabolic and neurotransmitter imbalance; interactions with resident immune cells in the brain, leading to release of toxic cytokines and chemokines. We also review the mechanisms underlying neuronal damage caused by the factors mentioned above. We have attempted to bring together recent findings in these areas to help appreciate the viral and host factors that bring about neurological dysfunction. In addition, we review host factors and viral genotypic differences that affect phenotypic pathological outcomes, as well as recent advances in treatment options to specifically address the neurotoxic mechanisms in play.

Introduction

HIV associated neurocognitive disorders (HAND) are a potential consequence of HIV-1 infection, and about half of all adults with AIDS suffer from neurological complications related to HIV-1 [1]. HIV-1 infection plays a pivotal role in HAND by generating products that lead to neurological damage in the central nervous system (CNS). HAND includes a spectrum of neurological disorders ranging from asymptomatic neurocognitive impairment (ANI), an intermediate form termed mild neurocognitive disorder (MND) and the severe form, HIV associated dementia (HAD) [2]. The relationship between the prevalence of these forms to each other and their occurrence in the overall population of HIV-1-infected individuals can be depicted in a pyramidal form, with the total number of HIV-1-infected individuals forming the base, with the upper layers having progressively fewer numbers of patients exhibiting ANI, MND and HAD. As the availability of highly active anti-retroviral therapy (HAART) has become more widespread worldwide, HIV-1-infected individuals are living longer. Although the incidence and prevalence of HAD have been reduced in the era of HAART, the prevalence of HAND overall is actually increasing worldwide. The increased lifespan of treated patients results in a chronic exposure of the brain to HIV-1 virions and viral proteins leading to inflammation, as well as a concomitant chronic inflammation in the peripheral immune system, leading to the accumulation of neurological damage [3]. The success of HAART in controlling peripheral viral load is not necessarily accompanied by reduction in the immune activation in the brain [4].

* Correspondence: vinayaka.prasad@einstein.yu.edu
†Equal contributors
Department of Microbiology and Immunology, Albert Einstein College of Medicine, 1300 Morris Park Avenue, Bronx, NY 10461, USA

Overview of HIV neuropathogenesis

Before embarking on delineating the viral and host factors that play central roles in HAND, it is helpful to have an understanding of the current working model for a mechanistic basis of HIV neuropathogenesis. Infiltration of monocytes into the brain is a hallmark of HAND [5]. Monocyte-derived macrophages (MDM) are one of the major types of cell that are infected by HIV-1 ($CD4^+$ T lymphocytes and dendritic cells being the other two cell types). Once the HIV-1-infected macrophages have established residence in the CNS, they secrete chemokines that establish a chemotaxis gradient across the blood–brain barrier (BBB), which recruits more monocytic cells from the peripheral compartment into the CNS [6]. This influx of HIV-1-infected monocytic cells leads to the infection of other CNS-resident monocytic cells, namely perivascular macrophages and microglia [7], which in turn results in greater BBB damage and accelerates the rate at which HIV-1-infected and uninfected monocytic cells can enter the brain. Neurons do not support HIV-1-infection or replication, but they do express several cell-surface receptors (CCR5, CXCR4, NMDAR etc.) that render them sensitive to insults by viral proteins (e.g. Tat, gp120), inflammatory cytokines (e.g. TNF-α, IL1β) and small metabolites (e.g. nitric oxide, arachidonic acid, etc.) secreted by immune cells in the brain [8]. The key events that contribute to HAND include direct neuronal apoptosis, dysregulation of key neuronal support cells, and the loss of dendritic arbor.

HIV-1 infection of Macrophages

The process of HIV-1 infection begins by HIV-1 binding to CD4 receptor on the target cell surface, through the viral envelope protein gp120 [9]. This binding induces a conformational change in gp120 that exposes a CD4-binding induced (CD4i) co-receptor binding site, which subsequently binds to either CCR5 or CXCR4 coreceptor [10]. The binding of gp120 to a co-receptor then exposes the fusion peptide in viral protein gp41, which is inserted into the cell membrane and drives fusion of the viral and cell membranes [11]. The co-receptor preference, which is determined primarily by the V3 loop in gp120 [12], designates a given HIV-1 isolate as either an R5 or X4 virus depending upon whether it uses CCR5 or CXCR4 coreceptor. Based on the fact that CCR5Δ32 mutation confers resistance to HIV-1 transmission [13], the field has come to the conclusion that only R5 viruses are transmissible and are the type of viruses detected systemically early in infection. However, later as the disease progresses, the predominant tropism switches to CXCR4-usage [14], at least in some of the cases (approximately 50%). CXCR4 usage is associated with faster viral replication and a more rapid $CD4^+$ T-cell decline [14]. However, this switch is not obligatory for disease progression, as exceptions are observed in some parts of the world where non-B subtypes of HIV-1 are prevalent [15].

HIV-1 can productively infect both $CD4^+$ T lymphocytes and monocytic cells/macrophages. Infection of monocytic/macrophage cells is primarily by M-tropic viruses driving fusion through the CCR5 coreceptor, but infection by T-tropic viruses through the CXCR4 coreceptor has also been observed [16]. While dendritic cells can also be infected by HIV-1, they do not support robust HIV-1 replication. However, they do play a crucial role in the systemic spread of HIV-1 due to their strategic presence in lymph nodes [17]. HIV-infection leads to a progressive decline in the population of $CD4^+$ T cells, which is due to loss of both infected $CD4^+$ T cells and uninfected cells (bystander killing) [18]. However, there is no systemic loss of monocytic cells, either infected or uninfected. It has been reported that monocytic/macrophage-tropic viruses, in addition to bearing gp120 that is able to recognize and bind CCR5 coreceptor, have evolved the capability to infect cells with a lower density of CD4 receptors on the cell surface and a greater fusion activity [19]. Furthermore, macrophages are also characterized by the budding of virions into internal multivesicular bodies, which are vacuoles within the cells, rather than budding through the plasma membrane directly to the external medium. This mechanism allows HIV-1 to 'hide' inside the infected macrophages, making macrophages one of the latent reservoirs of HIV-1 [20].

The predominant route of CNS exposure to HIV-1 is through peripheral blood monocytic cells/macrophages that have been infected by virus and transmigrate across the blood–brain barrier (BBB) [5]. Peripheral blood monocytes are categorized into classical "resting" monocytes that express only CD14 ($CD14^{++}CD16^-$), intermediate monocytes that maintain high levels of CD14, while gaining CD16 positivity ($CD14^{++}$ $CD16^+$), and non-classical "activated" monocytes that express high CD16 levels and lower levels of CD14 ($CD14^+CD16^{++}$) [21]. The $CD16^{++}$ subset, while comprising only about 5-10% of the total circulating monocyte population, is overrepresented in the brains of patients with HIV encephalopathy [22,23]. $CD16^{++}$ monocytes are more susceptible to HIV infection and support higher levels of viral replication [24]. Additionally, infected $CD16^{++}$ monocytes have been shown to transmigrate more efficiently across the BBB in response to a chemokine gradient [25]. While $CD4^+$ T lymphocytes have been suggested to play a role in trafficking HIV into the CNS, the vast majority of HIV-1 isolates derived from CNS tissue appear to be of macrophage-tropic lineage [26].

CNS invasion: disruption of the blood brain barrier

The BBB is located at all points of interaction between the brain tissue and blood vessels and consists of astrocytic end feet and human brain microvascular endothelial cells (HBMEC). In addition to the barrier created by HBMECs and astrocytes, pericytes envelope the abluminal side of endothelium and increase the selectivity of the barrier [27]. Pericyte density in the brain is much higher than that observed in other organs, thereby constituting an additional barrier [28]. The BBB maintains the sanctity of the brain's internal environment and provides an important physiologic and immunologic separation between the CNS and the peripheral circulation. HIV-1 infiltrates the BBB early after infection [29] using HIV-infected monocytic cells as a "Trojan horse" for entry into brain [30]. While low numbers of monocytes routinely enter the CNS as part of "immune surveillance" to replenish the population of resident macrophages, infection by HIV-1 increases the adherence of monocytes to endothelial cells, increasing their transmigration across the BBB [31]. The HIV-infected macrophages in the vicinity of the BBB secrete inflammatory cytokines and viral products that damage HBMECs, induce cellular oxidative stress and they also produce chemokines like CCL2 [32] that facilitate the build-up of additional immune cells near the barrier. The interplay between the secreted cytokines, viral products and HBMECs activates endothelial cells and increases surface expression of adhesion molecules on endothelial cells – which in turn accelerates the transmigration of infected macrophages across the BBB.

HIV-1 proteins Tat and gp120 both directly damage the BBB (Figure 1). Tat is a non-structural viral protein secreted by infected cells [33]. Tat mRNA [34], Tat protein [35] and antibodies to Tat [36] are detectable in the CNS of HIV-infected patients. Brain endothelial cells, when exposed to HIV-1 Tat, have been shown to alter the expression and distribution of tight junction proteins (claudins & occludins) [37]. Tat treatment of HBMECs *in vitro* up-regulates matrix metallopeptidase-9 (MMP-9), which in turn increases the permeability of brain endothelial cells by degrading occludins [38]. *In vitro* two-chamber models with HBMECs and astrocytes have also shown HIV-1 Tat causes dysregulation of nitric oxide production in brain endothelial cells [39] and induces secretion of CCL2, a key chemokine responsible for migration of immune cells [40].

Even though brain endothelial cells that line the BBB are not productively infected, several *in vivo* and *in vitro* studies have demonstrated that envelope glycoprotein gp120 causes a functional impairment at the BBB. The gp120 protein is found on the surface of virions and on infected cells as a homo-trimer, but gp120 is also shed from infected cells and found in soluble form as a monomer [41]. Studies involving HIV-1 gp120 transgenic mice, in which gp120 was expressed in thymocytes and the CNS, revealed that the permeability of the brain capillaries in mice is severely impaired [42]. Kanmogne *et al.* demonstrated, using a two-chamber BBB model, that the exposure of HBMECs to recombinant HIV-1 gp120 protein (from either X4 and R5 HIV-1 isolates) led to activation of proinflammatory and interferon-inducible genes, increased leukocyte adhesion, decreased trans-endothelial electrical resistance (TEER) and increased migration of monocytes across the barrier [43,44]. Removal of gp120 resulted in complete restoration of TEER and significant improvement in permeability. Exposure of HBMECs to

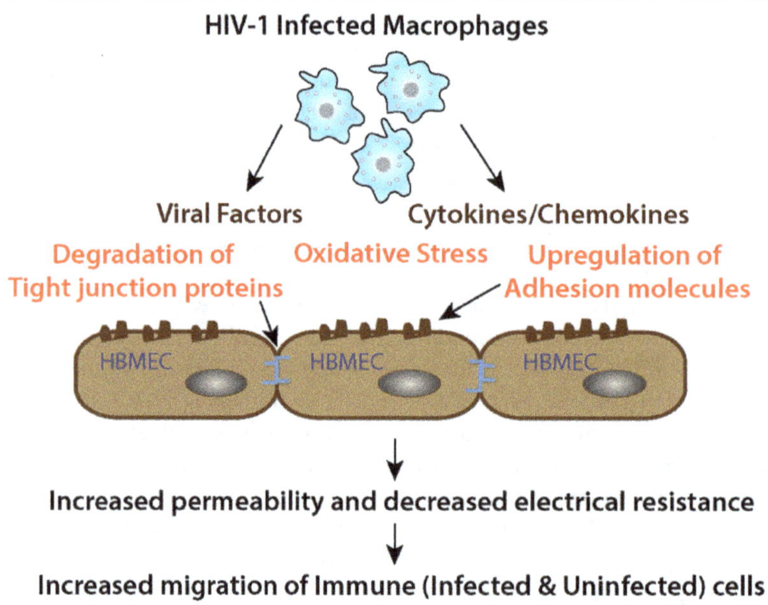

Figure 1 Invasion of the blood brain barrier. HIV-1 infected immune cells release toxic viral products and inflammatory cytokines leading to degradation of tight junction proteins, oxidative stress and up-regulation of adhesion molecules. This results in the increased permeability of the blood brain barrier and increased migration of immune cells across the barrier. HIV-1 infiltrates the BBB early after infection [29] using HIV-infected monocytic cells as a "Trojan horse" for entry into brain [30].

gp120 *in vitro* resulted in increased expression of adhesion molecules (ICAM and VCAM), damage to the barrier and a consequent increase in monocyte migration across the monolayer of endothelial cells [45]. There was a dose dependent increase in cytotoxicity of HBMECs when exposed to recombinant gp120, and gp120-mediated HBMEC cytotoxicity has been shown to involve the p38 mitogen-activated protein (MAP) kinase pathway [46].

Thus, both HIV-1 proteins gp120 and HIV-1 Tat have been implicated in perturbing the blood–brain barrier. Delineating the precise roles of additional viral and host factors that directly perturb the BBB as well as identifying reliable biomarkers of BBB damage would be crucial to furthering our understanding of the mechanisms driving the pathology specific to the BBB in HAND. Such knowledge will accelerate the development of innovative treatment strategies, specifically aimed at preventing damage to the BBB and reducing the CNS invasion of infected macrophages.

Mechanisms of neuropathogenesis

Although neurons cannot be infected by HIV-1, neuronal damage is a key feature in the development of HAND [47] Neurons are vulnerable to direct damage by several viral proteins. This vulnerability is mainly mediated through the presence of several neuronal cell surface receptors: the *N-methyl-D-Aspartate* receptors (NMDAR), the low-density lipoprotein receptor related protein (LRP), chemokine receptors CCR5 and CXCR4, and the dopamine transporter. Glutamate is the most abundant neurotransmitter in the brain, and it is responsible for propagating excitatory signal transmission by binding to NMDAR and opening cation specific channels in the cell membrane, allowing ingress of sodium and calcium ions and the egress of potassium ions [48]. LRP is a receptor involved in cholesterol trafficking in neurons, and also plays a role in signal transmission and inhibition of neuronal apoptosis [49]. Dopamine receptors and transporters are less widespread than NMDAR, but are importantly found in areas of the brain that are prone to high levels of HIV-1 infection, such as the striatum and substantia nigra, which are involved in executive function and the behavioral reward system [50], and there are lower expression levels of dopamine transporter in the striata of HIV patients with cognitive deficits [51].

The two major viral proteins that interact with the above receptors to cause neuronal injury are gp120 and Tat. Both monomeric and oligomeric gp120 have neurotoxic capabilities [52], and transgenic mice expressing gp120 have a spectrum of neuronal and glial changes resembling abnormalities in brains of HIV-1-infected humans [53]. HIV-1 gp120 directly binds NMDAR on human embryonic neurons and can cause a lethal influx of calcium ions [54] (Figure 2). HIV-1 gp120 can bind to either CCR5 or CXCR4 and induce death in neuroblastoma cells [52,55] (Figure 2). This apoptosis apparently takes place through a p38-MAPK-mediated signaling cascade [56]. Cognitive testing of gp120 transgenic mice showed age-dependent deficits in open field activity and spatial reference memory tests [57]. The natural ligands of both CCR5 (eg. CCL5, CCL3) and CXCR4 (CXCL12) were found to be neuroprotective against gp120 neurotoxicity [52,55,58,59]. However, CXCL12 displays neurotoxicity [56] after the N-terminal cleavage of a tetrapeptide in CXCL12 by MMP-2 [60]. Another factor up-regulated by the interaction of gp120 with CXCR4 is the neuronal nicotinic receptor α7, which increases cellular permeability to $[Ca^{2+}]$ influx and contributes to cell death [61].

The viral protein Tat also causes neurotoxicity via multiple pathways. Similar to gp120, Tat can activate NMDA receptors and drive the toxic influx of Ca^{2+} ions [62] (Figure 3). In addition to calcium dysregulation through the NMDAR, Tat can induce the phospholipase C-driven activation of inositol 1,4,5-triphosphate, which increases the intracellular levels of $[Ca^{2+}]$ by mobilizing stores in the endoplasmic reticulum and contributes to calcium toxicity and cell death [63]. Tat also binds LRP in neurons, causing LRP internalization and a decrease in uptake of natural LRP ligands such as amyloid-β peptide and Apolipoprotein E [64] (Figure 3). The interaction of Tat with LRP can lead to the formation of an apoptosis-promoting complex including postsynaptic density protein-95 (PSD-95), NMDA receptors and neuronal nitric oxide synthase (nNOS) [65]. Tat has been found to interfere with the expression of miRNAs in neurons, increasing the levels of CREB-targeting miR-34a and leading to neuronal dysfunction [66]. Tat can also interfere with the ability of dopamine transporter to reuptake dopamine [67]. This likely contributes to the particularly severe damage rendered to dopaminergic-rich regions in the brains of patients with severe HAND [51].

Other toxic viral proteins which have been found to activate caspases in neurons include Vpr [68] and Nef [69]. Vpu has been found to form cation-selective ion channels in a lipid bilayer membrane [70], though this effect has not been observed in neurons. Recently, stress pathways and accumulation of amyloid beta (Aβ) fibrils have been reported to be important in causing neuronal dysfunction. It has been suggested that an integrated stress response (ISR) pathway involving specific ISR proteins may underlie the neuroinflammatory processes observed in HAND [71]. It has also been reported that individuals with HIV encephalitis display a higher levels of intraneuronal Aβ accumulation in comparison with controls, suggesting that HIV impacts the clearance of Aβ in the brain [72].

Targeting the above discussed mechanisms of neuronal toxicity could yield therapies that can alleviate the

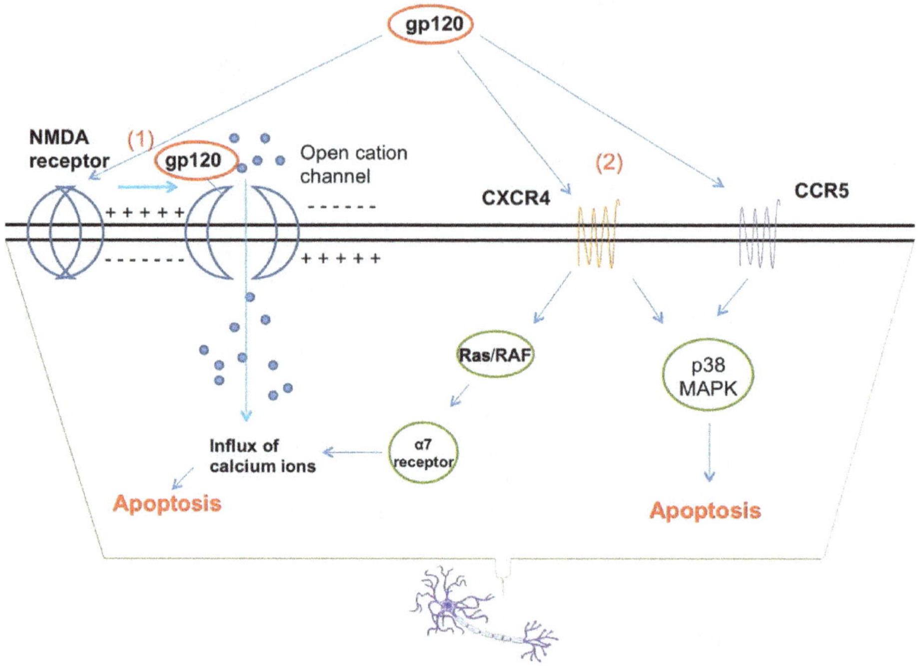

Figure 2 Mechanisms of gp120 neurotoxicity. (1) gp120 can bind to the NMDA receptor and lead to excessive opening of NMDAR-gated cation channels, allowing the influx of calcium ions to toxic levels [54]. (2) gp120 can directly bind to either CCR5 or CXCR4, activating an p38-MAPK mediated signaling cascade that leads to neuronal apoptosis [56]. The gp120-CXCR4 binding also up-regulates the expression of the nicotinic receptor α7, which increases cellular permeability to $[Ca^{2+}]$ influx and contributes to cell death [61].

symptoms and improve the quality of life for patients suffering from HAND.

Macrophage and microglial activation

In addition to toxic viral proteins, HIV-1-infected macrophages and microglia release a variety of neurotoxic host factors that contribute to neuronal injury. These can be broadly categorized as proinflammatory cytokines, chemokines, and small molecules. The proinflammatory cytokines induced by HIV-1-infection of macrophages include TNF-α, IL-1β, IL-6, IL-8 and IFN-α. TNF-α has been shown to also inhibit glutamate uptake by astrocytes, leading to a extracellular buildup of glutamate that can lead to neuronal excitotoxicity [73]. TNF-α has also been found to have a neuroprotective role, through the TNFR2 mediated activation of NF-κB through a PI3 kinase [74], so its role is more complicated than simply that of a neurotoxin. IL-1β is released from macrophages in response to protein kinases induced by gp120 [75], and both IL-1β and TNF-α were found to dysregulate glutamate production in neurons through the induction of glutaminase [76]. IL-6 is also directly induced in macrophages by gp120, and leads to the formation of large cytoplasmic vacuoles in neurons that disrupt neuronal function [77]. Excess levels of IFN-α have been correlated with severity of HIV dementia [78]. Treatment of MDM with IFN-α (or HIV-1 infection) has been reported to increase glutaminase (GLS1) expression through phosphorylation of STAT1, which was shown to act through GLS1 promoter [79]. In addition to inflammatory cytokines, small molecules released by HIV-1-infected macrophages such as platelet activating factor (PAF) and quinolinic acid play a key role in neurotoxicity via NMDAR dysregulation [80,81].

Microglia are mesoderm-derived cells whose population is established in the brain perinatally. They are responsible for immune surveillance of the CNS, and are the primary source of inflammatory cytokines in the brain [82]. Infected microglia are thought to be the main source of giant multinucleated cells, which are a hallmark of HIV associated dementia and an important source of inflammatory cytokines in the CNS of HIV-1 patients [83]. Microglia are a major source of neuronal excitotoxicity, releasing glutamate in response to HIV-1 infection [84]. Even in patients who are able to effectively control HIV infection via ART, increased microglial activation has been shown to correlate with poorer executive performance [85]. Treatment of fetal human microglia with recombinant Tat induces the production of a number of chemokines, such as CCL2 and CCL5, involved in the development of HAND [86]. Dysregulated chemokines released from microglia have an especially potent impact on neurons, due to the presence of several chemokine receptors on neuronal cell surface, including

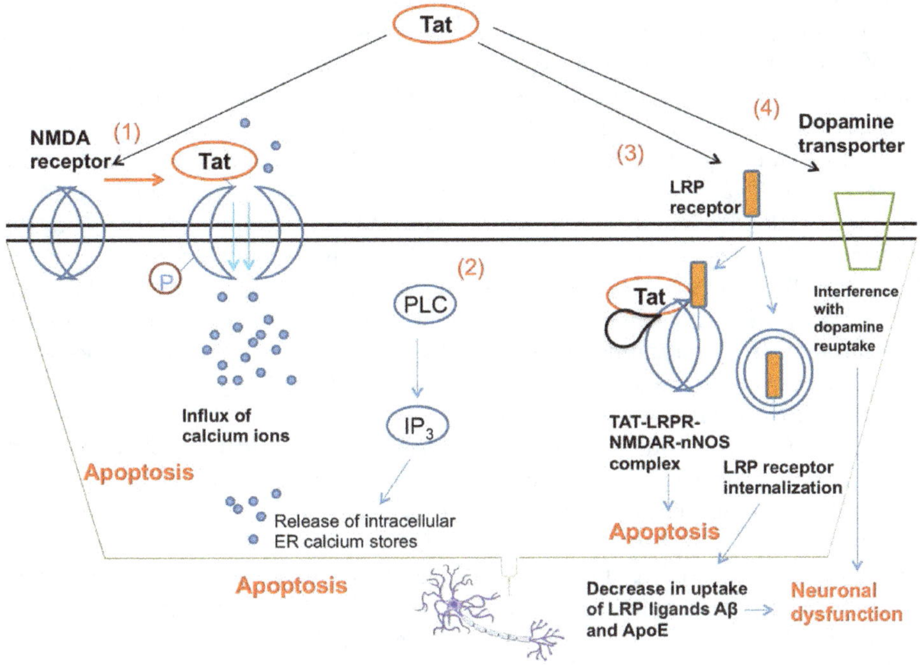

Figure 3 Mechanisms of Tat neurotoxicity. (1) Tat binds to the NMDA receptor and drives the phosphorylation of an intracellular NMDAR subunit, causing excess opening of cation channels and toxic accumulation of calcium [62]. (2) When applied to neurons, Tat is able to induce the activation of PLC and drive the IP3-mediated release of intracellular calcium from ER stores, further contributing to calcium toxicity and apoptosis [63]. (3) Tat can bind to LRP receptors, and be taken up as part of a macromolecular complex including NMDAR and neuronal nitric oxide synthase (nNOS) that induces cellular apoptosis [65]. Tat can also drive the internalization of the LRP receptor, reducing the uptake of LRP receptor ligands amyloid-β peptide and Apolipoprotein E, which may contribute to systemic neuronal dysfunction [64]. (4) Tat interferes with the activity of dopamine transporter, diminishing the reuptake of dopamine by pre-synaptic neurons and interfering with signal transmission [67].

CCR1, CCR4, CCR5, CCR9/10, CXCR2, CXCR4, and CX3CR1 [87].

Astrocytes: no longer a passive bystander

Over the past 10 years, a significant amount of research has gone into understanding the extensive role played by astrocytes in the CNS, overturning their previous status as merely space holders, structural scaffolding, and scavengers. Their newly described roles include uptake of neurotransmitters, modulation of synaptic transmission, BBB maintenance, vaso-modulation, and long-term potentiation. The new concept of neuronal-glial intercommunication, where astrocytes play a dynamic role by integrating neuronal inputs and modulating synaptic activity, has helped us better comprehend astrocyte dysfunction in the context of HAND [88,89].

It has been recently shown that astrocytes can be infected by HIV-1 *in vitro*, and additionally that infected astrocytes can impair BBB function [90], but the infected astrocytes are rarely seen in patient brain autopsies (although one recent study has shown 20% of the astrocytes are infected in patients with HAD [91]). Furthermore, recombinant Tat protein has been shown to be responsible for the induction of chemokines [92], cytokines [93] and nitric oxide synthetase [94] in cultured primary human astrocytes. For example, Tat has been shown to induce astrocytes to produce platelet-derived growth factor BB (PDGF-BB), which in turn induces the production of CCL2 [95]. HIV-1 Tat can also up-regulate the expression of MMP-9 via MAPK-NF-κB-dependent mechanism, and MMP-9, in turn, disrupts the BBB [96].

Exposure of astrocytes to gp120 causes up-regulation of IL-6 and TNF-α [97], and increases the release of glutamate and potassium, which leads to toxic increases in calcium in neurons and astrocytes [98]. Using Affymetrix microarray analysis, Wang *et al.* showed that primary human astrocytes, when exposed to HIV-1 or gp120 *in vitro*, have an impaired ability to transport L-glutamate, and the authors ascribed this defect to transcriptional inhibition of the EAAT2 glutamate transporter gene [99]. More recently, Fernandes *et al.* have used an animal model to show that gp120 prevents the uptake of extracellular glutamate by astrocytes, leading to a disruption of glutamate-glutamine homeostasis and a consequent impairment of memory [100]. Release of toxic cytokines, inability to take up excess glutamate and damage to the BBB make astrocytes a central offender in the pathogenesis of HAND.

Neuroprotective factors

Macrophages, microglia and even neurons themselves produce a number of neuroprotective mediators of inflammation. Neurotoxicity seen in HAND is the net result of the effects of neurotoxic insults and the action of neuroprotective host factors. In the quest to define neurotoxic agents responsible for HAND, the neuroprotective processes often go unnoticed. Platelet derived growth factor (PDGF) confers neuroprotection against gp120 toxicity by stimulating the PI3K/Akt pathway [101], and the pretreatment of neuronal cells with PDGF-CC abrogated Tat-mediated neurotoxicity by mitigating apoptosis and neurite loss [102]. Astrocytes exposed to HIV-1 or chronically infected with HIV-1 express the tissue inhibitor of metalloproteinases-1 (TIMP-1), which is shown to have a neuroprotective role when primary human neurons are exposed to HIV-1 [103]. It has also been reported that exposure of astrocytes to HIV-1 gp120 induces the expression of nuclear factor erythroid-derived 2-related factor 2 (Nrf2), which plays a role in the stimulation of antioxidant defensive enzymes [104].

Fractalkine (FKN/CX3CL1) is a chemokine produced by neurons, and it plays an important role in communication with microglia, which abundantly expresses the FKN receptor CX3CR1 (neurons also express this receptor but less abundantly). FKN plays an important role in neuroprotection and helps reduce gp120 toxicity via activation of ERK1/2 and CREB (this effect was seen both in the presence and absence of co-cultivated glial cells) [105]. Increased levels of FKN were found in the neurons of patients with HIV encephalitis, and FKN was found to potently drive the migration of monocytes across an *in vitro* trans-well system, as well as inhibit the neurotoxic effects of Tat protein in rat cerebellar neurons [106]. Also the chemokine CCL3L1 protects against gp120 neurotoxicity by phosphorylation of CREB, which promotes the transcription of the cell-survival gene bcl-2 [107]. The routes of action of these host mediators against viral neurotoxins may offer potential avenues of therapeutic intervention that capitalize on existing pathways of neuroprotection.

Host genetic determinants of neurotoxicity

Several important host gene polymorphisms have been associated with an effect on the transmission of HIV-1 and/or AIDS disease progression (e.g., CCR5-Δ32 [108], CCL31 [109]). Similarly, several host gene polymorphisms have been linked with effects on the susceptibility to neurocognitive impairment. A point mutation identified in CCR2 (V64I) that had been associated with slower immunosuppressive disease progression [110], has also been shown to be specifically associated with a slower progression of neurocognitive impairment [111]. This V64I variant was not associated with a difference in plasma or CSF viral load, suggesting that its impact could be mediated through a mis-regulation of the inflammatory response rather than through differences in viral replication. A polymorphism in the TNF-α gene increases its production in response to bacterial LPS, and this allele has been found in an increased frequency of patients with HAD [112]. An allele of CCL2, 2578G confers a 50% reduction in risk of acquiring HIV-1 infection. However, the same allele, subsequent to HIV infection, was also associated with a 4.5 fold increased risk of HAD [113]. This 2578G allele resulted in a greater transcriptional output of CCL2, which could exacerbate the development of HAND by increasing the influx of monocytic cells in response to CNS infection.

HAND co-morbidity with drugs of abuse

Neurocognitive disease in HIV-patients can be greatly exacerbated by abuse of drugs such as opiates, methamphetamine and cocaine. Injection drug users (IDUs) are at particular risk, as injection drug use remains an important route of HIV-1 transmission [114]. In addition, HIV-patients addicted to drugs of abuse are less likely to adhere to antiretroviral drug regimens. Opioid abuse is associated with faster HIV-1 disease progression, including increased risks of neurocognitive problems. While the "typical" opioid abuser has previously been perceived as a heroin IDU, there is a growing problem with the rising numbers of people abusing prescription opiates – a 2008 report indicated that while 400,000 Americans used heroin within one year, an estimated 12 million Americans abused prescription opiates within the same timeframe [115]. The mechanisms of opioid-mediated injury in conjunction with HIV-CNS infection are well documented. μ-opiod receptor (MOR) is one of the primary routes of opiod signaling [116]. While morphine itself leads to the down-regulation of MOR in cultured microglia, treatment of microglia with morphine and Tat reverses this down-regulation, providing a potential feed-forward mechanism of higher numbers of MOR at the cell-surface available to propagate further morphine-Tat mediated neurotoxicity [117]. Doxycycline-inducible Tat transgenic mice (that express HIV-1 Tat in astrocytes) that were administered both doxycycline and morphine showed a marked decrease in the density of dendritic spines in the striatum, compared with mice given either doxycycline or morphine alone [118]. PDGF-BB was also able to protect human neurons from synergistic Tat/morphine damage by inhibiting production of ROS and caspase-3 through the activation of the PI3K pathways [119].

Morphine also acts synergistically with gp120 to promote neuronal death through p38 MAP kinase signaling [120]. Mice that were transgenic for gp120 and subjected to morphine withdrawal failed to normalize oxidative capacity compared with non-transgenic mice subjected to morphine withdrawal. The same study also found failure to recover from synaptic damage in gp120-transgenic mice experiencing withdrawal compared with non-transgenic mice [121]. Tat-induced release of CCL2 from astrocytes is further enhanced by morphine, and can increase the chemotactic migration of a microglial cell line towards affected astrocytes [122]. HIV-1 patients using opiates were found to have higher levels of microglial activation in their brains [123]. There is also evidence of opioid use having an effect on HIV-1 infection and replication: morphine significantly enhanced the infectivity of human macrophages, possibly by an increase in CCR5 expression [124]. A more recent study showed that treatment of monocytes with morphine down-regulated several anti-HIV-1 microRNAs, which rendered the monocytes more susceptible to infection [125]. Administration of morphine to rhesus macaques before infection with SIV resulted in a higher viral set point compared with a non-morphine control group [126].

Methamphetamine (METH) use has been found to exacerbate brain injury and neuronal loss in HIV-1 patients, particularly in populations of interneurons in dopaminergeric areas (DA) where the drug acts on the behavioral reward system [127]. METH potentiates a Tat-mediated decrease in dopaminergic release in the cultured human fetal neurons [128]. In the human neuroblastoma cell line SH-SY5Y, treatment with both METH and Tat produced significantly higher levels of both apoptosis and formation of autophagosomes than either factor by itself [129]. In cultured human astrocytes, METH was found to potentiate the gp120-mediated release of the pro-inflammatory cytokine IL-6, mediated through the PI3K/Akt and NF-κB pathways [130]. Treatment of METH on astroglioma cells transfected with a Tat expression construct exacerbated Tat-induced down-regulation of the neuroprotective factor β-catenin [131]. Furthermore, HIV-patients using METH were found to have significantly higher viral loads than non-METH users. This was found to be a result of the interference of METH with antiretroviral therapy [132]. METH also interferes with the normal antigen processing and phagocytic functions of macrophages [133], enhances the susceptibility of macrophages to HIV-1 infection by up-regulation of CCR5 [134] and increases HIV-1 replication in CD4 T cells and monocytes [135].

Cocaine is also known to accelerate the pathology of HAND. The drug binds the dopamine transporter and reduces the rate of dopamine uptake. Cocaine potentiates Tat-mediated neurotoxicity through the action at D1 receptors [136], Cocaine administration to SHIV-infected simian macrophages enhanced viral replication through increases in NF-κB signaling and IL-10 [137], and cultured human endothelial cells exposed to cocaine experienced an up-regulation in adhesion molecules, resulting in increased monocyte transmigration across the BBB [138].

Interestingly, according to recent studies cannabinoids (CB) appear to actually mediate a degree of neuroprotection in the context of CNS-HIV-1 damage. Synthetic CBs acting on the CB2 receptor (CB2-R) were able to mitigate gp120-induced damage in both human dopaminergic neurons and CB-2R expressing microglia [139], and a CB2 agonist was found to rescue deficits in neurogenesis seen in gp120-expressing transgenic mice [140].

Viral genetic determinants

HIV-1 is phylogenetically divided into four groups: M, N, O and P, each representing a successful zoonotic event from primates – group M being the most widespread. Group M is further divided into subtypes A, B, C, D, F, G, H, J, K as well as a number of circulating recombinant forms (CRFs) of these subtypes. The global distribution of HIV-1 subtypes is region-specific, with a given geographical region correlating with the presence of a distinct subtype, a CRF or a particular combination of subtypes and CRFs [141]. Such a highly region-specific distribution is thought to be due either to a founder effect, to host-population genetics selecting for specific subtypes of HIV-1, or a combination of both [142]. Region-specific subtype-distribution has allowed researchers to correlate region-specific disease severity to subtype-specific viral gene polymorphisms, as documented in clinical studies. For example, reports from India, where HIV-1 subtype C is the predominant subtype, pointed to a lower incidence (0 - 4%) of severe forms of HAD [143,144], in contrast to geographic regions where subtype B HIV-1 is prevalent, which reported pre-HAART incidence levels of 15 - 30% [145,146].

Our laboratory previously investigated whether genetic differences between the circulating isolates are responsible for the wide variation in incidence of HAD in different geographic regions. We reported that a majority (88%) of HIV-1 subtype C isolates worldwide have a Tat protein with a Cys31Ser polymorphism that disrupts a dicysteine motif, which is a key element of Tat protein's homology to β-chemokines [147] (Figure 4). In contrast, the Tat proteins encoded by 99% of non-subtype C HIV-1 isolates maintained a C31 residue at that position. We demonstrated that Tat protein of subtype C HIV-1 isolates with a C31S polymorphism is defective for monocyte chemotaxis function in vitro [147]. As the infiltration of monocytic cells to the brain is a hallmark of HAD and plays a central role in triggering the inflammatory onslaught on neurons, we hypothesized that the C31S polymorphism in Tat protein of subtype C HIV-1 isolates contributes to the mechanistic basis for low incidence of HAD reported in India, as fewer monocytic cells would migrate to brain and result in little neuronal damage.

In subsequent studies, several other groups have showed that recombinant subtype C Tat protein has a decreased potential for direct neurotoxicity [149,152] and a decreased

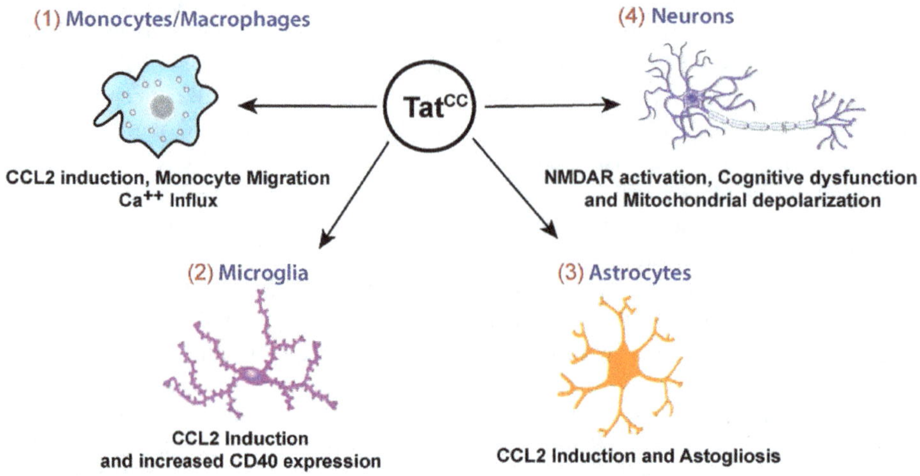

Figure 4 Contribution of the dicysteine motif in Tat to neuropathogenesis. (1) Tat is secreted by infected macrophages and microglia in the vincity of the blood brain barrier resulting in damage to the integrity of the barrier. Dicysteine Tat can act as a ligand on certain chemokine receptors expressed by circulating monocytes (i.e. CCR2, CCR3, CCR5), and promote monocyte migration across the BBB into the CNS [148]. Clade C Tat lacking the intact dicysteine motif fails to attract monocytes in a two chamber migration assay [149]. (2) Dicysteine Tat (TatB but not TatC) also induces higher expression of CCL2 and activation marker CD40 in microglial cells than non-dicysteine Tat [150]. (3) When applied to astrocytes, dicysteine Tat induces higher levels of CCL2 [149] and in HIVE SCID Mouse model astrogliosis is more pronounced in the presence of HIV-1 with an intact dicysteine motif [151]. (4) In neurons, it has been proposed that the Cys31 in the Tat dicysteine motif specifically disrupts the disulfide bond between Cys 744 and Cys 798 on the NR1 subunit of the NMDA receptor, leading to persistent activation of the NMDA receptor [152]. The increase in Tat-mediated apoptosis in dicysteine Tat is also seen in human primary neurons (mediated by increased levels of cleaved caspase-3), in addition to higher levels of ROS and increased levels of mitochondrial depolarization [149]. Primary Human neurons exposed to viral supernatants from HIV-1 with intact dicysteine motif exhibit neuronal apoptosis and HIV-1 SCID mice exposed to the same supernatants have cognitive dysfunction [151].

ability to induce inflammatory chemokine and cytokines [153-155]. In order to examine whether the C31S polymorphism is associated with biological differences in neuropathogenesis, we compared cognitive dysfunction and pathological changes induced by representative subtype C and B isolates in a SCID mouse HIV encephalitis (SCID-HIVE) model [155]. This allowed us to compare two genetically distinct HIV-1 isolates employing a single host genetic background. These studies revealed that subtype C isolates with a C31S polymorphism have lower potential to cause neuropathology and cognitive dysfunction [155] (Figure 4). In primary monocytes, subtype B Tat was found to induce higher amounts of pro-inflammatory factors than subtype C Tat, such as TNF, IL-6, CCL2, and IDO (an enzyme in the kynurenine pathway that leads to production of neurotoxic quinolinic acid) [153]. HIV-1 TatB has also been shown to disrupt the integrity of brain microvascular endothelial cells to a greater extent compared to Tat C [156]. Also, TatB, compared with TatC, can induce higher levels of IDO in human primary astrocytes [157], and TatB also induces higher levels of CCL2 in microglia [150] and primary astrocytes than TatC (this higher CCL2 induction was specifically associated with the presence of the dicysteine motif) [149] (Figure 4). Astroglioma cells that were either transfected with a Tat expression construct or treated with recombinant Tat showed a decrease in β-catenin, a transcriptional co-activator in the Wnt signaling pathway involved in neuroprotection. This β-catenin decrease was specific to the dicysteine motif in Tat, as neither TatC nor a TatB mutant with a disrupted dicysteine motif (C30G) were able to bring about this decrease [158].

The low incidence of HAD caused by subtype C HIV-1 in India was further corroborated by the absence of HAD in Ethiopia, as measured by neurocognitive tests using International HIV Dementia (IHD) scale. Subtype C HIV-1 is also widespread in the Southern African countries. Interestingly, however, recent cohort studies in South Africa and Botswana, where C is the predominant subtype, showed that the incidence of HAD is much higher than that in India at 25 and 38% respectively [159-162]. In light of our earlier findings indicating reduced neuropathogenicity for subtype C HIV-1 [155], we were intrigued by the increased incidence data reported for subtype C HIV-1 cohorts in Southern Africa. While it may be generally assumed that subtype C HIV-1 from different regions of the world are highly related, studies on the phylogenetic and molecular clock analysis of gp120 sequences of Indian HIV-1 isolates have shown that their origin in India occurred much later than that of South African subtype C HIV-1 [163,164]. Therefore, we initiated a multi-site study to investigate phylogenetic differences between Southern African (South Africa and Zambia) and South Asian (India and Bangladesh) subtype C HIV-1 isolates. Our results showed that, with respect to both the whole virus genome sequence as well as sequences encoding Tat protein, the Indian HIV-1C isolates are genetically distinct from those in Southern Africa. More importantly, HIV-1C isolates with an intact dicysteine motif in Tat protein (C31) were quite rare (2 - 3%) in India, while they were significantly more frequent in the Southern African countries (11 - 26%). Thus, the frequency of HIV-1C isolates with a C31 in Tat broadly paralleled the incidence of HAD in these countries. Neurocognitive tests in SCID-HIVE mice, using a representative subtype C from Southern Africa (HIV-1_{1084i}) with an intact dicysteine motif in Tat (C31) and comparing it to subtype C from India (HIV-$1_{IndieC1}$) lacking an intact dicysteine motif in Tat (C31S), showed that mice exposed to subtype C from Southern Africa exhibited significantly greater cognitive dysfunction compared to subtype C from India [151], especially when the testing paradigm presented a higher level of memory load. These findings lead to three main conclusions. One, intra-subtype variation exists and such variation can involve viral genes in HIV-1 that play a direct role in neurotoxicity. Two, it is more accurate to correlate differential disease outcomes in two geographical regions being compared, to differences in neurovirulence signatures rather than to differences in subtypes as a whole. Three, once further confirmed in a clinical study, it should be possible to perform a genetic screening in a subtype C HIV-1 epidemic for Tat genotype to gauge the risk of neurological dysfunction at the time of initial diagnosis.

Additional genetic determinants in Tat, other than C31, that play a crucial role in the pathogenesis of HAND are unknown, but are likely to exist. Further studies on differential neuropathogenesis potential of HIV-1 variants in different geographic regions will be informative. Similarly, considering the fact that gp120 causes neuropathogenesis via multiple pathways, it is also possible that there are genetic differences in gp120 between viral variants in their ability to cause HAND via gp120-mediated neurotoxicity. Identification of such variants and their impact on the pathogenesis of HAND will help dissect the various types of neurotoxic insults involving different cellular receptors and develop better therapeutics and/or diagnostics.

Treatment modalities for HAND

HAART significantly lowers the viral load in both the periphery and the CNS, and has been crucial in significantly decreasing the incidence and prevalence of severe forms of HAND [165]. However, recent clinical studies and a meta-analysis [1,166,167] in patients on HAART revealed milder forms of neurological dysfunction (ANI & MND) in greater than half of HIV-positive patients. In studies examining individuals with ART-controlled HIV viremia, HIV DNA in PBMCs correlated with regional brain atrophy highlighting the contribution of peripheral viral reservoirs to CNS pathology [168]. Even the modified HAART regimens that include drugs with better CNS penetration effectiveness (CPE) scores, termed neuro-HAART, have had limited success among patients [169-171]. Researchers have suggested various approaches to targeting latent CNS HIV reservoirs and sources of neuroinflammation such as cytokines, chemokines and oxidative stress that are in play inside the CNS and are refractory to antiretrovirals. Use of anti-inflammatory and anti-excitotoxic drugs like Minocycline (second-generation tetracycline derivative) [172] and Memantine (voltage-dependent, open channel NMDAR blocker) [173], that can cross the BBB at substantial levels and that have been shown to be neuroprotective in SCID HIVE mice and SIV models, are currently being investigated as adjuvants to treat HAND. Several neuroprotective factors, both endogenous (as discussed above) and exogenous (e.g., pDING; [174]) are also being proposed as alternate treatments, with a focus towards eliminating neuroinflammation caused by exposure to HIV-1 [101-103]. Intranasal delivery of neurotropic protective factors such as insulin, IGF-1 and neurotrophin has been shown to mitigate many of the behavioral and pathological deficits in gp120 transgenic mice [175]. *In vitro* studies, using innovative delivery techniques such as gold and lipid based nano-particles, have been shown to be effective in delivering HAART and anti-inflammatory/anti-excitotoxic agents across the blood brain barrier [176] to specifically target CNS reservoirs. NanoART treatments in humanized mice reduced viral loads and protected CD4 T-cell populations [177]. Natalizumab, a monoclonal antibody against alpha-4-integrin known to block trafficking of leukocytes across the blood–brain barrier, has been shown to be effective in preventing HIV-1 infected cells from breaching the BBB in a SIV model by Campbell and colleagues [178]. These new and innovative treatments, in combination with Neuro-HAART, could be useful in treating HAND in the aging at-risk HIV-1 infected population. Thus, current approaches to intervention of HAND include not only the careful choice of antiretrovirals with better CNS penetration and efficacy, but also the future use of neuroprotective agents or the modulation of neuroprotective host factors.

Conclusions

Our precise understanding of host factors that mediate the neurotoxic insult launched by exposure of CNS to HIV-1-infected cells, HIV-1 or specific HIV-1 proteins has increased in the recent past. In addition to increased knowledge about the pathways of neurotoxicity, we are also learning about the regional genetic variations in viral genes leading to intra-clade, region specific differences in disease severity. The discussion above clearly indicates that numerous opportunities exist to specifically block the neurotoxicity of viral and host proteins as well as potential neuroprotective factors that could be augmented to help alleviate the negative impact of HIV-1 on the brain.

Abbreviations

CNS: Central nervous system; HAND: HIV-1 associated neurological disorders; ANI: Asymptomatic neurocognitive impairment; MND: Mild neurocognitive disorder; HAD: HIV-1 associated dementia; HAART: Highly active anti-retroviral therapy; ART: Anti-retroviral therapy; BBB: Blood-brain barrier; HBMEC: Human brain microvascular endothelial cells; MAP: Mitogen-activated protein; NMDAR: N-methyl-D-Aspartate receptors; LRPR: Lipoprotein receptor related protein receptors; PAF: Platelet activating factor; PDGF: Platelet derived growth factor; CRFs: Circulating recombinant forms; SCID-HIVE: SCID mouse HIV-1 encephalitis; CPE: CNS penetration effectiveness.

Competing interests

The authors declare that they have no competing interests.

Authors' contributions

All three authors wrote sections of the manuscript. VRR developed the arrangement of the various sections and VRP was responsible for the integration of the sections. All authors read and approved the final manuscript.

Acknowledgements

The authors would like to thank Eliseo Eugenin (Rutgers University) and Lisa Baker for critically reading the manuscript. VRP would like to acknowledge support from NIH R01 MH083579.

References

1. Heaton RK, Franklin DR, Ellis RJ, McCutchan JA, Letendre SL, Leblanc S, Corkran SH, Duarte NA, Clifford DB, Woods SP, Collier AC, Marra CM, Morgello S, Mindt MR, Taylor MJ, Marcotte TD, Atkinson JH, Wolfson T, Gelman BB, McArthur JC, Simpson DM, Abramson I, Gamst A, Fennema-Notestine C, Jernigan TL, Wong J, Grant I, Group C, Group H: **HIV-associated neurocognitive disorders before and during the era of combination antiretroviral therapy: differences in rates, nature, and predictors.** *J Neurovirol* 2011, **17**(1):3–16.
2. Antinori A, Arendt G, Becker JT, Brew BJ, Byrd DA, Cherner M, Clifford DB, Cinque P, Epstein LG, Goodkin K, Gisslen M, Grant I, Heaton RK, Joseph J, Marder K, Marra CM, McArthur JC, Nunn M, Price RW, Pulliam L, Robertson KR, Sacktor N, Valcour V, Wojna VE: **Updated research nosology for HIV-associated neurocognitive disorders.** *Neurology* 2007, **69**(18):1789–1799.
3. Canizares S, Cherner M, Ellis RJ: **HIV and Aging: Effects on the Central Nervous System.** *Semin Neurol* 2014, **34**(1):27–34.
4. Airoldi M, Bandera A, Trabattoni D, Tagliabue B, Arosio B, Soria A, Rainone V, Lapadula G, Annoni G, Clerici M, Gori A: **Neurocognitive impairment in HIV-infected naive patients with advanced disease: the role of virus and intrathecal immune activation.** *Clin Dev Immunol* 2012, **2012**:467154.
5. Gendelman HE, Orenstein JM, Baca LM, Weiser B, Burger H, Kalter DC, Meltzer MS: **The macrophage in the persistence and pathogenesis of HIV infection.** *AIDS (London, England)* 1989, **3**(8):475–495.
6. Ho WZ, Cherukuri R, Douglas SD: **The macrophage and HIV-1.** *Immunol Ser* 1994, **60**:569–587.
7. Resnick L, Berger JR, Shapshak P, Tourtellotte WW: **Early penetration of the blood–brain-barrier by HIV.** *Neurology* 1988, **38**(1):9–14.
8. Gendelman HE, Lipton SA, Tardieu M, Bukrinsky MI, Nottet HS: **The neuropathogenesis of HIV-1 infection.** *J Leukoc Biol* 1994, **56**(3):389–398.
9. Matthews TJ, Weinhold KJ, Lyerly HK, Langlois AJ, Wigzell H, Bolognesi DP: **Interaction between the human T-cell lymphotropic virus type IIIB envelope glycoprotein gp120 and the surface antigen CD4: role of carbohydrate in binding and cell fusion.** *Proc Natl Acad Sci U S A* 1987, **84**(15):5424–5428.
10. Moore JP, Trkola A, Dragic T: **Co-receptors for HIV-1 entry.** *Curr Opin Immunol* 1997, **9**(4):551–562.
11. Gallo SA, Finnegan CM, Viard M, Raviv Y, Dimitrov A, Rawat SS, Puri A, Durell S, Blumenthal R: **The HIV Env-mediated fusion reaction.** *Biochim Biophys Acta* 2003, **1614**(1):36–50.
12. Xiao L, Owen SM, Goldman I, Lal AA, de Jong JJ, Goudsmit J, Lal RB: **CCR5 coreceptor usage of non-syncytium-inducing primary HIV-1 is independent of phylogenetically distinct global HIV-1 isolates: delineation of consensus motif in the V3 domain that predicts CCR-5 usage.** *Virology* 1998, **240**(1):83–92.
13. Huang Y, Paxton WA, Wolinsky SM, Neumann AU, Zhang L, He T, Kang S, Ceradini D, Jin Z, Yazdanbakhsh K, Kunstman K, Erickson D, Dragon E, Landau NR, Phair J, Ho DD, Koup RA: **The role of a mutant CCR5 allele in HIV-1 transmission and disease progression.** *Nat Med* 1996, **2**(11):1240–1243.
14. Connor RI, Sheridan KE, Ceradini D, Choe S, Landau NR: **Change in coreceptor use correlates with disease progression in HIV-1–infected individuals.** *J Exp Med* 1997, **185**(4):621–628.
15. Ping LH, Nelson JA, Hoffman IF, Schock J, Lamers SL, Goodman M, Vernazza P, Kazembe P, Maida M, Zimba D, Goodenow MM, Eron JJ Jr, Fiscus SA, Cohen MS, Swanstrom R: **Characterization of V3 sequence heterogeneity in subtype C human immunodeficiency virus type 1 isolates from Malawi: underrepresentation of X4 variants.** *J Virol* 1999, **73**(8):6271–6281.
16. Yi Y, Isaacs SN, Williams DA, Frank I, Schols D, De Clercq E, Kolson DL, Collman RG: **Role of CXCR4 in cell-cell fusion and infection of monocyte-derived macrophages by primary human immunodeficiency virus type 1 (HIV-1) strains: two distinct mechanisms of HIV-1 dual tropism.** *J Virol* 1999, **73**(9):7117–7125.
17. Wu L, KewalRamani VN: **Dendritic-cell interactions with HIV: infection and viral dissemination.** *Nat Rev Immunol* 2006, **6**(11):859–868.
18. Finkel TH, Tudor-Williams G, Banda NK, Cotton MF, Curiel T, Monks C, Baba TW, Ruprecht RM, Kupfer A: **Apoptosis occurs predominantly in bystander cells and not in productively infected cells of HIV- and SIV-infected lymph nodes.** *Nat Med* 1995, **1**(2):129–134.
19. Thomas ER, Dunfee RL, Stanton J, Bogdan D, Taylor J, Kunstman K, Bell JE, Wolinsky SM, Gabuzda D: **Macrophage entry mediated by HIV Envs from brain and lymphoid tissues is determined by the capacity to use low CD4 levels and overall efficiency of fusion.** *Virology* 2007, **360**(1):105–119.
20. Orenstein JM, Meltzer MS, Phipps T, Gendelman HE: **Cytoplasmic assembly and accumulation of human immunodeficiency virus types 1 and 2 in recombinant human colony-stimulating factor-1-treated human monocytes: an ultrastructural study.** *J Virol* 1988, **62**(8):2578–2586.
21. Ziegler-Heitbrock L, Ancuta P, Crowe S, Dalod M, Grau V, Hart DN, Leenen PJ, Liu YJ, MacPherson G, Randolph GJ, Scherberich J, Schmitz J, Shortman K, Sozzani S, Strobl H, Zembala M, Austyn JM, Lutz MB: **Nomenclature of monocytes and dendritic cells in blood.** *Blood* 2010, **116**(16):e74–e80.
22. Fischer-Smith T, Croul S, Sverstiuk AE, Capini C, L'Heureux D, Regulier EG, Richardson MW, Amini S, Morgello S, Khalili K, Rappaport J: **CNS invasion by CD14+/CD16+ peripheral blood-derived monocytes in HIV dementia: perivascular accumulation and reservoir of HIV infection.** *J Neurovirol* 2001, **7**(6):528–541.
23. Pulliam L, Gascon R, Stubblebine M, McGuire D, McGrath MS: **Unique monocyte subset in patients with AIDS dementia.** *The Lancet* 1997, **349**(9053):692–695.
24. Ellery PJ, Tippett E, Chiu YL, Paukovics G, Cameron PU, Solomon A, Lewin SR, Gorry PR, Jaworowski A, Greene WC, Sonza S, Crowe SM: **The CD16+ monocyte subset is more permissive to infection and preferentially harbors HIV-1 in vivo.** *J Immunol* 2007, **178**(10):6581–6589.
25. Williams DW, Calderon TM, Lopez L, Carvallo-Torres L, Gaskill PJ, Eugenin EA, Morgello S, Berman JW: **Mechanisms of HIV entry into the CNS: increased sensitivity of HIV infected CD14 + CD16+ monocytes to CCL2 and key roles of CCR2, JAM-A, and ALCAM in diapedesis.** *PLoS One* 2013, **8**(7):e69270.
26. Schnell G, Spudich S, Harrington P, Price RW, Swanstrom R: **Compartmentalized human immunodeficiency virus type 1 originates from long-lived cells in some subjects with HIV-1-associated dementia.** *PLoS Pathog* 2009, **5**(4):e1000395.
27. Zlokovic BV: **Neurodegeneration and the neurovascular unit.** *Nat Med* 2010, **16**(12):1370–1371.
28. Aguilera KY, Brekken RA: **Recruitment and retention: factors that affect pericyte migration.** *Cell Mol Life Sci: CMLS* 2014, **71**(2):299–309.
29. An SF, Groves M, Gray F, Scaravilli F: **Early entry and widespread cellular involvement of HIV-1 DNA in brains of HIV-1 positive asymptomatic individuals.** *J Neuropathol Exp Neurol* 1999, **58**(11):1156–1162.
30. Meltzer MS, Skillman DR, Gomatos PJ, Kalter DC, Gendelman HE: **Role of mononuclear phagocytes in the pathogenesis of human immunodeficiency virus infection.** *Annu Rev Immunol* 1990, **8**:169–194.
31. Nottet HS, Persidsky Y, Sasseville VG, Nukuna AN, Bock P, Zhai QH, Sharer LR, McComb RD, Swindells S, Soderland C, Gendelman HE: **Mechanisms for the**

transendothelial migration of HIV-1-infected monocytes into brain. *J Immunol* 1996, **156**(3):1284–1295.

32. Toborek M, Lee YW, Pu H, Malecki A, Flora G, Garrido R, Hennig B, Bauer HC, Nath A: **HIV-Tat protein induces oxidative and inflammatory pathways in brain endothelium.** *J Neurochem* 2003, **84**(1):169–179.
33. Ensoli B, Buonaguro L, Barillari G, Fiorelli V, Gendelman R, Morgan RA, Wingfield P, Gallo RC: **Release, uptake, and effects of extracellular human immunodeficiency virus type 1 Tat protein on cell growth and viral transactivation.** *J Virol* 1993, **67**(1):277–287.
34. Hudson L, Liu J, Nath A, Jones M, Raghavan R, Narayan O, Male D, Everall I: **Detection of the human immunodeficiency virus regulatory protein tat in CNS tissues.** *J Neurovirol* 2000, **6**(2):145–155.
35. Johnson TP, Patel K, Johnson KR, Maric D, Calabresi PA, Hasbun R, Nath A: **Induction of IL-17 and nonclassical T-cell activation by HIV-Tat protein.** *Proc Natl Acad Sci U S A* 2013, **110**(33):13588–13593.
36. Bachani M, Sacktor N, McArthur JC, Nath A, Rumbaugh J: **Detection of anti-tat antibodies in CSF of individuals with HIV-associated neurocognitive disorders.** *J Neurovirol* 2013, **19**(1):82–88.
37. Andras IE, Pu H, Deli MA, Nath A, Hennig B, Toborek M: **HIV-1 Tat protein alters tight junction protein expression and distribution in cultured brain endothelial cells.** *J Neurosci Res* 2003, **74**(2):255–265.
38. Xu R, Feng X, Xie X, Zhang J, Wu D, Xu L: **HIV-1 Tat protein increases the permeability of brain endothelial cells by both inhibiting occludin expression and cleaving occludin via matrix metalloproteinase-9.** *Brain Res* 2012, **1436**:13–19.
39. Kim TA, Avraham HK, Koh YH, Jiang S, Park IW, Avraham S: **HIV-1 Tat-mediated apoptosis in human brain microvascular endothelial cells.** *J Immunol* 2003, **170**(5):2629–2637.
40. Eugenin EA, Osiecki K, Lopez L, Goldstein H, Calderon TM, Berman JW: **CCL2/monocyte chemoattractant protein-1 mediates enhanced transmigration of human immunodeficiency virus (HIV)-infected leukocytes across the blood–brain barrier: a potential mechanism of HIV-CNS invasion and NeuroAIDS.** *J Neurosci* 2006, **26**(4):1098–1106.
41. Moore JP, McKeating JA, Weiss RA, Sattentau QJ: **Dissociation of gp120 from HIV-1 virions induced by soluble CD4.** *Science* 1990, **250**(4984):1139–1142.
42. Toneatto S, Finco O, van der Putten H, Abrignani S, Annunziata P: **Evidence of blood–brain barrier alteration and activation in HIV-1 gp120 transgenic mice.** *Aids* 1999, **13**(17):2343–2348.
43. Chaudhuri A, Duan F, Morsey B, Persidsky Y, Kanmogne GD: **HIV-1 activates proinflammatory and interferon-inducible genes in human brain microvascular endothelial cells: putative mechanisms of blood–brain barrier dysfunction.** *J Cerebr Blood Flow Metabol* 2008, **28**(4):697–711.
44. Kanmogne GD, Schall K, Leibhart J, Knipe B, Gendelman HE, Persidsky Y: **HIV-1 gp120 compromises blood–brain barrier integrity and enhances monocyte migration across blood–brain barrier: implication for viral neuropathogenesis.** *J Cereb Blood Flow Metab: Official J Int Soc Cereb Blood Flow Metab* 2007, **27**(1):123–134.
45. Stins MF, Shen Y, Huang SH, Gilles F, Kalra VK, Kim KS: **Gp120 activates children's brain endothelial cells via CD4.** *J Neurovirol* 2001, **7**(2):125–134.
46. Khan NA, Di Cello F, Stins M, Kim KS: **Gp120-mediated cytotoxicity of human brain microvascular endothelial cells is dependent on p38 mitogen-activated protein kinase activation.** *J Neurovirol* 2007, **13**(3):242–251.
47. Everall IP, Luthert PJ, Lantos PL: **Neuronal number and volume alterations in the neocortex of HIV infected individuals.** *J Neurol Neurosurg Psychiatry* 1993, **56**(5):481–486.
48. Cull-Candy S, Brickley S, Farrant M: **NMDA receptor subunits: diversity, development and disease.** *Curr Opin Neurobiol* 2001, **11**(3):327–335.
49. Hayashi H, Campenot RB, Vance DE, Vance JE: **Apolipoprotein E-containing lipoproteins protect neurons from apoptosis via a signaling pathway involving low-density lipoprotein receptor-related protein-1.** *J Neurosci* 2007, **27**(8):1933–1941.
50. Girault JA, Greengard P: **The neurobiology of dopamine signaling.** *Arch Neurol* 2004, **61**(5):641–644.
51. Chang L, Wang GJ, Volkow ND, Ernst T, Telang F, Logan J, Fowler JS: **Decreased brain dopamine transporters are related to cognitive deficits in HIV patients with or without cocaine abuse.** *Neuroimage* 2008, **42**(2):869–878.
52. Bardi G, Sengupta R, Khan MZ, Patel JP, Meucci O: **Human immunodeficiency virus gp120-induced apoptosis of human neuroblastoma cells in the absence of CXCR4 internalization.** *J Neurovirol* 2006, **12**(3):211–218.
53. Toggas SM, Masliah E, Rockenstein EM, Rall GF, Abraham CR, Mucke L: **Central nervous system damage produced by expression of the HIV-1 coat protein gp120 in transgenic mice.** *Nature* 1994, **367**(6459):188–193.
54. Lannuzel A, Lledo PM, Lamghitnia HO, Vincent JD, Tardieu M: **HIV-1 envelope proteins gp120 and gp160 potentiate NMDA-induced [Ca2+]i increase, alter [Ca2+]i homeostasis and induce neurotoxicity in human embryonic neurons.** *Eur J Neurosci* 1995, **7**(11):2285–2293.
55. Catani MV, Corasaniti MT, Navarra M, Nistico G, Finazzi-Agro A, Melino G: **gp120 induces cell death in human neuroblastoma cells through the CXCR4 and CCR5 chemokine receptors.** *J Neurochem* 2000, **74**(6):2373–2379.
56. Kaul M, Lipton SA: **Chemokines and activated macrophages in HIV gp120-induced neuronal apoptosis.** *Proc Natl Acad Sci U S A* 1999, **96**(14):8212–8216.
57. D'Hooge R, Franck F, Mucke L, De Deyn PP: **Age-related behavioural deficits in transgenic mice expressing the HIV-1 coat protein gp120.** *Eur J Neurosci* 1999, **11**(12):4398–4402.
58. Chalasani SH, Baribaud F, Coughlan CM, Sunshine MJ, Lee VM, Doms RW, Littman DR, Raper JA: **The chemokine stromal cell-derived factor-1 promotes the survival of embryonic retinal ganglion cells.** *J Neurosci* 2003, **23**(11):4601–4612.
59. Khan MZ, Brandimarti R, Musser BJ, Resue DM, Fatatis A, Meucci O: **The chemokine receptor CXCR4 regulates cell-cycle proteins in neurons.** *J Neurovirol* 2003, **9**(3):300–314.
60. Zhang K, McQuibban GA, Silva C, Butler GS, Johnston JB, Holden J, Clark-Lewis I, Overall CM, Power C: **HIV-induced metalloproteinase processing of the chemokine stromal cell derived factor-1 causes neurodegeneration.** *Nat Neurosci* 2003, **6**(10):1064–1071.
61. Ballester LY, Capo-Velez CM, Garcia-Beltran WF, Ramos FM, Vazquez-Rosa E, Rios R, Mercado JR, Melendez RI, Lasalde-Dominicci JA: **Up-regulation of the neuronal nicotinic receptor alpha7 by HIV glycoprotein 120: potential implications for HIV-associated neurocognitive disorder.** *J Biol Chem* 2012, **287**(5):3079–3086.
62. Nath A, Psooy K, Martin C, Knudsen B, Magnuson DS, Haughey N, Geiger JD: **Identification of a human immunodeficiency virus type 1 Tat epitope that is neuroexcitatory and neurotoxic.** *J Virol* 1996, **70**(3):1475–1480.
63. Haughey NJ, Holden CP, Nath A, Geiger JD: **Involvement of inositol 1,4,5-trisphosphate-regulated stores of intracellular calcium in calcium dysregulation and neuron cell death caused by HIV-1 protein tat.** *J Neurochem* 1999, **73**(4):1363–1374.
64. Liu Y, Jones M, Hingtgen CM, Bu G, Laribee N, Tanzi RE, Moir RD, Nath A, He JJ: **Uptake of HIV-1 tat protein mediated by low-density lipoprotein receptor-related protein disrupts the neuronal metabolic balance of the receptor ligands.** *Nat Med* 2000, **6**(12):1380–1387.
65. Eugenin EA, King JE, Nath A, Calderon TM, Zukin RS, Bennett MV, Berman JW: **HIV-tat induces formation of an LRP-PSD-95- NMDAR-nNOS complex that promotes apoptosis in neurons and astrocytes.** *Proc Natl Acad Sci U S A* 2007, **104**(9):3438–3443.
66. Chang JR, Mukerjee R, Bagashev A, Del Valle L, Chabrashvili T, Hawkins BJ, He JJ, Sawaya BE: **HIV-1 Tat protein promotes neuronal dysfunction through disruption of microRNAs.** *J Biol Chem* 2011, **286**(47):41125–41134.
67. Zhu J, Ananthan S, Mactutus CF, Booze RM: **Recombinant human immunodeficiency virus-1 transactivator of transcription1-86 allosterically modulates dopamine transporter activity.** *Synapse (New York, NY)* 2011, **65**(11):1251–1254.
68. Patel CA, Mukhtar M, Pomerantz RJ: **Human Immunodeficiency Virus Type 1 Vpr induces apoptosis in human neuronal cells.** *J Virol* 2000, **74**(20):9717–9726.
69. Trillo-Pazos G, McFarlane-Abdulla E, Campbell IC, Pilkington GJ, Everall IP: **Recombinant nef HIV-IIIB protein is toxic to human neurons in culture.** *Brain Res* 2000, **864**(2):315–326.
70. Ewart GD, Sutherland T, Gage PW, Cox GB: **The Vpu protein of human immunodeficiency virus type 1 forms cation-selective ion channels.** *J Virol* 1996, **70**(10):7108–7115.
71. Akay C, Lindl KA, Shyam N, Nabet B, Goenaga-Vazquez Y, Ruzbarsky J, Wang Y, Kolson DL, Jordan-Sciutto KL: **Activation status of integrated stress response pathways in neurones and astrocytes of HIV-associated neurocognitive disorders (HAND) cortex.** *Neuropathol Appl Neurobiol* 2012, **38**(2):175–200.

72. Achim CL, Adame A, Dumaop W, Everall IP, Masliah E, Neurobehavioral Research C: **Increased accumulation of intraneuronal amyloid beta in HIV-infected patients.** *J Neuroimmune Pharmacol* 2009, **4**(2):190–199.
73. Fine SM, Angel RA, Perry SW, Epstein LG, Rothstein JD, Dewhurst S, Gelbard HA: **Tumor necrosis factor alpha inhibits glutamate uptake by primary human astrocytes. Implications for pathogenesis of HIV-1 dementia.** *J Biol Chem* 1996, **271**(26):15303–15306.
74. Marchetti L, Klein M, Schlett K, Pfizenmaier K, Eisel ULM: **Tumor necrosis factor (TNF)-mediated neuroprotection against glutamate-induced excitotoxicity is enhanced by N-methyl-D-aspartate receptor activation. Essential role of a TNF receptor 2-mediated phosphatidylinositol 3-kinase-dependent NF-kappa B pathway.** *J Biol Chem* 2004, **279**(31):32869–32881.
75. Cheung R, Ravyn V, Wang L, Ptasznik A, Collman RG: **Signaling mechanism of HIV-1 gp120 and virion-induced IL-1beta release in primary human macrophages.** *J Immunol* 2008, **180**(10):6675–6684.
76. Ye L, Huang Y, Zhao L, Li Y, Sun L, Zhou Y, Qian G, Zheng JC: **IL-1β and TNF-α induce neurotoxicity through glutamate production: a potential role for neuronal glutaminase.** *J Neurochem* 2013, **125**(6):897–908.
77. Yeung MC, Pulliam L, Lau AS: **The HIV envelope protein gp120 is toxic to human brain-cell cultures through the induction of interleukin-6 and tumor necrosis factor-alpha.** *AIDS (London, England)* 1995, **9**(2):137–143.
78. Rho MB, Wesselingh S, Glass JD, McArthur JC, Choi S, Griffin J, Tyor WR: **A potential role for interferon-alpha in the pathogenesis of HIV-associated dementia.** *Brain Behav Immun* 1995, **9**(4):366–377.
79. Zhao L, Huang Y, Tian C, Taylor L, Curthoys N, Wang Y, Vernon H, Zheng J: **Interferon-alpha regulates glutaminase 1 promoter through STAT1 phosphorylation: relevance to HIV-1 associated neurocognitive disorders.** *PLoS One* 2012, **7**(3):e32995.
80. Kerr SJ, Armati PJ, Guillemin GJ, Brew BJ: **Chronic exposure of human neurons to quinolinic acid results in neuronal changes consistent with AIDS dementia complex.** *AIDS (London, England)* 1998, **12**(4):355–363.
81. Gelbard HA, Nottet HS, Swindells S, Jett M, Dzenko KA, Genis P, White R, Wang L, Choi YB, Zhang D: **Platelet-activating factor: a candidate human immunodeficiency virus type 1-induced neurotoxin.** *J Virol* 1994, **68**(7):4628–4635.
82. Rock RB, Gekker G, Hu S, Sheng WS, Cheeran M, Lokensgard JR, Peterson PK: **Role of microglia in central nervous system infections.** *Clin Microbiol Rev* 2004, **17**(4):942–964. table of contents.
83. Ghorpade A, Persidsky Y, Swindells S, Borgmann K, Persidsky R, Holter S, Cotter R, Gendelman HE: **Neuroinflammatory responses from microglia recovered from HIV-1-infected and seronegative subjects.** *J Neuroimmunol* 2005, **163**(1–2):145–156.
84. Huang Y, Zhao L, Jia B, Wu L, Li Y, Curthoys N, Zheng JC: **Glutaminase dysregulation in HIV-1-infected human microglia mediates neurotoxicity: relevant to HIV-1-associated neurocognitive disorders.** *J Neurosci* 2011, **31**(42):15195–15204.
85. Garvey LJ, Pavese N, Politis M, Ramlackhansingh A, Brooks DJ, Taylor-Robinson SD, Winston A: **Increased microglia activation in neurologically asymptomatic HIV-infected patients receiving effective ART.** *Aids* 2014, **28**(1):67–72.
86. D'Aversa TG, Yu KO, Berman JW: **Expression of chemokines by human fetal microglia after treatment with the human immunodeficiency virus type 1 protein Tat.** *J Neurovirol* 2004, **10**(2):86–97.
87. Meucci O, Fatatis A, Simen AA, Miller RJ: **Expression of CX3CR1 chemokine receptors on neurons and their role in neuronal survival.** *Proc Natl Acad Sci U S A* 2000, **97**(14):8075–8080.
88. Perez-Alvarez A, Araque A: **Astrocyte-neuron interaction at tripartite synapses.** *Curr Drug Targets* 2013, **14**(11):1220–1224.
89. Navarrete M, Perea G, Maglio L, Pastor J, Garcia de Sola R, Araque A: **Astrocyte calcium signal and gliotransmission in human brain tissue.** *Cereb Cortex* 2013, **23**(5):1240–1246.
90. Eugenin EA, Clements JE, Zink MC, Berman JW: **Human immunodeficiency virus infection of human astrocytes disrupts blood–brain barrier integrity by a gap junction-dependent mechanism.** *J Neurosci* 2011, **31**(26):9456–9465.
91. Churchill MJ, Wesselingh SL, Cowley D, Pardo CA, McArthur JC, Brew BJ, Gorry PR: **Extensive astrocyte infection is prominent in human immunodeficiency virus-associated dementia.** *Ann Neurol* 2009, **66**(2):253–258.
92. Conant K, Garzino-Demo A, Nath A, McArthur JC, Halliday W, Power C, Gallo RC, Major EO: **Induction of monocyte chemoattractant protein-1 in HIV-1 Tat-stimulated astrocytes and elevation in AIDS dementia.** *Proc Natl Acad Sci U S A* 1998, **95**(6):3117–3121.
93. Nath A, Conant K, Chen P, Scott C, Major EO: **Transient exposure to HIV-1 Tat protein results in cytokine production in macrophages and astrocytes. a hit and run phenomenon.** *J Biol Chem* 1999, **274**(24):17098–17102.
94. Liu X, Jana M, Dasgupta S, Koka S, He J, Wood C, Pahan K: **Human immunodeficiency virus type 1 (HIV-1) tat induces nitric-oxide synthase in human astroglia.** *J Biol Chem* 2002, **277**(42):39312–39319.
95. Bethel-Brown C, Yao H, Hu G, Buch S: **Platelet-derived growth factor (PDGF)-BB-mediated induction of monocyte chemoattractant protein 1 in human astrocytes: implications for HIV-associated neuroinflammation.** *J Neuroinflammation* 2012, **9**:262.
96. Ju SM, Song HY, Lee JA, Lee SJ, Choi SY, Park J: **Extracellular HIV-1 Tat up-regulates expression of matrix metalloproteinase-9 via a MAPK-NF-kappaB dependent pathway in human astrocytes.** *Exp Mol Med* 2009, **41**(2):86–93.
97. Yeung MC, Pulliam L, Lau AS: **The HIV envelope protein gp120 is toxic to human brain-cell cultures through the induction of interleukin-6 and tumor necrosis factor-alpha.** *Aids* 1995, **9**(2):137–143.
98. Holden CP, Haughey NJ, Nath A, Geiger JD: **Role of Na+/H + exchangers, excitatory amino acid receptors and voltage-operated Ca2+ channels in human immunodeficiency virus type 1 gp120-mediated increases in intracellular Ca2+ in human neurons and astrocytes.** *Neuroscience* 1999, **91**(4):1369–1378.
99. Wang Z, Trillo-Pazos G, Kim SY, Canki M, Morgello S, Sharer LR, Gelbard HA, Su ZZ, Kang DC, Brooks AI, Fisher PB, Volsky DJ: **Effects of human immunodeficiency virus type 1 on astrocyte gene expression and function: potential role in neuropathogenesis.** *J Neurovirol* 2004, **10**(Suppl 1):25–32.
100. Fernandes SP, Edwards TM, Ng KT, Robinson SR: **HIV-1 protein gp120 rapidly impairs memory in chicks by interrupting the glutamate-glutamine cycle.** *Neurobiol Learn Mem* 2007, **87**(1):1–8.
101. Peng F, Dhillon N, Callen S, Yao H, Bokhari S, Zhu X, Baydoun HH, Buch S: **Platelet-derived growth factor protects neurons against gp120-mediated toxicity.** *J Neurovirol* 2008, **14**(1):62–72.
102. Peng F, Yao H, Akturk HK, Buch S: **Platelet-derived growth factor CC-mediated neuroprotection against HIV Tat involves TRPC-mediated inactivation of GSK 3beta.** *PLoS One* 2012, **7**(10):e47572.
103. Ashutosh, Chao C, Borgmann K, Brew K, Ghorpade A: **Tissue inhibitor of metalloproteinases-1 protects human neurons from staurosporine and HIV-1-induced apoptosis: mechanisms and relevance to HIV-1-associated dementia.** *Cell Death Dis* 2012, **3**:e332.
104. Reddy PV, Gandhi N, Samikkannu T, Saiyed Z, Agudelo M, Yndart A, Khatavkar P, Nair MP: **HIV-1 gp120 induces antioxidant response element-mediated expression in primary astrocytes: role in HIV associated neurocognitive disorder.** *Neurochem Int* 2012, **61**(5):807–814.
105. Meucci O, Fatatis A, Simen AA, Bushell TJ, Gray PW, Miller RJ: **Chemokines regulate hippocampal neuronal signaling and gp120 neurotoxicity.** *Proc Natl Acad Sci U S A* 1998, **95**(24):14500–14505.
106. Tong N, Perry SW, Zhang Q, James HJ, Guo H, Brooks A, Bal H, Kinnear SA, Fine S, Epstein LG, Dairaghi D, Schall TJ, Gendelman HE, Dewhurst S, Sharewr LR, Gelbard HA: **Neuronal fractalkine expression in HIV-1 encephalitis: roles for macrophage recruitment and neuroprotection in the central nervous system.** *J Immunol* 2000, **164**(3):1333–1339.
107. Chun H, Hao W, Honghai Z, Ning L, Yasong W, Chen D: **CCL3L1 prevents gp120-induced neuron death via the CREB cell signaling pathway.** *Brain Res* 2009, **1257**:75–88.
108. Dean M, Carrington M, Winkler C, Huttley GA, Smith MW, Allikmets R, Goedert JJ, Buchbinder SP, Vittinghoff E, Gomperts E, Donfield S, Vlahov D, Kaslow R, Saah A, Rinaldo C, Detels R, O'Brien SJ: **Genetic restriction of HIV-1 infection and progression to AIDS by a deletion allele of the CKR5 structural gene. Hemophilia Growth and Development Study, Multicenter AIDS Cohort Study, Multicenter Hemophilia Cohort Study, San Francisco City Cohort, ALIVE.** *Sci (New York, NY)* 1996, **273**(5283):1856–1862.
109. Gonzalez E, Kulkarni H, Bolivar H, Mangano A, Sanchez R, Catano G, Nibbs RJ, Freedman BI, Quinones MP, Bamshad MJ, Murthy KK, Rovin BH, Bradley W, Clark RA, Anderson SA, O'Connell RJ, Agan BK, Ahuja SS, Bologna R, Sen L,

Dolan MJ, Ahuja SK: **The influence of CCL3L1 gene-containing segmental duplications on HIV-1/AIDS susceptibility.** *Sci (New York, NY)* 2005, **307**(5714):1434–1440.
110. Smith MW, Dean M, Carrington M, Winkler C, Huttley GA, Lomb DA, Goedert JJ, O'Brien TR, Jacobson LP, Kaslow R, Buchbinder S, Vittinghoff E, Vlahov D, Hoots K, Hoots K, Hilgartner MW, O'Brien SJ: **Contrasting genetic influence of CCR2 and CCR5 variants on HIV-1 infection and disease progression. Hemophilia Growth and Development Study (HGDS), Multicenter AIDS Cohort Study (MACS), Multicenter Hemophilia Cohort Study (MHCS), San Francisco City Cohort.** *Sci (New York, NY)* 1997, **277**(5328):959–965.
111. Singh KK, Ellis RJ, Marquie-Beck J, Letendre S, Heaton RK, Grant I, Spector S: **CCR2 polymorphisms affect neuropsychological impairment in HIV-1-infected adults.** *J Neuroimmunol* 2004, **157**(1–2):185–192.
112. Quasney MW, Zhang Q, Sargent S, Mynatt M, Glass J, McArthur J: **Increased frequency of the tumor necrosis factor-alpha-308 A allele in adults with human immunodeficiency virus dementia.** *Ann Neurol* 2001, **50**(2):157–162.
113. Gonzalez E, Rovin BH, Sen L, Cooke G, Dhanda R, Mummidi S, Kulkarni H, Bamshad MJ, Telles V, Anderson SA, Walter EA, Stephan KT, Deucher M, Mangano A, Bologna R, Ahuja SS, Dolan MJ, Ahuja SK: **HIV-1 infection and AIDS dementia are influenced by a mutant MCP-1 allele linked to increased monocyte infiltration of tissues and MCP-1 levels.** *Proc Natl Acad Sci U S A* 2002, **99**(21):13795–13800.
114. El-Bassel N, Shaw SA, Dasgupta A, Strathdee SA: **Drug use as a driver of HIV risks: re-emerging and emerging issues.** *Curr Opin HIV AIDS* 2014, **9**(2):150–155.
115. Substance Abuse and Mental Health Services Administration: *Results from the 2007 National survey on drug use and health: National findings. (Office of Applied Studies, NSDUH series H-34*, DHHS Publication No. SMA 08–4343). Rockville, MD: Substance Abuse and Mental Health Services Administration, Office of Applied Studies - U.S. Department of Health and Human Services; 2008.
116. Pert CB, Snyder SH: **Opiate receptor: demonstration in nervous tissue.** *Science* 1973, **179**(4077):1011–1014.
117. Turchan-Cholewo J, Dimayuga FO, Ding Q, Keller JN, Hauser KF, Knapp PE, Bruce-Keller AJ: **Cell-specific actions of HIV-Tat and morphine on opioid receptor expression in glia.** *J Neurosci Res* 2008, **86**(9):2100–2110.
118. Fitting S, Xu R, Bull C, Buch SK, El-Hage N, Nath A, Knapp PE, Hauser KF: **Interactive comorbidity between opioid drug abuse and HIV-1 Tat: chronic exposure augments spine loss and sublethal dendritic pathology in striatal neurons.** *Am J Pathol* 2010, **177**(3):1397–1410.
119. Malik S, Khalique H, Buch S, Seth P: **A growth factor attenuates HIV-1 Tat and morphine induced damage to human neurons: implication in HIV/AIDS-drug abuse cases.** *PLoS One* 2011, **6**(3):e18116.
120. Hu S, Sheng WS, Lokensgard JR, Peterson PK: **Morphine potentiates HIV-1 gp120-induced neuronal apoptosis.** *J Infect Dis* 2005, **191**(6):886–889.
121. Bandaru W, Patel N, Ewaleifoh O, Haughey NJ: **A failure to normalize biochemical and metabolic insults during morphine withdrawal disrupts synaptic repair in mice transgenic for HIV-gp120.** *J Neuroimmune Pharmacol* 2011, **6**(4):640–649.
122. El-Hage N, Wu G, Wang J, Ambati J, Knapp PE, Reed JL, Bruce-Keller AJ, Hauser KF: **HIV-1 Tat and opiate-induced changes in astrocytes promote chemotaxis of microglia through the expression of MCP-1 and alternative chemokines.** *Glia* 2006, **53**(2):132–146.
123. Arango JC, Simmonds P, Brettle RP, Bell JE: **Does drug abuse influence the microglial response in AIDS and HIV encephalitis?** *Aids* 2004, **18**(Suppl 1):S69–S74.
124. Guo CJ, Li Y, Tian S, Wang X, Douglas SD, Ho WZ: **Morphine enhances HIV infection of human blood mononuclear phagocytes through modulation of beta-chemokines and CCR5 receptor.** *J Investig Med* 2002, **50**(6):435–442.
125. Wang X, Ye L, Zhou Y, Liu MQ, Zhou DJ, Ho WZ: **Inhibition of anti-HIV microRNA expression: a mechanism for opioid-mediated enhancement of HIV infection of monocytes.** *Am J Pathol* 2011, **178**(1):41–47.
126. Kumar R, Torres C, Yamamura Y, Rodriguez I, Martinez M, Staprans S, Donahoe RM, Kraiselburd E, Stephens EB, Kumar A: **Modulation by morphine of viral set point in rhesus macaques infected with simian immunodeficiency virus and simian-human immunodeficiency virus.** *J Virol* 2004, **78**(20):11425–11428.
127. Langford D, Adame A, Grigorian A, Grant I, McCutchan JA, Ellis RJ, Marcotte TD, Masliah E: **Patterns of selective neuronal damage in methamphetamine-user AIDS patients.** *J Acquir Immune Defic Syndr* 2003, **34**(5):467–474.
128. Maragos WF, Young KL, Turchan JT, Guseva M, Pauly JR, Nath A, Cass WA: **Human immunodeficiency virus-1 Tat protein and methamphetamine interact synergistically to impair striatal dopaminergic function.** *J Neurochem* 2002, **83**(4):955–963.
129. Qi L, Gang L, Hang KW, Ling CH, Xiaofeng Z, Zhen L, Wai YD, Sang PW: **Programmed neuronal cell death induced by HIV-1 tat and methamphetamine.** *Microsc Res Tech* 2011, **74**(12):1139–1144.
130. Shah A, Silverstein PS, Kumar S, Singh DP, Kumar A: **Synergistic cooperation between methamphetamine and HIV-1 gsp120 through the P13K/Akt pathway induces IL-6 but not IL-8 expression in astrocytes.** *PLoS One* 2012, **7**(12):e52060.
131. Sharma A, Hu XT, Napier TC, Al-Harthi L: **Methamphetamine and HIV-1 Tat down regulate beta-catenin signaling: implications for methampetamine abuse and HIV-1 co-morbidity.** *J Neuroimmune Pharmacol* 2011, **6**(4):597–607.
132. Ellis RJ, Childers ME, Cherner M, Lazzaretto D, Letendre S, Grant I: **Increased human immunodeficiency virus loads in active methamphetamine users are explained by reduced effectiveness of antiretroviral therapy.** *J Infect Dis* 2003, **188**(12):1820–1826.
133. Talloczy Z, Martinez J, Joset D, Ray Y, Gacser A, Toussi S, Mizushima N, Nosanchuk JD, Goldstein H, Loike J, Sulzer D, Santambrogio L: **Methamphetamine inhibits antigen processing, presentation, and phagocytosis.** *PLoS Pathog* 2008, **4**(2):e28.
134. Liang H, Wang X, Chen H, Song L, Ye L, Wang SH, Wang YJ, Zhou L, Ho WZ: **Methamphetamine enhances HIV infection of macrophages.** *Am J Pathol* 2008, **172**(6):1617–1624.
135. Toussi SS, Joseph A, Zheng JH, Dutta M, Santambrogio L, Goldstein H: **Short communication: Methamphetamine treatment increases in vitro and in vivo HIV replication.** *AIDS Res Hum Retroviruses* 2009, **25**(11):1117–1121.
136. Aksenov MY, Aksenova MV, Nath A, Ray PD, Mactutus CF, Booze RM: **Cocaine-mediated enhancement of Tat toxicity in rat hippocampal cell cultures: the role of oxidative stress and D1 dopamine receptor.** *Neurotoxicology* 2006, **27**(2):217–228.
137. Dhillon NK, Williams R, Peng F, Tsai YJ, Dhillon S, Nicolay B, Gadgil M, Kumar A, Buch SJ: **Cocaine-mediated enhancement of virus replication in macrophages: implications for human immunodeficiency virus-associated dementia.** *J Neurovirol* 2007, **13**(6):483–495.
138. Yao H, Kim K, Duan M, Hayashi T, Guo M, Morgello S, Prat A, Wang J, Su TP, Buch S: **Cocaine hijacks sigma1 receptor to initiate induction of activated leukocyte cell adhesion molecule: implication for increased monocyte adhesion and migration in the CNS.** *J Neurosci* 2011, **31**(16):5942–5955.
139. Hu S, Sheng WS, Rock RB: **CB2 Receptor agonists protect human dopaminergic neurons against damage from HIV-1 gp120.** *PLoS One* 2013, **8**(10):e77577.
140. Avraham HK, Jiang S, Fu Y, Rockenstein E, Makriyannis A, Zvonok A, Masliah E, Avraham S: **The cannabinoid CB2 receptor agonist AM1241 enhances neurogenesis in GFAP/Gp120 transgenic mice displaying deficits in neurogenesis.** *Br J Pharmacol* 2014, **171**(2):468–479.
141. Hemelaar J, Gouws E, Ghys PD, Osmanov S: **Isolation W-UNfH, Characterisation: Global trends in molecular epidemiology of HIV-1 during 2000–2007.** *Aids* 2011, **25**(5):679–689.
142. Tebit DM, Nankya I, Arts EJ, Gao Y: **HIV diversity, recombination and disease progression: how does fitness "fit" into the puzzle?** *AIDS Rev* 2007, **9**(2):75–87.
143. Gupta JD, Satishchandra P, Gopukumar K, Wilkie F, Waldrop-Valverde D, Ellis R, Ownby R, Subbakrishna DK, Desai A, Kamat A, Ravi V, Rao BS, Satish KS, Kumar M: **Neuropsychological deficits in human immunodeficiency virus type 1 clade C-seropositive adults from South India.** *J Neurovirol* 2007, **13**(3):195–202.
144. Satishchandra P, Nalini A, Gourie-Devi M, Khanna N, Santosh V, Ravi V, Desai A, Chandramuki A, Jayakumar PN, Shankar SK: **Profile of neurologic disorders associated with HIV/AIDS from Bangalore, south India (1989–96).** *Indian J Med Res* 2000, **111**:14–23.
145. Langford TD, Letendre SL, Larrea GJ, Masliah E: **Changing patterns in the neuropathogenesis of HIV during the HAART era.** *Brain Pathol* 2003, **13**(2):195–210.
146. Sacktor N, Lyles RH, Skolasky R, Kleeberger C, Selnes OA, Miller EN, Becker JT, Cohen B, McArthur JC: **HIV-associated neurologic disease incidence changes: multicenter AIDS Cohort Study, 1990–1998.** *Neurology* 2001, **56**(2):257–260.
147. Ranga U, Shankarappa R, Siddappa NB, Ramakrishna L, Nagendran R, Mahalingam M, Mahadevan A, Jayasuryan N, Satishchandra P, Shankar SK,

Prasad VR: **Tat protein of human immunodeficiency virus type 1 subtype C strains is a defective chemokine.** *J Virol* 2004, **78**(5):2586–2590.

148. Albini, Ferrini S, Benelli R, Sforzini S, Giunciuglio D, Aluigi MG: **HIV-1 Tat protein mimicry of chemokines.** *Proc National Academy of Sciences - PNAS* 1998, **95**(22):13153–13158.
149. Mishra M, Vetrivel S, Siddappa NB, Ranga U, Seth P: **Clade specific differences in neurotoxicity of human immunodeficiency virus-1 B and C Tat of human neurons: significance of dicysteine C30C31 motif.** *Ann Neurol* 2008, **63**(3):366–376.
150. Campbell GR, Watkins JD, Singh KK, Loret EP, Spector SA: **Human immunodeficiency virus type 1 subtype C Tat fails to induce intracellular calcium flux and induces reduced tumor necrosis factor production from monocytes.** *J Virol* 2007, **81**(11):5919–5928.
151. Rao VR, Neogi U, Talboom JS, Padilla L, Rahman M, Fritz-French C, Gonzalez-Ramirez S, Verma A, Wood C, Ruprecht RM, Ranga U, Azim T, Joska J, Eugenin E, Shet A, Bimonte-Nelson H, Tyor WR, Prasad VR: **Clade C HIV-1 isolates circulating in Southern Africa exhibit a greater frequency of dicysteine motif-containing Tat variants than those in Southeast Asia and cause increased neurovirulence.** *Retrovirology* 2013, **10:**61.
152. Li W, Huang Y, Reid R, Steiner J, Malpica-Llanos T, Darden TA, Shankar SK, Mahadevan A, Satishchandra P, Nath A: **NMDA receptor activation by HIV-Tat protein is clade dependent.** *J Neurosci* 2008, **28**(47):12190–12198.
153. Gandhi N, Saiyed Z, Thangavel S, Rodriguez J, Rao KV, Nair MP: **Differential effects of HIV type 1 clade B and clade C Tat protein on expression of proinflammatory and antiinflammatory cytokines by primary monocytes.** *AIDS Res Hum Retroviruses* 2009, **25**(7):691–699.
154. Wong JK, Campbell GR, Spector SA: **Differential induction of interleukin-10 in monocytes by HIV-1 clade B and clade C Tat proteins.** *J Biol Chem* 2010, **285**(24):18319–18325.
155. Rao VR, Sas AR, Eugenin EA, Siddappa NB, Bimonte-Nelson H, Berman JW, Ranga U, Tyor WR, Prasad VR: **HIV-1 clade-specific differences in the induction of neuropathogenesis.** *J Neurosci* 2008, **28**(40):10010–10016.
156. Gandhi N, Saiyed ZM, Napuri J, Samikkannu T, Reddy PV, Agudelo M, Khatavkar P, Saxena SK, Nair MP: **Interactive role of human immunodeficiency virus type 1 (HIV-1) clade-specific Tat protein and cocaine in blood–brain barrier dysfunction: implications for HIV-1-associated neurocognitive disorder.** *J Neurovirol* 2010, **16**(4):294–305.
157. Samikkannu T, Saiyed ZM, Rao KV, Babu DK, Rodriguez JW, Papuashvili MN, Nair MP: **Differential regulation of indoleamine-2,3-dioxygenase (IDO) by HIV type 1 clade B and C Tat protein.** *AIDS Res Hum Retroviruses* 2009, **25**(3):329–335.
158. Henderson LJ, Sharma A, Monaco MC, Major EO, Al-Harthi L: **Human immunodeficiency virus type 1 (HIV-1) transactivator of transcription through its intact core and cysteine-rich domains inhibits Wnt/beta-catenin signaling in astrocytes: relevance to HIV neuropathogenesis.** *J Neurosci* 2012, **32**(46):16306–16313.
159. Joska JA, Fincham DS, Stein DJ, Paul RH, Seedat S: **Clinical correlates of HIV-associated neurocognitive disorders in South Africa.** *AIDS Behav* 2010, **14**(2):371–378.
160. Joska JA, Westgarth-Taylor J, Myer L, Hoare J, Thomas KG, Combrinck M, Paul RH, Stein DJ, Flisher AJ: **Characterization of HIV-Associated Neurocognitive Disorders among individuals starting antiretroviral therapy in South Africa.** *AIDS Behav* 2011, **15**(6):1197–1203.
161. Lawler K, Mosepele M, Ratcliffe S, Seloilwe E, Steele K, Nthobatsang R, Steenhoff A: **Neurocognitive impairment among HIV-positive individuals in Botswana: a pilot study.** *J Int AIDS Soc* 2010, **13:**15.
162. Modi G, Hari K, Modi M, Mochan A: **The frequency and profile of neurology in black South African HIV infected (clade C) patients - a hospital-based prospective audit.** *J Neurol Sci* 2007, **254**(1–2):60–64.
163. Bachu M, Yalla S, Asokan M, Verma A, Neogi U, Sharma S, Murali RV, Mukthey AB, Bhatt R, Chatterjee S, Rajan RE, Cheedarla N, Yadavalli VS, Mahadevan A, Shankar SK, Rajagopalan N, Shet A, Saravanan S, Balakrishnan P, Solomon S, Vajpayee M, Satish KS, Kundu TK, Jeang KT, Ranga U: **Multiple NF-kappaB sites in HIV-1 subtype C long terminal repeat confer superior magnitude of transcription and thereby the enhanced viral predominance.** *J Biol Chem* 2012, **287**(53):44714–44735.
164. Shankarappa R, Chatterjee R, Learn GH, Neogi D, Ding M, Roy P, Ghosh A, Kingsley L, Harrison L, Mullins JI, Gupta P: **Human immunodeficiency virus type 1 env sequences from Calcutta in eastern India: identification of features that distinguish subtype C sequences in India from other subtype C sequences.** *J Virol* 2001, **75**(21):10479–10487.
165. Dore GJ, McDonald A, Li Y, Kaldor JM, Brew BJ, National HIVSC: **Marked improvement in survival following AIDS dementia complex in the era of highly active antiretroviral therapy.** *Aids* 2003, **17**(10):1539–1545.
166. Alkali NH, Bwala SA, Nyandaiti YW, Danesi MA: **NeuroAIDS in sub-Saharan Africa: a clinical review.** *Ann Afr Med* 2013, **12**(1):1–10.
167. Heaton RK, Clifford DB, Franklin DR Jr, Woods SP, Ake C, Vaida F, Ellis RJ, Letendre SL, Marcotte TD, Atkinson JH, Rivera-Mindt M, Vigil OR, Taylor MJ, Collier AC, Marra CM, Gelman BB, McArthur JC, Morgello S, Simpsons DM, McCutchan JA, Abramson I, Gamst A, Fennema-Notestine C, Jernigan TL, Wong J, Grant I: **HIV-associated neurocognitive disorders persist in the era of potent antiretroviral therapy: CHARTER Study.** *Neurology* 2010, **75**(23):2087–2096.
168. Kallianpur KJ, Shikuma C, Kirk GR, Shiramizu B, Valcour V, Chow D, Souza S, Nakamoto B, Sailasuta N: **Peripheral blood HIV DNA is associated with atrophy of cerebellar and subcortical gray matter.** *Neurology* 2013, **80**(19):1792–1799.
169. McManus H, Li PC, Nolan D, Bloch M, Kiertiburanakul S, Choi JY, Mulhall B, Petoumenos K, Zhou J, Law M, Brew BJ, Wright E: **Does use of antiretroviral therapy regimens with high central nervous system penetration improve survival in HIV-infected adults?** *HIV Med* 2011, **12**(10):610–619.
170. Dahl V, Lee E, Peterson J, Spudich SS, Leppla I, Sinclair E, Fuchs D, Palmer S, Price RW: **Raltegravir treatment intensification does not alter cerebrospinal fluid HIV-1 infection or immunoactivation in subjects on suppressive therapy.** *J Infect Dis* 2011, **204**(12):1936–1945.
171. Vassallo M, Durant J, Biscay V, Lebrun-Frenay C, Dunais B, Laffon M, Harvey-Langton A, Cottalorda J, Ticchioni M, Carsenti H, Pradier C, Dellamonica P: **Can high central nervous system penetrating antiretroviral regimens protect against the onset of HIV-associated neurocognitive disorders?** *Aids* 2014, **28**(4):493–501.
172. Follstaedt SC, Barber SA, Zink MC: **Mechanisms of minocycline-induced suppression of simian immunodeficiency virus encephalitis: inhibition of apoptosis signal-regulating kinase 1.** *J Neurovirol* 2008, **14**(5):376–388.
173. Nath A, Haughey NJ, Jones M, Anderson C, Bell JE, Geiger JD: **Synergistic neurotoxicity by human immunodeficiency virus proteins Tat and gp120: protection by memantine.** *Ann Neurol* 2000, **47**(2):186–194.
174. Darbinian N, Khalili K, Amini S: **Neuroprotective activity of pDING in response to HIV-1 Tat.** *J Cell Physiol* 2014, **229**(2):153–161.
175. Kang YJ, Digicaylioglu M, Russo R, Kaul M, Achim CL, Fletcher L, Masliah E, Lipton SA: **Erythropoietin plus insulin-like growth factor-I protects against neuronal damage in a murine model of human immunodeficiency virus-associated neurocognitive disorders.** *Ann Neurol* 2010, **68**(3):342–352.
176. Mahajan SD, Aalinkeel R, Law WC, Reynolds JL, Nair BB, Sykes DE, Yong KT, Roy I, Prasad PN, Schwartz SA: **Anti-HIV-1 nanotherapeutics: promises and challenges for the future.** *Int J Nanomedicine* 2012, **7:**5301–5314.
177. Dash PK, Gendelman HE, Roy U, Balkundi S, Alnouti Y, Mosley RL, Gelbard HA, McMillan J, Gorantla S, Poluektova LY: **Long-acting nanoformulated antiretroviral therapy elicits potent antiretroviral and neuroprotective responses in HIV-1-infected humanized mice.** *Aids* 2012, **26**(17):2135–2144.
178. Spudich SS, Ances BM: **Neurologic complications of HIV infection: highlights from the 2013 Conference on Retroviruses and Opportunistic Infections.** *Top Antivir Med* 2013, **21**(3):100–108.

8

Collective patient behaviours derailing ART roll-out in KwaZulu-Natal: perspectives of health care providers

Janet Michel[1*], Christina Matlakala[3], Rene English[4], Richard Lessells[1] and Marie-Louise Newell[1,2]

Abstract

Background: Antiretroviral therapy (ART) roll-out is fraught with challenges, many with serious repercussions. We explored and described patient behaviour-related challenges from the perspective of health care providers from non-governmental organisations involved in ART programmes in KwaZulu-Natal, South Africa.

Methods: A descriptive case study design using qualitative approach was applied during this study. Data was collected from nine key informants from the three biggest NGOs involved in ART roll-out using in-depth semi-structured interviews. Transcribing and coding for emergent themes was done by two independent reviewers. Ethical approval for the study was granted by the UNISA research ethics committee of The Faculty of Health Sciences. Written consent was obtained from directors of the three NGOs involved and individual audio taped informed consent was obtained from all study participants prior to data collection.

Results: Findings revealed six broad areas of patient behaviour challenges. These were patient behaviour related to socio-economic situation of patient (skipping of medication due to lack of food, or due to lack of transport fees), belief systems (traditional and religious), stigma (non- disclosure), sexual practices (non-acceptability of condoms, teenage pregnancies), escapism (drug and alcohol abuse) and opportunism (skipping medication in order to access disability grant, teenage pregnancies in order to access child grant).

Conclusion: New programmes need to address patient behaviour as a complex phenomenon requiring a multi-pronged approach that also addresses social norms and institutions. In the face of continued ART scale up, this is further evidence for the need for multi-sectoral collaboration to ensure successful and sustainable ART roll-out.

Keywords: Patient behaviour, ART roll-out, Health care provider perspective, Non-governmental organisation, KwaZulu-Natal

Background

The HIV epidemic has had a major impact on the lives of people in Africa and understanding behavioural responses to HIV is crucial for predicting the future path of the epidemic, for preventing its future spread and maximizing efficient use of limited resources [1-5]. Human behaviour refers to a range of actions exhibited by humans and influenced among other things by culture, attitudes, emotions, values, ethics, authority, rapport, hypnosis, persuasion, coercion and genetics [6]. In the absence of an effective government response in South Africa, many NGOs were established solely to address HIV treatment and care. In KwaZulu-Natal (KZN) province, three major non-governmental organisations (NGOs) led the roll-out of HIV antiretroviral treatment (ART), some independently and others in partnership with the Department of Health [7]. These NGO's are thus of interest for exploring the challenges experienced in the delivery of ART. ART aims to reduce morbidity and mortality and improve quality of life, through durable suppression of viral replication and restoration of immunologic function, [8,9]. Anything that hinders any of the above processes, and in particular interferes with adherence to the therapy, poses challenges to ART roll-

* Correspondence: jmichel@africacentre.ac.za
[1]Africa Centre for Health and Population Studies, University of KwaZulu-Natal, Somkhele, PO Box 198, Mtubatuba, KwaZulu-Natal 3935, South Africa

out. Successful administration of ART requires the patient to adhere for life for at least 95% of the treatment prescribed. ART adherence has been found to be influenced by health service- and patient-related factors [10,11] and multiple patient behaviours can collectively enhance risks of HIV infection acquisition, transmission and treatment non-adherence [12,13]. Suboptimal adherence leads to incomplete viral suppression, continued destruction of the immune system, disease progression, emergence of resistant viral strains, and thus limits future treatment options [3,8,14].

In South Africa, ART scale up started in 2004 and in 2010 the South African Department of Health embarked on a large scale ART roll-out programme providing HIV treatment and care to all citizens who need it free of charge [15], with need defined by specific eligibility criteria. Because patient behaviour and adherence is crucial to the success of ART roll-out, we explored and described patient behaviour-related challenges reported from the perspective of non-governmental organisations in KwaZulu-Natal. Much has been written on sexual behaviour, especially sexual disinhibition and the inconsistent use, or unacceptability, of condoms derailing the success of ART [16-18] and there has been mention, but no collective summary, of patient behaviour-related challenges derailing ART from the health provider perspective and this study attempts to address this gap in the knowledge base.

Results

Participants revealed different patient behaviours they considered detrimental to ART roll-out. Six broad areas emerged as patient behaviour related to socio-economic situation, belief systems, stigma, sexual practices, escapism and opportunism. A summary list of identified themes is given in Table 1.

Table 1 Summary of findings using classification by theme and category

Theme	Category	Meaning unit
Socio-economic situation of patient	**Poverty**	• Lack of food • Lack of transport fees
Belief system	**Religious ideological/ traditional**	• Self-ordained religious prophets • Use of traditional medicine.
Stigma	**Non-disclosure**	• Non-disclosure by women • Non-disclosure of parents to their teenage children who are HIV positive. • Non-disclosure of mothers when they leave the children in the care of grandmothers/ baby minders
Sexual practice	**Culture/ psychosocial factors**	• Unacceptability of condom use. • Teenage pregnancies
Escapism	**Substance abuse**	• Alcohol abuse • Drug abuse (whoonga)
Opportunism	**Abuse**	• SASSA guidelines. • Child grant

Socio-economic situation related behaviour

Socio-economic problems of the patients were indicated as presenting a real challenge to the successful roll-out of ART. Factors related to the socio-economic situation of the patients were identified as aspects such as skipping of medication doses when food is unavailable and inability to collect medication due to lack of transport fees. The following were some of the narratives from the participants in relation to skipping medication:

"Socio-economic problems lead patients to skip doses of medication when food is unavailable". (Professional nurse 1)

"Social problems lead to defaulting treatment. Many patients lack support at home. They miss review dates due to lack of transport fee and they do not take medicine when they do not have food. They say the tablets make one very sick when taken on an empty stomach". (Professional nurse 3)

The findings concur with research done elsewhere [19] that revealed food insecurity as a common and important barrier to accessing medical care and ARV adherence.

"Patients discontinue treatment when there is lack of money for transport to collect medication supplies". (Programme coordinator 1)

The findings are also in line with Du Preez [20] who indicated that some of the problems hindering the fight against HIV/AIDS are unemployment and poverty; and that despite HIV treatment being free, transport costs are a major obstacle for people on ART.

Belief systems

All participants mentioned how patients' belief systems are interfering with ART use. A belief system can be religious, philosophical, ideological or a combination of these. It is a way of life, basis of culture, identity and moral values [21]. All the participants mentioned use of traditional medicine and religious prophets as systems people frequently fall back on to regain wellness and equilibrium. Cultural traditions help participants cope with illness, physical disability, economic hardship, and face oppression and discrimination [22]. The participants revealed the following:

"60-70% of the patients mix traditional herbal medicine and ART". (Professional nurse 1)

"Enemas given to children impair the absorption of ART". (ART Doctor 2)

"We had cases of inpatients that died clearly from muti [African traditional medicine] *over-dose. One had this blackish thing that got stuck in his throat and was pulled out during resuscitation".* (ART Doctor 3)

Use of traditional medicine is not the only belief system the participants identified as posing a challenge to ART roll-out as revealed by the following further quotes:

"A patient disappeared to visit one of the prophets in Mpumalanga and later came back with a very low CD4 cell count and died a few days later". (Professional nurse 2)

"One patient was doing very well on treatment. She asked for leave to go home and was granted. Her CD4 cell count was 520 when she left. She returned some weeks later after having spent most of that time at a prophet"s shrine in Johannesburg with a CD4 cell count of 28. We tried all we could but she died within a week". (Professional nurse 3)

Stigma

Non-disclosure for fear of stigma was highlighted as a challenge by most of the participants. One professional nurse explained the fear of stigma as follows:

"Patients refuse to be referred to local clinic. We have staff members working here in an organisation that rolls out ART but people are unwilling to go present themselves at the clinic to get ART. Someone said I would rather die than to go to any of these clinics because the nurses know me". (Programme coordinator 1)

"Most patients do not want to be referred to local clinic, something that could help considering their financial problems. They would rather travel 50 km every month to take supplies than be seen at their local clinic". (ART Doctor 3)

The above statement indicates that health care providers perceive stigma as still deep despite public sector campaigns [23]. Health care workers working in ART programmes seem themselves not to have gotten over stigma let alone patients seeking care from these providers as revealed above. The participants mentioned that stigma manifested in the form of non-disclosure of different groups like women not disclosing to men. One ART doctor made the following comments:

"Most women who are dependent on their boyfriends do not disclose for fear of loss of income". (ART Doctor 3)

Non-disclosure of mothers to baby-minders like grandmothers was cited by most participants. One professional nurse described this as follows:

"Baby dumping at grandmothers who are oblivious to the baby's HIV status especially in teenage pregnancies is a problem. If they did not know the status of the baby, how on earth do you expect them to have understood the importance [of ART] and adhered to the treatment as required?" (Professional nurse 2)

Non-disclosure of parents to their (teenage) children who are HIV positive was mentioned by most participants as a real concern exacerbated by the very fact that puberty itself is a phase fraught with its own challenges.

"Parents do not disclose to their HIV positive teenagers making it difficult to explain to this group what medication they are taking". (Professional nurse 1)

Sexual behaviour

Sexual behaviour is defined as the manner in which humans experience and express their sexuality. People engage in a variety of sexual acts from time to time, and for a wide variety of reasons. Teenage pregnancies and unacceptability of condoms were cited by most participants. One of the ways of preventing HIV is through the use of condoms. The participants cited this as a big challenge especially in light of the amount of money that has been poured into making condoms freely available. Condom use seemed not to have been embraced in KwaZulu-Natal. One Doctor commented:

"Use of condoms has not been widely accepted in this community. They come back with STIs and yet claim to use condoms". (ART Doctor 1)

Teenage pregnancies were cited as a huge challenge by most participants:

"70-80% of the pregnant women are teens. The children do not see the importance of education". (Professional nurse 1)

"Desperation amongst teenage mothers is overwhelming. Crisis centre in Pinetown is full and cannot accommodate more desperate teenagers". (Programme coordinator 1)

The problem of teenage pregnancies pose additional challenges to ART roll out as put in by one participant:

"Post-delivery, girls go back to school. They seldom come back for review, losing both mother and baby as loss to follow up". (Professional nurse 3)

The health workers highlighted that the interactions between schooling, sexual debut, pregnancy, child grant and social desirability of having a baby, especially since it is common for girls to continue school after the birth of a child, is not understood adding to the complexity.

Escapism

Most participants mentioned that some patients try to escape reality through substance abuse. Escapism is defined as the tendency to seek distraction and relief from unpleasant realities, especially by seeking entertainment or engaging in fantasy [24]. This could be a sign of failing to cope with their situation or status. Alcoholism was cited as one of the escape routes patients were using as revealed below:

"A number of males patients often abuse alcohol. They say it helps them forget about their problems". (ART Doctor 2)

"We have some patients who come to pick up their supplies totally drunk. One wonders how they can adhere to such a strict treatment". (Programme coordinator 2)

Drug abuse, particularly 'whoonga', was cited by all the participants as a new challenge that has crept into the ART arena. 'Whoonga' is a highly addictive substance incorporating efavirenz, a commonly used antiretroviral drug usually mixed with marijuana or other illicit drugs [25]. In KwaZulu-Natal, drug dealers are now enticing AIDS patients into selling their life-saving antiretrovirals [26]. Drug abuse was cited as the other escape route as revealed by the following statements from participants:

"Many patients come back to claim more drugs after allegedly having been robbed. In some settings spouses share one month's supply and sell the other supply to drug dealers. They then come back with an affidavit from the police and demand another drug supply". (Programme coordinator 3)

"Some patients have been mugged. They were followed from the hospital and when they alighted from the taxi, they were told to hand over their hand bags for something important was in there. All the muggers took out were ARVs". (Professional nurse 1)

"They stand at the gate and scout for candidates that are likely coming for ART supply. The thin and sickly are targeted and followed". (ART Doctor 2)

Opportunism

All the participants mentioned that South African Social Security Agency (SASSA) guidelines were fuelling poor adherence as the patients were eager to access the grant. SASSA guidelines stipulate the criteria to be used for an HIV positive patient to receive a grant. One criterion used previously was a CD4 cell count of 200 and below (it should be noted that the criterion has now changed as explained below). An opportunist is defined as a person who adapts his actions to take advantage of the circumstances with little regard for consequences for others [27]. The study revealed that in order to access a perceived benefit, patients do not always act in their own best interests [28]. Participants also revealed what has been shown in research elsewhere that most patients say: "It is better to die from AIDS than to die of hunger [29].

The following statements came from participants:

"Patients skip their medication in order to keep the CD4 count low thereby making them eligible for the SASSA grant. SASSA guidelines are fuelling non adherence". (Professional nurse 2)

"Patients threaten us with unspecified consequences if we do not recommend them to receive a grant. Alternatively, they simply stop taking medication until the CD4 cell count has dropped below 200". (Professional nurse 3)

The grant eligibility criteria have since changed to the clinical picture of the patient irrespective of CD4 count. The discretion is now in the hands of the doctor and they still report pressure from patients to recommend them for a grant.

Teenage pregnancies were also cited as an opportunistic practice, demonstrating the complex nature of patient behaviour in ART as well as making it difficult to define where opportunistic behaviour or any another patient behaviour like sexual begins or ends. It was further speculated that the child grant could be peddling this trend of teenage pregnancies. Some participants mentioned the following about teenage pregnancies:

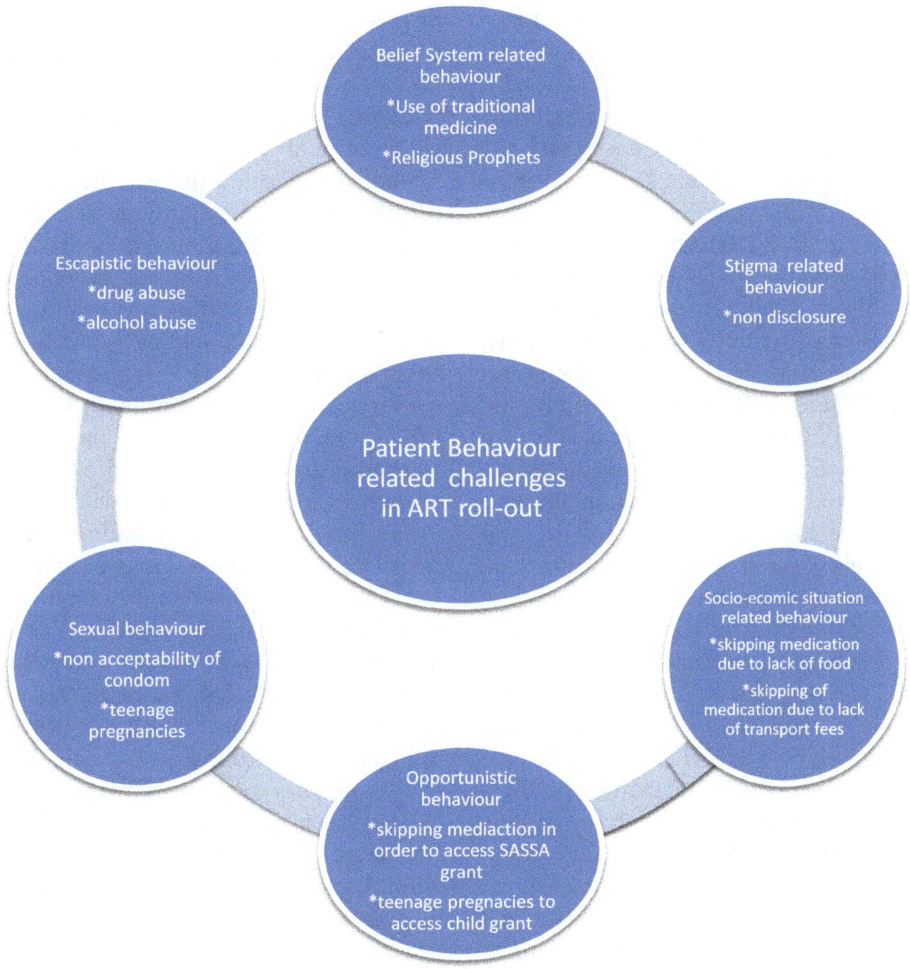
Belief System related behaviour
*Use of traditional medicine
*Religious Prophets
Stigma related behaviour
*non disclosure
Socio-ecomic situation related behaviour
*skipping medication due to lack of food
*skipping of medication due to lack of transport fees
Opportunistic behaviour
*skipping mediaction in order to access SASSA grant
*teenage pregnacies to access child grant
Sexual behaviour
*non acceptability of condom
*teenage pregnancies
Escapistic behaviour
*drug abuse
*alcohol abuse
Patient Behaviour related challenges in ART roll-out

Figure 1 **Diagrammatic summary of findings.**

> *"There are fifteen year old girls coming for the third pregnancy. They say with three kids you can get a decent amount of support grant to live on".*
> (Professional nurse 1)

It is worth mentioning that Makiwane and Udjo (2006) [30] found no link between teenage fertility and child support grant. More research is called for into this area since little is known about what is enticing teenagers to fall pregnant despite knowledge and free availability of family planning methods (Figure 1).

Discussion

Studies on patient behaviour to date have mostly dwelt on sexual behaviour in ART roll-out [31-35]. This study revealed that patient-related behaviours undermining ART roll-out are not only confined to sexual practices like unacceptability of condoms, but go beyond that and that these behaviours are heavily influenced by broader socioeconomic, cultural, and environmental factors [12].

Findings indicated that the socio-economic situation of patients has a bearing on the success or otherwise of ART programmes. Patients skip medication doses when they do not have food because ARVs increase appetite and lead to hunger in the absence of food, the side effects of ARVs are exacerbated in the absence of food and doses are skipped or ARVs not started at all if there is added nutritional burden. In addition patients do not pick up their monthly medical supplies if they do not have transport fees. Taking the socio-economic aspects of the population or community into consideration before rolling out any programme is of utmost importance to ensure efficiency and effectiveness. Measures to ensure food security and strategies like mobile ART teams that bring the service into the community should be taken into consideration before the actual roll-out of ART begins.

Findings indicated that use of traditional medicine and religious prophets are systems people frequently fall back on to regain wellness and equilibrium. The results support previous research that revealed that cultural traditions help participants cope with illness, physical disability, economic hardship, and face oppression and discrimination [22,36]. According to the World Health Organisation, 80% of Africa's population uses traditional medicine for primary health care [37]. Considering the proportion of the native population that seeks help from traditional healers, this challenge is of utmost importance in ART roll-out. Van Dyk (2001) [38] mentions the need to take into consideration ancestors, witches, sorcerers, importance of having children, perception of condoms, the importance of community life and traditional healers when planning HIV and AIDS programmes keeping in mind that these patients may not fully disclose other therapies[39] . Of concern to the health care providers are toxicities as has been demonstrated in other studies [36,40]. Findings revealed that belief systems, religious and ideological being rooted in and intertwined with culture, pose challenges to health care workers as health education on the dangers of mixing ART and traditional medicine goes unheeded and self-ordained religious prophets tell patients that they have been prayed for and are now healed and need not take medication putting themselves, close contacts and family at risk especially with MDR TB [41]. The health care workers could not ascertain whether patients take traditional medicine as a result of their socio- economic situation (financial and transport barrier) or do they do so because traditional and complementary medicine is so embedded in culture. In light of this we recommend the integration of traditional healers and faith institutions into the health system as partners in HIV treatment and care. The South African government has recognized this need with the Draft National Policy on African traditional medicine in 2008 but the integration of TM/CAM into public and private facilities and the reimbursement by medical schemes is far behind [42].

Stigma was also cited as a challenge, concurring with previous research that revealed that HIV related stigma and discrimination remain a key concern in South Africa despite the multitude of HIV awareness campaigns by government and civil society organizations [23,43]. The intimate nature in which HIV is transmitted has contributed to the extreme levels of stigma and discrimination surrounding those infected by the virus [35].) The situation is compounded if children are involved [43]. The economic dependency of women on men and threat or fear or rejection could be to blame [44,45]. This is further evidence to show that if the women do not disclose their status, protected sex or condom use is most likely not going to be considered, increasing the chances of HIV transmission. This underscores the importance of promoting and improving the status of women [46] in the community through education, skills training and creation of employment opportunities. Non-disclosure of parents to their (teenage) children who are HIV positive was revealed to be of concern to the health care providers as this group is in the stage of exploring sexual relations, bringing to the fore the need to address the whole issue of 'positive prevention [47,48].

Findings indicated that the health care providers perceive condom acceptability to be low in the community. This is in line with other studies that revealed that despite millions of Rand having been poured into promoting the use of condoms to prevent the spread of HIV, condom use is still relatively low [16-18]. The current approach to reduce HIV transmission through condom use appears to have borne little fruit [16,49]. What makes it complex is that in other studies, food insecurity was found to decrease control over condom use and increased high risk sexual behaviour among HIV-infected individuals [19,50] demonstrating complex links between sexual behaviour and socio-economic and cultural environments. Could this be further evidence to the premise that behaviour is so rooted in social contexts, so inflected by social differences and so at the mercy of social resources that behaviours must be thought of as primarily social subject to individual variations at the margins only? Is this a suggestion that there are therefore more insidious and powerful determinants of behaviour that need addressing [12,51]? It is important that organisations in ART roll-out take into consideration the fact that condom availability does not necessarily translate to condom acceptance let alone use. This calls for a combination of strategies in HIV prevention including programs targeting individual behaviour; broad-based efforts to alter social norms and address the underlying drivers of the epidemic; and effective use of biomedical or technological tools, such as treatment of sexually transmitted infections (STIs), medical male circumcision and Treatment as Prevention [52]. Combination prevention is essential since HIV prevention is neither simple nor simplistic [12].

Results suggested that some providers think that patients try to escape reality through substance abuse, a sign of failing to cope with their situation or status. Health care providers think that these patients see their situation to be so beyond what they can deal with so much so that they see an exit from this state as the only way to bring relief hence they resort to alcohol and drugs. Persons living with HIV have high rates of comorbid depression, estimated to be between 20-50%, and according to literature, depression predisposes to risky behaviour [39,53]. The findings suggest that it is most likely during this period of distorted perception of risk that HIV is transmitted, re-infections occur and medication get forgotten. This is further evidence to the importance of screening HIV infected people for depression and mental health. Department of Health and organisations involved in ART roll-out need to be aware of the importance of routine screening patients for depression [53-55] and the detrimental vicious cycle this can cause in ART, a gap the current ART tools have not filled. While the health care workers invest in teaching the importance of protected sex, a depressed patient on the other hand due to his illness, might not even see the risk the health care worker is talking about as a result of the impaired risk perception [35,56]. We conclude that it is this sense of hopelessness that makes them not only prone to risky behaviour but also makes them not to adhere to treatment for nothing seems to matter anymore, be it their life or some-one else's life. The critical staff shortage in the health system [35,36] and the fact that most clinics in South Africa do not provide mental health services, compound this challenge for health providers. Many patients according to the health care providers are dying for care, love and hope. Unfortunately they search in the wrong places. Heavy alcohol use and stimulants remain major drivers of HIV transmission in many places and in many groups of people [12]. Drug and alcohol abuse are factors that threaten adherence in ART [57].

Over and above the issues of adherence, health care providers are concerned by the fact that alcohol increases susceptibility to some infections. Infections associated with both alcohol and AIDS include tuberculosis, pneumonia, hepatitis C, which is a leading cause of death among people living with HIV. Alcohol may also increase the severity of AIDS -related brain damage which is characterised in its severest form by profound dementia and a high death rate [58,59]. The patients drink to forget their problems but they tend to forget their medication too, a major challenge in ART where at least 95% of adherence is required for treatment to be successful. Religiosity may foster values, beliefs, and norms that reduce avoidant coping behaviours such as drinking denial and withdrawal [60]. Studies have shown that more religious individuals are less likely to engage in negative health behaviours such as drinking and smoking [61,62]. Faith organisations could play a critical role in ART roll-out by providing hope, re -emphasizing the value and sanctity of every life and most of all providing love and care the health care workers cannot provide due to staff shortages [60].

The problem of drug abuse (whoonga) was revealed as being rife in and around Pinetown, near Durban. This problem was also expressed in the media and a documentary film was recorded by local television [25] and radio [63] which reported that more and more children as young as 11 are smoking whoonga no longer to get high, but to avoid the pain experienced when the drug levels drop. High HIV prevalence rates have resulted in large numbers of children growing without parents [64,65]. Lack of parental support, monitoring and communication, psychosocial factors like family environment, a common feature in communities ravaged by HIV and AIDS could be contributing [46,66]. In light of this, the involvement of community, politicians, leaders, business people and social institutions is called for to deal with this challenge comprehensively and synergistically in a way that is suitable and sustainable in the South African context.

The study also revealed that in order to access a perceived benefit, patients do not always act in their own best interests [28]. SASSA guidelines stipulate the criteria to be used for an HIV positive patient to receive a grant. One of the criteria previously was a CD4 cell count of 200 and below or recently serious clinical disease. It seems to defy the logic of the health care providers that patients forego their health in-order to access a monetary good (grant). This concurs with findings elsewhere that revealed that TB-ridden residents in Khayelitsha charge R50 to R100 for sputum samples to desperate unemployed people to dupe doctors into getting them onto the social grant system [67]. The struggle seems to focus on surviving the day and hopefully see tomorrow. Many participants reported what has been found elsewhere in research that patients say "It is better to die from AIDS than to die of hunger [29]. Talking about a disease that can kill one after 5 or so years seems not taken heed of when the patient is concerned about whether or not he/she can have a meal today. The results are consistent with recent findings that found that unmet subsistence needs are stronger predictors of poor health and adherence to ART [68]. Telling them to preserve a life one does not have becomes a useless exercise. Once again the health care workers found it difficult to define where socio-economic, sexual or opportunistic patient behaviour begins or ends. These behaviours seem interconnected at many levels. Providing free ART does not mean treatment adherence. Multi-pronged approach to deal with the socio- economic context of the patients to meet subsistence needs is needed in order to restore dignity and hope. A hopeful generation is apt to plan for the future, their health and lives including HIV prevention and treatment. Once again faith organisations have a role to play in ART roll-out. Intervention components that enhance spiritual peace can counteract negative effects of stigma and depression in PLWHA [69,70]. There is a gap the health care workers cannot fill hence the need to integrate faith organisations in the health system.

The findings of the current study need to be considered within several constraints and limitations. A study such as this is limited by virtue of a small sample. Data was collected from nine individuals from three organisations which mean that the findings of this study may not be generalized to other NGOs. An additional and important limitation is that due to the qualitative nature of the study, the quality of the research is heavily dependent upon the prior knowledge and experience of the researcher. Only health care provider perspectives were explored and further research could shed light on patient perspectives.

Conclusion

In summary, our study revealed that health care workers are confronted by different patient behaviours they fear are undermining ART roll out. Individual or patient behaviour is often thought of as rationale and predictable but the findings revealed that it is heavily influenced by broader socioeconomic, cultural, and environmental factors. New programmes need to address patient behaviour as a complex phenomenon that needs a multi thronged approach encompassing the socio-economic and cultural context of the patient [52]. More validated ART program models are needed that affect social norms and institutions including the integration of traditional medicine and faith based organisations hence our results draw attention to the need for multi-sectoral collaboration between the Department of Health and other departments such as trade and commerce, social welfare, agriculture and public works to ensure a concerted, comprehensive and sustainable ART programme [12,19,69].

Methods

Study setting

Three major non-governmental organizations led ART roll-out programmes in KwaZulu-Natal from an early stage: the Southern African Catholic Bishops Conference (SACBC), Hlabisa HIV Treatment and Care Programme (a partnership between the Africa Centre for Health and Population Studies and the Department of Health) and Amangwe village. The SACBC AIDS programme was created as part of the Catholic Church's response to HIV and AIDS in KZN, South Africa. It was the front runner in ensuring universal access to ART, before the South African Government had made a pledge to ensure universal access to ART [71]. The Africa Centre for Health and Population Studies was established in 1998 with the objective of conducting population research in an ethical manner and to enhance local research capacity. The centre responded in 2004 to the high HIV prevalence by engaging in a partnership with the Department of Health in the delivery of safe, effective, efficient, equitable and sustainable ART to all who needed it in the Hlabisa subdistrict, KZN. Staff from both the Department of Health and the Africa Centre worked together to provide HIV treatment and care services in one district hospital and 17 primary health care clinics [72]. Amangwe village was established as a response to the HIV epidemic by the industrial and business community of Richards Bay. The Zululand Chamber of Business Foundation Health and Welfare portfolio recognized the devastating effects of HIV and, after research and consultation with stakeholders, established Amangwe village, an HIV and AIDS intervention that addresses a broad spectrum of HIV-related problems. These are, Ethembeni Care Centre for inpatient and outpatient care of HIV infected patients, an orphan and vulnerable children programme and an outreach, education and training programme. The Centre works alongside the Department of Health, receiving referrals for HIV care and treatment as well as a subsidy [73].

Study participants

The participants consisted of programme leaders, doctors and professional nurses working in the three above-named NGOs. These groups were selected as they are the cadres that dealt directly with ART patients from assessment, initiation, monitoring, and management of complications to adherence support. A sample, representative of these sub-groups, was selected by targeting specific sectors [74]. A purposive sample of nine participants was included in the form of three programme leaders who directed and supervised the ART programme, three doctors who were responsible for prescribing, monitoring and dealing with ART complications and three professional nurses who were responsible for monitoring, referring and providing nursing care to patients on ART from the three NGOs. The sample size depended on the saturation of data.

Ethical approval for the study was granted by the UNISA research ethics committee of the faculty of health sciences. Written consent was obtained from directors of the three NGOs involved (Ethembeni Care Centre, Africa Centre and SACBC) and individual audio taped informed consent was obtained from all study participants prior to data collection. Participants were also assured that they could withdraw from the study at any time if they so wished, without penalty.

Data collection

A qualitative approach was utilised in an attempt to understand the challenges experienced by NGOs from the subjective perspective of project coordinators, doctors and nurses involved in the roll-out of ART. The complexities, richness and diversity of their work can only be captured by describing what really goes on in their day-to-day work, incorporating the context in which they operate as well as their frame of reference [75]. Data was collected by means of individual face-to-face interviews with participants. The interviews took place in eThekwini, uThungulu and uMkhanyakude districts of KZN in offices on the premises of the relevant NGOs or at clinics between 1 February 2011 and 10 April 2011. None of the professional nurses interviewed had a NIMART qualification nor was initiating ART at the time of interviews despite Department of Health task shifting recommendations having been passed in 2010.

The interview schedule was developed according to Reysoo and Heldens (2007) [76], steps for guide development that include selecting the topic, defining all the aspects of the topic, formulating initial (open ended) questions, determining the kind of questions, determining the logical order of the topics/questions, preparing the introduction and the end and preparing the interview technical indications. Individual face-to-face interviews were held in English in the afternoon between 14.00 and 16.00 when the clinics would be less busy. A semi-structured format was followed and each interview lasted about 20 minutes [77]. The central question was the same, with probes and clarifications, while recording was uniform [74]. The interviews were recorded on an audio recorder with the permission of the interviewees. The central question was "*What are the challenges you experience with regards to patient behaviour in the roll-out of* ART?" This question was followed by probing questions based on the initial response from the participant. Notes were written down on the interview schedule during the interview and written up during the transcription to capture the researcher's own observations. The observations made during data collection assisted the researcher during data analysis in providing additional insight into emergent themes and sub-themes.

Each taped interview was typed by the researcher in the form of a verbatim transcript. The researcher typed the transcripts within two days of the interview and completed the transcripts of one NGO before interviews with the next one.

Coding and analysis

Transcribed interviews were entered into ATLAS/ti [78]. The transcribed data was independently coded by two investigators who were trained in qualitative data methods. Content analysis was done to explore in detail for common themes and these were then established into units of meaning or codes [75]. Following the traditions of qualitative analyses, the investigators read the transcripts multiple times to identify major themes and then discussed identified themes and came to consensus on coding.

Member checking was also done by having research participants review, validate and verify researcher's interpretations and conclusion [79]. In addition, triangulation which denotes the use of more than one data source that is programme coordinators, doctors and nurses was also utilised [80].

Competing interests

The authors declare that they have no competing interests.

Authors' contributions

JM, CM, RE, RL and MLN contributed to conception and design, drafting and critical revision of the article. JM, CM and RL undertook acquisition, analysis and interpretation of data. All authors read and approved the final manuscript.

Acknowledgements

We would like to acknowledge the staff from Africa Centre, Southern African Catholic Bishops Conference and Amangwe village for support and participation in the study.

Source of funding

The Africa Centre for Health and Population Studies, University of KwaZulu-Natal, is supported by a grant from Wellcome Trust (082384/Z/07/Z). The Hlabisa HIV Treatment and Care Programme is funded by the generous support of the American people through the United States Agency for International Development (USAID) and the President's Emergency Plan (PEPFAR) under the terms of Award No. 674-A-00-08-0001-00. None of the funding organisations had any role in the design and conduct of the study, in the collection, analysis, and interpretation of the data, or in the preparation, review or approval of the manuscript.

Author details

[1]Africa Centre for Health and Population Studies, University of KwaZulu-Natal, Somkhele, PO Box 198, Mtubatuba, KwaZulu-Natal 3935, South Africa. [2]Faculty of Medicine, University of Southampton, Southampton, UK. [3]University of South Africa, Preller St., Pretoria 0002, South Africa. [4]Health Systems Trust, Westville, South Africa.

References

1. Haacker M: *The Impact on the Social Fabric and the Economy. The Macroeconomics of HIV/AIDS International Monetary Fund*; 2004.
2. Oster E: *HIV and Sexual Behaviour Change: Why not Africa?.* NBER Working; 2007a. From: http://www.nber.org/papers/w13049 (accessed 21 July 2013).
3. Tawfik Y, Kinoti S, Blain C: *Introducing Antiretroviral Therapy on a large scale. 2002 Hope and Caution: AED. Global Health, Population and Nutrition group.* Washington, DC: Academy for Educational Development; 2002.
4. Venter WDF: **What is the optimal CD4 count to start anti retrovirals in HIV infected adults.** *Southern African Journal of Epidemiology and Infection* 2009, **24**(4):3.
5. *WHO Country Cooperation Strategy 2008–2013.* South Africa: World Health Organisation. From: http://www.who.int/countryfocus/cooperation_strategy/ccs_zaf_en.pdf (accessed 21 July 2013).
6. *Human Behavior Representation in Constructive Simulation.* RTO TECHNICAL REPORT. Final Report of Task Group 128, consolidating the Findings of Task Group 143; 2009. http://www.cso.nato.int/abstracts.aspx (accessed 21 July 2013).
7. Aids Foundation South Africa: *Current Situation*; 2010. http://www.unaids.org/en/media/unaids/contentassets/documents/unaidspublication/2011/20111130_ua_report_en.pdf (accessed 21 July 2013).
8. Nyambura AW: *Factors that influence non adherence to antiretroviral therapy among HIV and AIDS patients in Central Province, Kenya*, MPH thesis. School of Health Sciences. Nairobi: Kenyatta University; 2009.
9. Maenza J, Flexner C: **Combination antiretroviral therapy for HIV infection.** *Fam Physician* 1998, **57**(Suppl 11):2789–2798.
10. Ehlers VJ, Van der Wal DM: **Nurses perceptions about Botswana patients' antiretroviral therapy adherence.** *Health SA Gesondheid* 2009, **14**(Suppl 1):1–8.
11. Castro A: **Adherence to Antiretroviral Therapy: Merging the Clinical and Social Course of AIDS.** *PlosMed* 2005, **2**(12):e338. doi:101371/jounal.pmed.0020338.
12. Coates TJ, Richter L, Caceres C: **HIV Prevention Behavioural strategies to reduce HIV transmission: how to make them work better.** *Lancet* 2008, **372**:669–684.

13. Vanable PA, Carey MP, Blair DC, Littlewood RA: **Impact of HIV related stigma on health behaviours and psychological adjustment among HIV positive men and women.** *AIDS Behaviour* 2006, **10**(Suppl 5):473–482.
14. HIV Care & ART: *A Course for Pharmacists.* Reference Manual for Trainers. MinistryofHealthEthiopia; 2005. http://www.go2itech.org/HTML/TT06/toolkit/curricula/print/HIVTrainingPharmacists/PharmRefManual.pdf (accessed 21 July 2013).
15. *The South African Anti Retroviral Treatment Guidelines*; 2010. http://www.doh.gov.za/docs/policy/2013/ART_Treatment_Guidelines_Final_25March2013.pdf (accessed 21 July 2013).
16. Chimbindi N: **Youth not scared of HIV. Africa centre for health and population studies.** *The Open AIDS Journal* 2010, **4**:88–95.
17. MacPhail C, Campbell C: **I think condoms are good but, aai, I hate those things': condom use among adolescents and young people in a Southern African township.** *Soc Sci Med* 2001, **52**(Suppl 11):1613–1627.
18. Burgard SA, Kusunoki Y: **Gender and condom use among black South African young people.** *Population Studies Center Research Report* 2009:09–683. http://www.psc.isr.umich.edu/pubs/pdf/rr09-683.pdf (accessed 21 July 2013).
19. Weiser SD, Tuller DM, Frongiloo EA, Senkungu J, Bangsberg DR: **Food insecurity is associated with poor virologic response among HIV infected patients receiving antiretroviral medications.** *J Gen Intern Med* 2011, **26**(Suppl 9):1012–1018.
20. Du Preez CJ: *Living and Care arrangements of non -urban households in KwaZulu-Natal, South Africa in the context of HIV and AIDS*, PhD thesis. Wageningen: Wageningen University; 2010.
21. Cohen R, Kennedy P: *Global Sociology.* Palgrave Macmillan Publishers Limited; 2000.
22. Shambley-Ebron DZ, Boyle JS: **In Our Grandmothers' Footsteps: Perceptions of Being Strong in African American Women with HIV/AIDS.** *Advances in Nursing Practice* 2006, **29**(Suppl 3):195–206.
23. Palitza K: *HIVstigmapersists.* http://www.ipsnews.net/2010/01/south-africa-hiv-stigma-persists/ 2009; (accessed 21 July 2013).
24. *Oxford English Dictionary.* 2nd edition. Oxford: Clarendon Press; 1989.
25. Donna B, Donna B: *"'Whoonga' drug: a new twist in S.Africa's AIDS war".* Associated Press. E-News: Third Degree; 2011. 25 January 2011 at 21.30hrs.
26. Ramsamy R, Ramsamy R: *Deadly gamble.* Zululand Observer; 2010. From: http://en.wikipedia.org/wiki/Whoonga (accessed 21 July 2013).
27. *Collins English Dictionary.* Millenium Edition. Harper Collins Glasgow; 1998.
28. Coetzee B, Kagee A, Vermuelen N: **Structural barriers to adherence to antiretroviral therapy in a resource- constrained setting: the perspectives of health care providers.** *AIDS Care: Psychological and Socio- medical Aspects of AIDS/HIV* 2011, **23**(Suppl 2):146–151.
29. KoKotka A, Tanya: *It's better to die of AIDS than hunger.* New Internationalist Magazine; 2005. From: http://newint.org/features/2005/04/01/harare-zimbabwe/ (accessed 21 July 2013).
30. Makiwane M, Udjo E: *Is the child support grant associated with an increase in teenage fertility in South Africa?: evidence from national surveys and administrative data*; 2006. Final report December, accessed on 21 July 2013 from: http://www.info.gov.za/view/Download FileAction?id=129451.
31. Fisher JD, Fisher W, Cornman DH, Amico RK, Bryan A, Friedland GH: **Clinician delivered intervention during routine clinical care reduces unprotected sexual behaviour among HIV Infected Patients.** *J Acquir Immune Defic Syndr* 2006, **41**(Suppl 1):44–52.
32. Bandawe CR: **Revisiting Human behaviour in relation to HIV AIDS.** *Malawi Medical Journal. Malawi Med J* 2004, **14**(2):27–28.
33. Museveni Y: **Behavioural Change is the only way to fight AIDS.** *Wall Street Journal* 2004. From: http://www.ph.ucla.edu/epi/seaids/behavioralchange.html (accessed 21 July 2013).
34. Lovelife: *Impending Catastrophe revisited. An update on the HIV/AIDS epidemic in South Africa.* Parklands: Lovelife; 2006.
35. Morrison CC: *Promotion: a needs analysis for the antiretroviral rollout at the University of KwaZulu-Natal. Master's thesis.* Durban: Faculty of Humanities, Development and Social Sciences University of KwaZulu-Natal; 2005.
36. Ojikutu B, Jack C, Ramjee G: *Provision of Antiretroviral therapy in South Africa: Unique challenges and remaining obstacles.* Harvard Medical School Boston, Massachusetts: Division of AIDS; 2007.
37. WHO: *Global Atlas of Traditional, Complimentary and Alternative Medicine.* Kobe: WHO Centre for health development; 2005.
38. Van Dyk AC: **Traditional African beliefs and customs: implications for aids education and prevention in Africa.** *South African Journal Of Psychology* 2001, **31**(Suppl 2):110–130.
39. Peltzer K, Friend du Preez N, Ramalgan S, Anderson J: **Antiretroviral treatment adherence among HIV patients in KwaZulu-Natal, South Africa.** *BMC Public Health Journal* 2010, **2010**(10):111–112.
40. Stewart MJ, Steenkamp V, Van Der Merwe S, Zuckerman M, Crowther NJ: **The cytotoxic effects of a traditional Zulu remedy, impila (Callilepis laureola).** *Hum Exp Toxicol* 2002, **21**(Suppl 12):643–647.
41. Vuvu V: *Treatment Action Campaign face -off over healing claims.* http://www.tac.org.za/community/node/3009. 2011 (accessed 21 July 2013).
42. Gqaleni N, Moodley I, Kruger H, Ntuli A, McLeod H: **Traditional and complementary medicine.** In *South African Health Review.* Edited by Harrison S, Bhana R, Ntuli A. Durban, South Africa: Health Systems Trust; 2007.
43. Kiapi EM: *No laws to fight HIV stigma in schools.* http://ngonewsafrica.org/archives/737 2009; (accessed 21 July 2013).
44. Mucheto T, Chadambuka A, Shambara G, Mufuta T, Gombe N, Nyamayaro W: *Determinants of non-disclosure of HIV status among women attending the Prevention of Mother to Child Transmission Programme.* Makonde District, Zimbabwe; 2009.
45. Soul City and Khomanani: *HIV and AIDS: Prevention, Care and Treatment.* South Africa: Jacana Media; 2004.
46. Nyirenda M, Newell ML: *Orphan hood and HIV risk in rural KwaZulu Natal. State of the population of KwaZulu Natal: Demographic Profile and Development Indicators Book.* 9th edition; 2010:175.
47. Mkwanazi NB, Rochat TJ, Bland RM: *The Importance of Counselling Around Disclosure in Preparation for Parental Disclosure to Children. Africa Centre for Health and Population Studies.* UKZN Poster Presentation at the 5th SA AIDS Conference 2011.
48. Zuurmond M: *Adherence to ARVS- Challenges and Successes.* Zambia: CAFOD; 2008. From: http://catalogue.safaids.net/publications/adherence-arvs-challenges-and-successes (accessed 21 July 2013).
49. Bandawe CR, Foster D: **AIDS-related beliefs, attitudes and intentions among Malawian students in three secondary schools.** *AIDS Care* 1996, **8**:223–232.
50. Vogenthaler NS, Hadley C, Rodriguez AE, Valverde EE, del Rio C, Metsch LR: **Depressive Symptoms and Food Insufficiency Among HIV-Infected Crack Users in Atlanta and Miami.** *AIDS Behav* 2011, **15** (Suppl 7):1520–1526. http://www.researchgate.net/publication/41124398_Depressive_symptoms_and_food_insufficiency_among_HIV-infected_crack_users_in_Atlanta_and_Miami (accessed 21 July 2013).
51. Desjarlais R, Eisenberg GB, Kleinman A: *World Mental Health Problems and Priorities in Low income Countries.* New York: Oxford University press; 1995.
52. *Behavior Change and HIV Prevention.* Global HIV Prevention Working Group August; 2008. Re Considerations for the 21st Century; 2008. From: http://www.globalhivprevention.org/pdfs/HIV_Prevention_Strategies_0604.pdf (accessed 21 July 2013).
53. Schumacher JE, McCullumsmith C, Mugavero MJ, Ingle-Pang PE, Raper JL, Willig JH, You Z, Batey DS, Crane H, Lawrence ST, Wright C, Treisman G, Saag MS: *Routine Depression Screening in an HIV Clinic Cohort Identifies Patients with Complex Psychiatric Co-morbidities who show significant response to treatment. AIDS and Behaviour.* New York: Springer Science + Business Media; 2012.
54. Joska JA, Fincham DS, Stein DJ, Paul RH, Seedat S: **Clinical Correlates of HIV-Associated Neurocognitive Disorders in South Africa.** *AIDS Behav* 2010, **14**:371–378. http://www.ncbi.nlm.nih.gov/pubmed/19326205 (accessed 21 July 2013).
55. Akena D, Stein DJ, Joska J: *Does Screening HIV-Positive Individuals in Uganda for Major Depressive Disorder Improve Case Detection Rates and Antidepressant Prescription?.* AIDS and Behavior© Springer Science + Business Media New York; 2012. http://www.researchgate.net/profile/Dickens_Akena/publications/ (accessed 21 July 2013).
56. Diamond J: *Gender and Depression: Typical and Atypical Symptoms and Suicide Risk.* TUI University; 2008. From: http://www.scribd.com/doc/19054412/Depression-Gender-and-Suicide-A-Research-Study-on-Male Female-Differences-in-Depression (accessed 21 July 2013).
57. Cook RT: **Alcohol abuse, alcoholism, and damage to the immune system: a review.** *Alcoholism: Clinical and Experimental Research* 1998, **9**:1927–1942.
58. Reda AA, Biadgilign R, Biadgilign S: **Determinants of adherence to antiretroviral therapy among HIV Infected Patients in Africa.** *AIDS Research and Treatment* 2012. http://www.hindawi.com/journals/art/2012/574656/ (accessed 21 July 2013).
59. Meyerhoff DJ: **Effects of alcohol and HIV infection on the central nervous system.** *Alcohol Res Health* 2001, **25**(Suppl 4):288–298.

60. Steglitz J, Ng R, Mosha JS, Divinity and distress: **The Impact of Religion and spirituality on Mental Health of HIV Positive Adults in Tanzania.** *AIDS and Behaviour* 2012, **16:**2392–2398.
61. Wallace JM, Forman TA: **Religion's role in promoting health and reducing risk among American youth.** *Health Education & Behaviour* 1998, **25**(Suppl 6):721–741.
62. Strawbridge WJ: **Frequent attendance at religious services and mortality over 28 years.** *Am J Public Health* 1997, **87**(Suppl 6):957–961.
63. East Coast Radio: *Talk at 8:30. 2011. More children using whoonga.*
64. Connolly M, Monasch R: *Africa's orphaned generation.* New York: UNICEF; 2003.
65. Leyanaar JK: **HIV/AIDS and African Orphan crisis.** *Paediatric Child Health* 2005, **10**(Suppl 5):259–260.
66. Andrew JA, Hops H, Ary D: **Parental Influence on early adolescent substance use.** *Specific and non-specific effects. Journal of Early Adolescents* 1993, **13**(Suppl 3):285–310.
67. Nkuna B: *South African TB patients sell sputum to grant fraudsters*; 2010. http://westcapenews.com/?p=1066http://westcapenews.com/?p=1066 (accessed 21 July 2013).
68. Riley ED, Moore K, Sorensen JL, Tulsky JP, Bangsberg DR, Neidlands TB: **Basic subsistence needs and overall health among human immunodeficiency virus infected homeless and unstably housed women.** *Am J Epidemiol* 2011, **174**(Suppl 5):515–522.
69. Orach SO: **ART in Ugandan Catholic Health Services. Opportunities and challenges.** *UMU Press* 2005, **3:**21–27.
70. Chaudoir SR, Norton WE, Earnshaw VA, Monetham L, Mugavero MJ, Hiers KM, Coping with HIV stigma: **Do proactive Coping and Spiritual peace buffer the effect of Stigma on Depression.** *AIDS Behav* 2012, **8:**2382–2391. http://www.ncbi.nlm.nih.gov/pubmed/21956644 (accessed 21 July 2013).
71. Munro A: *Belated, but powerful: The response of the catholic church to HIV/AIDS in Five Southern African Countries. Southern African Catholic Bishops Conference Office.* Pretoria: South Africa; 2002.
72. Houlihan CF, Bland RM, Mutevedzi PC, Lessells RJ, Ndirangu J, Thulare H, Newell ML: **Cohort Profile: Hlabisa HIV treatment and care programme.** *Int J Epidemiol* 2010:1–9. http://www.ncbi.nlm.nih.gov/pubmed/20154009 (accessed 21 July 2013).
73. *Amangwe Village.* http://www.ethembenicc.org.za/ (accessed 21 July 2013).
74. Katzellenbogen JM, Joubert G, Karim A: *Epidemiology. A Manual for South Africa.* Cape Town: Oxford University Press Southern Africa; 2007.
75. Mouton J: *How to succeed in your Master's and Doctoral studies. A South African guide and Resource Book.* Pretoria: Van Schaik Publishers; 2008.
76. Reysoo F, Heldens J: *Qualitative interview*; 2007. http://www.slideserve.com/jerod/focus-group (accessed 21 July 2013).
77. Holloway I: **The status of method: flexibility, consistency and coherence.** *Qual Res* 2003, **3**(Suppl 3):345–357.
78. Muhr I: *Atlas .ti.* Berlin: Scientific Software development; 2008. http://www.atlasti.com (accessed 21 July 2013).
79. Brink HI: *Fundamentals of Research Methodology For Health Care Professionals.* 3rd edition. Cape Town: Juta & Company LTD; 2011.
80. De Vos AS, Strydom H, Fouche CB, Delport CSL: *Research at Grass roots. For the Social Sciences and Human Service Profession.* 3rd edition. Pretoria: Van Schaik Publishers; 2007.

The effects of opioids on HIV reactivation in latently-infected T-lymphoblasts

Johannes Prottengeier[1*], Eleni Koutsilieri[2] and Carsten Scheller[2]

Abstract

Background: Opioids may have effects on susceptibility to HIV-infection, viral replication and disease progression. Injecting drug users (IDU), as well as anyone receiving opioids for anesthesia and analgesia may suffer the clinical consequences of such interactions. There is conflicting data between *in vitro* experiments showing an enhancing effect of opioids on HIV replication and clinical data, mostly showing no such effect. For clarification we studied the effects of the opioids heroin and morphine on HIV replication in cultured CD4-positive T cells at several concentrations and we related the observed effects with the relevant reached plasma concentrations found in IDUs.

Methods: Latently-infected ACH-2 T lymphoblasts were incubated with different concentrations of morphine and heroine. Reactivation of HIV was assessed by intracellular staining of viral Gag p24 protein and subsequent flow cytometric quantification of p24-positive cells. The influence of the opioid antagonist naloxone and the antioxidants N-acetyl-cysteine (NAC) and glutathione (GSH) on HIV reactivation was determined. Cell viability was investigated by 7-AAD staining and flow cytometric quantification.

Results: Morphine and heroine triggered reactivation of HIV replication in ACH-2 cells in a dose-dependent manner at concentrations above 1 mM (EC_{50} morphine 2.82 mM; EC_{50} morphine 1.96 mM). Naloxone did not interfere with heroine-mediated HIV reactivation, even at high concentrations (1 mM). Opioids also triggered necrotic cell death at similar concentrations at which HIV reactivation was observed. Both opioid-mediated reactivation of HIV and opioid-triggered cell death could be inhibited by the antioxidants GSH and NAC.

Conclusions: Opioids reactivate HIV *in vitro* but at concentrations that are far above the plasma levels of analgesic regimes or drug concentrations found in IDUs. HIV reactivation was mediated by effects unrelated to opioid-receptor activation and was tightly linked to the cytotoxic activity of the substances at millimolar concentrations, suggesting that opioid-mediated reactivation of HIV was due to accompanying effects of cellular necrosis such as activation of reactive oxygen species and NF-κB.

Keywords: HIV, Reactivation, Opioids, Heroine, Morphine, Naloxone, ACH-2

Introduction

Many of the HIV-infected individuals who inject intravenous drugs consume morphine, heroin or related substances. There is conflicting data on the impact of opioids on HIV disease progression. Whereas in vitro studies suggest a potential link between opioid exposure and elevated virus replication or decreased immune function [1-5], most of epidemiological and clinical studies do not find a correlation between opioid intake and progression of HIV infection [6-12]. In order to reconcile these conflicting data, we performed *in vitro* experiments studying the effects of opioids (heroin and morphine) on HIV replication in the chronically-infected CD4-positive T cell line ACH-2 [13]. CD4-positive T cells represent the cellular reservoir in which HIV is harbored predominantly in the body and they contribute to most of the viral replication detected in the blood plasma [14-16].

* Correspondence: Johannes.Prottengeier@kfa.imed.uni-erlangen.de
[1]Department of Anesthesiology, Erlangen University Hospital, Krankenhausstrasse 12, 91054 Erlangen, Germany
Full list of author information is available at the end of the article

Results

Morphine and heroine reactivate HIV in ACH-2 cells

In order to investigate the effects of the opioids heroine and morphine on reactivation of proviral HIV in latently-infected T cells, we incubated ACH-2 cells with different concentrations of morphine-sulfate and heroine. After incubation for 24 h we measured intracellular HIV-p24 protein expression by flow cytometry. We found a dose-dependent reactivation of HIV for morphine (Figure 1A) and heroine (Figure 1B). The EC_{50} concentrations for the two substances were 2.82 mM and 1.96 mM, respectively (Figure 1). Figures 1C and D display representative dot-plots analyzing p24-expression (y-axis) of untreated (Figure 1C) or 4 mM heroin-treated (D) cells. The background expression visible in Figure 1C is typical for ACH-2 cells and originates from intrinsic stimulation of the cells. We also tested the effects of heroin on HIV replication at very low concentrations, similar to the plasma concentrations found in IDUs and found no activating effects (Figure 1D).

Naloxone does not inhibit heroine-mediated reactivation of HIV

Opioid receptor signaling has been described on lymphocytes [1] and opioid receptors that bind the opioid antagonist naloxone have been identified on T cells (reviewed in [17]). We therefore investigated whether the observed HIV-activating effect of opioids was mediated by opioid-specific receptor stimulation. For that we triggered HIV reactivation with heroine in the absence or presence of different concentrations of naloxone. As depicted

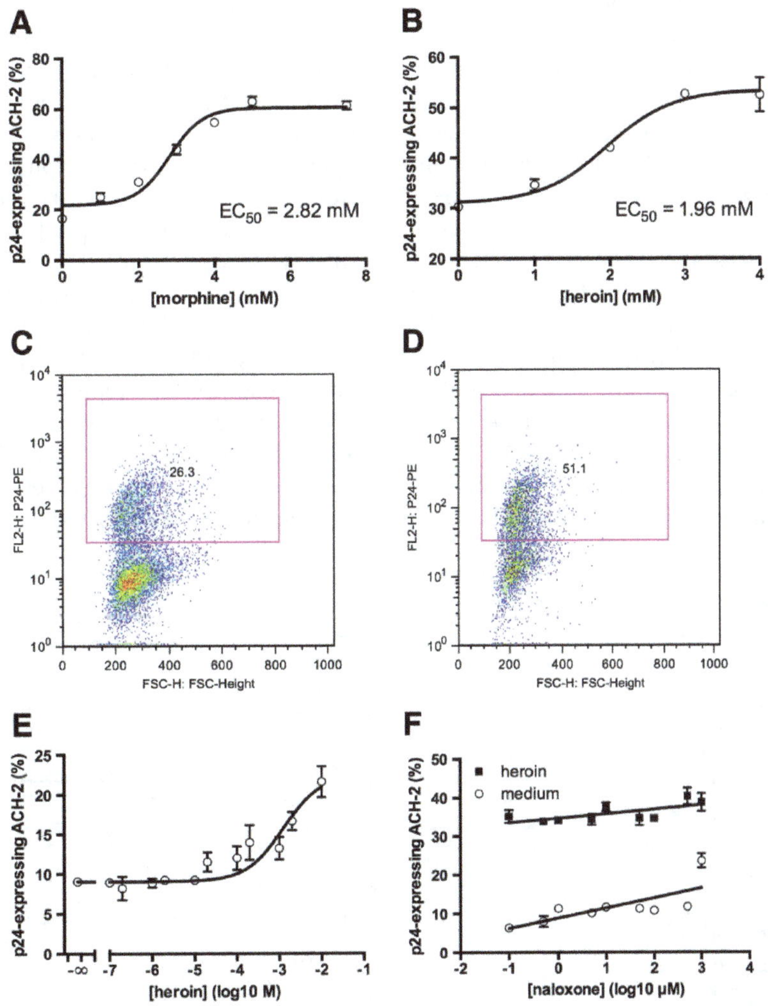

Figure 1 Opioids activate HIV replication in vitro. Latently-HIV-infected ACH-2 T lymphoblasts were cultured for 24 hours in the presence of different concentrations of morphine **(A)** or heroin **(B)**. HIV replication was quantified by intracellular staining of HIV p24-antigen and flow cytometry. **C, D**: representative dot-plot analyses of ACH-2 cells left untreated **(C)** or treated with 4 mM heroin **(D)**. The x-axis displays the forward scatter, the y-axis displays p24-expression. Pink rectangles represent the gates for p24-positive cells and the small numbers within indicate the proportion (%) of p24-positive cells from the total number of events. **E**: Heroin has no effects on HIV reactivation at concentrations found in plasma of IDUs (1-10 μM). **F**: Latently-HIV-infected ACH-2 T lymphoblasts were cultured for 24 hours in the presence of 5 mM heroin, together with different concentrations of naloxone (0 μM and 0.1μM – 1 mM). HIV replication was quantified by intracellular staining of HIV p24-antigen and flow cytometry. Data as mean ± S.E.M. from duplicates and linear regression. The slopes of both regressions are positive and significantly differ from = zero (p = 0.0008 for medium and p = 0.0152 for heroin).

in Figure 1F, naloxone did not interfere with heroine-mediated HIV reactivation, indicating that opioid receptor-independent mechanisms account for the observed effects.

NAC and GSH inhibit opioid-mediated HIV reactivation

Heroin- and morphine-mediated activation of HIV replication was completely prevented by the antioxidants N-acetylcystein (NAC) or reduced glutathione (GSH) (Figure 2), indicating that oxidative stress might be involved in opioid-mediated reactivation of HIV. The relatively high opioid concentrations needed to stimulate HIV replication were also associated with induction of necrotic cell death. A3.01 T cells, the uninfected parental cell line of ACH-2 cells, showed a significant amount of necrosis induction following treatment with 2.5 mM heroin as assessed by staining with the cell dye 7-AAD (Figure 3A). This necrosis induction could again be completely prevented by the antioxidant N-acetylcystein (Figure 3A). We used for this experiment the uninfected parental cell line because the 7-AAD dye requires non-fixated cells, which in case of the HIV-infected ACH-2 cells we could not subject to our flow cytometer for safety reasons. In order to demonstrate that ACH-2 cells react in a similar way to opioids as A3.01 cells, we analyzed cell death in ACH-2 cells by a characteristic shift of the cell population in the forward-scatter/sideward-scatter dot plot analysis, which correlates with 7-AAD-staining. This shift is depicted in Figure 3C from representative analyses for different heroin concentrations. The corresponding p24-expression profiles are depicted in Figure 3D. As shown in Figure 3B, activation of HIV in ACH-2 cell completely paralleled with opioid-triggered necrosis. We reported earlier that necrotic signaling triggers NF-κB and HIV-reactivation in ACH-2 T lymphoblasts [18]. These data indicate that the observed opioid-mediated activation of HIV replication was secondary to the opioid-triggered necrosis observed at high concentrations.

Discussion

Opioid-mediated reactivation of latent HIV infection in our model was observed at concentrations in the lower millimolar range. Since opioids are common in the HIV-risk group of injecting drug users (IDUs), this activity might influence the pathogenesis of HIV infection in this group of patients. However, plasma concentrations of heroine in IDUs are in the range of 1–10 μM [19] and even maximum plasma concentrations are only in the range of 1500–3900 ng/ml (reviewed in [20]), which corresponds to 4.1-10.7 μM (calculated with a molar weight of 369.41 g/mol). Secondly plasma-concentrations of medically administered morphine and its modern derivates for means of analgesia remain well below those ranges of reactivating effects [21-23]. These *in vivo* concentrations are 2–3 orders of magnitude lower than the *in vitro* concentration at which we observed a stimulating effect. It therefore seems very unlikely that the here-described opioid-mediated reactivation of HIV may have any influence on HIV replication *in vivo*.

Opioid-triggered reactivation of HIV replication in latently-infected cells has been described in the monocytic cell line U1 [3]. HIV reactivation after treatment with morphine was observed in the picomolar (10^{-12})

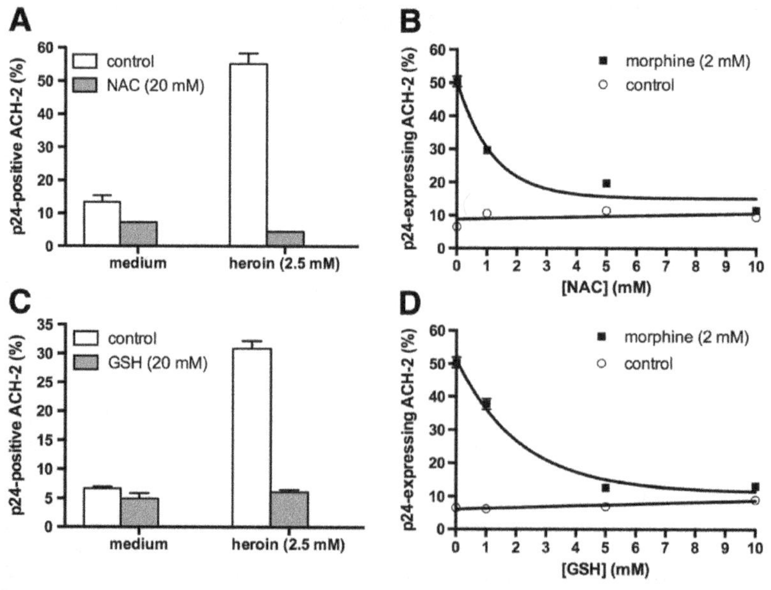

Figure 2 Antioxidants inhibit opioid-mediated reactivation of HIV. Latently-HIV-infected ACH-2 T lymphoblasts were cultured for 24 hours with of heroin **(A, C)** or morphine **(B, D)** in the presence or absence of the antioxidants N-acetylcystein (NAC) **(A, B)** or glutathione **(C, D)**. HIV replication was quantified by intracellular staining of HIV p24-antigen and flow cytometry.

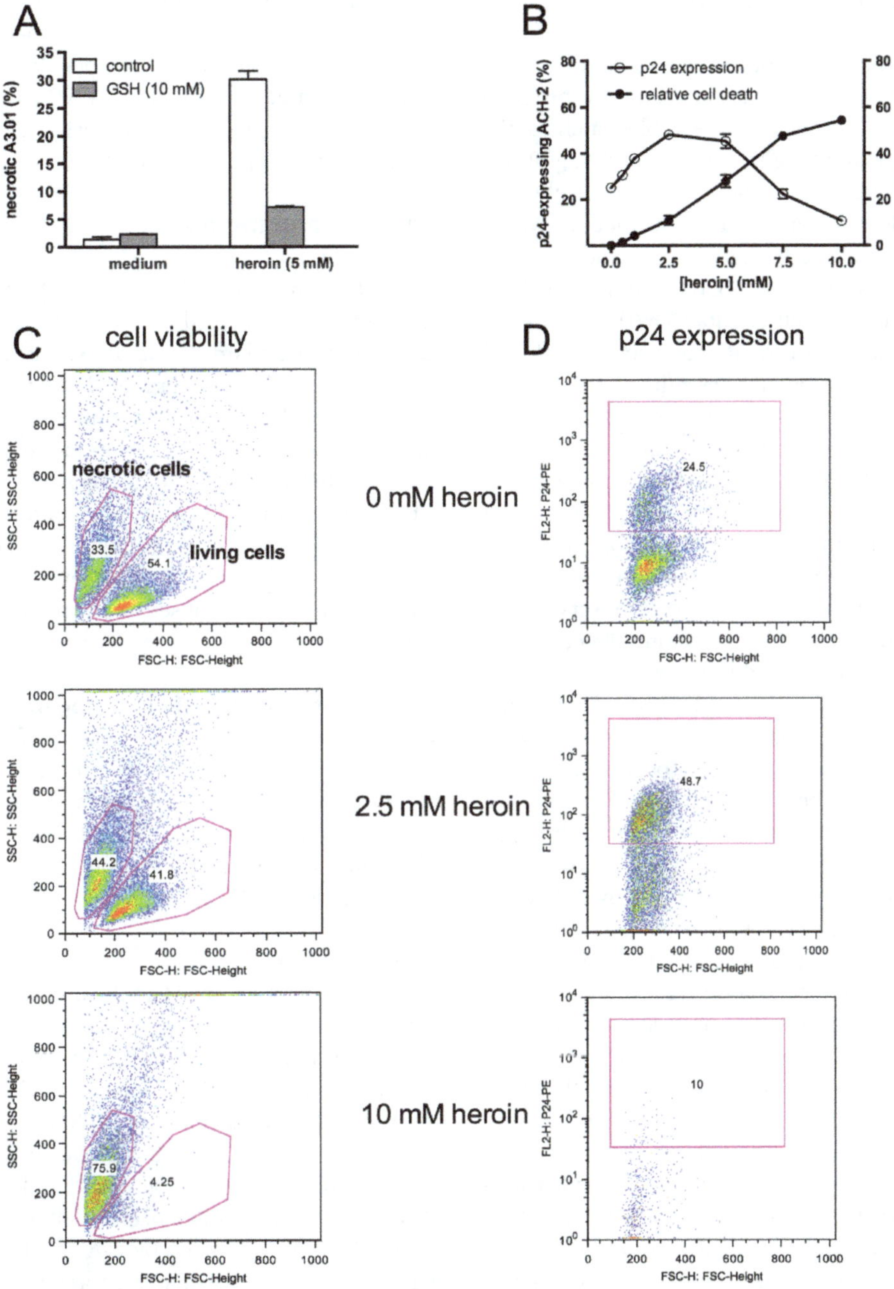

Figure 3 Opioid-mediated reactivation of HIV is tightly linked to cellular necrosis. Latently-HIV-infected ACH-2 T lymphoblasts were cultured for 24 hours with of heroin in the presence or absence of glutathione. HIV replication was quantified by intracellular staining of HIV p24-antigen and flow cytometry **(A)**. Cell viability was assessed by FSC/SSC-analysis in flow cytometry **(B)**. Representative dot plots of cell viability analysis **(C)** and p24-expression **(D)** at different heroin concentrations. Pink rectangles on the right represent the gates for p24-positive cells and the small numbers within indicate the proportion (%) of p24-positive cells from the total number of events. Pink regions on the left represent the gates for living and necrotic cells and the small numbers within indicate the proportion (%) of events within the region from the total number of events.

range but not at higher concentrations. Especially at micromolar concentrations – the concentration range of plasma levels found in drug abusers - no effects were observed [3]. Similar effects were reported from the same group when studying productive infection in cultured peripheral blood lymphocytes [4]. In studies with experimental SHIV-infection in the rhesus macaque model, elevated viral load was reported in morphine-treated animals (n = 6) versus untreated animals (n = 3) [2]. Recently, a decrease in anti-HIV microRNA expression was reported in monocytes following treatment with morphine and heroin [5], suggesting a potential explanation for the increased viral replication found in *in vitro* studies.

In contrast, the majority of epidemiological studies does not show negative effects of drug abuse on HIV progression [8-12], but many confounding variables such as the pattern of drug use may make it difficult to clearly interpret this data. To address this, a prospective clinical study with a total of 1148 participants was performed, in which the effects of hard drug use (opioids or cocaine) on HIV disease parameters was studied [6]. Drug use had no effect on HIV viral load or CD4 cell counts (n = 613 versus n = 535). In line with this, no effects of drug use on viral load have been observed in a seroconverter study with 60 injection drug users in a total of 149 participants [7].

The literature therefore seems to be divided into experimental and *in vitro* studies reporting enhancement of HIV infection following treatment with opioids and *in vivo* studies not finding such a correlation. We suggest that this difference, at least in parts, relates to the concentration range at which effects were observed: All *in vitro* studies reporting an HIV-activating effect of opioids in cell culture found these effects at very low concentrations and no activity was observed at relevant plasma concentrations [3-5]. Moreover, all so-far reported *in vitro* data were generated in monocytes [3,5] (or in PBMC containing monocytes [4]), whereas more than 99% of HIV particles detected in the human plasma originate from T-lymphocytes [15,24,25]. Hence, effects found in monocytes *in vitro* may not be representative for the lymphocyte-driven plasma viral load *in vivo*. Our *in vitro*-results indicate that there is an HIV-stimulating effect of opioids also in T cells, but only at concentrations that are far above relevant *in vivo*-concentrations. The molecular mechanism of HIV latency in the ACH-2 cell line used in our study is caused by a defect in the Tat/TAR axis [26] and the same mechanism of latency is also frequently found in latently-infected primary T cells isolated from HIV patients [27].

Taken together, the literature seems to be divided into *in vitro* studies reporting enhancement of HIV infection following treatment with opioids and *in vivo* studies not finding such a correlation. Our *in-vitro* results indicate that there is an HIV-stimulating effect of opioids in latently-infected T cells, but only at concentrations that are far beyond relevant *in vivo*-concentrations and our findings may therefore contribute to reconcile the apparently conflicting data of *in vitro* and *in vivo* research. Our data provides no evidence that the medical use of opioids for indications of anesthesia and analgesia in HIV-infected patients may have any side effects on HIV replication.

Conclusion

Opioids reactivate HIV *in vitro* but at concentrations that are far above the plasma levels of analgesic regimes or drug concentrations found in IDUs. HIV reactivation is mediated by effects unrelated to opioid-receptor activation and seems tightly linked to the cytotoxic activity of these substances at a millimolar level, suggesting that opioid-mediated reactivation of HIV is due to accompanying effects of cellular necrosis such as activation of reactive oxygen species and NF-κB.

Materials and methods

Cell culture

A3.01 (human CD4 + –T-lymphoblasts, NIAID) and ACH-2 (latently HIV-infected A3.01, Folks 1989, NIAID) were cultured in standard tissue flasks using RPMI-medium (Invitrogen, Karlsruhe, Germany) supplemented with 10% FCS (Linaris, Bettingen, Germany) at 37°C and 5% CO2 atmosphere. Peripheral blood mononuclear cells (PBMC) were isolated by Ficoll/Paque density-separation centrifugation from human whole blood donated by healthy volunteers. For the different experiments 10^5 cells per well were cultured in flat-bottom 96 well plates in a total volume of 200 μl for 24 h in the absence or presence of the indicated substances.

Opioids, antagonists and other reagents

Morphine and Heroine were obtained from the University of Wurzburg's Department of Forensic Medicine. The Use and Discard of those substances were documented in accordance with the German Narcotics Act. Naloxone, Glutathion and N-Acetylcysteine were purchased through Sigma, St.Lewis, MO.

Flow cytometry

Reactivation of HIV in ACH-2 cells was quantified by the expression of viral p24-antigen detected by flow cytometry (Becton-Dickinson, Heidelberg, Germany). Cells were fixated for 20 min with 4% formalin in PBS and later permeabilized with 0.5% saponin in PBS/5%BSA. The following antibodies were used: 183-H12-5C-anti-HIV-p24-mouse-antibody and goat-anti-mouse antibodies conjugated with FITC or PE (BD Biosciences). Cell death in uninfected A3.01 cells was quantified by 7-AAD staining according to the instructions of the manufacturer (BD Biosciences). Besides staining with 7-AAD, necrotic cells also displayed a characteristic shift in a forward-scatter (FSC)/sideward scatter (SSC) dot plot. This shift was used to quantify necrotic cells also for HIV-infected ACH-2 cells, for which a 7-AAD staining was not possible for safety reasons (7-AAD staining requires nonfixated cells which in case of ACH-2 cells would contaminate the flow cytometer with HIV).

Competing interests

All of the authors declare that they have no competing interests.

Authors' contributions

CS conceived of the study and helped to draft the manuscript. JP conducted the study, performed the statistical analysis and is the main author of the manuscript. EK participated in the study's design and helped to draft the manuscript. All authors read and approved the final manuscript.

Acknowledgements
We thank Ingeborg Euler-König for excellent technical assistance. The following agents were obtained through National Institutes of Health – AIDS Research and Reference Reagent Program: A3.01 and ACH-2 cells by T. Folks; p24-HIV-Hybridoma (183-H12-5C) by B.Chesebro and H.Chen. The study was supported by a grant from the Bundesministerium für Bildung und Forschung (BMBF 01 KI 9479).

Author details
[1]Department of Anesthesiology, Erlangen University Hospital, Krankenhausstrasse 12, 91054 Erlangen, Germany. [2]Institute of Virology and Immunobiology, University of Würzburg, Würzburg, Germany.

References

1. Nair MP, Schwartz SA, Polasani R, Hou J, Sweet A, Chadha KC: **Immunoregulatory effects of morphine on human lymphocytes.** *Clin Diagn Lab Immunol* 1997, **4**(2):127–132.
2. Perez-Casanova A, Husain K, Noel RJ Jr, Rivera-Amill V, Kumar A: **Interaction of SIV/SHIV infection and morphine on plasma oxidant/antioxidant balance in macaque.** *Mol Cell Biochem* 2008, **308**(1–2):169–175.
3. Peterson PK, Gekker G, Hu S, Anderson WR, Kravitz F, Portoghese PS, Balfour HH Jr, Chao CC: **Morphine amplifies HIV-1 expression in chronically infected promonocytes cocultured with human brain cells.** *J Neuroimmunol* 1994, **50**(2):167–175.
4. Peterson PK, Sharp BM, Gekker G, Portoghese PS, Sannerud K, Balfour HH Jr: **Morphine promotes the growth of HIV-1 in human peripheral blood mononuclear cell cocultures.** *AIDS* 1990, **4**(9):869–873.
5. Wang X, Ye L, Zhou Y, Liu MQ, Zhou DJ, Ho WZ: **Inhibition of anti-HIV microRNA expression: a mechanism for opioid-mediated enhancement of HIV infection of monocytes.** *Am J Pathol* 2011, **178**(1):41–47.
6. Thorpe LE, Frederick M, Pitt J, Cheng I, Watts DH, Buschur S, Green K, Zorrilla C, Landesman SH, Hershow RC: **Effect of hard-drug use on CD4 cell percentage, HIV RNA level, and progression to AIDS-defining class C events among HIV-infected women.** *J Acquir Immune Defic Syndr* 2004, **37**(3):1423–1430.
7. Lyles CM, Dorrucci M, Vlahov D, Pezzotti P, Angarano G, Sinicco A, Alberici F, Alcorn TM, Vella S, Rezza G: **Longitudinal human immunodeficiency virus type 1 load in the italian seroconversion study: correlates and temporal trends of virus load.** *J Infect Dis* 1999, **180**(4):1018–1024.
8. Prins M, Veugelers PJ: **Comparison of progression and non-progression in injecting drug users and homosexual men with documented dates of HIV-1 seroconversion. European Seroconverter Study and the Tricontinental Seroconverter Study.** *AIDS* 1997, **11**(5):621–631.
9. Biggar RJ: **AIDS incubation in 1891 HIV seroconverters from different exposure groups. International Registry of Seroconverters.** *AIDS* 1990, **4**(11):1059–1066.
10. Spijkerman IJ, Langendam MW, Veugelers PJ, van Ameijden EJ, Keet IP, Geskus RB, van den Hoek A, Coutinho RA: **Differences in progression to AIDS between injection drug users and homosexual men with documented dates of seroconversion.** *Epidemiology* 1996, **7**(6):571–577.
11. Carre N, Deveau C, Belanger F, Boufassa F, Persoz A, Jadand C, Rouzioux C, Delfraissy JF, Bucquet D: **Effect of age and exposure group on the onset of AIDS in heterosexual and homosexual HIV-infected patients. SEROCO Study Group.** *AIDS* 1994, **8**(6):797–802.
12. Pehrson P, Lindback S, Lidman C, Gaines H, Giesecke J: **Longer survival after HIV infection for injecting drug users than for homosexual men: implications for immunology.** *AIDS* 1997, **11**(8):1007–1012.
13. Folks TM, Clouse KA, Justement J, Rabson A, Duh E, Kehrl JH, Fauci AS: **Tumor necrosis factor alpha induces expression of human immunodeficiency virus in a chronically infected T-cell clone.** *Proc Natl Acad Sci U S A* 1989, **86**(7):2365–2368.
14. Psallidopoulos MC, Schnittman SM, Thompson LM 3rd, Baseler M, Fauci AS, Lane HC, Salzman NP: **Integrated proviral human immunodeficiency virus type 1 is present in CD4+ peripheral blood lymphocytes in healthy seropositive individuals.** *J Virol* 1989, **63**(11):4626–4631.
15. Schnittman SM, Psallidopoulos MC, Lane HC, Thompson L, Baseler M, Massari F, Fox CH, Salzman NP, Fauci AS: **The reservoir for HIV-1 in human peripheral blood is a T cell that maintains expression of CD4.** *Science* 1989, **245**(4915):305–308.
16. McElrath MJ, Pruett JE, Cohn ZA: **Mononuclear phagocytes of blood and bone marrow: comparative roles as viral reservoirs in human immunodeficiency virus type 1 infections.** *Proc Natl Acad Sci U S A* 1989, **86**(2):675–679.
17. Sharp BM: **Multiple opioid receptors on immune cells modulate intracellular signaling.** *Brain Behav Immun* 2006, **20**(1):9–14.
18. Scheller C, Sopper S, Chen P, Flory E, Koutsilieri E, Racek T, Ludwig S, ter Meulen V, Jassoy C: **Caspase inhibition activates HIV in latently infected cells. Role of tumor necrosis factor receptor 1 and CD95.** *J Biol Chem* 2002, **277**(18):15459–15464.
19. Rook EJ, Huitema AD, van den Brink W, van Ree JM, Beijnen JH: **Population pharmacokinetics of heroin and its major metabolites.** *Clin Pharmacokinet* 2006, **45**(4):401–417.
20. Rook EJ, Huitema AD, van den Brink W, van Ree JM, Beijnen JH: **Pharmacokinetics and pharmacokinetic variability of heroin and its metabolites: review of the literature.** *Curr Clin Pharmacol* 2006, **1**(1):109–118.
21. Martini C, Olofsen E, Yassen A, Aarts L, Dahan A: **Pharmacokinetic-pharmacodynamic modeling in acute and chronic pain: an overview of the recent literature.** *Expert Rev Clin Pharmacol* 2011, **4**(6):719–728.
22. Lotsch J: **Pharmacokinetic-pharmacodynamic modeling of opioids.** *J Pain Symptom Manage* 2005, **29**(5 Suppl):S90–S103.
23. Zollner C, Schafer M: **[Opioids in anesthesia].** *Anaesthesist* 2008, **57**(7):729–740. quiz 741–722.
24. Perelson AS, Neumann AU, Markowitz M, Leonard JM, Ho DD: **HIV-1 dynamics in vivo: virion clearance rate, infected cell life-span, and viral generation time.** *Science* 1996, **271**(5255):1582–1586.
25. Ho DD, Neumann AU, Perelson AS, Chen W, Leonard JM, Markowitz M: **Rapid turnover of plasma virions and CD4 lymphocytes in HIV-1 infection.** *Nature* 1995, **373**(6510):123–126.
26. Emiliani S, Van Lint C, Fischle W, Paras P Jr, Ott M, Brady J, Verdin E: **A point mutation in the HIV-1 Tat responsive element is associated with postintegration latency.** *Proc Natl Acad Sci U S A* 1996, **93**(13):6377–6381.
27. Yukl S, Pillai S, Li P, Chang K, Pasutti W, Ahlgren C, Havlir D, Strain M, Gunthard H, Richman D, Rice AP, Daar E, Little S, Wong JK: **Latently-infected CD4+ T cells are enriched for HIV-1 Tat variants with impaired transactivation activity.** *Virology* 2009, **387**(1):98–108.

10

A possible role for CCR5 in the progression of atherosclerosis in HIV-infected patients

Laura Fernández-Sender[1], Carlos Alonso-Villaverde[1,2], Anna Rull[1], Esther Rodríguez-Gallego[1], Marta Riera-Borrull[1], Anna Hernández-Aguilera[1], Jordi Camps[1], Raúl Beltrán-Debón[1], Gerard Aragonès[1], Javier A Menendez[3] and Jorge Joven[1*]

Abstract

Background: Chemokines can block viral entry by interfering with HIV co-receptors and are recognised mediators of atherosclerosis development. A number of experimental drugs that inhibit HIV entry arrest the development of atherosclerosis in animal models. We hypothesised that the expression of chemokine receptors in circulating leukocytes is associated with the rate of atherosclerosis progression in HIV-infected patients.

Methods: The increase in intima-media thickness during a 2-year follow-up was used to classify HIV-infected patients (n = 178) as progressors (n = 142) or non-progressors (n = 36) with respect to atherosclerosis. Logistic regression was used to assess variables associated with atherosclerosis progression. Mutations in the CCR5Δ32, CCR2 64I, and CX3CR1 (T280M and V249I) co-receptors as well as the levels of CCR5, CXCR4, CX3CR1, and CCR2 mRNA expression in circulating leukocytes were analysed as independent variables.

Results: Among the baseline variables, only genetic variants explained the dichotomous outcome. The expression of CCR2 and CXCR4 did not discriminate between progressors and non-progressors. Conversely, CCR5 and CX3CR1 expression was higher in not only progressors but also patients with detectable viral load. The logistic regression, however, demonstrated a significant role for CCR5 expression as a predictor of atherosclerosis progression (B = 2.1, OR = 8.1, p = 0.04) and a negligible effect for CXC3R1 and CCR2 expression.

Conclusions: Available CCR5 antagonists should be investigated for their potential to delay the course of atherosclerosis in HIV-infected patients.

Keywords: Cardiovascular risk factors, Chemokine receptors, Genetic variants, Inflammation, Maraviroc

Background

Current therapies achieve long-term remission and/or prevent morbid conditions associated with human immunodeficiency virus-1 (HIV-1) infection. Despite the ineffective elimination of the virus, correct management is accompanied by a growing increase in life expectancy that involves age-related complications. For example, atherosclerosis and other non-communicable diseases develop earlier and more rapidly in HIV patients compared with non-infected individuals of a similar age with similar risk factors [1-3].

Persistent immune activation may be the reason for this phenomenon, likely through host gene variations in chemokine responses to non-infectious particles or viral proteins [4-6]. Chemokines and chemokine receptors play a significant role in atherosclerosis, may influence susceptibility to HIV infection, and may affect the course of both diseases [6,7]. The CC chemokines, which contain two adjacent cysteines near the amino terminus, are particularly important, and the role of CCL2, a ligand for CCR2, in the development of atherosclerosis has been substantiated in animal models and humans [5,8]. Furthermore, orally bioavailable agents that inhibit the

* Correspondence: jorge.joven@urv.cat
[1]Unitat de Recerca Biomèdica, Hospital Universitari Sant Joan, Institut d'Investigació Sanitaria Pere Virgili (IISPV), Universitat Rovira i Virgili, Reus, Spain, carrer Sant Llorenç 21, Reus 43201, Spain

chemotaxis of primary CCR2-expressing human monocytes towards CCL2 are currently in various clinical trials [9,10]. More recently, the chemokine receptor CCR5 and its ligands (CCL3, CCL4 and CCL5) have been implicated in the pathogenesis of atherosclerosis [11], and a relatively common mutation with a corresponding lack of function (CCR5 Δ32) confers relative resistance to HIV infection [12] and a reduction in susceptibility to coronary artery disease [13]. These and other findings have facilitated the development and further approval of CCR5 antagonists (maraviroc) as antiretroviral agents in patients infected with strains that do not use CXCR4 as the co-receptor [14]. It remains to be established whether maraviroc influences the development of atherosclerosis; however, we have recently identified the beneficial effects of both lipid metabolism and inflammation [15]. Fractalkine (CX3CL1) and its receptor, CX3CR1, have also been implicated as modulators of both HIV infection and atherosclerosis, and functional polymorphisms in CXC3R1 (V249I and T280M) are clinically relevant during the course of these conditions [16,17].

The available data are difficult to interpret because of the high redundancy of the chemokine system, conflicting results for the cardiovascular risk predictions, and effects from possible interactions among receptors, which could be confounding factors [16,17]. In this study, we investigated for the first time whether the expression of chemokine receptors in circulating leukocytes was relevant for the assessment of atherosclerosis progression in HIV-infected patients. We determined that CCR5 expression in these cells might be a strong predictor of atherosclerosis progression, indicating a further therapeutic target for CCR5 antagonists.

Methods

Study design, population and standardised ultrasound protocol

This report was prepared in accordance with the STROBE guidelines described at http://www.strobe-statement.org/. The procedures were performed in accordance with the Code of Ethics of the World Medical Association (Declaration of Helsinki) for experiments involving humans, and the study was approved by the ethics committee at the Hospital Universitari de Sant Joan de Reus. Patients who accepted the invitation to participate in the study provided full informed consent. HIV-infected patients who attended our outpatient clinic were routinely asked to be incorporated into a cohort (n = 523) in accordance with previously described procedures [1,6,18]. None of the included patients were treated with CCR5 antagonists. In a retrospective, longitudinal study, we sampled a cross-section of the patients to assess the intima-media thickness (IMT) at baseline (when incorporated into the cohort) and 2 years later.

We used the LOGIQ 700 ME system (General Electric) to obtain normalised values IMT [1,6]. We identified and digitally recorded the far wall of the common carotid artery (1 cm proximal to the bifurcation), the carotid bulb (in the bifurcation), and the internal carotid artery (1 cm distal from the bifurcation). The IMT measurements of each arterial segment were averaged and used in the statistical analyses as the combined IMT. We identified patients with a 2-year difference in the IMT value that was equal to or lower than the technical differences among examiners as non-progressors. This value was obtained via an intraclass correlation coefficient determined with 30 measurements ($r = 0.89$, $p < 0.001$) and established as 0.01 mm (standard deviation 0.02 mm). The progressors exhibited ΔIMT >0.01 mm and/or the presence of a previously unrecognised plaque in the second observation. The procedures were performed essentially as described previously [6,19,20]. To assess the reproducibility of the measurements, the images of 30 randomly selected patients were re-measured using the same protocol. The intraclass correlation coefficient between the 2 sets of measurements was 0.91, and the absolute difference in IMT was 0.007 mm (0.018). To assess the reproducibility of the rescanning and re-measurement, we also measured the inter-month correlation ($r = 0.95$; $n = 15$).

The other relevant data were collated from clinical records or obtained using standardised guidelines and routine laboratory methods [21,22]. The covariates used were obtained in the same time frame for each participant. To avoid sampling bias, we selected and presented data only from patients who did not exhibit changes in variables or episodes that were likely to contribute to the outcome during follow-up (n = 217). The patients were observed by their attending doctors every 3 months, and no major events were recorded. Changes in the clinical and laboratory markers of cardiovascular risk and/or HIV infection were considered not relevant (less than 5% of differences with respect to the normal inter-day coefficient of variation for each measurement). The resulting study population was used to determine whether chemokine receptor expression in blood cells was associated with atherosclerosis progression, and additional fasting venous blood samples were drawn immediately before the second IMT measurement under conditions that guaranteed RNA preservation (using TEMPUS blood RNA tubes from Applied Biosystems, Foster City, CA). Inappropriately documented IMT measurements (n = 16), inappropriately handled samples (n = 9), and changes in the antiretroviral treatment (n = 14) were detected and considered exclusion criteria. Therefore, the data for 178 patients are presented. This number was considered sufficiently higher than the minimum sample size obtained (n = 121) according to available data [6,19,20] and assuming a difference between groups exceeding 10%, an overall standard deviation of 20%, and 80% power with a two-sided 5% significance level.

DNA genotyping and mRNA expression

The methods used to isolate DNA and assess the presence of CCR-2 V64I, CCR-5 Δ32, and CX3CR-1 (V249I and T280M) variants have been described in detail [6,23] (see Additional file 1: Table S1 for additional information). RNA in circulating leukocytes was isolated using an ABI PRISM 6100 (Applied Biosystems), and the expression of selected receptors (CCR5, CCR2, CXCR4 and CX3CR1) was measured using the reagents and methods indicated in Table 1. The results were analysed using RQ Manager Software for automated data analysis. The expression values for the target genes were normalised to the values of a designated endogenous control (GAPDH), which was not affected by the HIV infection in our hands, and expressed in arbitrary units [24,25]. We hypothesised that there may be differences between the distribution of the mRNAs and the localisation of the actual proteins and that it was unlikely that surface cell receptors could be delivered to other tissues or undergo posttranslational rearrangements [26].

Statistical analyses

The data were presented as the means plus the standard error of the mean (in parentheses). The normality of the distributions was assessed using the Kolmogorov-Smirnov method. The groups were compared using Student's unpaired *t*-test or Kruskal–Wallis one-way analysis. There were no adjustments for multiple testing for genetic analyses because the variants were not rare and the correspondence for their phenotypes was absent according to the described procedures [27]. The χ^2 test was used to compare categorical variables. Multivariate logistic regression stepwise analyses were performed to detect factors associated with the condition of progressors. Odds ratios were included when necessary. Allelic frequency descriptions and Hardy-Weinberg equilibrium tests were performed using freely available software (http://bioinfo.iconcologia.net/SNPstats). To create a "quasi-randomised" experiment, we used the propensity score analyses described previously [28-30]. For other measurements, we used SPSS software version 18.0 (SPSS Inc., Chicago, IL).

Results and discussion

In accordance with our expectations, most of the patients included in the study were considered progressors (n = 142); however, a substantial number of patients demonstrated no evidence of increased IMT values during the 2-year study (n = 36). The patients who demonstrated progression of subclinical atherosclerosis were treated with either an efavirenz-based regimen (38%) or protease inhibitors (39%), and a number of patients were left untreated. The majority of the patients maintained a low viral load. The treatment regimens for patients who did not demonstrate progression were similar. We did not observe a between-group difference in the lipid-lowering and/or hypoglycaemic treatments, and to avoid confusion, none of the patients were taking CCR5 antagonists.

The treatment and other baseline clinical and laboratory variables (Table 2) did not allow the prediction of whether subclinical atherosclerosis would progress. However, this does not mean that any of these variables could be determinants of progression because according to our study design, only negligible changes were allowed. We appreciate that this is not feasible for normal clinical management procedures; however, we believe it would be helpful to search for other possible predisposing factors. Intervention and randomisation were not used in this study. The presence of bias was considered unlikely but could be a limitation of the study as discussed below. Despite these considerations, we reasonably excluded the robust influence of factors such as age, gender, smoking habits, lipoprotein disturbances, the presence of lipodystrophy (fat loss or accumulation perceived by the patient or the clinician) or HCV co-infection, inflammation and insulin resistance (Table 2).

Arguably, a 2-year follow-up might not be sufficient to evaluate the full effect of the variables. A longer follow-up to ascertain the role of host-related, genetically determined variants, however, is not feasible because the progression of carotid atherosclerosis in these patients is

Table 1 Summary of taqman® gene expression assays used in this study*

Gene symbol	Assay ID*	Context sequence	Amplicon length (bp)
CX3CR1	Hs00365842_m1	CAGTCCACGCCAGGCCTTCACCATG	84
CCR2	Hs00174150_m1	GGGGAGAAGTTCAGAAGCCTTTTTC	74
CXCR4	Hs00607978_s1	CCTGTCCTGCTATTGCATTATCATC	153
CCR5	Hs00152917_m1	GAAACTCTCCCCGGGTGGAACAAGA	98
GAPDH	Hs99999905_m1	TTGGGCGCCTGGTCACCAGGGCTGC	124

*Thermal cycling and fluorescence detection was performed on the Applied Biosystems ABI Prism 7900HT Detection System with ABI Prism 7900HT SDS Software 2.2. Forty cycles were run with the following parameters: 2 mins at 50°C and 10 mins at 94.5°C and for each cycle 30 secs at 97°C for denaturation and 1 min at 59.7°C for transcription. FAM was the reporter dye.

Table 2 Baseline participants' clinical and laboratory characteristics blindly collated from medical records at the end of the study

	Non-progressors (n = 36; 20%)	Progressors (n = 142; 80%)	p value
Age, years.	42.1 (1.5)	42.3 (8.2)	NS
Male, n (%)	22 (61.1)	105 (73.9)	NS
BMI, kg/m^2	22.9 (0.5)	23 (3.2)	NS
Current smokers, n (%)	27 (75.8)	92 (64.6)	NS
Systolic blood pressure, mm Hg	116 (2)	123 (2)	NS
Diastolic blood pressure, mm Hg	77 (1)	78 (1)	NS
Baseline IMT, mm	0.81 (0.03)	0.75 (0.02)	NS
Final IMT, mm	0.81 (0.02)	0.94 (0.02)	<0.0001
Δ IMT, mm	0 (0.01)	0.19 (0.02)	<0.0001
Total cholesterol, mmol/L	4.62 (0.21)	4.63 (0.14)	NS
HDL cholesterol, mmol/L	1.21 (0.05)	1.12 (0.04)	NS
LDL cholesterol, mmol/L	2.44 (0.14)	2.54 (0.12)	NS
Triglycerides, mmol/L	2.42 (0.33)	2.31 (0.29)	NS
Apolipoprotein A I, mmol/L	1.42 (0.04)	1.45 (0.04)	NS
Oxidized-LDL, ng/mL	86.4 (5.3)	98.6 (12.7)	NS
Lipodystrophy, n (%)	23 (63.9)	101 (71.1)	NS
HVC co-infection, n (%)	24 (66.7)	77 (54.2)	NS
hs-CRP, mg/L.	4.4 (0.7)	3.8 (0.7)	NS
Insulin, pmol/L	81.2 (10)	71 (8)	NS
Glucose, mmol/L.	5.4 (0.2)	5.2 (0.4)	NS
HIV-1 RNA < 50 copies/mL, n (%)	28 (77.2)	110 (77.5)	NS
CD4 cell count, cell/mm^3	575 (45)	485 (37)	NS
CD8 cell count, cell/mm^3	1020 (65)	994 (55)	NS
Δ CD4 cell count, cell/mm^3	37 (36)	36 (31)	NS

BMI, body mass index; HDL, high density lipoprotein; IMT, intima-media thickness; LDL, low density lipoprotein. Propensity scores calculated via regression analyses were close to 0 indicating that the probability of these variables affecting the progression in IMT is low.

faster than in non-infected patients, and the evaluation of non-classical factors requires shorter periods [19,20]. We have previously demonstrated non-concordance between subclinical atherosclerosis and the calculated Framingham risk score in HIV-infected patients [31]. However, the issue of non-concordance is under debate and in a recent study, increased Framingham risk scores were associated with abnormal early and late surrogate markers of atherosclerosis. However, low scores were also associated with significant subclinical atherosclerosis in these patients [32].

Despite the identification of several trends (Table 3), the distribution of selected chemokine-related genetic variants did not demonstrate significant differences between the progressors and non-progressors. Next, we measured the mRNA expression of chemokine receptors involved in HIV entry into leukocytes. The chemokine receptors were selected according to available data implicating these receptors in the course of atherosclerosis. Interestingly, we observed that the variant CCR5 Δ32 was responsible for the increased expression of these receptors, but only CCR2 and CCR5 reached statistical significance (Figure 1). Patients who expressed the CCR2 V62I gene variant also demonstrated a two-fold higher expression (p = 0.004) of CCR5 compared with non-carriers (data not shown). The expression of chemokine receptors, especially CCR5, did not correlate with increases in IMT. However, CX3CR1 expression demonstrated a marginal effect ($\rho = 0.21$, $P = 0.053$). The lack of significant correlations does not discard a quantitative relationship because

Table 3 Allelic frequency for selected polymorphisms as segregated according to the progression in IMT measurements during a two-year period

Allele	Non-progressors	Progressors	P-value
CXC3CR-1 249 V	0.61	0.50	NS
CXC3CR-1 280 M	0.10	0.12	NS
CCR2 62 I	0.07	0.08	NS
CCR5 Δ32	0.03	0.08	0.08

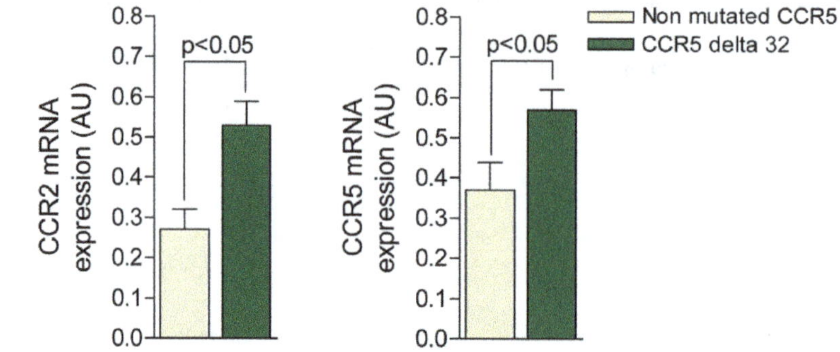

Figure 1 The presence of the CCR-5 Δ32 polymorphism in HIV-infected patients was associated with a significant increase in the expression of CCR2 and CCR5 in circulating leukocytes with respect to patients without the mutation. Similarly, the CCR2 V62I was also associated with a similarly higher CCR5 expression (data not shown).

the influence of high variability and the absence of normal distribution may mask the association between continuous variables.

We observed that the expression of CCR2 and CXCR4 did not discriminate between progressors and non-progressors, and the expression of CCR5 and CX3CR1 was significantly higher in the progressors (Figure 2). These results are plausible because the data obtained in humans and animal models indicate that CCR5 is crucial for monocyte recruitment, and CX3CR1 appears to sustain chronic monocyte adhesion and survival within the plaque in diseased arteries during atherosclerosis development [33,34]. Because the increase in CCR5 and CX3CR1 expression was higher in not only progressors but also the patients with detectable viral load, our data might support a role for the virus in determining the rapid development of atherosclerosis [35,36]. No differences were found in CXCR4; however, the expression of CCR2 was 3-fold higher in patients with a detectable viral load ($p = 0.007$), an effect that was considered independent of the condition of either progressors or non-progressors (Figure 3). Therefore, further studies will be needed to ascertain a relationship between relatively poor management of the infection and the development

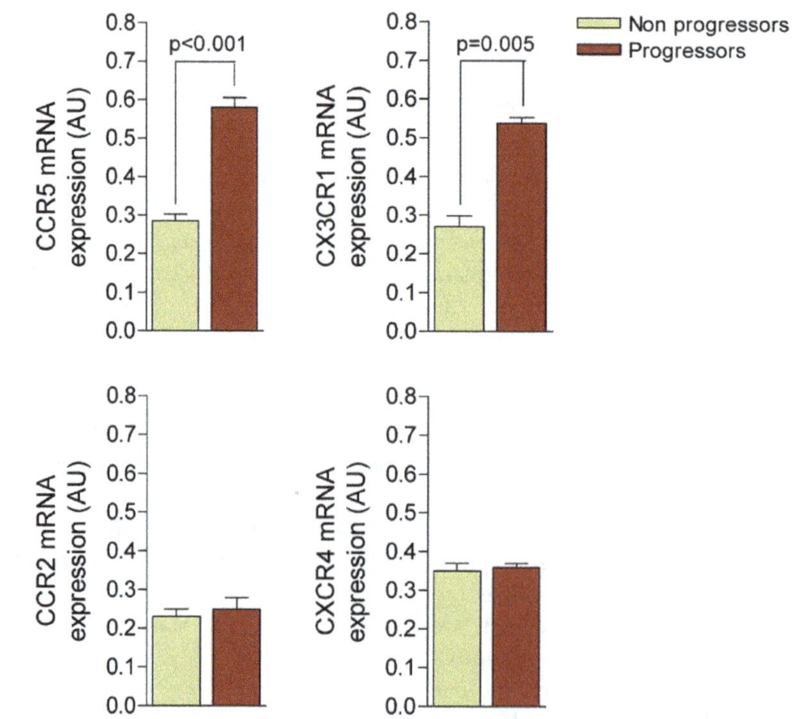

Figure 2 The expression of CCR2 and CXCR4 in circulating leukocytes from progressors and non-progressors was similar but there were a significant increase in CCR5 and CX3CR1 in patients who showed progression in intima-media thickness.

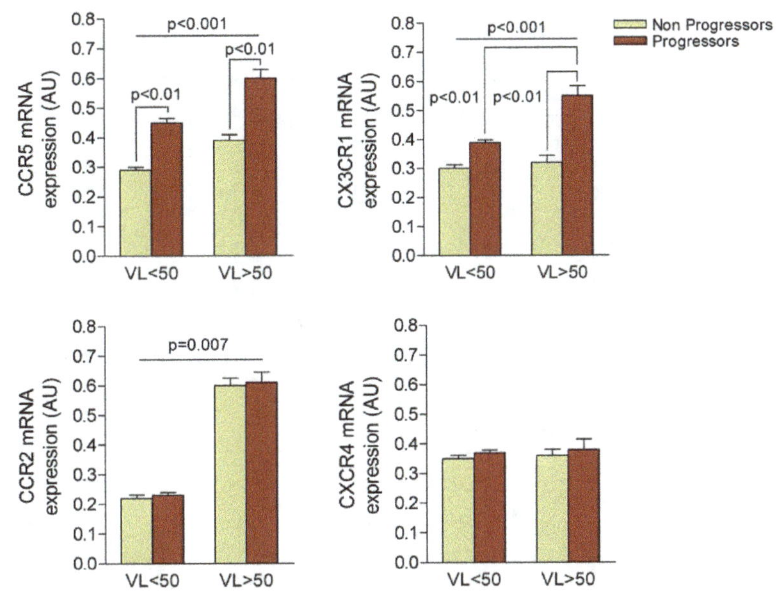

Figure 3 Detectable viral load (VL) was also a determinant factor in the rate of expression of chemokine receptors with the exception of CXCR4. The expression of CCR2 was higher in patients with detectable viral load but this difference was not related to the progression of atherosclerosis. Conversely, the increase in CCR5 and CX3CR1 expression was not only higher in progressors but also in those with detectable viral load.

of vascular lesions. This interpretation is substantiated by the observation that a number of chemokines block or delay viral entry by interfering with HIV co-receptors [37]. There are multiple plausible mechanisms underlying the interference between the retroviral life cycle and chemokines. First, endothelial cells line the entire cardiovascular system and are frequently in contact with memory CD4+ T cells, which provide signals to HIV-1 -infected CD4+ T cells to enhance HIV-1 production, an effect that persists despite antiretroviral therapy [36]. Second, infiltrating HIV-infected monocytes/macrophages promote proinflammatory effects *per se*. This process is important because HIV itself can infect vascular smooth muscle cells via a mechanism dependent on chemokine receptors, and this may partially explain the exacerbated atherosclerosis reported in infected individuals [37].

The course of HIV infection, however, may also be associated with other factors, such as body mass index (BMI), high-density lipoproteins (HDLs) or reverse cholesterol transport from macrophages, the amount of circulating oxidised low-density lipoproteins (LDL-ox) and the number of $CD8^+$ T cells in the blood [38-40]. We investigated this possibility and determined that when the values of these variables were divided into tertiles, a qualitatively similar effect on the expression of CCR5 and CX3CR1 was observed (Figure 4). The expression of both receptors was higher in patients with the highest BMI, LDL-ox and $CD8^+$ T cells. Additionally, patients with the lowest value for HDL cholesterol demonstrated a higher increase in CCR5 and CX3CR1 expression. These findings support the hypothesis that several modifiable factors cannot be excluded in the assessment of a possible association between the course of accelerated atherosclerosis and the course of HIV infection [31-33,41-43]. Univariate analyses suggested that these assumptions were correct, and multivariate logistic regression analyses determined that the dichotomous model was explained by only a small number of variables (Table 4). Logistic regression was used rather than discriminant function analysis to include predictors lacking normal distribution, and all predictors were used to determine group membership according to outcome (progressors and non-progressors).

Generally, we found that CCR5 expression is the best predictor of progression in atherosclerosis and that a number of host gene variants may have a significant effect. Although CCR2 and CX3CR1 are predisposing factors in atherosclerosis and inflammation [41,42], we also determined that under these conditions, the effects of the expression of these receptors appeared negligible. This is not surprising because the expression of chemokines in different tissues can change in response to multiple stimuli [44].

The predominant role of CCR5 expression in circulating leukocytes in HIV-infected patients as a predictive factor for the rate of progression of atherosclerosis suggests that drugs affecting chemokines should be investigated for their role not only as protective agents in HIV-infection but also in atherosclerosis-related complications. This suggestion is in accordance with the observation that a number of experimental drugs that inhibit HIV entry can

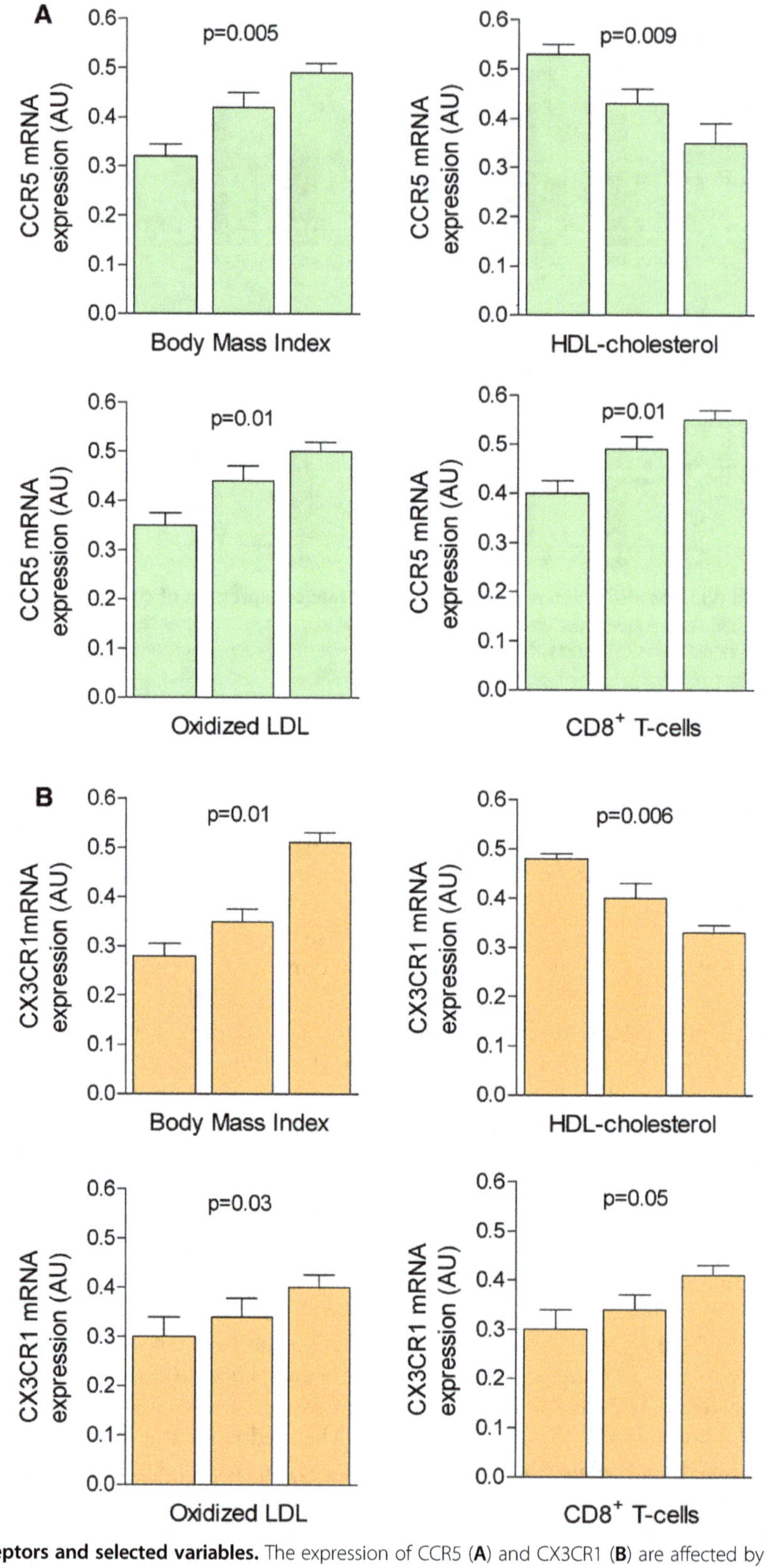

Figure 4 Chemokine receptors and selected variables. The expression of CCR5 (**A**) and CX3CR1 (**B**) are affected by modifiable factors and increased in patients with the highest values of body mass index, the concentration of oxidized LDL-ox, and the number of circulating CD8$^+$ T cells and the lowest value for HDL-cholesterol. The cutoff values for the first and second tertiles were respectively: BMI, 20.1 and 23.3; HDL-cholesterol, 0.84 and 1.11 mmol/L; ox-LDL, 51.1 and 80.2 ng/mL, and CD8, 592 and 920 cells/mm^3.

Table 4 Significant predictor variables found in multivariate logistic regression stepwise analysis used for the binary outcome (progressors and non-progressors) with respect to subclinical atherosclerosis

	B	Wald	p value	Odds ratio	CI 95% for OR	
					Lower	Upper
CCR5 expression	2.1	3.9	0.04	8.1	1	65
CCR5 Δ32	−2.2	4.9	0.02	0.1	0.01	0.71
CX3CR1 280 V	−2.9	7	0.008	0.05	0.005	0.462
CX3CR1 249 M	−1.4	3.5	0.05	0.24	0.05	1.05

arrest the progression of atheroma plaques in animal models [45-47] and that CCR5 antagonists can affect cardiovascular risk factors [48,49]. Therefore, we propose that available CCR5 antagonists that have been clinically validated should be considered as not only antiviral drugs but also potentially useful agents for the management of inflammation-related diseases.

Possible limitations of the study

Biases are particularly difficult to avoid in studies with these characteristics. However, in this study, recall bias and detection bias were essentially excluded from the design. We also excluded the possibility that the increase in the IMT measurement was sensitive to small, unmeasured confounders (hidden biases) because the patients were examined at least 8 times during the study according to a strict clinical protocol for the detection of the outcome and related variables. Additionally, covariate adjustment using propensity score analyses demonstrated good performance, with scores reflecting a low probability that the participant's baseline characteristics played a role in the increase in IMT. Finally, we appreciate that the length of the follow-up may be important and should be considered carefully when replicating our findings.

Competing interests

The authors declare that they have no competing interests and have no conflict of interest to declare.

Authors' contributions

All authors have contributed to the acquisition, analysis and interpretation of data and have been involved in drafting and revising the manuscript. The design was initially conceived by C A-V, L F-S and JJ. All authors have given final approval of the version to be published and may take public responsibility of the content.

Acknowledgements

The funding source and granting support played no role in the study design; in the collection, analysis and interpretation of data; in the writing of the manuscript; or in the decision to submit the manuscript for publication. The Unitat de Recerca Biomèdica is financially supported by the Instituto de Salud Carlos III (Ministerio de Sanidad y Consumo y Fondo de Investigación Sanitaria) through competitive grants PI11/00130, PI11/02187, PI08/01381 and PI08/01175.

Author details

[1]Unitat de Recerca Biomèdica, Hospital Universitari Sant Joan, Institut d'Investigació Sanitaria Pere Virgili (IISPV), Universitat Rovira i Virgili, Reus, Spain, carrer Sant Llorenç 21, Reus 43201, Spain. [2]Pressent address: Servei de Medicina Interna, Hospital Sant Pau i Santa Tecla, carrer Rambla Vella 14, Tarragona 43003, Spain. [3]Translational Research Laboratory, Catalan Institute of Oncology (ICO) and Girona Biomedical Research Institute (IdIBGi), Avda de França s/n 17007, Girona, Spain.

References

1. Alonso-Villaverde C, Coll B, Parra S, Montero M, Calvo N, Tous M, Joven J, Masana L: **Atherosclerosis in patients infected with HIV is influenced by a mutant monocyte chemoattractant protein-1 allele.** *Circulation* 2004, **110**:2204–9.
2. Önen NF, Overton ET: **A review of premature frailty in HIV-infected persons; another manifestation of HIV-related accelerated aging.** *Curr Aging Sci* 2011, **4**:33–41.
3. Piggott DA, Muzaale AD, Mehta SH, Brown TT, Patel KV, Leng SX, Kirk GD: **Frailty, HIV Infection, and Mortality in an Aging Cohort of Injection Drug Users.** *PLoS One* 2013, **8**(1):e54910.
4. Renga B, Francisci D, D'Amore C, Schiaroli E, Mencarelli A, Cipriani S, Baldelli F, Fiorucci S: **The HIV Matrix Protein p17 Subverts Nuclear Receptors Expression and Induces a STAT1-Dependent Proinflammatory Phenotype in Monocytes.** *PLoS One* 2012, **7**(4):e35924.
5. Coll B, Alonso-Villaverde C, Joven J: **Monocyte chemoattractant protein-1 and atherosclerosis: is there room for an additional biomarker?** *Clin Chim Acta* 2007, **383**:21–9.
6. Coll B, Parra S, Alonso-Villaverde C, Aragonés G, Montero M, Camps J, Joven J, Masana L: **The role of immunity and inflammation in the progression of atherosclerosis in patients with HIV infection.** *Stroke* 2007, **38**:2477–84.
7. Koenen RR, Weber C: **Chemokines: established and novel targets in atherosclerosis.** *EMBO Mol Med* 2011, **3**:713–25.
8. Kanzler I, Liehn EA, Koenen RR, Weber C: **Anti-inflammatory therapeutic approaches to reduce acute atherosclerotic complications.** *Curr Pharm Biotechnol* 2012, **13**(1):37–45.
9. Sullivan TJ, Dairaghi DJ, Krasinski A, Miao Z, Wang Y, Zhao BN, Baumgart T, Berahovich R, Ertl LS, Pennell A, Seitz L, Miao S, Ungashe S, Wei Z, Johnson D, Boring L, Tsou CL, Charo IF, Bekker P, Schall TJ, Jaen JC: **Characterization of CCX140-B, an orally bioavailable antagonist of the CCR2 chemokine receptor, for the treatment of type 2 diabetes and associated complications.** *J Pharmacol Exp Ther* 2012. doi:10.1124/jpet.111.190918.
10. Yadav A, Saini V, Arora S: **MCP-1: chemoattractant with a role beyond immunity: a review.** *Clin Chim Acta* 2010, **411**:1570–9.
11. Jones KL, Maguire JJ, Davenport AP: **Chemokine receptor CCR5: from AIDS to atherosclerosis.** *Br J Pharmacol* 2011, **162**:1453–69.
12. Samson M, Libert F, Doranz BJ, Rucker J, Liesnard C, Farber CM, Saragosti S, Lapoumeroulie C, Cognaux J, Forceille C, Muyldermans G, Verhofstede C, Burtonboy G, Georges M, Imai T, Rana S, Yi Y, Smyth RJ, Collman RG, Doms RW, Vassart G, Parmentier M: **Resistance to HIV-1 infection in Caucasian individuals bearing mutant alleles of the CCR-5 chemokine receptor gene.** *Nature* 1996, **382**:722–25.
13. Afzal AR, Kiechl S, Daryani YP, Weerasinghe A, Zhang Y, Reindl M, Mayr A, Weger S, Xu Q, Willeit J: **Common CCR5-del32 frameshift mutation associated with serum levels of inflammatory markers and cardiovascular disease risk in the Bruneck population.** *Stroke* 2008, **39**:1972–8.
14. Dorr P, Westby M, Dobbs S, Griffin P, Irvine B, Macartney M, Mori J, Rickett G, Smith-Burchnell C, Napier C, Webster R, Armour D, Price D, Stammen B, Wood A, Perros M: **Maraviroc (UK-427,857), a potent, orally bioavailable, and selective small-molecule inhibitor of chemokine receptor CCR5 with broad-spectrum anti-human immunodeficiency virus type 1 activity.** *Antimicrob Agents Chemother* 2005, **49**:4721–32.

15. Parra J, Portilla J, Pulido F, Sánchez-de la Rosa R, Alonso-Villaverde C, Berenguer J, Blanco JL, Domingo P, Dronda F, Galera C, Gutiérrez F, Kindelán JM, Knobel H, Leal M, López-Aldeguer J, Mariño A, Miralles C, Moltó J, Ortega E, Oteo JA: **Clinical utility of maraviroc.** *Clin Drug Investig* 2011, **31**:527–542.
16. Umehara H, Bloom ET, Okazaki T, Nagano Y, Yoshie O, Imai T: **Fractalkine in vascular biology: from basic research to clinical disease.** *Arterioscler Thromb Vasc Biol* 2004, **24**:34–40.
17. Mc Dermott DH, Halcox JPJ, Schenke WH, Waclawiw MA, Merrell MN, Epstein N, Quyyumi AA, Murphy PM: **Association between polymorphism in the chemokine receptor CX3CR1 and coronary vascular endothelial dysfunction and atherosclerosis.** *Circ Res* 2001, **89**:401–7.
18. Pineda JA, González J, Ortega E, Tural C, Macías J, Griffa L, Burgos A, Grafihco Study Team: **Prevalence and factors associated with significant liver fibrosis assessed by transient elastometry in HIV/hepatitis C virus-coinfected patients.** *J Viral Hepat* 2010, **17**:714–9.
19. Mangili A, Polak JF, Skinner SC, Gerrior J, Sheehan H, Harrington A, Wanke CA: **HIV infection and progression of carotid and coronary atherosclerosis: the CARE study.** *J Acquir Immune Defic Syndr* 2011, **58**(2):148–53.
20. Papasavvas E, Hsue P, Reynolds G, Pistilli M, Hancock A, Martin JN, Deeks SG, Montaner LJ: **Increased CD34(+)/KDR(+) cells are not associated with carotid artery intima-media thickness progression in chronic HIV-positive subjects.** *Antivir Ther* 2012, **17**(3):557–63.
21. Martinez E, Mocroft A, García-Viejo MA, Perez-Cuevas JB, Blanco JL, Mallolas J, Bianchi L, Conget I, Blanch J, Phillips A, Gatell JM: **Risk of lipodystrophy in HIV-1-infected patients treated with protease inhibitors: a prospective cohort study.** *Lancet* 2001, **357**:592–8.
22. Simó JM, Castellano I, Ferré N, Joven J, Camps J: **Evaluation of a homogeneous assay for high-density lipoprotein cholesterol: limitations in patients with cardiovascular, renal, and hepatic disorders.** *Clin Chem* 1998, **44**:1233–41.
23. Faaij CM, Willemze AJ, Révész T, Balzarolo M, Tensen CP, Hoogeboom M, Vermeer MH, van Wering E, Zwaan CM, Kaspers GJ, Story C, van Halteren AG, Vossen JM, Egeler RM, van Tol MJ, Annels NE: **Chemokine/chemokine receptor interactions in extramedullary leukaemia of the skin in childhood AML: differential roles for CCR2, CCR5, CXCR4 and CXCR7.** *Pediatr Blood Cancer* 2010, **55**(2):344–8.
24. Alonso-Villaverde C, Aragonès G, Beltrán-Debón R, Fernández-Sender L, Rull A, Rodríguez-Sanabria F, Marsillach J, Pardo-Reche P, Camps J, Joven J: **Host-pathogen interactions in the development of metabolic disturbances and atherosclerosis in HIV infection: the role of CCL2 genetic variants.** *Cytokine* 2010, **51**:251–8.
25. Alonso-Villaverde C, Aragonès G, Beltrán-Debón R, Fernández-Sender L, Rull A, Camps J, Alegret JM, Joven J: **Treatment of hypertriglyceridemia and HIV: fenofibrate-induced changes in the expression of chemokine genes in circulating leukocytes.** *AIDS Res Ther* 2009, **6**:26.
26. Mackness B, Beltran-Debon R, Aragones G, Joven J, Camps J, Mackness M: **Human tissue distribution of paraoxonases 1 and 2 mRNA.** *IUBMB Life* 2010, **62**(6):480–2.
27. Kang SJ, Gordon D, Finch SJ: **What SNP genotyping errors are most costly for genetic association studies?** *Genet Epidemiol* 2004, **26**:132–41.
28. Normand SL, Sykora K, Li P, Mamdani M, Rochon PA, Anderson GM: **Readers guide to critical appraisal of cohort studies: 3.** *Analytical strategies to reduce confounding. BMJ* 2005, **330**(7498):1021–3.
29. Weitzen S, Lapane KL, Toledano AY, Hume AL, Mor V: **Principles for modeling propensity scores in medical research: a systematic literature review.** *Pharmacoepidemiol Drug Saf* 2004, **13**(12):841–53.
30. Shah BR, Laupacis A, Hux JE, Austin PC: **Propensity score methods gave similar results to traditional regression modeling in observational studies: a systematic review.** *J Clin Epidemiol* 2005, **58**(6):550–9.
31. Parra S, Coll B, Aragonés G, Marsillach J, Beltrán R, Rull A, Joven J, Alonso-Villaverde C, Camps J: **Nonconcordance between subclinical atherosclerosis and the calculated Framingham risk score in HIV-infected patients: relationships with serum markers of oxidation and inflammation.** *HIV Med* 2010, **11**(4):225–31.
32. Falcone EL, Mangili A, Skinner S, Alam A, Polak JF, Wanke CA: **Framingham risk score and early markers of atherosclerosis in a cohort of adults infected with HIV.** *Antivir Ther* 2011, **16**(1):1–8.
33. Zernecke A, Shagdarsuren E, Weber C: **Chemokines in atherosclerosis: an update.** *Arterioscler Thromb Vasc Biol* 2008, **28**(11):1897–908.
34. Gautier EL, Jakubzick C, Randolph GJ: **Regulation of the migration and survival of monocyte subsets by chemokine receptors and its relevance to atherosclerosis.** *Arterioscler Thromb Vasc Biol* 2009, **29**(10):1412–8.
35. Vicenzi E, Biswas P, Mengozzi M, Poli G: **Role of pro-inflammatory cytokines and beta-chemokines in controlling HIV replication.** *J Leukoc Biol* 1997, **62**(1):34–40.
36. Choi J, Walker J, Talbert-Slagle K, Wright P, Pober JS, Alexander L: **Endothelial cells promote human immunodeficiency virus replication in nondividing memory T cells via Nef-, Vpr-, and T-cell receptor-dependent activation of NFAT.** *J Virol* 2005, **79**(17):11194–204.
37. Eugenin EA, Morgello S, Klotman ME, Mosoian A, Lento PA, Berman JW, Schecter AD: **Human immunodeficiency virus (HIV) infects human arterial smooth muscle cells in vivo and in vitro: implications for the pathogenesis of HIV-mediated vascular disease.** *Am J Pathol* 2008, **172**(4):1100–11.
38. Rose H, Hoy J, Woolley I, Tchoua U, Bukrinsky M, Dart A, Sviridov D: **HIV-infection and high density lipoprotein metabolism.** *Atherosclerosis* 2008, **199**(1):79–86.
39. Mujawar Z, Rose H, Morrow MP, Pushkarsky T, Dubrovsky L, Mukhamedova N, Fu Y, Dart A, Orenstein JM, Bobryshev YV, Bukrinsky M, Sviridov D: **Human immunodeficiency virus impairs reverse cholesterol transport from macrophages.** *PLoS Biol* 2006, **4**(11):e365.
40. Aragonès G, García-Heredia A, Guardiola M, Rull A, Beltrán-Debón R, Marsillach J, Alonso-Villaverde C, Mackness B, Mackness M, Pedro-Botet J, Pardo-Reche P, Joven J, Camps J: **Serum paraoxonase-3 concentration in HIV-infected patients.** *Evidence for a protective role against oxidation. J Lipid Res* 2012, **53**(1):168–74.
41. Postea O, Vasina EM, Cauwenberghs S, Projahn D, Liehn EA, Lievens D, Theelen W, Kramp BK, Butoi ED, Soehnlein O, Heemskerk JW, Ludwig A, Weber C, Koenen RR: **Contribution of platelet CX(3)CR1 to platelet-monocyte complex formation and vascular recruitment during hyperlipidemia.** *Arterioscler Thromb Vasc Biol* 2012, **32**(5):1186–93.
42. Suresh P, Wanchu A: **Chemokines and chemokine receptors in HIV infection: role in pathogenesis and therapeutics.** *J Postgrad Med* 2006, **52**(3):210–7.
43. Paul A, Calleja L, Camps J, Osada J, Vilella E, Ferré N, Mayayo E, Joven J: **The continuous administration of aspirin attenuates atherosclerosis in apolipoprotein E-deficient mice.** *Life Sci* 2000, **68**(4):457–65.
44. Tous M, Ferré N, Rull A, Marsillach J, Coll B, Alonso-Villaverde C, Camps J, Joven J: **Dietary cholesterol and differential monocyte chemoattractant protein-1 gene expression in aorta and liver of apo E-deficient mice.** *Biochem Biophys Res Commun* 2006, **340**(4):1078–84.
45. van Wanrooij EJ, Happé H, Hauer AD, de Vos P, Imanishi T, Fujiwara H, van Berkel TJ, Kuiper J: **HIV entry inhibitor TAK-779 attenuates atherogenesis in low-density lipoprotein receptor-deficient mice.** *Arterioscler Thromb Vasc Biol* 2005, **25**(12):2642–7.
46. Feng Y, Broder CC, Kennedy PE, Berger EA: **HIV-1 entry cofactor: functional cDNA cloning of a seven-transmembrane, G protein-coupled receptor.** *Science* 1996, **272**:872–6.
47. Wilen CB, Tilton JC, Doms RW: **Molecular Mechanisms of HIV Entry.** *Adv Exp Med Biol* 2012, **726**:223–42.
48. Funderburg N, Kalinowska M, Eason J, Goodrich J, Heera J, Mayer H, Rajicic N, Valdez H, Lederman MM: **Effects of maraviroc and efavirenz on markers of immune activation and inflammation and associations with CD4+ cell rises in HIV-infected patients.** *PLoS One* 2010, **5**(10):e13188.
49. Aukrust P, Yndestad A, Smith C, Ueland T, Gullestad L, Damås JK: **Chemokines in cardiovascular risk prediction.** *Thromb Haemost* 2007, **97**:748–54.

11

High virologic response rate after second-line boosted protease inhibitor-based antiretroviral therapy regimens in children from a resource limited setting

Thanyawee Puthanakit[1,2], Gonzague Jourdain[3], Piyarat Suntarattiwong[4], Kulkanya Chokephaibulkit[5], Umaporn Siangphoe[1], Tulathip Suwanlerk[1], Wasana Prasitsuebsai[1,5], Virat Sirisanthana[6], Pope Kosalaraksa[7], Witaya Petdachai[8], Rawiwan Hansudewechakul[9], Naris Waranawat[4] and Jintanat Ananworanich[1,10,11*] On behalf of the HIV-NAT 086 study team

Abstract

Background: Limited data exist for the efficacy of second-line antiretroviral therapy among children in resource limited settings. We assessed the virologic response to protease inhibitor-based ART after failing first-line non-nucleoside reverse transcriptase inhibitor (NNRTI)-based regimens.

Methods: A retrospective chart review was conducted at 8 Thai sites of children who switched to PI –based regimens due to failure of NNRTI –based regimens. Primary endpoints were HIV RNA < 400 copies/ml and CD4 change over 48 weeks.

Results: Data from 241 children with median baseline values before starting PI-based regimens of 9.1 years for age, 10% for CD4%, and 4.8 $\log_{10}$ copies/ml for HIV RNA were included; 104 (41%) received a single ritonavir-boosted PI (sbPI) with 2 NRTIs and 137 (59%) received double-boosted PI (dbPI) with/without NRTIs based on physician discretion. SbPI children had higher baseline CD4 (17% vs. 6%, $p < 0.001$), lower HIV RNA (4.5 vs. 4.9 $\log_{10}$ copies/ml, $p < 0.001$), and less frequent high grade multi NRTI resistance (12.4% vs 60.5%, $p < 0.001$) than the dbPI children. At week 48, 81% had HIV RNA < 400 copies/ml (sbPI 83.1% vs. dbPI 79.8%, $p = 0.61$) with a median CD4 rise of 9% (+7%vs. + 10%, $p < 0.005$). However, only 63% had HIV RNA < 50 copies/ml, with better viral suppression seen in sbPI (76.6% vs. 51.4%, p 0.002).

Conclusion: Second-line PI therapy was effective for children failing first line NNRTI in a resource-limited setting. DbPI were used in patients with extensive drug resistance due to limited treatment options. Better access to antiretroviral drugs is needed.

Keywords: Pediatric HIV, Drug resistance, Second-line antiretroviral therapy, Protease-inhibitors, Resource limited settings

* Correspondence: Jintanat.A@hivnat.org
[1]The HIV Netherlands Australia Thailand Research Collaboration (HIV-NAT), Bangkok, Thailand
[10]South East Asia Research Collaboration with Hawaii, Hawaii, Thailand
Full list of author information is available at the end of the article

Introduction

The most commonly used first-line antiretroviral therapy (ART) in HIV-infected children in resource-limited settings (RLS) is a non nucleoside reverse transcriptase inhibitor (NNRTI)-based treatment[1,2]. Data from individual cohorts in Thailand [3], Uganda [4] Cambodia [5] and those from a meta-analysis of 1457 children [1] showed that 70–81% had viral suppression after 1 year of first-line treatment. Several pediatric programs in RLS have begun to provide second-line therapy; 5.8% and 20% among cohorts of HIV-infected children in South Africa [6] and the TREAT Asia regional network [7], but treatment outcomes data are limited. The second-line regimen for children failing NNRTI-based treatment in all treatment guidelines is a low-dose ritonavir boosting protease inhibitors (boosted PI) in combination with 2 nucleoside reverse transcriptase inhibitors (NRTIs) [8,9] which was reasonably effective [10].

However, in RLS without routine virologic monitoring, the diagnosis of treatment failure is usually late, of which brings about concerns for multi-NRTI resistance [11]. Reported incidence rate of multi-NRTI drug resistance from cohort with routine viral load monitoring is only 8% [12] compared to 36% seen in settings in which treatment failure was detected by clinical or immunologic criteria [13]. In such cases in RLS, the only effective anti-retroviral (ARV) drug option available for second-line therapy is boosted PI with limited choices for effective NRTIs. Often times, double-boosted PI regimens are used to provide 2 active agents in the regimen. Double-boosted PIs is an alternative second-line therapy option in the Thai National Guideline; however, there have been limited data of its safety and efficacy in HIV-infected children [14].

The primary objective of this study is to describe the immunologic and virologic efficacy of second-line ARV regimens containing either single- or double-boosted PI over a 48-week period in children with NNRTI-based treatment failure in Thailand.

Material and methods

Study design and subjects

We formed a network of 8 large pediatric HIV centers in Thailand to retrospectively collect treatment outcome data of all children who failed NNRTI-based therapy and received ritonavir-boosted PI regimen as a second-line drug regimen. Immunologic treatment failure was defined according to the Thai guideline either CD4 percentage decline > 5 percentage point in a patient with CD4% less than 15, or CD4 cell count drop > 30% of baseline within 6 months [15]. Before 2006, the access to plasma HIV RNA monitoring was limited and it was performed after immunologic failure was suspected. Virological failure was defined as HIV RNA > 1000 copies/ml after at least 6 months of antiretroviral therapy. After 2006, annual HIV RNA was accessible through the national program. In some cases, genotypic resistance testing was performed before switching to second-line regimens, and the test was performed only if plasma HIV RNA was > 1,000 copies/ml.

Cases selected were HIV-infected children aged < 18 years, with a documented history of immunologic or virologic failure on NNRTI-based ART who received ritonavir-boosted PIs-based regimen for at least 24 weeks. They were excluded if they had previously received PIs treatment prior to the ritonavir-boosted PIs for longer than 30 days, or received second-line drugs not belonging to the NRTI, NNRTI, and PI classes. Standardized forms were used for retrospective hospital chart extraction: include demographics, CDC HIV clinical classification, history of ART, CD4 cell count and percentage, and genotypic resistance test result before switching to PI-based HAART. Follow up CD4, plasma HIV RNA and adverse events after switch to PI regimen were extracted and censored at last patient visit. After switching to second-line therapy, CD4 was uniformly monitored every 6 months and HIV RNA every 6–12 months. Single-boosted PI was defined as low dose ritonavir combined with one other PI drug. Double-boosted PI was defined as low dose ritonavir combined with another two PI drugs, or therapeutic dose ritonavir (350–400 mg/m^2/dose) combined with one other PI drug.

The HIV RNA testing was performed using 50 copies/ml as the limit of detection, except for some cases in the early 2000s which used 400 copies/ml as the detection limit. Genotypic resistance testing was performed by TrueGene HIV-1 Genotyping system (Visible Genetics, Inc., Toronto, Canada) at 5 sites, ViroSeq HIV-1 Genotyping System (Celera Diagnostics, Alameda, Calif.) at 1 site and with an in house method using Stanford and International AIDS society (IAS) database [16] at 2 sites. The study was approved by the Ethics Committees at all sites.

Statistical analysis

Primary endpoints were the proportion of children with plasma HIV RNA < 400 copies/ml at week 48 and the CD4 changes at 48 weeks after switching to second-line PI therapy. Secondary endpoints were the proportion of children with plasma HIV RNA < 50 copies/ml and the prevalence of adverse events. The analysis was performed using available data.

The cumulative probability of virologic treatment failure defined as HIV RNA > 400 copies/ml after at least 6 months of second-line boosted PI regimen was calculated using the Kaplan Meier estimates. The data included patients who had HIV RNA result at least once after 24 weeks of treatment and censored at 24 months or earlier in cases of discontinuation of the follow-up. The difference between single- and double -boosted PI was tested using the log rank test.

The predictors for treatment failure defined as HIV RNA < 400 copies/ml at week 48 were explored in a logistic regression model. Factors included CD4 cell count at time of switch to boosted PI regimen (dichotomized as > 100 cells/mm^3), plasma HIV RNA at time of switch to boosted PI regimen (dichotomized as > 10,000 copies/ml), ART regimen as single-boosted PI or double-boosted PI, use of lopinavir/ritonavir (LPV/r) –containing regimen, and grade of resistance mutations. Definition of high grade multi-NRTI resistance was defined as ≥ 4 thymidine analog mutations (TAMs) or the presence of Q151M or 69 insertion. Low grade multi-NRTI resistance was defined as 1 to 3 TAMs. Factors with p-value < 0.2 in the univariate analysis were tested in the multivariate analysis. Analyses were performed using SAS version 9.1(SAS Institute, Cary, NC, USA).

Results

Patient characteristics and antiretroviral regimen

Between September 2002 and June 2007, 241 children were enrolled, including 1, 11, 62, 63, 60, and 44 children per calendar year. There were 104 children who switched to single-boosted PI and 137 children who switched to double-boosted PI (137 children) at 8 HIV pediatric clinics. The baseline characteristics of the children are shown in Table 1. The medians (interquartile range [IQR]) were 9.1 (7.2-11.1) years for age and 2.2 (1.5-2.9) years for duration of NNRTI-based regimen. Among 203 children who had genotypic resistance testing performed, 195 children (96%) had the test result prior to switching to PI-based regimen and the remaining had the test done on stored samples at a later date. The ARV regimens were chosen by physician's discretion based on ARV treatment history, genotypic resistance pattern (if available), and the availability of ARV drugs. Indinavir has been available in national program, since 2002, while LPV/r has been available in national antiretroviral program since 2005. The median follow-up time was 26.0 months (IQR 12.7-36.8). Overall, at the time of switch to second line regimens, the children who were prescribed single-boosted PI were younger (median: 8.9 versus 9.4 years, P = 0.046), had a significantly higher baseline CD4% (17% versus 6%, p < 0.001), a lower baseline plasma HIV RNA (4.5 $\log_{10}$ versus 4.9 $\log_{10}$ copies/ml; p <0.001), and a lower proportion of genotypes with multi-NRTI resistance mutation (12.4% versus 60.5%, p < 0.001) compared with children who received double-boosted PI regimen.

The single-boosted PI regimens included 55 (53%) indinavir/r (IDV/r) and 49 (47%) lopinavir/r (LPV/r). The NRTI backbones used were 50 (48%) zidovudine (AZT) plus lamivudine (3TC), 29 (28%) AZT plus didanosine (ddI), 17 (16%) ddI plus 3TC and 8 (8%) miscellaneous. Among children in the double -boosted PI group, 77 (56%) did not receive any NRTI, 37 (27%) received 3TC as the only NRTI, and 23 (17%) received other NRTIs. The double-boosted PI regimens were LPV/r + IDV in 46 (34%) children, IDV/r + Nelfinavir (NFV) in 24 (18%), LPV/r + Saquinavir (SQV) in 20 (15%), LPV/r + NFV in 17(12%), IDV + RTV in 16(12%), IDV/r + SQV in 8 (6%) and other PIs in 6 (4%) children.

Efficacy of second-line boosted protease inhibitor regimens

At week 24, 223 had CD4 information and 190 had plasma HIV RNA information. The overall median (IQR) CD4% change was 5 (1–8) % with more CD4 rise in children who received double- compared to single-boosted PI (+5% vs. +4%, p < 0.016). Overall 78% achieved HIV RNA < 400 copies/ml. The proportion with HIV RNA < 400 copies/ml was not different between groups; 80.9% (72/89) in single- vs. 76.2% (77/101) in double-boosted PI regimens. The proportion with HIV RNA below 50 copies/ml was 59% overall with a higher proportion in single- compared to double-boosted PI groups: 66.7% (58/87) vs. 51.2% (44/86) p = 0.038).

The outcomes at week 48 after initiation of boosted PI regimens are shown in Table 2. The increase in CD4 percentage was significantly higher among children who received double-boosted PI. Overall, 81.3% had HIV RNA < 400 copies/ml (single-versus double-boosted PI: 83.1% vs. 79.8%, p = 0.61). Sixty-three percent had plasma HIV RNA < 50 copies/ml; a higher proportion of these were children who received single-boosted PI compared with those receiving double-boosted PI (76.6% vs. 51.4%, p = 0.002).

Subgroup analysis was performed for the outcome HIV RNA < 400 copies/ml at week 48. Among children in single-boosted PI group, 30/36 (83.3%) of children who received indinavir/r and 24/29 (82.8%) of children who received lopinavir/r had undetectable viral load (P-value 0.655). Among children in double boosted PI group, 47/57 (82.5%) of children who did not receive any NRTI and 16/22 (72.7%) of children who received NRTIs had undetectable viral load (p-value 0.252).

Adverse events

During the follow-up period, there were 31 adverse events that led to discontinuation or substitution of PI drugs. The median time of discontinuation or substitution were 13.3 months (IQR 7.1-26.0) after start PI-based regimen. There were 20 events for IDV-related toxicity (13% of children who used IDV)due to nephrotoxicity (n = 11), hyperbilirubinemia (n = 4), nausea

Table 1 Baseline Characteristics among 241 HIV-infected children who received second-line protease inhibitor -based antiretroviral therapy

Characteristics	All (n = 241)	Single-boosted PIRegimens[1] (n = 104)	Double-boosted PI regimens[1] (n = 137)	P-value
Gender: Male	117 (49)	55 (53)	62 (45)	0.24
Age, years	9.1 (7.2-11.1)	8.9 (6.1-11.1)	9.4 (7.6-11.2)	**0.046**
Prior to initiate NNRTI regimen				
CDC clinical staging				**0.04**
N	10 (4.2)	7 (6.7)	3 (2.2)	
A	58 (24.3)	29 (27.9)	29 (21.6)	
B	113 (47.3)	39 (37.5)	74 (54.8)	
C	58 (24.3)	29 (27.9)	29 (21.5)	
CD4 percentage	5 (1–10)	3.5 (1–11)	5 (2–10)	0.53
CD4 cell/mm^3	109 (27–410)	109 (21–395)	112 (28–413)	0.51
Prior to switch to second-line boosted -PI regimen				
Weight for age Z-score	−1.7 (−2.1 to −0.9)	−1.4 (−1.9 to −0.7)	−1.9 (−2.3 to −1.4)	**<0.001**
CD4% (n = 239)	10 (4–18)	17 (7–24)	6 (2–12)	**<0.001**
CD4 cell/mm^3 (n = 238)	195 (70–442)	379 (165–659)	123 (38–273)	**<0.001**
HIV RNA, log $_{10}$ copies/mL (n = 227)	4.8 (4.3-5.3)	4.5 (3.9-5.1)	4.9 (4.5-5.4)	**<0.001**
Antiretroviral treatment history				
Mono/dual NRTI exposure prior to NNRTI-based regimen	71 (29.5)	23 (22.1)	48 (35.0)	**0.03**
Duration on NNRTI-based treatment, years	2.2 (1.5-2.9)	2.3 (1.5-3.1)	2.0 (1.4-2.9)	**0.04**
NNRTI regimen				**0.01**
Nevirapine	167 (69.3)	81 (77.9)	86 (62.8)	
Efavirenz	74 (30.7)	23 (22.1)	51 (37.2)	
NRTI-backbone				
d4T/3TC	142(58.9)	71 (68.2)	71 (51.8)	**0.015**
AZT/3TC	60 (24.9)	25(24.0)	35(25.6)	
d4T/ddI	17 (7.1)	4 (3.9)	13(9.5)	
AZT/ddI	14(5.8)	3(2.9)	11(8.0)	
ddI/3TC	8 (3.3)	1 (1.0)	7 (5.1)	
Multi-NRTI resistance[2]				**<0.001**
No TAMs	45/203(22.2)	38/89 (42.7)	7/114 (6.1)	
Low grade multi-NRTI	78/203 (38.4)	40/89 (44.9)	38/114 (33.3)	
High grade multi-NRTI	80/203 (39.4)	11/89 (12.4)	69/114 (60.5)	

Data are presented in median (IQR) or number (%).
[1]Single boosted PI regimens include ritonavir-boosted Protease inhibitor plus 2 nucleoside reverse transcriptase. Double-boosted PI regimens included 2 protease inhibitors plus ritonavir with/without NRTI/NNRTI.
[2]Definition of multi NRTI resistance: high grade is defined as ≥ 4 thymidine analog associated mutations (TAMs) or the presence of Q151M or 69Insertion. Low grade multi NRTI resistance is defined as 1–3 TAMs and without Q151M and 69insertion.

vomiting (n = 2), intolerance (n = 1), blurred vision (n = 1), hypertriglyceridemia (n = 1); 5 events for full dose RTV (31% of children who used full dose of RTV) due to intolerance (n = 3), hyperbilirubinemia (n = 1) and hypertriglyceride (n = 1); 4 events for NFV (10% of children who used NFV) due to intolerance (n = 2), rash (n = 1) and diarrhea (n = 1); 1 event for SQV (4% of children who used SQV) due to intolerance and 1 event for LPV/r (0.8% of children who used LPV/r) due to dyslipidemia. Proportion of children with elevated low density lipoprotein was significantly more in the double-boosted compared to single-boosted PI groups (Table 2).

Table 2 Outcomes after 48 weeks of boosted protease inhibitor regimens

Outcomes	Week 48			
	Total	Single -boosted PI	Double-boosted PI	P-value
Median (IQR) CD4%	20 (15–26) (n = 200)	24 (18–30) (n = 83)	17 (14–22) (n = 117)	**< 0.001**
Median(IQR) CD4% gain	10(1–7) (n = 199)	7(2–12) (n = 83)	10(6–15) (n = 116)	0.002
% with HIV RNA < 400 copies/ml	81.3 (n = 144)	83.1 (n = 65)	79.8 (n = 79)	0.610
% with HIV RNA < 50 copies/ml	63.0 (n = 138)	76.6 (n = 64)	51.4 (n = 74)	**0.002**
% with Cholesterol > 200 mg/dl	42.5 (n = 162)	34.3 (n = 70)	48.9 (n = 92)	0.062
% with Triglyceride > 150 mg/dl	62.4 (n = 157)	61.8 (n = 68)	62.9 (n = 89)	0.882
% with Low density lipoprotein > 130 mg/dl	31.8 (n = 88)	16.2 (n = 37)	43.1 (n = 51)	**0.007**

Cumulative probability of virologic treatment failure

The cumulative probability of virologic treatment failure was analyzed by including data from 199 patients who had HIV RNA results at least once after 6 months of boosted PI regimens. The Kaplan Meier estimate is shown in Figure 1. The cumulative probabilities of having HIV RNA > 400 copies/ml at 24 months of treatment were 0.28 (95% CI 0.19-0.40) for children who received single-boosted PI and 0. 27 (95% CI 0.18-0.39) for children on double-boosted PI, p = 0.813 by log rank test.

Predictors for virologic suppression at week 48 after boosted PI regimen

The predictors for virologic suppression at week 48 were explored by multivariate logistic regression analysis as shown in Table 3. Male, young age and high weight for age z-score were significantly associated with virologic suppression. Male had a 2.9 times odds of achieving viral suppression compared to female. Chances for viral suppression were more likely in children younger than 9 years (3.6 times odds) and those with weight for age z-score > −1.7 (4.2 times odds). There was a trend for a better virologic suppression rate among children who switched to boosted PI regimen when their CD4 count was > 100 cell/mm^3 or plasma HIV RNA levels < 4 $\log_{10}$ copies/ml but these did not reach statistical significance ($p > 0.05$).

Discussion

Our study provides information on outcomes of second-line ART in NNRTI-failing children as part of a large multicenter observational study in a RLS. This study showed good virologic efficacy of second-line boosted PI regimens with 81% achieving HIV RNA < 400 copies/ml at 48 weeks of treatment. Children with more advanced HIV disease were preferentially treated with double-boosted PI versus single-boosted PI regimens. Both regimen types performed equally well in suppressing HIV

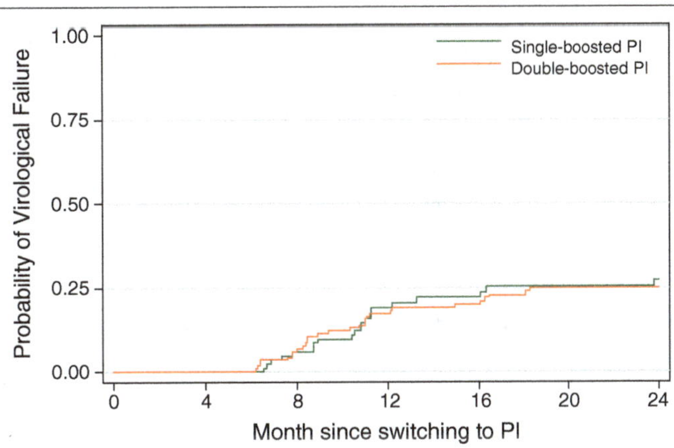

Single-boosted PI*	83	83	77	53	49	43	35
Double-boosted PI*	116	116	108	94	84	72	67

* No. patients at visits

P 0.813 by Log-Rank test

Figure 1 Kaplan Meier estimated for time to treatment failure, defined as HIV RNA > 400 copies/ml, after switching to second line PI regimen.

Table 3 The predictors for virological suppression defined as HIV viral load < 400 copies/ml at week 48 of boosted protease inhibitor-based antiretroviral regimens

	Proportion of children with viral suppression n(%)	Univariate analysis		Multivariate analysis	
		Odd Ratios (95%CI)	P-value	Odd Ratios (95%CI)	P-value
ARV regimens					
Single-boosted PI	54/65(83.1%)	1		1	
Double-boosted PI	63/79 (79.8%)	0.80 (0.34-1.88)	0.611	0.82 (0.27-2.42)	0.712
Gender					
Male	62/69 (89.9%)	3.22 (1.27-8.20)	0.014	2.85 (1.06-7.66)	0.018
Female	55/75 (73.3%)	1		1	
Age, years					
< 9.1	67/76 (88.2%)	2.68 (1.12-6.46)	0.028	3.60 (1.25-10.36)	0.038
≥ 9.1	50/68 (73.5%)	1		1	
Weight for age Z-score					
< −1.7	42/59 (71.2%)	1		1	
≥ −1.7	64/72 (88.9%)	3.24 (1.28-8.18)	0.013	2.42 (0.85-6.84)	0.097
CD4 at time of switch to second line regimen					
< 100 cell/mm3	30/42 (71.4%)	1		1	
≥100 cell/mm3	84/99 (84.9%)	2.24 (0.94-5.33)	0.068	2.12 (0.71-6.36)	0.178
Plasma HIV RNA at time of switch					
< 4 $\log_{10}$ copies/ml	25/29 (86.2%)	1.53 (0.48-4.86)		-	-
≥ 4 $\log_{10}$ copies/ml	25/111 (80.4%)	1	0.474		
Mono/dual NRTI exposure					
Yes	41/50 (82.0%)	1.08 (0.45-2.62)	0.867		
No	76/94 (80.9%)	1			
Duration on NNRTI-based					
< 2.2 year	69/84(82.1%)	1.15 (0.50-2.67)	0.745		
≤ 2.2 year	48/60(80.0%)	1			
NNRTI –based regimen					
NVP-based	81/96 (84.4%)	1.80 (0.77-4.23)	0.178	1.24 (0.43-3.55)	0.691
EFV-based	36/48 (75.0%)	1		1	
Multi-NRTI resistance			0.809	-	-
No TAMs	25/32 (78.1%)	1			
Low grade multi-NRTI	35/44 (79.6%)	1.09 (0.36-3.31)			
High grade multi-NRTI	36/43 (83.7%)	1.44 (0.45-4.62)			
LPV/r in the regimen					
Yes	60/71 (84.5%)	1.53 (0.66-3.58)	0.325		
No	57/73 (78.1%)	1			

below 400 copies/ml but further suppression to less than 50 copies/ml was significantly less with double-boosted PI.

This study supports recycling of 2NRTIs in combination with a potent boosted PI as second-line therapy in children. The 2010 WHO guideline recommend replacing AZT/3TC or d4T/3TC in the first line regimen with abacavir (ABC)/3TC or ABC/ddI [17]; however, that practice is rare in Thailand due to the high cost of ABC rendering it unavailable in the Thai national ARV program. Therefore, recycling of inactive or partially active 2NRTIs such as AZT/3TC, AZT/ddI or ddI/3TC was common in this study. At the time of the study, tenofovir (TDF) was not yet approved for adolescents nor was it available in Thailand. Similarly, LPV/r is the

PI of choice in the WHO guideline but it was in limited supply in Thailand before 2005, resulting in the use of a more toxic drug, IDV, in half of our children.

The virologic response to second-line single boosted PI regimen in our study compares favorably to reports from other countries [15-17]. In a French cohort, 92% on LPV/r second line regimens had HIV RNA < 400 copies/ml despite having lower CD4 (14.8%) and higher HIV RNA (4.8 $\log_{10}$ copies/ml) than our children. The Spanish multicenter retrospective observational study showed 71.5% of PI-experienced children on LPV/r-based having HIV RNA < 400 copies/ml [10]. A long term cohort of children treated with LPV/r-based regimen showed that 81% remained on therapy after more than 4 years; 75% of those children had HIV RNA < 400 copies/ml at their last visit. [18] In another pediatric study, patients tended to have better virologic outcome if they were on LPV/r as supposed to unboosted PI, nelfinavir [19]. We also saw a trend towards better virologic outcome among children who received LPV/r, but this did not reach statistical significance. In Malawi, 10% of adults died after initiating second-line regimen and 85% of the survivors had viral suppression at 12 months [20].

Double-boosted PI is an acceptable alternative second-line therapy option in Thailand for children with late treatment failure who have few or no fully active drugs aside from PIs [15]. The pediatric HIV-NAT 017 study which treated children with second-line SQV and LPV/r reported a viral suppression rate similar to that observed in our study with 64% having HIV RNA < 50 copies/ml at week 48 [21]. A non-randomized study in Thai adults showed that the double-boosted PI regimen was not as potent in suppressing HIV RNA to below 50 copies/ml when compared to the single-boosted PI regimen among patients with low grade multi- NRTI resistance mutations [22]. Of note is the inability of that study to compare the two regimen types among patients with high grade multi-NRTI resistance mutations. Our study showed that double-boosted PI had a higher rate of low level viremia, HIV RNA between 50 and 400 copies/ml, compared to single-boosted PI. This could possibly be confounded by indication that children with more advanced disease received double-boosted PI regimen or due to inferior potency of a PI mono-class regimen. A recent randomized study of second-line PIs in Thai adults showed mono LPV/r treatment to result in significantly more low level viremia than a 3-drug regimen with TDF, 3TC and LPV/r [23]. Another second-line study in Thai adults who received a single active drug, LPV/r, together with 3TC to reduce viral fitness also showed that only 67% achieved HIV RNA <50 copies/ml with 16% having low viremia between 50–400 copies/ml [24]. The recent review literature [25] and meta-analysis [26]on protease inhibitor monotherapy also showed a slightly inferior virological efficacy of protease inhibitor monotherapy than that of protease inhibitor plus nucleosides. However, failure of protease inhibitor monotherapy does not imply losing therapeutic options, usually reintroduction of nucleosides can lead to virologic suppression. [25,26] The higher rates of dyslipidemia with double-boosted PI and the higher pill burden further limits its use particularly if newer and more potent ARVs with favorable lipid profile e.g. atazanavir, darunavir, and raltegravir becomes available to children in RLS.

There is a lack of evidence to inform the optimum time to switch to second line regimens in RLS. The WHO guideline, relying heavily on a public health approach to care, recommends switching to second-line regimen when CD4 is < 100 cells/mm^3 or HIV RNA is > 5,000 copies/ml [27]. We demonstrated a trend towards better virologic suppression following second-line therapy in children who switched when their CD4 was > 100 cell/mm^3 or HIV RNA was < 10,000 copies/ml. Delayed in switching to second-line therapy may lead to resistance mutations accumulation which would be problematic in RLS where ARV options are limited. The PENPACT-1 study showed that children failing first-line NNRTI who were randomized to a delayed switch at HIV RNA > 30,000 copies/ml had more TAMs compared to those who switched at HIV RNA > 1,000 copies/ml [28] This however did not affect the overall virologic outcome after second-line therapy in that study likely due to several reasons: children who failed had low rates of NRTI resistance of 1-5%, they had no CD4 failure, and they had access to routine HIV RNA monitoring, genotyping and good ARV options. The situation in RLS may be quite different as switching occurs later with immunologic or clinical failure coupled with the lack of HIV RNA and genotyping monitoring, and limited ARV options.

This study has several limitations. First is incomplete data, which is an inherent limitation of a retrospective study design. The information of adherence to treatment is not captured. Second, the lack of randomization of single- versus double-boosted PI regimens hinders the ability to directly compare the outcome between these two regimens. Third, the duration of NNRTI-based first line regimen in our study was relatively short, around 2 years. Furthermore, we have access to laboratory monitoring including CD4, plasma HIV RNA and genotypic resistance testing to guide the design of the new regimens which may limit the applicability of our results to other resource-limtted settings where treatment failure is detected later and genotyping is unavailable. However, the constraint in available ARV choices in our population prohibited us to fully utilize genotyping information. Therefore, we believe that our data represent typical clinical care settings in most resource-limited countries.

In conclusion, this study provides security to clinicians in RLS to give children second-line treatment despite drug choice and laboratory monitoring constraints. Although we saw a good success rate in our study, one-fifth did not achieve viral suppression. Such children in RLS currently have no treatment option beyond second-line regimens. This emphasizes the urgent need to derive strategies to study, plan and procure new drugs and drug classes for children with treatment failure worldwide.

The HIV-NAT 086 study team

The HIV Netherlands Australia Thailand Research Collaboration (HIV-NAT), The Thai Red Cross AIDS Research Centre, Bangkok: T. Bunupuradah, C. Phasomsap, P. Kaew-on.

Institut de Recherche pour le Développement (IRD), UMI 174, Program for HIV Prevention and Treatment, Department of Medical Technology, Faculty of Associated Medical Sciences, Chiang Mai University, Chiang Mai, Thailand, The Global Fund to Fight AIDS, Malaria and Tuberculosis supported drug and laboratory monitoring for some children: S Kanjanavanit, Nakornping Hospital, Somdej Pranangchao Sirikit Hospital, Chonburi, Somdej Pranangchao Sirikit Hospital, Chonburi: T Hinjiranandana, Bhumibol Adulyadej Hospital, Bangkok: P Layangool, Somdej Prapinklao Hospital, Bangkok: N Kamonpakorn, Mae Chan Hospital, Chiang Rai: S Buranabanjasatean, Prapokklao Provincial Hospital, Chantaburi: C Ngampiyaskul.

Queen Sirikit National Institute of Child Health, Bangkok: T. Chotpitayasunondh, S. Chanpradub, P. Leawsrisuk. Department of Pediatrics, Faculty of Medicine, Siriraj Hospital, Mahidol University: S. Chearskul, N. Vanprapar, W. Phongsamart, K. Lapphra, P. Chearskul, O. Wittawatmongkol, W. Prasitsuebsai, K. Intalapaporn, N. Kongstan, N. Pannin, A. Maleesatharn, B. Khumcha.

Research Institute for Health Sciences (RIHES), Chiang Mai University, Chiang Mai: L. Aurpibul, N. Wongnum, R. Nadsasarn.

Department of Pediatrics, Faculty of Medicine, Khon Kaen University: P. Lumbiganon, P. Tharnprisan, T. Udompanich. Petchburi Hospital, Petchburi: M. Yentang.

Chiang Rai Regional Hospital, Chiang Rai: A. Khonponoi, N. Maneerat, S. Denjunta, S. Watanaporn, C. Yodsuwan, W. Srisuk, S. Somsri, K. Surapanichadul

Competing interests

All authors declare no conflict of interest and that member of their immediate families do not have a financial interest in or arrangement with any commercial organization that may have a direct interest in the subject matter of this article.

Authors's contribution

TP, GJ, KC, and JA designed the study, collected data, wrote the first draft, reviewed manuscript before submission. PS, TS,WP,VS, PK,WP,RH, NW collected data, reviewed and commented of manuscript before submission. US analyzed, reviewed and commented draft of manuscript before submission. All authors have read and approved the final manuscript.

Acknowledgements

The study was funded by the Commission on Higher Education, Ministry of Education in Thailand. The data were collected from the Pediatric PHPT cohort study (N = 74), Queen Sirikit National Institute of Child Health, Bangkok (N = 53), HIVNAT, Thai Red Cross AIDS Research Center, Bangkok (N = 44), Siriraj Hospital, Mahidol University, Bangkok (N = 28), Chiang Mai University hospital, Chiang Mai (N = 18), Khon Kaen University, Khon Kaen (N = 16), Petchburi Provincial Hospital, Petchburi (N = 4) and Chiang Rai Regional Hospital, Chiang Rai (N = 4). We would like to thank Frank Benjamin Steven, MD for his help in preparing the English manuscript.

Author details

[1]The HIV Netherlands Australia Thailand Research Collaboration (HIV-NAT), Bangkok, Thailand. [2]Department of Pediatrics, Faculty of Medicine, Chulalongkorn University, Bangkok, Thailand. [3]Institut de Recherche pour le Développement (IRD), UMI 174, Program for HIV Prevention and Treatment, Department of Medical Technology, Faculty of Associated Medical Sciences, Chiang Mai University, Chiang Mai, Thailand. [4]Queen Sirikit National Institute of Child Health, Bangkok, Thailand. [5]Department of Pediatrics, Faculty of Medicine Siriraj Hospital, Mahidol University, Bangkok, Thailand. [6]Research Institute for Health Sciences, Chiang Mai University, Chiang Mai, Thailand. [7]Department of Pediatrics, Faculty of Medicine, Khon Kaen University, Khon Kaen, Thailand. [8]Petchburi Hospital, Petchburi, Thailand. [9]Chiang Rai Regional Hospital, Chiang Rai, Thailand. [10]South East Asia Research Collaboration with Hawaii, Hawaii, Thailand. [11]Department of Medicine, Faculty of Medicine, Chulalongkorn University, Bangkok, Thailand.

References

1. Ciaranello AL, Chang Y, Margulis AV, Bernstein A, Bassett IV, Losina E, *et al*: **Effectiveness of pediatric antiretroviral therapy in resource-limited settings: a systematic review and meta-analysis.** *Clin Infect Dis* 2009 Dec 15, **49**(12):1915–27.
2. Kariminia A, Chokephaibulkit K, Pang J, Lumbiganon P, Hansudewechakul R, Amin J, *et al*: **Cohort profile: the TREAT Asia pediatric HIV observational database.** *Int J Epidemiol* 2011 Feb, **40**(1):15–24.
3. Puthanakit T, Oberdorfer A, Akarathum N, Kanjanavanit S, Wannarit P, Sirisanthana T, *et al*: **Efficacy of highly active antiretroviral therapy in HIV-infected children participating in Thailand's National Access to Antiretroviral Program.** *Clin Infect Dis* 2005 Jul 1, **41**(1):100–7.
4. Kamya MR, Mayanja-Kizza H, Kambugu A, Bakeera-Kitaka S, Semitala F, Mwebaze-Songa P, *et al*: **Predictors of long-term viral failure among ugandan children and adults treated with antiretroviral therapy.** *Journal of acquired immune deficiency syndromes* 2007, **46**(2):187–93.
5. Janssens B, Raleigh B, Soeung S, Akao K, Te V, Gupta J, *et al*: **Effectiveness of highly active antiretroviral therapy in HIV-positive children: evaluation at 12 months in a routine program in Cambodia.** *Pediatrics* 2007 Nov, **120** (5):e1134–40.
6. Jaspan HB, Berrisford AE, Boulle AM: **Two-year outcomes of children on non-nucleoside reverse transcriptase inhibitor and protease inhibitor regimens in a South African pediatric antiretroviral program.** *Pediatr Infect Dis J* 2008, **27**(11):993–8.
7. Prasitsuebsai W, Bowen AC, Pang J, Hesp C, Kariminia A, Sohn AH: **Pediatric HIV clinical care resources and management practices in Asia: a regional survey of the TREAT Asia pediatric network.** *AIDS Patient Care STDS* 2010, **24**(2):127–31.
8. PENTA 2009 guidelines for the use of antiretroviral therapy in paediatric HIV-1 infection. Available at: ≤http://www.pentatrials.org/guide09.pdf≥ (Accessed: July 31, 2009)
9. Working Group on Antiretroviral Therapy and Medical Managment of HIV-infected children: *Guidelines for the Use of Antiretroviral Agents in Pediatric HIV Infection, February 23, 2009.* US Department of Health and Human Services: Access; 2009. http://AIDSinfo.nih.gov/.
10. Resino S, Bellon JM, Ramos JT, Navarro ML, Martin-Fontelos P, Cabrero E, *et al*: **Salvage lopinavir-ritonavir therapy in human immunodeficiency virus-infected children.** *Pediatr Infect Dis J* 2004, **23**(10):923–30.

11. Sungkanuparph S, Manosuthi W, Kiertiburanakul S, Piyavong B, Chumpathat N, Chantratita W: **Options for a second-line antiretroviral regimen for HIV type 1-infected patients whose initial regimen of a fixed-dose combination of stavudine, lamivudine, and nevirapine fails.** *Clin Infect Dis* 2007 Feb 1, **44**(3):447–52.
12. Jittamala P, Puthanakit T, Chaiinseeard S, Sirisanthana V: **Predictors of virologic failure and genotypic resistance mutation patterns in thai children receiving non-nucleoside reverse transcriptase inhibitor-based antiretroviral therapy.** *Pediatr Infect Dis J* 2009, **28**(9):826–30.
13. Puthanakit T, Jourdain G, Hongsiriwon S, Suntarattiwong P, Chokephaibulkit K, Sirisanthana V, *et al*: **HIV-1 drug resistance mutations in children after failure of first-line nonnucleoside reverse transcriptase inhibitor-based antiretroviral therapy.** *HIV medicine* 2010, **11**(9):565–72.
14. Bunupuradah T, van der Lugt J, Kosalaraksa P, Engchanil C, Boonrak P, Puthanakit T, *et al*: **Safety and efficacy of a double-boosted protease inhibitor combination, saquinavir and lopinavir/ritonavir, in pretreated children at 96 weeks.** *Antivir Ther* 2009, **14**(2):241–8.
15. Thai Ministry of Public Health: *Thai National guideline for managment of HIV-infected children and adults*; 2004. ISBN 974-297-2982.
16. Sirivichayakul S, Ruxrungtham K, Ungsedhapand C, Techasathit W, Ubolyam S, Chuenyam T, *et al*: **Nucleoside analogue mutations and Q151M in HIV-1 subtype A/E infection treated with nucleoside reverse transcriptase inhibitors.** *AIDS (London, England)* 2003, **17**(13):1889–96.
17. World Health Organization: *Antiretroviral therapy for HIV infection in infants and children: towards universal access.*: Recommendations for a public health approach; 2010.
18. Kline MW, Rugina S, Ilie M, Matusa RF, Schweitzer AM, Calles NR, *et al*: **Long-term follow-up of 414 HIV-infected Romanian children and adolescents receiving lopinavir/ritonavir-containing highly active antiretroviral therapy.** *Pediatrics* 2007 May, **119**(5):e1116–20.
19. De Luca M, Miccinesi G, Chiappini E, Zappa M, Galli L, De Martino M: **Different kinetics of immunologic recovery using nelfinavir or lopinavir/ritonavir-based regimens in children with perinatal HIV-1 infection.** *Int J Immunopathol Pharmacol* 2005, **18**(4):729–35.
20. Hosseinipour MC, Kumwenda JJ, Weigel R, Brown LB, Mzinganjira D, Mhango B, *et al*: **Second-line treatment in the Malawi antiretroviral programme: high early mortality, but good outcomes in survivors, despite extensive drug resistance at baseline.** *HIV medicine* 2010, **11**(8):510–8.
21. Kosalaraksa P, Bunupuradah T, Engchanil C, Boonrak P, Intasan J, Lumbiganon P, *et al*: **Double boosted protease inhibitors, saquinavir, and lopinavir/ritonavir, in nucleoside pretreated children at 48 weeks.** *Pediatr Infect Dis J* 2008, **27**(7):623–8.
22. Chetchotisakd P, Anunnatsiri S, Mootsikapun P, Kiertiburanakul S, Anekthananon T, Bowonwatanuwong C, *et al*: **Efficacy and tolerability of a double boosted protease inhibitor (lopinavir + saquinavir/ritonavir) regimen in HIV-infected patients who failed treatment with nonnucleoside reverse transcriptase inhibitors.** *HIV medicine* 2007, **8**(8):529–35.
23. Bunupuradah T, Chetchotisakd P, Ananworanich J, Munsakul W, Jirajariyavej S, Kantipong P, *et al*: **A randomized comparison of second-line lopinavir/ritonavir monotherapy vs. tenofovir/lamivudine/lopinavir/ritonavir in patients failing NNRTI-regimens: the HIV STAR study.** *Antivir Ther* 2012, **Jul 2 [Epub ahead of print]**.
24. Manosuthi W, Kiertiburanakul S, Amornnimit W, Prasithsirikul W, Thongyen S, Nilkamhang S, *et al*: **Treatment outcomes and plasma level of ritonavir-boosted lopinavir monotherapy among HIV-infected patients who had NRTI and NNRTI failure.** *AIDS Res Ther* 2009, **6**:30.
25. Perez-Valero I, Arribas JR: **Protease inhibitor monotherapy.** *Curr Opin Infect Dis*, **24**(1):7–11.
26. Mathis S, Khanlari B, Pulido F, Schechter M, Negredo E, Nelson M, *et al*: **Effectiveness of protease inhibitor monotherapy versus combination antiretroviral maintenance therapy: a meta-analysis.** *PLoS One* 2011, **6**(7): e22003.
27. ***Antiretroviral therapy for HIV infection in infants and children towards universal access Recommendation for public health approach: 2010 revision***; **Available at: ≤ http://www.who.int/hiv/topics/paediatric/en/index.html ≥ (Access September 2, 2010).**
28. Babiker A, Castro nee Green H, Compagnucci A, Fiscus S, Giaquinto C, Gibb DM, *et al*: **First-line antiretroviral therapy with a protease inhibitor versus non-nucleoside reverse transcriptase inhibitor and switch at higher versus low viral load in HIV-infected children: an open-label, randomised phase 2/3 trial.** *Lancet Infect Dis* 2011, (4):273–83.

12

HCV RNA viral load is independent from CD4 cell count and plasma HIV RNA viral load in immunocompetent HIV-HCV co-infected patients: a 3-years follow-up study

Monica Basso[1], Marzia Franzetti[1], Renzo Scaggiante[1], Andrea Sattin[1], Carlo Mengoli[1], Mario Cruciani[2], Marta Fiscon[1], Giorgio Palù[1] and Saverio Giuseppe Parisi[1*]

Abstract

Background: HCV RNA viral load is an important predictor of sustained virological response and, recently, a significant correlation with liver fibrosis was described. We investigated on possible influence of clinical and viro-immunological variables on HCV viral load in HIV-HCV co-infected patients over a study time of three years (2009-2012).

Methods: We retrospectively enrolled 98 adult patients with a diagnosis of chronic HIV infection in 2009, a diagnosis of chronic HCV infection with a detectable plasma HCV RNA in 2009 and 2012, HCV therapy-naïve or with failed and stopped antiviral treatment before June 2008. The following variables were recorded: age, gender, HCV genotype, IL28B rs12979860 CC genotype, HCV treatment status, advanced liver fibrosis diagnosis, antiretroviral therapy, CD4+ cell count, HCV viral load, HIV RNA (plasma HIV-1 RNA levels were measured from blood samples every three months at least). The correlation was established using linear regression analysis, analysis of variance and Fisher's exact test. Comparisons between groups were performed using Fisher's exact test, the independent samples t-test and the t-test for paired data, as appropriate, for continuous variables. A mixed mode (ME) maximum likelihood linear regression model was constructed to evaluate the dependence of HCV viral load.

Results: HCV RNA levels did not change significantly from 2009 to 2012 (from 3924650 ± 5320177 IU/ml to 3085128 ± 3372347 IU/ml, $p = 0.13$); the CD4+ count increased significantly (from a mean of 576 to a mean of 654, $p = 0.003$). Using linear regression, a positive correlation was observed for HCV load and genotype 1 ($p = 0.002$), nonresponder status ($p = 0.04$) and with interleukin 28B CC allele ($p = 0.05$). Other studied covariates failed to reach a significant correlation.

Conclusions: The HCV RNA load, a known pretreatment predictor of response to antiviral therapy, was independent of the two main parameters of HIV disease, plasma HIV RNA and CD4 cell count, over an observation time of 3 years in patients with recovered or spontaneously maintained immunocompetence.

Keywords: HIV RNA, HCV RNA, Follow-up, Interleukin 28B CC allele, HCV genotype 1

Background

Hepatitis C virus (HCV) is the cause of a significant proportion of cases of chronic liver disease. In human immunodeficiency virus (HIV)-HCV co-infected patients effectively treated with HAART (highly active antiretroviral therapy), HCV-related morbidity and mortality has increased alarmingly in recent years [1]. The treatment of HCV disease with pegylated interferon and ribavirin is challenging in HIV-positive patients, but reductions in liver-related and liver-independent mortality have been demonstrated in patients who achieved sustained virological response (SVR) [2]. The efficacy of therapy with pegylated interferon and ribavirin is lower than in mono-infected patients; the SVR rates are 38% in naïve patients and 28% with retreatment [3,4]. Ideally, the timing of HIV and HCV therapies must be individualized and tailored

* Correspondence: saverio.parisi@unipd.it
[1]Department of Molecular Medicine, University of Padova, Via Gabelli 63, 35100 Padova, Italy

based on personal patient clinical characteristics, which can change with time; this approach is especially recommended for HIV patients with HCV genotype 1 infection, who may be candidates for antiviral treatment, including direct-acting antiviral drugs (DAAs) [5].

A low pretreatment HCV RNA load is a known positive factor of SVR [6]. The recently published European AIDS Clinical Society Guidelines stated that a low pretreatment HCV RNA value is 400,000-600,000 IU/mL [7]. A pretreatment HCV RNA viral load < 600,000 IU/ml is significantly associated with SVR in co-infected patients treated with pegylated interferon and ribavirin ($p < 0.001$) [8], even in subjects with compensated cirrhosis ($p = 0.01$) [9]; conversely, a value higher than this threshold is a predicting factor for relapse ($p = 0.02$) in the study by Rivero-Juarez et al. [10]. The HCV RNA viral load is thought to play a role in fields other than antiviral treatment; Kirk et al. [11] reported a significant correlation between liver fibrosis and HCV RNA load ($p < 0.001$) in a cohort of 1176 HCV-positive subjects (34% with HIV coinfection).

Studies on clinical and viro-immunological correlates of HCV RNA load in HIV patients reported conflicting results. In a cross-sectional study by Collazos et al. [12], HCV RNA load was lower in subjects with undetectable HIV viremia (6.17 $\log_{10}$ IU/mL versus 6.08 $\log_{10}$ IU/mL, $p = 0.03$), whereas Grint et al. [13] demonstrated that only ongoing HAART is a predictive factor of HCV viral load stability over time, with an increase of 2.6% per year compared to 27.6% in untreated subjects ($p = 0.009$). Plasma HIV viremia is a dynamic variable; patients taking antiretroviral therapy (ART) may develop virological breakthrough or experience side effects leading to treatment interruption, and untreated subjects may start antiretroviral drugs.

In this work, we investigate whether HCV viral load (quantified at the beginning and at the end of the study) is associated with the demographic, clinical and virological characteristics of HIV-HCV-co-infected patients. We performed HCV RNA analysis, both as a continuous value and as a discrete variable (low HCV RNA when viral load was lower than 600,000 IU/ml).

Results

A total of 1497 patients with HIV infection were followed at the Infectious Disease Unit of Padova Hospital in Italy in 2012. In 373 subjects, a diagnosis of HCV co-infection was reported. A complete description of the selection process is summarized in Figure 1.

The majority of the patients were Caucasian (80/82, 97.6%). Genotype 3 infection was the most frequent non-type 1 infection (20 patients, 24.4%), 12 patients (14,6%) had genotype 4 and only 2 subjects had genotype 2 (2.4%). The diagnosis of advanced liver fibrosis was based on clinical and not invasive evaluation in most patients; Overall a liver biopsy was performed in only 10 patients (12.2%). The diagnosis of advanced liver fibrosis was performed by invasive evaluation only in one patient, liver stiffness data were available for 8 out the 19 patients (42.1%). Among the 17 patients who did not achieve an SVR, 8 (47%) had an HCV genotype 1 infection. The baseline characteristics of the included patients are described in Table 1.

At the end of the study period, 73 patients were on ART. In 63 subjects (86.3%), no treatment interruption was reported. Among subjects who never stopped ART, successful HIV viremia suppression was observed in 37/63 (58.7%) A total of 14/82 (17.1%) patients showed HIV RNA suppression in only one of the two periods included in the IFU. Among these 14 patients, 9 of the 11 subjects with ongoing ART achieved successful HIV RNA suppression during FFU; thus, the overall percentage of treated subjects with successful suppression at the end of the study period was .46/63 (73%). A detailed description of the 2012 antiviral regimen is reported in Figure 2.

The CD4+ count increased significantly from T1 to T2, with a mean increase of 78 cells/mm3 (from 576 to 654 cells/mm3, $p = 0.003$), and the T2 value correlated positively with the T1 count ($p = 0.0001$). Undetectable plasma HIV viremia at IFU predicted HIV RNA suppression at FFU ($p = 0.0001$) and was positively correlated with the CD4+ cell count at T2 ($p = 0.03$). Undetectable plasma HIV viremia at IFU was correlated with the CD4+ cell count at T1 ($p = 0.04$). The HCV RNA level did not change significantly during the observation period ($p = 0.71$). In 11 (13.4%) patients a low HCV RNA viral load was reported both at T1 and T2 and in 22 (26.8%) subjects only at T1. Low HCV RNA viral load at T1 had a positive association with low HCV RNA at T2 ($p = 0.001$) and a negative correlation with the CD4+ cell count at T2 ($p = 0.01$).

The ME linear regression revealed significant positive correlations between $\log_{10}$ HCV RNA and HCV genotype 1 ($p = 0.002$), previous failed HCV treatment ($p = 0.04$) and harboring the IL28B CC allele ($p = 0.05$). All other explanatory covariates failed to reach significant P values, including the successful suppression of HIV viremia or persistent ongoing viral replication (irrespective of the study period analyzed) and ongoing ART at the end of follow-up (Table 2). The predicted HCV viremia margins after ME linear regression were calculated, including the three significant predictors of high HCV viral load (Table 3).

Discussion

The objective of this longitudinal study was to analyze the possible influences of clinical and virological parameters on plasma HCV replication evaluated at the beginning and at the end of a time interval of 3 years. Our data indicate that age, gender, a diagnosis of advanced

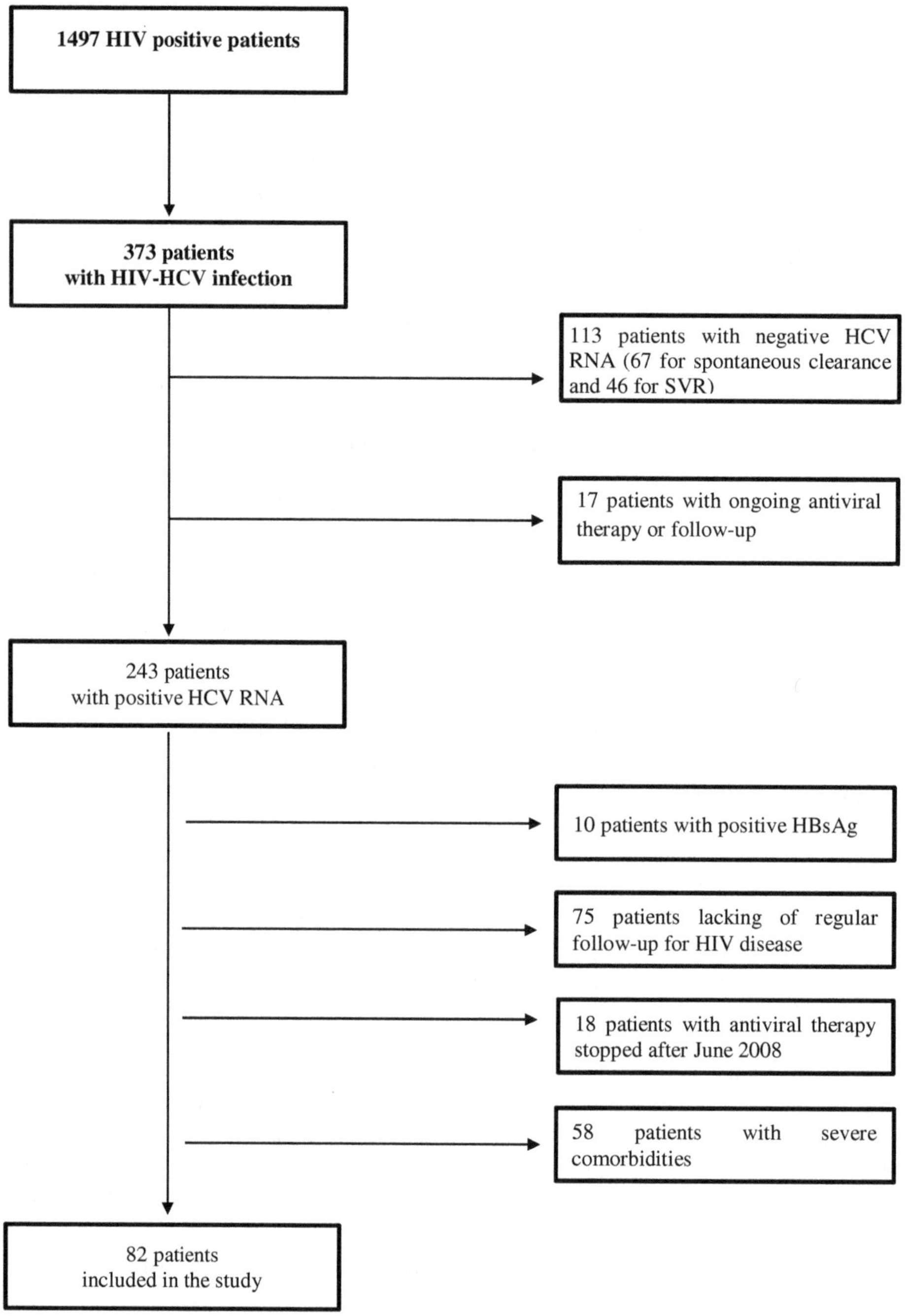

Figure 1 Flow chart describing the selection of the study patients.

liver fibrosis, CD4+ cell count and successful HIV therapy, leading to undetectable plasma viremia, failed to exhibit significant effects on HCV RNA levels.

Furthermore, we focused our interest on the characteristics of HIV-HCV-co-infected patients with persistent serum HCV RNA levels lower than 600,000 IU/ml. Co-infected patients with persistent low HCV RNA levels are typically infected with non-genotype 1 viruses and represent a small proportion (13.4%) of our population of HIV-HCV-co-infected subjects. However, when only baseline data are considered, the proportion of co-infected patients increased to 26.8%, a figure comparable to the 25% reported in the study by Rallon et al. [14] in a cohort of 196 co-infected patients. The association between HCV genotype 1 and the IL28B C allele with higher HCV RNA values is described in HIV-HCV-co-infected patients [11,15]; these findings demonstrated that no unintended selection bias occurred.

Table 1 Demographic, clinical and virological features of the 82 HIV-HCV co-infected patients who fulfilled the inclusion criteria

Variables	Results
Age (years)[1]	48 (±6)
Male, n (%)[2]	62 (75.6)
HCV Genotype 1, n (%)[2]	48 (58.5)
Previous HCV therapy, n (%)[2]	17 (20.7)
Advanced liver fibrosis, n (%)[2]	19 (23.2)
CD4 cell count at T1[1] (cells/mm^3)	576 (±280)
CD4 cell count at T2[1] (cells/mm^3)	654 (±351)
HCV RNA at T1[1] (IU/ml)	3924650 (±5320177)
HCV RNA at T2[1] (IU/ml)	3085128 (±3372347)
Ongoing ART at T2[2], n (%)	73 (89)
Clean IFU, n (%)[2]	39 (47.6)
Clean FFU[5], n (%)[2]	57 (69.5)
Discordant HIV RNA suppression at IFU[4], n (%)	14 (17.1)
IL 28B CC genotype, n (%)[2]	20 (31.7)

[1]mean and SD; [2]absolute number and percentage respect to all included patients.
ART: Anti Retroviral Therapy; Clean IFU: HIV viremia undetectable during initial follow-up (0-24 months from T1), regardless of being on ART; Clean FFU: HIV viremia undetectable during final follow-up (24-36 months from T1), regardless of being on ART.
Data on IL28B genotype were available for the 63 patients (76.8%).

Barreiro et al. [16] stated that subjects with HIV-HCV co-infection are more likely than HIV-negative subjects to experience variations in HCV RNA load greater than 0.5 log over a mean period of 43 months. The number of patients surveyed was greater than that in our study (644 versus 82), but the proportion of patients on ART was similar to ours (82% and 86.7%, respectively). Only two HCV RNA controls were available in our study because there was no clinical indication to prompt more frequent measurements. Nevertheless, increases of 0.5 log IU/ml of both the baseline and the final mean HCV RNA values for the patients categorized as having low-level viremia would correspond to values below 800,000 IU/ml, the threshold accepted as "low" [17]; therefore, our patients maintained their virological classification throughout the study period.

Most included patients (76.8%) were on ART, but a persistent undetectable HIV RNA load with a cut-off of 50 copies/ml was observed in only 58.7% of patients. At a comparable end point (144 weeks of follow-up), the cross-study analysis by Hua et al. [18] on 279 HIV-HCV-naïve co-infected patients described a rate of virological failure (defined as plasma HIV viremia > 200 copies/ml) of 10.5% (4 patients out of 38 evaluable patients). Of note, HCV status was defined only serologically and not by the presence of detectable HCV RNA, and HBsAg-positive patients were included, albeit the percentage was low (4.3%). ART efficacy was not the purpose of our work; nevertheless, we can report an interesting finding on the long-term efficacy in a small but homogeneous cohort of all HCV patients positive for HCV RNA, with no HBV coinfection and of Caucasian ethnicity who were treated according to the updated HIV guidelines.

Grint et al. [13] described HCV viral load changes in 1541 patients selected from the EuroSIDA study cohort: the median follow-up was five years, and the only factor able to stabilize HCV viral load was ART. In this study, 1148 subjects (74.5%) were on ART at baseline, with undetectable HIV RNA levels in 657 patients (57.2%); 393 subjects were not taking ART (88.2% with a detectable HIV RNA). Despite this virological picture, the absence or presence of detectable plasma HIV viremia has no significant influence on HCV RNA viral load. Successful ART and undetectable HIV plasma viremia are obviously strictly related if we exclude long-term non-progressing patients. We considered our patients to be responders to therapy when viral replication was lower

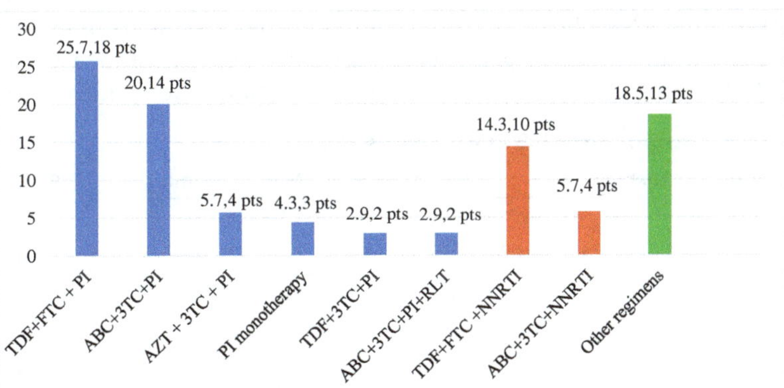

Figure 2 Antiretroviral drug regimens of the 73 co-infected patients treated in 2012 (data available for 70/73 patients, 95.6%): for each drug combination are reported both percentage respect to the number of treated patients and absolute number. Legend: ABC = abacavir; AZT = zidovudine; FTC = emtricitabine; MVC = maraviroc; NNRTI = non-nucleoside reverse transcriptase inhibitors; PI = protease inhibitor; RLT = raltegravir; TDF = tenofovir; 3TC = lamivudine.

Table 2 Mixed mode (ME) maximum likelihood linear regression model test with log_{10} HCV RNA as dependent variable

Log_{10} HCV RNA	Coef.	Std. Err.	z	P	95% Conf.	Interval
Age	0.011	0.021	0.50	0.614	-0.030	0.051
Gender	0.068	0.194	0.35	0.727	-0.313	0.448
HCV genotype 1	0.543	0.178	3.04	0.002	0.194	0.893
Advanced liver fibrosis	-0.183	0.205	-0.89	0.372	-0.585	0.219
ART	-0.175	0.284	-0.62	0.537	-0.731	0.381
CD4 cell count/mm3	0.000	0.000	-0.21	0.831	-0.001	0.000
Previous HCV therapy	0.378	0.185	2.05	0.041	0.016	0.740
IL28B CC genotype	0.331	0.168	1.96	0.050	0.001	0.660
_cons	5.229	1.047	5.00	0.000	3.178	7.281

Log likelihood = -95.223521, Wald $chi^2(8)$ = 18.96, P = 0.0151.
ART: Anti Retroviral Therapy; Clean IFU: HIV viremia undetectable follow-up, regardless of being on ART.

than 50 copies/ml (400 copies/ml in the study by Grint et al.); however, such a threshold identifies a clinically successful suppression but does not indicate definitively absent plasma HIV replicative activity. There is mounting evidence on the prognostic role of HIV residual viremia (2.5-50 copies/ml) [19], and we cannot exclude the possibility that residual viremia may influence HCV RNA viral load, as could greater HIV burden. No correlation was observed between CD4+ cell count and HCV RNA values as previously described [12]; CD4+ cell count increased from T1 to T2 (mean increase of 78 cells/mm^3, $p = 0.003$). The baseline immunocompetence in our enrolled patients was greater than that reported for subjects in the study by Grint et al. 576 cells/mm3 versus 340 cells/mm^3 in the subjects on ART [13].

Interestingly, low HCV RNA viral load at T1 was negatively correlated with CD4+ cell count at T2 ($p = 0.01$). This finding does not contradict our other data because it was described in a selected population of patients: those with low HCV RNA viral load. This report is the first to describe this correlation, and only speculative hypotheses can be made, including the inverse correlation between CD4 cell apoptosis and serum HCV RNA [20].

There is a growing evidence of a low rate of prescription of antiviral treatment in co-infected patients. The study by Ioannou et al. [21] reported that only 994 out of 5999 (18%) HIV-HCV-co-infected patients assisted by the Veterans Affairs healthcare system received an interferon-based regimen. This percentage rises to 25.3% in the EuroSIDA cohort but is accompanied by a reduction in treatment incidence in 2009 [22]. The proper timing at which to begin pegylated interferon and ribavirin treatment, associated with DAA when indicated, must take HIV disease status into account, but such coordination is not an easy task. Concomitant ART may be a risk factor for the development of side effects even in the case of therapy with pegylated interferon and ribavirin without DAA; However, a CD4+ cell number greater than 450/mmc predicts SVR in co-infected patients with HCV genotype 1 [23,24].

Conclusions

The strengths of this study can help treating physicians to tailor the beginning of HCV disease treatment because we demonstrated that HCV RNA value, a known pretreatrment predictor of response to antiviral therapy, remain independent of the two main parameters of HIV disease, plasma HIV RNA detectability and CD4+ cell count, over an observation time of 3 years and in patients with recovered or spontaneously maintained immunocompetence.

Table 3 Predicted HCV viremia, margins after ME linear regression

HCV genotype 1	Previous HCV therapy	IL28B CC	Margin (IU/ml)	95% Conf. interval (IU/ml)	
No	No	No	$5.16x10^5$	$2.55x10^5$	$1.04x10^6$
No	No	Yes	$9.13x10^5$	$3.90x10^5$	$2.14x10^6$
No	Yes	No	$1.02x10^6$	$4.34x10^5$	$2.42x10^6$
No	Yes	Yes	$2.95x10^6$	$8.78x10^5$	$9.94x10^6$
Yes	No	No	$1.66x10^6$	$9.61x10^5$	$2.87x10^6$
Yes	No	Yes	$3.36x10^6$	$1.68x10^6$	$6.71x10^6$
Yes	Yes	No	$3.86x10^6$	$1.70x10^6$	$8.74x10^6$
Yes	Yes	Yes	$7.46Ex10^6$	$3.08x10^6$	$1.81x10^7$

Three predictors were included, HCV genotype 1, previous anti HCV therapy, and IL28=CC, in all combinations.

Methods

HIV-HCV co-infected patients

We retrospectively enrolled patients into the study on the basis of the following eligibility criteria: 1) older than 18 years; 2) diagnosis of chronic HIV infection in 2009; 3) diagnosis of chronic HCV infection with a detectable plasma HCV RNA in 2009 and 2012; 4) hepatitis B serum antigen (HBsAg)-negative in 2009 and 2012; 5) HCV therapy-naïve or with failed and stopped antiviral treatment before June 2008; 6) regular viro-immunological follow-up of HIV disease from 2009 to 2012; 7) no pregnancy at the time of enrollment and throughout the time of the study; and 8) no severe comorbidities.

Severe comorbidities were defined as any pathological condition reported to increase HCV RNA load (i.e., intravenous drug use or alcohol abuse).

The enrolled subjects gave informed consent for all procedures and for the use of their blinded data for scientific evaluation and publication. This study was conducted in accordance with the Helsinki Declaration and local legislation and was approved by the local Ethics Committee.

Throughout the study period, the patients were untreated for HIV infection or received antiretroviral treatment according to the current international guidelines. Decisions on HIV therapy were at the discretion of the treating physician; there were no restrictions on CD4+ cell counts in 2009 and 2012.

Study time

Two time periods were identified: Initial Follow-Up (IFU) and Final Follow-Up (FFU). IFU started at T1 (in 2009) and lasted 2 years. The end of IFU coincided with the start of FFU, a one-year period closer to the end of the study, which finished at T2, in 2012 (Figure 3).

Study of HIV infection

Plasma HIV-1 RNA levels were measured from blood samples at all visits (every three months at least). The lower limit of detection of the commercial test changed over the course of the study from 20 to 40 copies/mL, but we considered plasma HIV viremia as undetectable when the viral load was below the limit of 50 copies/ml [25].

Patients were classified as having undetectable HIV viremia if no plasma value exceeded 50 copies/ml; only a single viral blip throughout every year (an increase in the HIV RNA plasma viral load above 50 copies/ml but lower than 500 copies/ml and followed by undetectable HIV RNA) was tolerated [26].

HIV viremia was classified as detectable if any other result occurred. The detectability of HIV viremia was analyzed for each period of 12 months and was categorized as successful suppression or no suppression. Patients who reported different results in the HIV viremia control during the two 12-month periods included in IFU were considered to exhibit no HIV RNA suppression, with the aim of clearly identifying the cohort of HIV-HCV-co-infected patients with persistent plasma HIV RNA levels < 50 copies/ml.

Patients were classified as taking ART in 2012 when the HCV RNA was measured if the treatment had been ongoing for at least three months.

Study of HCV infection

A diagnosis of advanced liver fibrosis was made when a liver biopsy revealed a result corresponding to Metavir scores F3 and F4 or when liver stiffness measured by a transient elastography by FibroScan (Echosens, Paris, France) had a value higher than 9.5 Kpa [27]. If these data were not available the estimation of hepatic fibrosis was made on clinical, laboratory and ultrasound data as described by Pineda et al. [28]. Therapy with pegylated interferon and ribavirin was not started during the study time because of the lack of urgent indication or due to patient refusal. Previously failed antiviral treatment included therapy with interferon (standard or pegylated) as monotherapy or with ribavirin according to the current international guidelines at the moment of treatment start. Any virological response different from SVR was classified as no response to antiviral treatment.

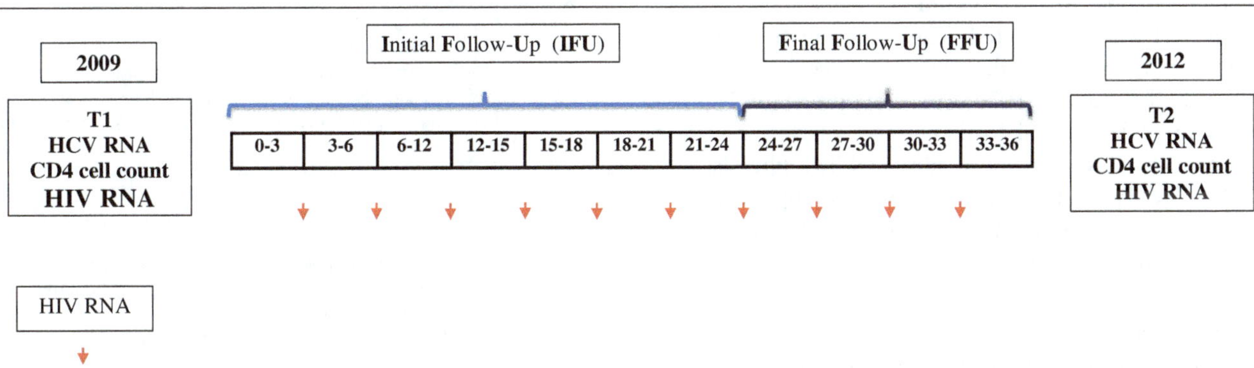

Figure 3 Study design overview. Initial Follow-Up (IFU) started at T1 (in 2009) and lasted 2 years, Final Follow-Up (FFU) started at the end of IFU, lasted one year and finished at T2, in 2012.

Virological methods

HCV RNA genotypes were determined using the VERSANT® HCV genotype 2.0 assay (INNOLiPA, Innogenetics, Belgium). HIV and HCV plasma viral loads (copies/ml) were evaluated using different platforms: until July 2011 with the COBAS TaqMan assay (Roche, Basel, Switzerland) and thereafter using the Abbott RealTime assay (Abbott RT), (Abbott Molecular Inc., Des Plaines, IL).

Interleukin (IL)28B polymorphism genotyping at single-nucleotide polymorphism locus rs12979860 was conducted using a validated in-house method. The IL28B allele was classified as CC or not CC (including CT and TT) for statistical analysis.

Statistical analysis

The following variables were recorded: age, gender, HCV genotype 1 (binary, HCV genotype 1 versus non-genotype 1), IL28B CC genotype (binary, CC genotype versus CT/TT genotypes), previously failed anti-HCV treatment versus naïve to antiviral therapy (binary, yes versus no), advanced liver fibrosis (binary, presence versus absence of advanced liver fibrosis), antiretroviral therapy (binary, ongoing versus no antiretroviral therapy ongoing at T2), CD4+ cell count at T1 and at T2, HCV viral load at T1 and at T2, IFU HIV RNA levels (binary, bad versus good HIV RNA suppression) and final follow-up HIV RNA levels (binary, bad versus good HIV RNA suppression).

Moreover, the following derived variables were obtained: $\log_{10}$ HCV RNA at T1 and $\log_{10}$ HCV RNA at T2 after $\log_{10}$ transformation of T1 HCV RNA and T2 HCV RNA, respectively.

The variables were submitted to pairwise correlation analysis to outline the underlying pattern in the evaluated population. The correlation was established using linear regression analysis, analysis of variance (ANOVA) and Fisher's exact test. Comparisons between groups were performed using Fisher's exact test, the independent samples t-test and the t-test for paired data, as appropriate, for continuous variables.

A mixed mode (ME) maximum likelihood linear regression model was constructed. The following time-varying covariates were obtained: CD4+ cell count, logHCV viremia and successful HIV viremia suppression. The dependence of HCV viral load on a set of time-invariant (age, gender, HCV genotype 1, advanced liver fibrosis, previous failed HCV therapy) and time-varying covariates was established. The limit of significance for all analyses was established at $p < 0.05$.

Ethical approval

The local government, which was represented by the Veneto Regional Health Authority, approved the study and provided funding (Regional Government Decrees 3643/2004 and 3499/2008). This study was conducted in accordance with the Helsinki Declaration and local legislation (Ethics Committee of Padova University Hospital, prot. 2606-12P).

Abbreviations

ART: Antiretroviral therapy; DAAs: Direct-acting antiviral drugs; FFU: Final follow-up; HAART: Highly active antiretroviral therapy; HCV: Hepatitis C virus; HIV: Human immunodeficiency virus; IFU: Initial follow-up; SVR: Sustained virological response.

Competing interests

The authors declare that they have no competing interests.

Authors' contributions

MB collected the data, interpreted the findings, and wrote the paper; MF managed the patients and interpret the findings; RS managed the patients and wrote the paper; AS managed the patients and helped to interpret the findings; CM interpreted the data and performed the statistical analysis; MC helped to interpret the findings and wrote the paper; MF helped to interpret the findings and write the paper; GP helped to design the study and write the paper; SGP designed and coordinated the study, interpreted the findings, and wrote the paper. All authors read and approved the final manuscript.

Acknowledgements

This work was supported by MURST ex 60% 2012 and 2013 (to MB).
This work will be presented in part to the 24th European Congress of Clinical Microbiology and Infectious Diseases in Barcelona, Spain, 10 – 13 May 2014 (Abstract Reference No: ECCMI-2802).

Author details

[1]Department of Molecular Medicine, University of Padova, Via Gabelli 63, 35100 Padova, Italy. [2]Center of Community & Medicine and HIV Outpatient Clinic, Verona, Italy.

References

1. Andreoni M, Giacometti A, Maida I, Meraviglia P, Ripamonti D, Sarmati L: **HIV-HCV co-infection: epidemiology, pathogenesis and therapeutic implications.** *Eur Rev Med Pharmacol Sci* 2012, **16:**1473–1483.
2. Berenguer J, Rodríguez E, Miralles P, Von Wichmann MA, López-Aldeguer J, Mallolas J, Galindo MJ, Van Den Eynde E, Téllez MJ, Quereda C, Jou A, Sanz J, Barros C, Santos I, Pulido F, Guardiola JM, Ortega E, Rubio R, Jusdado JJ, Montes ML, Gaspar G, Esteban H, Bellón JM, González-García J: **Sustained virological response to interferon plus ribavirin reduces non–liver-related mortality in patients coinfected with HIV and Hepatitis C virus.** *Clin Infect Dis* 2012, **55:**728–736.
3. Davies A, Singh KP, Shubber Z, Ducros P, Mills EJ, Cooke G, Ford N: **Treatment outcomes of treatment-naïve Hepatitis C patients co-infected with HIV: a systematic review and meta-analysis of observational cohorts.** *PLoS One* 2013, **8:**e55373.
4. Basso M, Parisi SG, Mengoli C, Gentilini V, Menegotto N, Monticelli J, Nicolè S, Cruciani M, Palù G: **Sustained virological response and baseline predictors in HIV-HCV coinfected patients retreated with pegylated interferon and ribavirin after failing a previous interferon-based therapy: systematic review and meta-analysis.** *HIV Clin Trials* 2013, **14:**127–139.
5. Sulkowski MS: **Current management of Hepatitis C Virus infection in patients With HIV co-infection.** *J Infect Dis* 2013, **207:**S26–S32.
6. Zeuzem S, Rodríguez-Torres M, Rajender Reddy K, Marcellin P, Diago M, Craxi A, Pockros P, Rizzetto M, Bernstein D, Shiffman ML, Lin A, Tatsch F, Hadziyannis S: **Optimized threshold for serum HCV RNA to predict treatment outcomes in hepatitis C patients receiving peginterferon alfa-2a/ribavirin.** *J Viral Hepat* 2012, **19:**766–774.
7. **European Guidelines for treatment of HIV-infected adults in Europe.** In *English online version 7.0* www.eacsociety.org/Portals/0/Guidelines_Online_131014.pdf.
8. Rallón NI, Naggie S, Benito JM, Medrano J, Restrepo C, Goldstein D, Shianna KV, Vispo E, Thompson A, McHutchison J, Soriano V: **Association of a single**

nucleotide polymorphism near the interleukin-28B gene with response to hepatitis C therapy in HIV/hepatitis C virus-coinfected patients. *AIDS* 2010, **24:**F23–F29.

9. Mira JA, García-Rey S, Rivero A, de los Santos-Gil I, López-Cortés LF, Girón-González JA, Téllez F, Márquez M, Merino D, Ríos-Villegas MJ, Macías J, Rivero-Juárez A, Pineda JA: **Response to pegylated interferon plus ribavirin among HIV/hepatitis C virus-coinfected patients with compensated liver cirrhosis.** *Clin Infect Dis* 2012, **55:**1719–1726.
10. Rivero-Juarez A, Mira JA, Camacho A, Neukam K, Perez-Camacho I, Caruz A, Macias J, Torre-Cisneros J, Pineda JA, Rivero A: **Baseline risk factors for relapse in HIV/HCV co-infected patients treated with PEG-IFN/RBV.** *Infection* 2013, **41:**21–26.
11. Kirk GD, Mehta SH, Astemborski J, Galai N, Washington J, Higgins Y, Balagopal A, Thomas DL: **HIV, age, and the severity of hepatitis C virus-related liver disease: a cohort study.** *Ann Intern Med* 2013, **158:**658–666.
12. Collazos J, Cartón JA, Asensi V: **Evaluation of the possible influence of hepatitis C virus and liver fibrosis on HIV type 1 immunological and virological outcomes.** *HIV Med* 2011, **12:**308–315.
13. Grint D, Peters L, Reekie J, Soriano V, Kirk O, Knysz B, Suetnov O, Lazzarin A, Ledergerber B, Rockstroh JK, Mocroft A: **Stability of hepatitis C virus (HCV) RNA levels among interferon-naïve HIV/HCV-coinfected individuals treated with combination antiretroviral therapy.** *HIV Med* 2013, **14:**370–378.
14. Rallón NI, Soriano V, Naggie S, Restrepo C, Goldstein D, Vispo E, McHutchison J, Benito JM: **IL28B gene polymorphisms and viral kinetics in HIV/hepatitis C virus-coinfected patients treated with pegylated interferon and ribavirin.** *AIDS* 2011, **25:**1025–1033.
15. Labarga P, Soriano V, Caruz A, Poveda E, Di Lello FA, Hernandez-Quero J, Moreno S, Bernal E, Miró JM, Leal M, Gutierrez F, Portilla J, Pineda JA: **Association between IL28B gene polymorphisms and plasma HCV-RNA levels in HIV/HCV-co-infected patients.** *AIDS* 2011, **25:**761–766.
16. Barreiro P, Labarga P, Fernández-Montero JV, Poveda E, de Mendoza C, Sánchez C, Vispo E, Soriano V: **Longitudinal changes in viral RNA concentration in patients with chronic hepatitis C and/or HIV infection in the absence of antiviral therapy.** *J Clin Virol* 2013, **58:**391–395.
17. Sulkowski MS, Sherman KE, Dieterich DT, Bsharat M, Mahnke L, Rockstroh JK, Gharakhanian S, McCallister S, Henshaw J, Girard PM, Adiwijaya B, Garg V, Rubin RA, Adda N, Soriano V: **Combination therapy with telaprevir for chronic Hepatitis C Virus Genotype 1 infection in patients with HIV: a randomized trial.** *Ann Intern Med* 2013, **159:**86–96.
18. Hua L, Andersen JW, Daar ES, Glesby MJ, Hollabaugh K, Tierney C: **Hepatitis C virus/HIV coinfection and responses to initial antiretroviral treatment.** *AIDS* 2013, **27:**2725–2734.
19. Parisi SG, Andreis S, Mengoli C, Scaggiante R, Ferretto R, Manfrin V, Cruciani M, Giobbia M, Boldrin C, Basso M, Andreoni M, Palù G, Sarmati L: **Baseline cellular HIV DNA load predicts HIV DNA decline and residual HIV plasma levels during effective antiretroviral therapy.** *J Clin Microbiol* 2012, **50:**58–63.
20. Laskus T, Kibler KV, Chmielewski M, Wilkinson J, Adair D, Horban A, Stańczak G, Radkowski M: **Effect of hepatitis C infection on HIV-induced apoptosis.** *PLoS One* 2013, **8:**e75921.
21. Ioannou GN, Bryson CL, Weiss NS, Miller R, Scott JD, Boyko EJ: **The prevalence of cirrhosis and hepatocellular carcinoma in patients with HIV infection.** *Hepatology* 2013, **58:**249–257.
22. Grint D, Peters L, Schwarze-Zander C, Beniowski M, Pradier C, Battegay M, Jevtovic D, Soriano V, Lundgren JD, Rockstroh JK, Kirk O, Mocroft A: **Temporal changes and regional differences in treatment uptake of hepatitis C therapy in EuroSIDA.** *HIV Med* 2013, **14:**613–623.
23. Funk EK, Shaffer A, Shivakumar B, Sneller M, Polis MA, Masur H, Heytens L, Nelson A, Kwan R, Kottilil S, Kohli A: **Short communication: Interferon/ Ribavirin treatment for HCV Is associated with the development of Hypophosphatemia in HIV/Hepatitis C Virus-Coinfected patients.** *AIDS Res Hum Retroviruses* 2013, **29:**1190–1194.
24. Avidan NU, Goldstein D, Rozenberg L, McLaughlin M, Ferenci P, Masur H, Buti M, Fauci AS, Polis MA, Kottilil S: **Hepatitis C viral kinetics during treatment with peg IFN-alpha-2b in HIV/HCV coinfected patients as a function of baseline CD4+ T-cell counts.** *J Acquir Immune Defic Syndr* 2009, **52:**452–458.
25. Thompson MA, Aberg JA, Hoy JF, Telenti A, Benson C, Cahn P, Eron JJ, Günthard HF, Hammer SM, Reiss P, Richman DD, Rizzardini G, Thomas DL, Jacobsen DM, Volberding PA: **Antiretroviral treatment of adult HIV infection: 2012 recommendations of the International Antiviral Society-USA panel.** *JAMA* 2012, **308:**387–402.
26. Grennan JT, Loutfy MR, Su D, Harrigan PR, Cooper C, Klein, Machouf N, Montaner JS, Rourke S, Tsoukas C, Hogg B, Raboud J: **Magnitude of virologic blips is associated with a higher risk for virologic rebound in HIV-infected individuals: a recurrent events analysis.** *J Infect Dis* 2012, **205:**1230–1238.
27. Blanco F1, Barreiro P, Ryan P, Vispo E, Martín-Carbonero L, Tuma P, Labarga P, Medrano J, González-Lahoz J, Soriano V: **Risk factors for advanced liver fibrosis in HIV-infected individuals: role of antiretroviral drugs and insulin resistance.** *J Viral Hepat* 2011, **18:**11–16.
28. Pineda JA, Aguilar-Guisado M, Rivero A, Giron-Gonzalez JA, Ruiz-Morales J, Merino D, Ríos-Villegas MJ, Macías J, López-Cortés LF, Camacho A, Merchante N, Del Valle J: **Natural history of compensated hepatitis C virus-related cirrhosis in human immunodeficiency virus-infected patients.** *Clin Infect Dis* 2009, **49:**1274–1282.

13

Sexual risk behaviour, marriage and ART: a study of HIV-positive people in Papua New Guinea

Wing Young Nicola Man[1,2], Angela Kelly[1,3*], Heather Worth[1], Andrew Frankland[1], Patti Shih[1], Martha Kupul[3], Thiri Lwin[1], Agnes Mek[3], Barbara Kepa[3], Rebecca Emori[3], Frances Akuani[3], Brenda Cangah[3], Lucy Walizopa[3], Lawrencia Pirpir[3], Somu Nosi[3] and Peter M Siba[3]

Abstract

Background: The prevention of intimate partner transmission of HIV remains an important component of comprehensive HIV prevention strategies. In this paper we examine the sexual practices of people living with HIV on antiretroviral therapy (ART) in Papua New Guinea (PNG).

Method: In 2008, a total of 374 HIV-positive people over the age of 16 and on ART for more than two weeks were recruited using a non-probability, convenience sampling methodology. This accounted for around 18% of adults on ART at the time. A further 36 people participated in semi-structured interviews. All interviews were thematically analysed using NVivo qualitative data analysis software.

Results: Less than forty per cent (38%) of participants reported having had sexual intercourse in the six months prior to the survey. Marital status was by far the most important factor in determining sexual activity, but consistent condom use during vaginal intercourse with a regular partner was low. Only 46% reported consistent condom use during vaginal intercourse with a regular partner in the last six months, despite 77% of all participants reporting that consistent condom use can prevent HIV transmission. Consistent condom use was lowest amongst married couples and those in seroconcordant relationships. The vast majority (91.8%) of all participants with a regular heterosexual partner had disclosed their status to their partner. Qualitative data reinforced low rates of sexual activity and provided important insights into sexual abstinence and condom use.

Conclusions: Considering the importance of intimate partner transmission of HIV, these results on the sexual practices of people with HIV on ART in PNG suggest that one-dimensional HIV prevention messages focussing solely on condom use fail to account for the current practices and needs of HIV-positive people, especially those who are married and know their partners' HIV status.

Keywords: HIV, Papua New Guinea, Sexual Behaviour, Antiretroviral Therapy

Background

Papua New Guinea (PNG) reported its first person diagnosed with HIV in 1987. Although more recent national adult prevalence estimates suggest the epidemic is progressing less rapidly than previously feared with less than 1% (0.9% 2009 estimate and 0.8% 2010 estimate) of the adult population currently estimated to be infected [1,2], HIV prevalence in PNG however remains among the highest in the Asia-Pacific Region. PNG's HIV epidemic has been, and continues to be, heterosexually transmitted with more women than men diagnosed as HIV-positive [2]. The epidemic exhibits substantial geographic heterogeneity, with nearly 90% of diagnoses coming from the seven Highlands provinces, the National Capital District and Morobe Province [2]. It is widely recognised from within PNG and from international agencies that innovative strategies for the treatment and care of people living with HIV and of HIV prevention are urgently needed to address the complex public health issue that HIV poses in a country with unparalleled geographical, linguistic and cultural diversity

* Correspondence: a.kelly@unsw.edu.au
[1]School of Public Health and Community Medicine, UNSW Medicine, University of New South Wales, Sydney, Australia
[3]Sexual & Reproductive Health Unit, Papua New Guinea Institute of Medical Research, Goroka, Papua New Guinea

[3]. PNG is home to more culturally diverse groups and languages than any other country in the world; for example, it is reported that there are more than 800 living languages [4].

Following a global effort towards universal access to lifesaving antiretroviral drugs in developing countries, PNG began its first pilot project of ART in 2004. As a result of efforts to universalize access to ART, treatment has now been rolled out throughout PNG. At the time of the study there were around 38 sites offering ART and fewer than 7,000 people (adults and children) had been registered for treatment [1]. By the end of 2010, 78 sites were offering ART in 20 provinces with 11,244 adults and 610 children registered for treatment since 2004. Of these, 71% of adults and 88.2% of children had commenced treatment [2].

At the time of this study CD4 cell count testing was available only at the central laboratory in Port Moresby and in one other site and thus not widely accessible. Since the time of this study, and as a result of the work of the Clinton Health Access Initiative and the Central Public Health Laboratory, CD4 cell count testing, although not available throughout the country as part of routine clinical management, has now become far more accessible. At the time of writing this paper, viral load testing was still not used as part of the clinical management of HIV in PNG.

It is well documented that ART has dramatically altered the lives of people living with HIV in both developed and developing countries. The impacts of ART have been many and one such area is the realm of sexual behaviour. At the time treatment were becoming widely accessible there was a public health concern that treatments would see an increase in sexual activity, specifically a reduction in safe sex among those living with HIV cf.[5-7]. An early meta-analysis of sexual behaviour and ART with studies, largely drawn from United States of America-based studies and of studies exclusively about or including men who have sex with men, concluded that unprotected sexual behaviour was elevated in people who had less concern regarding unsafe sex as a result of the widespread availability of ART [8].

Until recently the majority of research on the sexual behaviours and practices of people on ART were drawn from developed countries and populations such as men who have sex with men [6,7,9-13]. In more recent years there has been an important and growing body of work emerging from developing countries, particularly from sub-Saharan Africa. These studies suggest there has not been a reduction in reported rates of consistent condom use by HIV-positive people on treatment [12,14-20]. These findings suggest that ART has not led to sexual risk compensation (the abandonment of condoms and other changes to sexual behaviour such as increased number of partners) as was previously feared; thus the gains made in HIV prevention appear to be maintained. Indeed, much evidence now suggests that there are high rates of sexual abstinence in developing countries by those on treatment [5,14,17,18,20-24]. In a recent meta-analysis of cross-sectional and longitudinal studies conducted in sub-Saharan Africa, it was found that individuals on ART were significantly less likely to have unprotected sex or to have multiple sexual partners compared with when they were ART-naïve, but there were no significant differences in sexual activity [25]. Drawn from a larger study of the social experiences of people on ART in PNG [26,27], this paper focuses on sexual behaviour and condom use. Furthermore, set in the country with the greatest HIV epidemic in the Pacific, our wider study was the first known behavioural study of people living with HIV (PLHIV) in the region and provides the only published quantitative data on PLHIV sexual behaviour in the region to date.

Results

Table 1 presents the socio-demographic characteristics for the entire sample and for men and women separately. Of the 374 study participants, 147 (39%) were men and 227 (61%) were women. The majority (72%) of the sample was aged 35 years or younger, with a median age of 30 years, and a range from 16 to 69 years. The men in the study were significantly older than the women, with median ages of 35 and 28 respectively. Three-quarters of the sample reported having never been to school (21%), or been educated up to elementary (9%) or primary school only (43%). Overall, men reported having attained a higher level of education than women with a significantly greater proportion of men having completed secondary or higher education (39%) compared with women (19%). One-fifth of the overall sample (20%) reported that they drink alcohol, and significantly more men drink (27%) compared with women (17%).

Almost half the participants (47%) were married or engaged (of these, only three were engaged), about one-fifth were separated or divorced (22%), almost a quarter were widowed (24%) and a small proportion were never married (7%). Overall, 38% (95% CI: 33% - 43%) of participants had sexual intercourse, and 32% (95% CI: 27% - 37%) of participants had sexual intercourse with a regular partner in the last six months. Men were significantly more likely to be married or engaged (58%) compared with women (40%). Men were also more likely to have had sexual intercourse in the last six months with a regular partner of the opposite sex (39%, 95% CI: 31% - 47%) compared with women (28%, 95% CI: 22% - 34%). Of those who were engaged or married, 58% (95% CI: 51% - 66%) had sexual intercourse with a regular opposite-sex partner, whereas only 9% (95% CI: 5% - 14%) of those who were never married, separated or divorced had sex with a regular opposite

Table 1 Sample characteristics

	Male (n = 147)	Female (n = 227)	Total (N = 374)	p (χ^2)[a]
Age in years[b]	35 (30–42)	28 (24–33)	30 (26–37)	**<0.001**
Marital status				**<0.001 (23.048)**
Never married	10% (15)	4% (10)	7% (25)	
Married / engaged	58% (85)	40% (90)	47% (175)	
Separated / divorced	18% (26)	25% (57)	22% (83)	
Widowed	14% (21)	31% (70)	24% (91)	
Education				**<0.001 (17.916)**
None	18% (26)	23% (53)	21% (79)	
Elementary / primary	44% (64)	58 % (131)	52% (195)	
Secondary or higher	39% (57)	19% (43)	27% (100)	
Drinks alcohol	27% (39)	16% (37)	20% (76)	**0.017 (5.666)**
Had any sex in the last six months	45% (66)	34% (77)	38% (143)	**0.033 (4.552)**
Had sex with regular partner in the last six months	39% (57)	28% (63)	32% (120)	**0.026 (4.974)**
Had sex with casual partner in the last six months	7% (10)	7% (16)	7% (26)	0.927 (0.008)
Knew HIV can be transmitted by having sex with another person	96% (141)	95% (215)	95% (356)	0.595 (0.283)
Knew consistent condom use prevent HIV transmission	87% (128)	78% (178)	82% (306)	**0.034 (4.499)**
Knew HIV cannot be transmitted via mosquito bites	77% (113)	78% (176)	77% (289)	0.881 (0.022)
Knew a HIV-infected person on ART may still infect their sexual partner	90% (132)	86% (195)	87% (327)	0.267 (1.231)
Knew ART medication can suppress HIV	88% (129)	81% (183)	83% (312)	0.070 (3.288)
Knew ART medication cannot get rid of HIV from the body	70% (103)	77% (175)	74% (278)	0.129 (2.307)

[a] Numbers in bold indicate that there is a statistically significant difference in the characteristic between males and females ($p < 0.05$).
[b] Median (lower and upper quartile) and p-value from Mann–Whitney U test for difference in age between males and females were given for age. Five participants did not report their age.

sex partners (not shown in table). Small and similar proportions of men and women (both 7%) had sexual intercourse with casual opposite-sex partners in the last six months.

Data from the interviews reinforced the behavioural data on high levels of sexual abstinence. While reasons for sexual abstinence were not asked in the behavioural survey, in the interviews participants discussed a number of motivating factors for why they were not sexually active. These included social and individual responsibility to avoid further transmission of the virus, a fear of super infection and a lack of sexual desire since being diagnosed with HIV. Examples of these motivators are suggested in the following narratives from study participants:

> I encourage other people not to dream about sex. You should abstain completely...It's people living with the virus who decide whether this virus goes on or not. So if everyone is really honest and takes responsibility and abstain from sexual behaviours the virus will die with them. (*Woman living with HIV)*

> What we should be preaching and telling people is don't do it...I think that condoms are not the answer. The answer is no sex and that is it. *(Man living with HIV)*

> Now that I am on medication I just don't want to sleep with men. What if I give them my disease and they give me theirs? Like I will get double sickness or something. *(Woman living with HIV)*

> Before I felt like having sex with anyone at anytime but now that I am on ART it has decreased my sexual drive. *(Man living with HIV)*

Abstinence from sexual intercourse was also the result of health education messages and the directives given from health care workers. These directives while posited within a type of positive living discourse entailed the incitement of fear and destruction. The following narrative examples illustrate this:

> They told me not to eat greasy food and stopped me from having sex with men. Don't get married...You can go and get married but you will destroy yourself again so don't get married. *(Woman living with HIV)*

> ...when I go for trainings they say that the dirt is below and the clean water is on top and when you shake this water the dirt and the clean water will mix like when you have sex with a man the virus of the

> man and the woman will work hard and it will make you feel weak and symptoms will quickly appear and you will lose weight, feel very sick and die. That's why my thoughts on not sleeping with a man is strong...I must stay by myself and the disease will just live in me without any strength. *(Woman living with HIV)*

Almost all participants reported that HIV can be sexually transmitted (95%), and over 80% knew that a HIV-positive person on ART may still infect their sexual partner (87%), that ART medication can reduce viral load (83%) and that consistent condom use prevents HIV transmission (82%). Comparatively fewer participants knew that HIV cannot be transmitted via mosquito bites (77%) and that ART medication cannot cure a person of HIV (74%). Significantly more men (compared with women) knew that consistent condom use prevents HIV transmission. Those with a higher level of education were more likely to know that HIV can be sexually transmitted (linear trend $p = 0.002$) and that HIV cannot be transmitted via mosquito bites (linear trend $p < 0.001$; not shown in table).

Table 2 shows the sexual behaviour of the 143 participants who had sexual intercourse in the last six months, of whom 66 were men and 77 were women. The majority of the 143 respondents had sex with a regular sexual partner only (77%), 7% had sex with both regular and casual sexual partners, 11% had sex with casual sexual partners only, and the rest (5%) comprised four women who did not report the type of sexual intercourse they had with their sex partner(s) and three men who only had sex with sex workers. There was no significant difference in consistent condom use amongst men and women during vaginal intercourse with either regular or casual sexual partners. Overall, 11 (17%) men reported that they had anal intercourse in the past six months, of whom one had anal intercourse with opposite-sex casual sexual partners only, one with both opposite-sex casual and regular sexual partners, four with opposite-sex regular sexual partners only and five had anal intercourse

Table 2 Sex practice of the participants who had sex in the last six months

	Male (n = 66)	Female (n = 77)	Overall (N = 143)	p (χ^2) [c]
Had sex with regular partner	86% (57)	81% (63)	84% (120)	0.461 (0.544)
Consistent condom use during vaginal sex with regular partner [a]				0.088 (2.936)
Yes	54% (31)	39% (24)	46% (55)	
No	46% (26)	61% (38)	54% (64)	
Condom use at last vaginal sex with regular partner [a]				0.085 (2.971)
Yes	70% (40)	55% (34)	62% (74)	
No	30% (17)	45% (28)	38% (45)	
Had opposite-sex anal sex with regular partner [b]				0.887 (0.020)
Yes	9% (5)	10% (6)	9% (11)	
No	91% (52)	90% (57)	91% (109)	
Had sex with casual partner	15% (10)	21% (16)	18% (26)	0.384 (0.757)
Consistent condom use during vaginal sex with casual partner				0.646 [c]
Yes	33% (2)	50% (8)	45% (10)	
No	67% (4)	50% (8)	55% (12)	
Condom use at last vaginal sex with casual partner				0.631 [c]
Yes	67% (4)	62% (10)	64% (14)	
No	33% (2)	38% (6)	36% (8)	
Had opposite-sex anal sex with casual partner				0.538 [c]
Yes	20% (2)	6% (1)	12% (3)	
No	80% (8)	94% (15)	89% (23)	
Had same-sex anal sex with casual partner				–
Yes	50% (5)	–	50% (5)	
No	50% (5)	–	50% (5)	
Had any anal sex	17% (11)	9% (7)	13% (18)	0.173 (1.854)

[a] One female participant did not answer the question on frequency of condom use during vaginal sex with regular partner in the last six months.
[b] As none had sex with same-sex regular partners in the last six months, only opposite-sex anal sex was reported with regular partner.
[c] Pearson chi-square test was used for all variables except consistent condom use and having had opposite-sex anal sex with casual partner for which Fisher exact test was used.

with same-sex casual sexual partners only. Only 11 (9%) women reported that they had anal intercourse with a regular sexual partner.

Table 3 shows the factors associated with having had sexual intercourse in the last six months. Significantly fewer women had sex in the last six months in the unadjusted bivariate analysis, but this is not significant after adjusting for marital status in a Mantel-Haenszel test (OR_{MH} = 0.86; 95%CI = 0.53 - 1.39; $\chi_{MH}^2 = 0.37$; p = 0.543; not shown in table) or for a combination of other factors in the logistic regression model. Those who were married, with a higher level of education, who drink alcohol, who were resident in the Southern region (i.e. Port Moresby) and who knew that HIV cannot be transmitted via mosquito bites were more likely to have had sexual intercourse in the last six months in both the bivariate and regression analyses.

Table 4 shows the factors associated with consistent condom use during vaginal intercourse with a regular sexual partner in the last six months. After adjustment for other factors, women were significantly less likely to use a condom compared with men. Having an HIV-negative regular sexual partner was associated with more consistent condom use, although this was not significant. This non-significance is possibly due to the lack of power as only a small number of participants (n = 26)

Table 3 Factors associated with having had sex in the last six months (N = 374)

	% (count)					
	Did not have sex (n = 231)	Had sex (n = 143)	Crude OR (95% CI)	p[a]	Adj. OR (95% CI)	p[a]
Female (versus Male)	65% (150)	54% (77)	**0.63 (0.41, 0.96)**	**0.033**	1.03 (0.60, 1.77)	0.918
Age [b]				0.482		-
16-25	24% (55)	25% (36)	1.00		-	
26-35	45% (103)	50% (71)	1.05 (0.63, 1.77)	0.845	-	-
>35	30% (69)	25% (35)	0.77 (0.43, 1.39)	0.394	-	-
Marital status				**<0.001**		**<0.001**
Never married	9% (20)	4% (5)	**0.15 (0.05, 0.42)**	**<0.001**	**0.08 (0.02, 0.24)**	**<0.001**
Married / engaged	29% (66)	76% (109)	1.00		1.00	
Separated / divorced	27% (63)	14% (20)	**0.19 (0.11, 0.35)**	**<0.001**	**0.15 (0.08, 0.29)**	**<0.001**
Widowed	36% (82)	6% (9)	**0.66 (0.03, 0.14)**	**<0.001**	**0.05 (0.02, 0.12)**	**<0.001**
Education				**<0.001**[c]		**0.041**
None	25% (58)	15% (21)	1.00		1.00	
Elementary / primary	55% (128)	47% (67)	1.45 (0.81, 2.58)	0.213	1.20 (0.59, 2.42)	0.616
Secondary or higher	20% (45)	39% (55)	**3.37 (1.79, 6.38)**	**<0.001**	**2.43 (1.09, 5.41)**	**0.030**
Region of residence				0.064		**0.015**
Southern	25% (58)	34% (49)	1.00		1.00	
Highlands	67% (154)	62% (89)	0.68 (0.43, 1.09)	0.106	0.57 (0.31, 1.03)	0.063
Momase	8% (18)	4% (5)	**0.33 (0.11, 0.97)**	**0.034**	**0.18 (0.05, 0.62)**	**0.007**
Drinks alcohol (versus Does not drink alcohol)	16% (38)	27% (38)	**1.83 (1.10, 3.04)**	**0.020**	**2.04 (1.08, 3.87)**	**0.029**
Knew HIV can be transmitted by having sex with another person	95% (219)	96% (137)	1.25 (0.46, 3.42)	0.661	-	-
Knew consistent condom use prevent HIV transmission	81% (188)	83% (118)	1.08 (0.63, 1.86)	0.783	-	-
Knew HIV cannot be transmitted via mosquito bites	72% (166)	86% (123)	**2.41 (1.37, 4.22)**	**0.002**	**2.60 (1.31, 5.13)**	**0.006**
Knew a HIV-infected person on ART may still infect their sexual partner	85% (198)	90% (129)	1.54 (0.79, 2.99)	0.203	-	-
Knew ART medication can suppress HIV	83% (191)	85% (121)	1.15 (0.65, 2.03)	0.626	-	-
Knew ART medication cannot get rid of HIV from the body	71% (164)	80% (114)	1.61 (0.97, 2.65)	0.061	1.23 (0.66, 2.28)	0.509

[a] Numbers in bold indicate that there is a statistically significant association with having sex in the last six months (p < 0.05).
[b] Five participants did not report their age.
[c] There was a significant linear trend (p < 0.001) of increase in having had sex in the last six months with higher education level with crude OR (95% CI) of 1.85 (1.37, 2.51).

Table 4 Consistent condom use during vaginal sex with regular sex partner (N = 119)

	% (count)					
	Inconsistent condom use (n = 64)	Consistent condom use (n = 55)	Crude OR (95% CI)[a]	p[a]	Adj OR (95% CI)[a]	p[a]
Female (versus Male)	59% (38)	44% (24)	0.53 (0.25, 1.11)	0.088	**0.39 (0.17, 0.88)**	**0.023**
Age [b]				0.183		-
16-25	30% (19)	20% (11)	1.00		–	
26-35	51% (32)	47% (26)	1.40 (0.56, 3.50)	0.465	–	–
>35	19% (12)	33% (18)	2.59 (0.88, 7.63)	0.073	–	–
Married/ engaged (versus Not married / engaged)	91% (58)	78% (43)	0.37 (0.13 , 1.09)	0.060	0.34 (0.10, 1.13)	0.078
HIV sero-concordance				0.195		–
Concordant (i.e. partner is HIV positive)	64% (41)	56% (31)	1.00		–	
Disconcordant (i.e. partner is HIV negative)	16% (10)	29% (16)	2.12 (0.83, 5.39)	0.108	–	–
Unknown (i.e. partner's status is unknown)	20% (13)	15% (8)	0.81 (0.30, 2.22)	0.687	–	–
HIV positive status disclosed to partner	92% (59)	87% (48)	0.58 (0.17, 1.97)	0.377	–	–
Education				0.110 [c]		–
None	17% (11)	9% (5)	1.00		–	
Elementary / primary	50% (32)	40% (22)	1.51 (0.46, 5.03)	0.496	–	–
Secondary or higher	33% (21)	51% (28)	2.93 (0.85, 10.13)	0.074	–	–
Region of residence				0.751		–
Southern	33% (21)	27% (15)	1.00		–	
Highlands	63% (40)	69% (38)	1.33 (0.60, 2.97)	0.485	–	-
Momase	5% (3)	4% (2)	0.93 (0.14, 6.44)	0.944	–	-
Drinks alcohol (versus Does not drink alcohol)	16% (10)	35% (19)	**2.85 (1.16, 7.01)**	**0.017**	**2.76 (1.05, 7.21)**	**0.039**
Knew HIV can be transmitted by having sex with another person	94% (60)	98% (54)	3.60 (0.38, 33.98)	0.232	–	–
Knew consistent condom use prevent HIV transmission	84% (54)	82% (45)	0.83 (0.32, 2.19)	0.711	–	–
Knew HIV cannot be transmitted via mosquito bites	84% (54)	89% (49)	1.51 (0.51, 4.50)	0.454	–	–
Knew a HIV-infected person on ART may still infect their sexual partner	86% (55)	96% (53)	4.34 (0.87, 21.71)	0.051	4.88 (0.76, 31.27)	0.094
Knew ART medication can suppress HIV	84% (54)	89% (49)	1.51 (0.51, 4.50)	0.454	–	–
Knew ART medication cannot cure HIV	70% (45)	89% (49)	**3.45 (1.22, 9.71)**	**0.013**	**3.89 (1.30, 11.62)**	**0.015**

[a] Numbers in bold indicate that there is a statistically significant association with consistent condom use during vaginal sex with regular sex partner ($p < 0.05$).
[b] One participant did not report his age.
[c] There was a significant linear trend ($p = 0.038$) of increase in consistent condom use with higher education level with crude OR (95% CI) of 1.74 (1.03, 2.94).

identified that their regular sexual partner was HIV-negative (i.e. they were in a serodiscordant relationship). Almost all of the participants with a regular sexual partner had disclosed their HIV status to them (90%) and disclosure was significantly higher amongst those who reported they were married or engaged (94%) compared with those who were not married or engaged (67%; p = 0.003 from Fisher's exact test). Disclosure of an HIV-positive status was also not significantly associated with consistent condom use. Of the 12 participants who did not disclose, one knew their partner was HIV-positive and another knew their partner was HIV-negative. Those who drank alcohol were more likely to consistently use a condom, compared with those who did not drink alcohol and those who knew that ART could not cure a person with HIV were over three times more likely to use a condom than those who did not in both the bivariate and regression analyses.

From the interviews it is evident that for people in sero-discordant sexual relationships, and where HIV status was disclosed, the use of condoms was something that was negotiated and entailed intimate partner communication. This was particularly the case for women with HIV. Women reported that they had initially started to use condoms with their regular HIV-negative partner but that as the relationship continued condom used discontinued. For example, one woman said the following about her HIV-negative husband:

> 'He told me, I love you and we will live together. In my own belief your sickness will not get me' he said... We stayed with condoms for six months but after six months he told me 'How long are we going to use condoms? Will we use them until we die?'

There was no data in the qualitative interviews as to whether or not women would rather have continued using condoms but were unable to counter their husband's preference. The qualitative interviews from married women and men whose partners were HIV-positive indicated that condoms were not needed as a result of concordant serostatus.

Discussion

Overall, the level of sexual activity amongst the sample in this study was low. The overall percentage of both women and men on ART who reported sexual activity (38%) is much lower than the proportions found by some studies in developing country contexts see for example [28-32]. For example, the proportion of women in this study reporting sexual activity in the last six months is lower than that found among women in a three-country study of Brazil, South Africa and Uganda [5] where almost half had sexual intercourse in the last month (46%).

Not surprisingly there was a relationship between sexual intercourse in the past six months and a person's marital status with married people more likely to have had sexual intercourse. Among those that have never married, were separated/divorced or widowed, 9% reported that they had sexual intercourse with a regular partner, but this is significantly less than those who reported themselves as married or engaged (58%). This finding on the relationship between sexual intercourse and marital status concurs with data from other developing countries with heterosexually driven epidemics. For example, married people with HIV in Kenya were significantly more likely to report sexual intercourse than those who were not [22]. Similarly, in Uganda, compared with HIV-positive people who were widowed, those who identified as married were also significantly more likely to be sexually active [16,17]. Likewise, a three-country study by Kaida et al. [5] showed that recent sexual activity for HIV-positive women in Brazil, South Africa and Uganda was significantly associated with being married.

Marital status was similarly important, although not statistically significant, in relation to consistent condom use. Those who reported not being married or engaged reported higher rates of consistent condom use compared with those who were married. HIV-positive people on ART who were married or engaged were more likely to be sexually active with a regular partner but were at the same time less likely to consistently use condoms, irrespective of a partner's HIV status cf. [27].

The high level of sexual abstinence by women in this study suggests that although the literature to date has shown little to no control by women over their sexual and reproductive lives, the women in this study, and in particular those who were not married, were not devoid of power to control their sexual life as is indicated elsewhere. And merely because a woman with HIV does not use a condom with her husband does not automatically and unequivocally equate with disempowerment, as suggested by the qualitative interviews. The qualitative data from this study offers some insights into this particular aspect of the behavioural data and involves intangible issues associated with long-term relationships, intimate communication and love. Rather, condom use is negotiated in light of knowledge of a partner's HIV status, long-term commitment and love. For those women with HIV-negative partners inconsistent condom use appears to be the initiated by their regular male partners. As one of the quotes used in the Results section of this paper illustrates, it appears that their regular partners (husbands) had accepted their HIV status and were not afraid of becoming infected. International research supports this inference, especially research in serodiscordant couples where it has been shown that the HIV-negative partner has been the principal initiator of unsafe sex [33,34]. One reading of this could be that men had a poor understanding of their risk for HIV acquisition. Another reading of the data is that women were not able to counter their partners' wishes to discontinue using condoms. A more likely scenario from an detailed reading of that data suggests that this absence of fear was based on elusive aspects of a relationships including acceptance of HIV, understanding and experience of risk and other relationship issues such as duration of the relationship, love and intimacy [27]. Furthermore, what it means to be in a serodiscordant relationship is context-specific and it cannot then be assumed that risk-management and decisions about sexual practices will be and indeed should be the same globally [35].

Women were not questioned about lifetime sexual or physical violence or about sexual relationship power, so we cannot therefore postulate about their ability to have control in their sexual and reproductive lives more generally, as is possible in other studies cf. [36]. There is however some research in PNG that does link HIV status with lifetime intimate partner violence [37]. Unlike other studies that link HIV risk to intimate partner violence amongst newly diagnosed women with HIV, this study was of women who were already diagnosed with HIV. Furthermore, of the women with HIV-negative partners, all were in relationships that had been initiated following their diagnosis and therefore we cannot comment of the relationship between violence and HIV risk as others have done.

It is true that in PNG women are subjugated to much gender-based violence and have been reported to have minimal to no control over their sexual and reproductive lives [38,39]. Furthermore, international research has consistently reported that women's vulnerability to HIV is linked to an absence of power, ability to negotiate sexual relationships and experiences of intimate partner violence cf. [36,40]. Moreover, it has long been posited that gender-based power differentials between women and men often compromises a woman's ability to negotiate condoms cf. [41,42]. Although it may well be possible that women in this study were unable to counter their HIV-negative partners' desire to discontinue using condoms, this is not what the data suggested. This is an interesting finding and warrants further scrutiny especially in light of the long history of research on gender, HIV and vulnerably that suggests otherwise. It would however appear that it is possible that this data contributes to a recent and increasing recognition within PNG that women can and indeed are exhibiting agency in choosing sexual and lifetime partners [43], with some becoming involved in polygamous marriages in the desire to obtain status through money and items of modernity such as cars and expensive mobile phones [44].

In countries where viral load testing is part of routine clinical care and management, informed choices about viral suppression and risk of HIV transmission are possible. To date this is not the situation in PNG. And although in other settings there is an awareness of the low risk of sexual transmission while on ART (for example the Swiss Statement) there is no such discourse or health messaging in PNG. In fact, there is evidence in PNG that PLHIV whose partner is also positive are recommended to still use condoms for fear of 'super-infection' [45]. Therefore, it is unlikely that such knowledge about viral load and infectivity can account for unprotected sex between sero-discordant partners for whom condoms play a greater role than where both partners are HIV-positive.

Although people living with HIV are increasingly making active choices to have children as a recent qualitative study of prevention of mother-to-child transmission in PNG has found [45], it is our informed opinion in this study that the low use of condoms was not reflective of a desire on behalf of HIV-positive women to conceive or of HIV-positive men to father a child. In 2008, when this study was conducted, ART was not widely available, and there was little to no discussion of HIV-positive women actively choosing to reproduce (as opposed to testing HIV-positive while pregnant) and prevention of mother to child transmission programs were still in their infancy. No women in the qualitative arm of our study reported wanting to have children after being diagnosed with HIV and neither did any men report wanting to have children. Furthermore, the qualitative data suggests that we can be confident that participants' low rates of reported sexual activity was not an artefact of social desirability or indeed a discrepancy in what is constituted as sexual intercourse. Rather the qualitative data suggests that in the early stages of ART availability in PNG, many PLHIV were against the notion of both themselves and any other PLHIV from having sex. At the time of this study participants were reporting that reasons for sexual abstinence included a personal and social responsibility not to transmit HIV to another person and a fear of becoming re-infected with HIV. There was no gender difference in reported reasons for sexual abstinence. Additionally, the role of others, particularly health care workers, influencing a person's beliefs and therefore decisions about sexual behaviour were also deemed important. This is not surprising since adherence to ART was also related to following instruction from the doctor/health care worker [46]. As people stay on treatment and as people live longer it will be important to chart if and how sexual behaviour changes and if the meanings ascribed to sexual intercourse and condom use similarly alter.

Since much of the HIV prevention message in PNG focuses on reducing extra-marital relationships and being faithful to one's partner, it appears that safe sex within marriages of people living with HIV may need to be emphasised. Condoms have traditionally been seen in PNG as something used outside of a marriage; sex within a marriage is perceived to be safe and this is suggested by the 'one faithful partner concept' [47-50]. However in this study of HIV-positive people, those who were married or engaged were proportionally more likely to report having an HIV-positive partner than those who were not, and for those with HIV-positive partners, the need for consistent condom use to prevent transmission is lessened [48]. Though not statistically significant, proportionally less of those with a HIV-positive partner (43%) or of those who did not know the status of their regular partner (38%) consistently used condoms compared with those whose partner was HIV-negative (62%). In other words, consistent condom use was much higher (OR 2.12) among participants whose partners were known to be HIV-negative. Others have similarly identified that the HIV status of one's partner affects condom use [27,51].

Almost all of the participants with a regular sexual partner had disclosed their HIV status to them and disclosure was significantly higher amongst those who were married or engaged compared with those who were not. This rate of disclosure to a sexual partner was much higher than that found in other studies, which report disclosure rates to regular partners ranging between 62 - 80% [52-55]. Similarly this data suggests that compared with positive people in other settings who report barriers to disclosure of serostatus cf. [56], people in PNG experienced fewer obstacles in the disclosure of HIV in intimate sexual relationships.

Consistent use of condoms was not significantly associated with HIV knowledge. Knowledge about the preventative nature of condoms against the sexual transmission of HIV was high (77%), indicating, as others have found, that there was a discrepancy between knowledge and behaviour. Among those that reported vaginal intercourse in the last six months, less than half (46%) reported consistent condom use. However, knowing that ART cannot cure a person of HIV was significantly associated with consistent condom use (OR 3.89). In other words, people with living HIV who were well-informed about their ART were using condoms more consistently. This contrasts with South African data which found that HIV and ART knowledge was not associated with condom use [19]. The association between education level and knowledge that HIV can be transmitted via sexual intercourse, but not via mosquito bites indicates that there could be some confusion about transmission of HIV which may be different from other commonly known blood-borne pathogens such as malaria amongst people who are less educated. This suggests that educational materials targeting this confusion may be beneficial.

Our study found that there was a strong association between having sexual intercourse in the last six months and consuming alcohol. On the other hand, there was a strong association between consistent condom use and consuming alcohol. While other behavioural studies have shown a relationship amongst HIV-positive people between drinking alcohol and high risk sexual behaviour [14,32,57,58] this was not the case in this study of Papua New Guineans on ART.

Conclusions

Given that inconsistent condom use is more frequent in married and engaged relationships and in relationships where HIV status is undisclosed, structural prevention efforts that prioritise and increase access to couple testing and support safe HIV disclosure are likely to play an important role in the prevention of intimate partner transmission in PNG. As people's health continues to improve on ART it may well be that people currently single or widowed may re-engage in sexual relationships and will need support and education to do so in a safe manner. Results from this study show that people living with HIV who are well-informed about ART are more consistent in their use of condoms. It thus appears that health care services play an important role as a structural facilitator for HIV prevention cf. [59] where health education during a person's preparation with a health care worker to initiate ART plays an important role in the prevention of HIV through the use of condoms. Therefore, positive prevention needs to take a holistic view to preventing secondary transmission of HIV through wider HIV education such as ART rather than messages that simply chant to always use a condom. It also reinforces the wider health benefits of access to ART and good clinical education about the use of ART. Continuing to engage people with HIV in positive prevention, of discussing serostatus mixing and HIV disclosure will be important in preventing the secondary transmission of HIV in PNG and are likely to play a far greater role than a one-dimensional HIV prevention message of always using a condom. Moreover, as greater numbers of people are diagnosed with HIV; HIV-positive people are prescribed ART; survival rates increase and biomedical markers such as CD4 count and possibly viral load become part of standard clinical practice then, the sexual lives of PLHIV in PNG are likely to have changed and further research is warranted.

Methods

The data were collected as part of a mixed-method study undertaken in six provinces throughout PNG between February and July 2008. The purpose of the study was to explore the social experience of HIV-positive men and women on ART.

A total of 374 HIV-positive people over the age of 16 and had been on ART for more than two weeks were recruited using a non-probability, convenience sampling methodology. As of December 2007, just prior to the commencement of this study there were 2,250 people enrolled on ART (185 of whom were children [60]). This survey therefore accounted for around 18% of adults on ART. Participants were recruited through a number of sites including ART prescribing sites, PLHIV drop-in centres and support groups in six provinces: Southern Highlands Province, National Capital District, Eastern Highlands Province, Morobe Province, Chimbu Province and Western Highlands Province.

Participants were invited by a third party (other PLHIV or health care workers) to participate in the study. All potential participants were explicitly informed that they were under no obligation to participate, and their access to ART or any form of treatment or support would not be affected should they decide not to participate in the study. Health care workers often gave a large 'toksave' (public notice) to PLHIV at the ART clinic waiting to be seen by a health care worker rather than individually inviting participants to participate.

After potential participants provided initial consent, they were directed to a nominated researcher. Once they had made contact, the researcher explained the purpose of the study and outlined what participation would entail. Upon providing informed consent, the participant completed an interviewer-administered questionnaire in either *Tok Pisin*, a PNG lingua franca, or English.

The interviewers were Papua New Guineans undergoing an intensive HIV social research training cadetship, coordinated by the PNG Institute of Medical Research and the University of New South Wales. In addition, a person living with HIV was employed as a member of the research team and trained in the methodologies of the study. Analysis of the data was undertaken by the lead authors.

The survey included items on socio-demographics, knowledge and beliefs around HIV and treatment, stigma and discrimination, health and well-being, disclosure, food security, alcohol use, ART adherence, sexual practices, and access to services. Standardised scales were used and piloted prior to study. At the end of the questionnaire one qualitative question on the meaning of ART in people's lives was also asked.

No names were recorded on the questionnaire. All questionnaires were coded by province and recruitment site. A sub-sample of 36 participants also participated in a semi-structured qualitative interview. Qualitative data was used to triangulate behavioural data. The results reinforced key quantitative findings and provided socio-cultural and gendered context to the meaning of the behavioural data.

Ethical considerations

Ethics approval for this study was granted by the Papua New Guinea Medical Research Advisory Committee, the Research Advisory Committee of the National AIDS Council Secretariat of Papua New Guinea, the Papua New Guinea Institute of Medical Research Internal Review Board and the Human Ethics Committee of the University of New South Wales.

Questions and variables on sex practice

All participants were asked whether they had sexual intercourse in the last six months. Those participants who had sexual intercourse in the last six months were then asked whether they had sexual intercourse with a regular and/or a casual opposite sex partner in the last six months and whether they had vaginal and/or anal intercourse with these partners. Men were asked an additional question on whether or not they had sexual intercourse with another man in the past six months. Of those who had vaginal intercourse in the last six months with a regular or casual sex partner, participants were asked whether they never used a condom, or sometimes, almost every time or always used a condom during vaginal intercourse. Consistent condom use during vaginal intercourse was dichotomised into "yes" for using a condom every time versus "no" for all other answers (i.e. never, sometimes, almost every time or no response). Participants were also asked whether they used a condom during the last vaginal or anal intercourse with their regular or casual sex partner.

Statistical analysis

All categorical variables were analysed using the $\chi 2$ test for bivariate association. All continuous variables were analysed using the Mann–Whitney U test. Variables with $p < 0.10$ in the bivariate analyses were entered into a logistic regression model to estimate adjusted odds ratios and 95% confidence intervals for further examining factors associated with sexual practice and condom use with regular partners. As none of the men had anal intercourse with a regular male partner in the last six months, the analyses on intercourse and condom use with regular sex partners comprises only regular partners of the opposite-sex. All analyses were carried out using Stata v11 [61].

Qualitative analysis

All interviews were digitally recorded, transcribed and translated into English. All identifiable information was removed. All interviews were managed and analysed using Nvivo 9 qualitative analysis software. Analysis of interviews was based on a grounded theory approach to data [62]. After initial reading of all of the interviews, memo writing and data comparison, a codebook was developed by two of the researchers. Interviews were double coded and where a discrepancy emerged the two researchers discussed the data and a decision on the final code made. Data saturation was reached with no new themes emerging. Preliminary data analysis was presented at team meetings and discussed during the writing up of the study report and subsequent publications.

Competing interests

The authors declare that they have no competing interests.

Authors' contributions

WYNM led the analysis of quantitative data and drafting of the paper. AK designed the study, secured funding, oversaw data collection and data analysis, led the analysis of qualitative data, contributed to the drafting of the manuscript and revising it critically for important intellectual content and gave final approval of the version to be submitted. AF oversaw the first stages of data analysis of the study and contributed to the drafting of the manuscript. PS contributed to the drafting of the manuscript. HW assisted in securing funding for the study and overseeing the implementation of it and contributed to the drafting of the manuscript. MK, AM, BK, RE, FA, BC, LW, LP and SN collected data and participated in data analysis for the manuscript. TL assisted in data analysis for this manuscript. PMS assisted in securing funding for the study, oversaw the implementation of the study and contributed to the drafting of the manuscript. All authors read and approved the final manuscript.

Acknowledgements
The authors would like to acknowledge the Papua New Guinea National AIDS Council Secretariat who funded the study from which this manuscript is drawn from and acknowledge the contribution and support of people living with HIV in PNG.

Author details
[1]School of Public Health and Community Medicine, UNSW Medicine, University of New South Wales, Sydney, Australia. [2]Faculty of Health Sciences, University of Sydney, Sydney, New South Wales, Australia. [3]Sexual & Reproductive Health Unit, Papua New Guinea Institute of Medical Research, Goroka, Papua New Guinea.

References

1. Papua New Guinea National AIDS Council Secretariat: *Papua New Guinea HIV Prevalence: 2009 Estimates.* Port Moresby: PNG NACS; 2010.
2. Papua New Guinea National Department of Health: *The 2011 STI, HIV and AIDS Annual Surveillance Report.* Port Moresby: PNG NDoH; 2012.
3. Joint United Nations Programme on HIV/AIDS, World Health Organization: *Oceania AIDS Epidemic Update: Regional Summary.* Geneva, Switzerland: UNAIDS; 2007.
4. Smith GP: *Growing up with Tok Pisin: Contact, creolization, and change in Papua New Guinea's national language.* London, UK: Battlebridge Publications; 2002.
5. Kaida A, Gray G, Bastos FI, Andia I, Maier M, McIntyre J, Grinsztejn B, Strathdee SA, Bangsberg DR, Hogg R: **The relationship between HAART use and sexual activity among HIV-positive women of reproductive age in Brazil, South Africa, and Uganda.** *AIDS Care* 2008, **20**(1):21–25.
6. Stolte IG, Dukers NH, de Wit JB, Fennema JS, Coutinho RA: **Increase in sexually transmitted infections among homosexual men in Amsterdam in relation to HAART.** *Sex Transm Infect* 2001, **77**(3):184–186.
7. Katz MH, Schwarcz SK, Kellogg TA, Klausner JD, Dilley JW, Gibson S, McFarland W: **Impact of highly active antiretroviral treatment on HIV seroincidence among men who have sex with men: San Francisco.** *Am J Public Health* 2002, **92**(3):388–394.
8. Crepaz N, Hart TA, Marks G: **Highly active antiretroviral therapy and sexual risk behavior: A meta-analytic review.** *J Am Med Assoc* 2004, **292**(2):224–236.
9. Crepaz N, Marks G: **Towards an understanding of sexual risk behavior in people living with HIV: A review of social, psychological, and medical findings.** *AIDS* 2002, **16**(2):135–149.
10. Stolte IG, Dukers NH: **Response to 'High-risk sexual behaviour increases among London gay men between 1998 and 2001: what is the role of HIV optimism?'.** *AIDS* 2003, **17**(13):2011–2012. author reply 2012–2013.
11. Elford J: **Changing patterns of sexual behaviour in the era of highly active antiretroviral therapy.** *Curr Opin Infect Dis* 2006, **19**(1):26–32.
12. Diamond C, Richardson JL, Milam J, Stoyanoff S, McCutchan JA, Kemper C, Larsen RA, Hollander H, Weismuller P, Bolan R: **Use of and adherence to antiretroviral therapy is associated with decreased sexual risk behavior in HIV clinic patients.** *J Acquir Immune Defic Syndr* 2005, **39**(2):211–218.
13. Van Der Snoek EM, De Wit JBF, Mulder PGH, Van Der Meijden WI: **Incidence of sexually transmitted diseases and HIV infection related to perceived HIV/AIDS threat since highly active antiretroviral therapy availability in men who have sex with men.** *Sex Transm Dis* 2005, **32**(3):170–175.
14. Apondi R, Bunnell R, Ekwaru JP, Moore D, Bechange S, Khana K, King R, Campbell J, Tappero J, Mermin J: **Sexual behavior and HIV transmission risk of Ugandan adults taking antiretroviral therapy: 3 year follow-up.** *AIDS* 2011, **25**(10):1317–1327.
15. Bechange S, Bunnell R, Awor A, Moore D, King R, Mermin J, Tappero J, Khana K, Bartholow B: **Two-year follow-up of sexual behavior among HIV-uninfected household members of adults taking antiretroviral therapy in Uganda: No evidence of disinhibition.** *AIDS Behav* 2010, **14**(4):816–823.
16. Bunnell R, Ekwaru JP, Solberg P, Wamai N, Bikaako-Kajura W, Were W, Coutinho A, Liechty C, Madraa E, Rutherford G, *et al:* **Changes in sexual behavior and risk of HIV transmission after antiretroviral therapy and prevention interventions in rural Uganda.** *AIDS* 2006, **20**(1):85–92.
17. Bunnell R, Opio A, Musinguzi J, Kirungi W, Ekwaru P, Mishra V, Hladik W, Kafuko J, Madraa E, Mermin J: **HIV transmission risk behavior among HIV-infected adults in Uganda: Results of a nationally representative survey.** *AIDS* 2008, **22**(5):617–624.
18. Eisele TP, Mathews C, Chopra M, Lurie MN, Brown L, Dewing S, Kendall C: **Changes in risk behavior among HIV-positive patients during their first year of antiretroviral therapy in Cape Town South Africa.** *AIDS Behav* 2009, **13**(6):1097–1105.
19. Peltzer K, Ramlagan S: **Safer sexual behaviours after 1 year of antiretroviral treatment in KwaZulu-Natal, South Africa: A prospective cohort study.** *Sex Health* 2010, **7**(2):135–141.
20. Venkatesh KK, De Bruyn G, Lurie MN, Mohapi L, Pronyk P, Moshabela M, Marinda E, Gray GE, Triche EW, Martinson NA: **Decreased sexual risk behavior in the era of HAART among HIV-infected urban and rural South Africans attending primary care clinics.** *AIDS* 2010, **24**(17):2687–2696.
21. Eisele TP, Mathews C, Chopra M, Brown L, Silvestre E, Daries V, Kendall C: **High levels of risk behavior among people living with HIV initiating and waiting to start antiretroviral therapy in Cape Town South Africa.** *AIDS Behav* 2008, **12**(4):570–577.
22. Sarna A, Luchters SMF, Geibel S, Kaai S, Munyao P, Shikely KS, Mandaliya K, Van Dam J, Temmerman M: **Sexual risk behaviour and HAART: A comparative study of HIV-infected persons on HAART and on preventive therapy in Kenya.** *Int J STD AIDS* 2008, **19**(2):85–89.
23. Kennedy C, O'Reilly K, Medley A, Sweat M: **The impact of HIV treatment on risk behaviour in developing countries: A systematic review.** *AIDS Care - Psycho Socio-Med Aspects AIDS/HIV* 2007, **19**(6):707–720.
24. Bateganya M, Colfax G, Shafer LA, Kityo C, Mugyenyi P, Serwadda D, Mayanja H, Bangsberg D: **Antiretroviral therapy and sexual behavior: A comparative study between antiretroviral-naive and -experienced patients at an urban HIV/AIDS care and research center in Kampala.** *Uganda. AIDS Patient Care STDs* 2005, **19**(11):760–768.
25. Berhan A, Berhan Y: **Is the Sexual Behaviour of HIV Patients on Antiretroviral therapy safe or risky in Sub-Saharan Africa? Meta-Analysis and Meta-Regression.** *AIDS Res Ther* 2012, **9**(1):14.
26. Kelly A, Frankland A, Kupul M, Kepa B, Cangah B, Nosi S, Emori R, Walizopa L, Mek A, Pirpir L, *et al: The Art of Living: The Social Experience of Treatments for People Living With HIV in Papua New Guinea.* Goroka PNG: Papua New Guinea Institute of Medical Research; 2009.
27. Kelly A, Kupul M, Frankland A, Worth H, Nosi S, Mek A, Kepa B, Walizopa L, Emori R, Pirpir L, *et al:* **Living serodiscordantly in Papua New Guinea: Sexual practices of HIV-positive people on ART by serostatus of regular heterosexual partner.** *AIDS Care - Psycho Socio-Med Aspects AIDS/HIV* 2011, **23**(6):734–740.
28. Seeley J, Russell S, Khana K, Ezati E, King R, Bunnell R: **Sex after ART: Sexual partnerships established by HIV-infected persons taking anti-retroviral therapy in Eastern Uganda.** *Cult Health Sex* 2009, **11**(7):703–716.
29. Pearson CR, Cassels S, Kurth AE, Montoya P, Micek MA, Gloyd SS: **Change in sexual activity 12 months after ART initiation among HIV-positive mozambicans.** *AIDS Behav* 2011, **15**(4):778–787.
30. Wandera B, Kamya MR, Castelnuovo B, Kiragga A, Kambugu A, Wanyama JN, Easterbrook P, Sethi AK: **Sexual behaviors over a 3-year period among individuals with advanced HIV/AIDS receiving antiretroviral therapy in an Urban HIV clinic in Kampala, Uganda.** *J Acquir Immune Defic Syndr* 2011, **57**(1):62–68.
31. Lurie M, Pronyk P, De Moor E, Heyer A, De Bruyn G, Struthers H, McIntyre J, Gray G, Marinda E, Klipstein-Grobusch K, *et al:* **Sexual behavior and reproductive health among HIV-infected patients in urban and rural South Africa.** *J Acquir Immune Defic Syndr* 2008, **47**(4):484–493.
32. Venkatesh KK, Srikrishnan AK, Safren SA, Triche EW, Thamburaj E, Prasad L, Lurie MN, Kumar MS, Kumarasamy N, Solomon S, *et al:* **Sexual risk behaviors among HIV-infected South Indian couples in the HAART era: Implications for reproductive health and HIV care delivery.** *AIDS Care - Psycho Socio-Med Aspects AIDS/HIV* 2011, **23**(6):722–733.
33. Van Der Straten A, Vernon KA, Knight KR, Gómez CA, Padian NS: **Managing HIV among serodiscordant heterosexual couples: Serostatus, stigma and sex.** *AIDS Care - Psycho Socio-Med Aspects AIDS/HIV* 1998, **10**(5):533–548.
34. Kalichman SC: **Couples with HIV/AIDS.** In *The psychology of couples and illness.* Edited by Schmaling KB, Sher TG. Washington: American Psychological Association; 2000:171–190.

35. Persson A: **Notes on the concepts of "serodiscordance" and "risk" in couples with mixed HIV status.** *Global Public Health.* 2012 Oct 9; **8**(2):209-20.
36. Dunkle KL, Jewkes RK, Brown HC, Gray GE, McIntryre JA, Harlow SD: **Gender-based violence, relationship power, and risk of HIV infection in women attending antenatal clinics in South Africa.** *Lancet* 2004, **363**(9419):1415–1421.
37. Lewis I, Maruia B, Mills D, Walker S: *Final report on links between HIV transmission and violence against women in PNG.* Canberra, Australian Capital Territory: University of Canberra; 2007.
38. Australian Agency for International Development: *Violence against women in Melanesia and East Timor: Building on regional and global promising approaches.* Canberra, Australia: Office of Development Effectiveness; 2008.
39. Constitutional and Law Reform Commission of Papua New Guinea: *Final report on domestic violence. Report No 14.* Port Moresby, Papua New Guinea: Constitutional and Law Reform Commission of Papua New Guinea; 1992.
40. Maman S, Campbell J, Sweat MD, Gielen AC: **The intersections of HIV and violence: Directions for future research and interventions.** *Soc Sci Med* 2000, **50**(4):459–478.
41. Amaro H: **Love, sex, and power: Considering women's realities in HIV prevention.** *Am Psychol* 1995, **50**(6):437–447.
42. Amaro H, Raj A: **On the margin: Power and women's HIV risk reduction strategies.** *Sex Roles* 2000, **42**(7–8):723–749.
43. Spark C: **Gender trouble in town: Educated women eluding male domination, gender violence and marriage in PNG.** *Asia Pacific J Anthro* 2011, **12**(2):164–179.
44. Mek A, Kelly A, Wilson L, Siki R, Aeno H, Naketrumb R, Whittaker M, Fitzgerald L, Kaldor J, Vallely A: *Mi igris long koins bilong em (I was attracted to him for his money): The socio-cultural context of women's involvement and experiences of polygamous marriages in the highlands of PNG, conference paper presented at Sexualities, Sexual Rights and HIV in Papua New Guinea and the Pacific.* Canberra, Australia; 2012.
45. Kelly A, Worth H, Kupul M, Fiya V, Vallely L, Neo R, Ase S, Ofi P, Mola G, Kariwiga G, *et al*: *HIV, pregnancy and parenthood: A qualitative study of the prevention and treatment of HIV in pregnant women, parents and their infants in Papua New Guinea.* Sydney, Australia: PNG Institute of Medical Research and the University of New South Wales; 2013.
46. Kelly A, Worth H, Man N, Nosi S, Emori R, Mek A, Akuani F, Kupul M, Kepa B, Walizopa L, *et al*: **Barriers and facilitators for adherence to antiretroviral therapy in Papua New Guinea.** *Curr HIV Res* 2010, **8**(8):630–637.
47. Wardlow H: **"You have to understand: Some of us are glad AIDS has arrived": Christianity and condoms among the Huli, Papua New Guinea.** In *Making Sense of AIDS: Culture, Sexuality and Power in Melanesia.* Edited by Eves R, Butt L. Honolulu: University of Hawai'i Press; 2008:324–352.
48. Wardlow H: **Men's extramarital sexuality in rural Papua New Guinea.** *Am J Public Health* 2007, **97**(6):1006–1014.
49. Hammar L: **Fear and loathing in Papua New Guinea.** In *Making Sense of AIDS: Culture, Sexuality and Power in Melanesia.* Edited by Eves R, Butt L. Honolulu: University of Hawai'i Press; 2008:60–79.
50. Wilde C: **Acts of faith: Muscular christianity and masculinity among the Gogodala of Papua New Guinea.** *Oceania* 2004, **75**(1):32–48.
51. Kumarasamy N, Venkatesh KK, Srikrishnan AK, Prasad L, Balakrishnan P, Murugavel KG, Thamburaj E, Solomon S, Mayer KH: **Couples at risk for HIV infection in Southern India: Characteristics of HIV-infected patients in concordant and discordant heterosexual relationships.** *Int J STD AIDS* 2010, **21**(2):96–100.
52. Olley BO, Seedat S, Stein DJ: **Self-disclosure of HIV serostatus in recently diagnosed patients with HIV in South Africa.** *Afr J Reprod Health* 2004, **8**(2):71–76.
53. Skogmar S, Shakely D, Lans M, Danell J, Andersson R, Tshandu N, Odén A, Roberts S, Venter WDF: **Effect of antiretroviral treatment and counselling on disclosure of HIV-serostatus in Johannesburg, South Africa.** *AIDS Care - Psycho Socio-Med Aspects AIDS/HIV* 2006, **18**(7):725–730.
54. Nachega JB, Lehman DA, Hlatshwayo D, Mothopeng R, Chaisson RE, Karstaedt AS: **HIV/AIDS and antiretroviral treatment knowledge, attitudes, beliefs, and practices in HIV-infected adults in Soweto, South Africa.** *J Acquir Immune Defic Syndr* 2005, **38**(2):196–201.
55. Vu L, Andrinopoulos K, Mathews C, Chopra M, Kendall C, Eisele TP: **Disclosure of HIV Status to Sex Partners Among HIV-Infected Men and Women in Cape Town, South Africa.** *AIDS Behav* 2010, **16**(1):1–7.
56. Logie CH, James L, Tharao W, Loutfy MR: **HIV, gender, race, sexual orientation, and sex work: A qualitative study of intersectional stigma experienced by HIV-positive women in Ontario, Canada.** *PLoS Med* 2011, **8**(11).
57. Shuper PA, Joharchi N, Irving H, Rehm J: **Alcohol as a correlate of unprotected sexual behavior among people living with HIV/AIDS: Review and meta-analysis.** *AIDS Behav* 2009, **13**(6):1021–1036.
58. Theall KP, Clark RA, Powell A, Smith H, Kissinger P: **Alcohol consumption, art usage and high-risk sex among women infected with HIV.** *AIDS Behav* 2007, **11**(2):205–215.
59. Sumartojo E: **Structural factors in HIV prevention: Concepts, examples, and implications for research.** *AIDS* 2000, **14**(11 SUPPL.):S3–S10.
60. Papua New Guinea Nantional Department of Health: *The 2008 STI, HIV and AIDS annual surveillance report.* Port Moresby, Papua New Guinea: Papua New Guinea National Department of Health; 2009.
61. StataCorp: *Stata Statistical Software: Release 11.* College Station, Texas: StataCorp LP; 2009.
62. Charmaz K: **Grounded Theory: Objectivist and Constructivist Methods.** In *Handbook of Qualitative Research.* 2nd edition. Edited by Denzin NK, Lincoln YS. Thousand Oaks, California: Sage; 2000:509–535.

Mortality and loss to programme before antiretroviral therapy among HIV-infected children eligible for treatment in The Gambia, West Africa

Uduak Okomo[1*], Toyin Togun[1], Francis Oko[1], Kevin Peterson[2] and Assan Jaye[1,3]

Abstract

Background: HIV infection among children, particularly those under 24 months of age, is often rapidly progressive; as a result guidelines recommend earlier access to combination antiretroviral therapy (cART) for HIV infected children. Losses to follow-up (LTFU) and death in the interval between diagnosis and initiation of ART profoundly limit this strategy. This study explores correlates of LTFU and death prior to ART initiation among children.

Methods: The study is based on 337 HIV-infected children enrolled into care at an urban centre in The Gambia, including those alive and in care when antiretroviral therapy became available and those who enrolled later. Children were followed until they started ART, died, transferred to another facility, or were LTFU. Cox proportional hazards regression models were used to determine the hazard of death or LTFU according to the baseline characteristics of the children.

Results: Overall, 223 children were assessed as eligible for ART based on their clinical and/or immunological status among whom 73 (32.7%) started treatment, 15 (6.7%) requested transfer to another health facility, 105 (47.1%) and 30 (13.5%) were lost to follow-up and died respectively without starting ART. The median survival following eligibility for children who died without starting treatment was 2.8 months (IQR: 0.9 - 5.8) with over half (60%) of all deaths occurring at home. ART-eligible children less than 2 years of age and those in WHO stage 3 or 4 were significantly more likely to be LTFU when compared with their respective comparison groups. The overall pre-treatment mortality rate was 25.7 per 100 child-years of follow-up (95% CI 19.9 - 36.8) and the loss to programme rate was 115.7 per 100 child-years of follow-up (95% CI 98.8 - 137). In the multivariable Cox proportional hazard model, significant independent predictors of loss to programme were being less than 2 years of age and WHO stage 3 or 4. The Adjusted Hazard Ratio (AHR) for loss to programme was 2.06 (95% CI 1.12 – 3.83) for being aged less than 2 years relative to being 5 years of age or older and 1.92 (95% CI 1.05 - 3.53) for being in WHO stage 3 or 4 relative to WHO stage 1 or 2.

Conclusions: Earlier enrolment into HIV care is key to achieving better outcomes for HIV infected children in developing countries. Developing strategies to ensure early diagnosis, elimination of obstacles to prompt initiation of therapy and instituting measures to reduce losses to follow-up, will improve the overall outcomes of HIV-infected children.

Keywords: Paediatrics, HIV, Pre-antiretroviral therapy, Loss to follow-up, Mortality, Retention, Sub-Saharan Africa

* Correspondence: uokomo@mrc.gm
[1]Medical Research Council (UK) Laboratories, Atlantic Road, Fajara, P.O. Box 273, Banjul, The Gambia
Full list of author information is available at the end of the article

Background

Combination antiretroviral therapy (cART) has significantly improved the prognosis for HIV-infected children in resource-limited settings [1-4]. Eligibility for ART among children in resource-limited settings is based on either clinical and/or immunological criteria to start treatment at World Health Organization (WHO) clinical stage 3 or 4 disease, or at a CD4 T-cell count/percent below the age-appropriate immunological threshold [5]. However, because of the more rapid disease progression and significantly higher risk of mortality in the first two years of life among HIV-infected children in sub-Saharan Africa [6,7], WHO now recommends that all infants and children aged <24 months with confirmed HIV-infection start ART as soon as possible irrespective of clinical stage or immunological threshold [5,7,8]. Unfortunately, the majority of HIV-infected children in sub-Saharan Africa are diagnosed late with advanced clinical disease and immunosuppression, and are usually 5 years of age or older at initiation of therapy [2,4]. This is due to, among other reasons, the fact that health systems in resource limited settings still face considerable challenges in their efforts to scale-up access to early paediatric HIV diagnosis and treatment, particularly among children aged < 18 months in whom a definitive diagnosis requires sophisticated laboratory techniques. Another challenge that treatment programmes face is ensuring that all children who test HIV-positive are successfully linked to and retained in a Paediatric HIV/AIDS care programme such that they can initiate ART as soon as they are eligible [4,9]. Retention of patients in pre-ART care is of paramount importance in ensuring the success of ART programmes. Loss to care has been defined as "discontinuation of active engagement in pre-ART care for any reason, including death" [10]. Loss to follow-up (LTFU) from HIV care programmes in particular represents missed opportunities for the timely initiation of life-saving treatment. A systematic review of adult ART programmes in sub-Saharan Africa reported that retention is as low as 60% after 2 years [11], which is consistent with our observation of one-third of ART-eligible adults who died or were lost to follow-up prior to initiation of treatment [12]. However, there is a paucity of data on mortality and loss to follow-up experiences of ART-eligible HIV-infected children who fail to initiate treatment because this information is not routinely assessed as part of program evaluations [13-15].

In 2008, the prevalence of HIV-1 and HIV-2 in The Gambia was estimated to be 1.6% and 0.4%, respectively [16]. The prevalence of paediatric HIV/AIDS is amongst the lowest in sub-Saharan Africa with less than 1000 children below the age of 15 years known to be living with HIV/AIDS [17]. Approximately one-third of these are receiving life-saving ART though the proportion that are eligible but are yet to initiate ART is unknown. This study aims to investigate, and determine factors associated with, pre-ART loss to follow-up and mortality among ART-eligible HIV-infected children at the Paediatric HIV clinic of the Medical Research Council (MRC) Unit in Fajara, The Gambia – West Africa.

Results

Enrolment, follow-up and ART eligibility

A total of 411 HIV infected children attended the MRC paediatric HIV clinic at least once between June 1993 and January 2010; of these, 74 were excluded from the analysis because they had either died or were LTFU prior to June 2004 when pre-ART sensitization and screening began (Figure 1).

Among the 337 children in care between June 2004 and January 2010 and included in the analysis were 318 (94%) HIV-1 infected, 16 (5%) HIV-2 and 3 (1%) HIV-1/HIV-2 dually infected children. Their median age at diagnosis of HIV infection was 23 months (IQR: 12 – 71 months). Of these children, 126 (37%) were aged less than 18 months, 119 (35.3%) aged between 18 – 59 months and 92 (27.3%) 5 years or older at the time of diagnosis. HIV-2 infected children were older at the time of HIV diagnosis (median 65.6 months; IQR: 26 - 98) than HIV-1 (23.3 months; IQR: 12 – 62) and HIV-1/HIV-2 dually infected children (10.2 months; IQR: 7.6 - 21.8) but this was not statistically significant. 164 (49%) children were female. Overall, 114 (34%) children did not meet ART initiation criteria over this period while 223 (66%) children were found to be eligible for treatment (Figure 1).

Characteristics of ART-eligible patients

The majority of children in the cohort were enrolled after January 2006 with eligibility based on the 4-stage 2006 revision of the WHO paediatric treatment guidelines (Table 1). 177 (80%) of the children were eligible to start cART at presentation or within 6 months of their being diagnosed with HIV infection; 60% of the children were 2 years of age or older at eligibility. Information on parental vital status was available for 173 of the 223 children, of which half were orphaned: 70 (41%) had lost one parent and 16 (9%) had lost both parents. Only 99 (44%) children had documentation of their parents HIV status - 76 had at least one HIV-positive parent, 17 had both parents HIV-positive and 6 had both parents HIV-negative. Gender, HIV type, CD4% and the vital status of the parents were not significantly associated with the outcomes of survival or retention but there were significant differences by age and WHO clinical status (Table 2); children less than 2 years of age and those in WHO stage 3 or 4 at ART eligibility were significantly more likely to be LTFU when compared with their respective comparison groups.

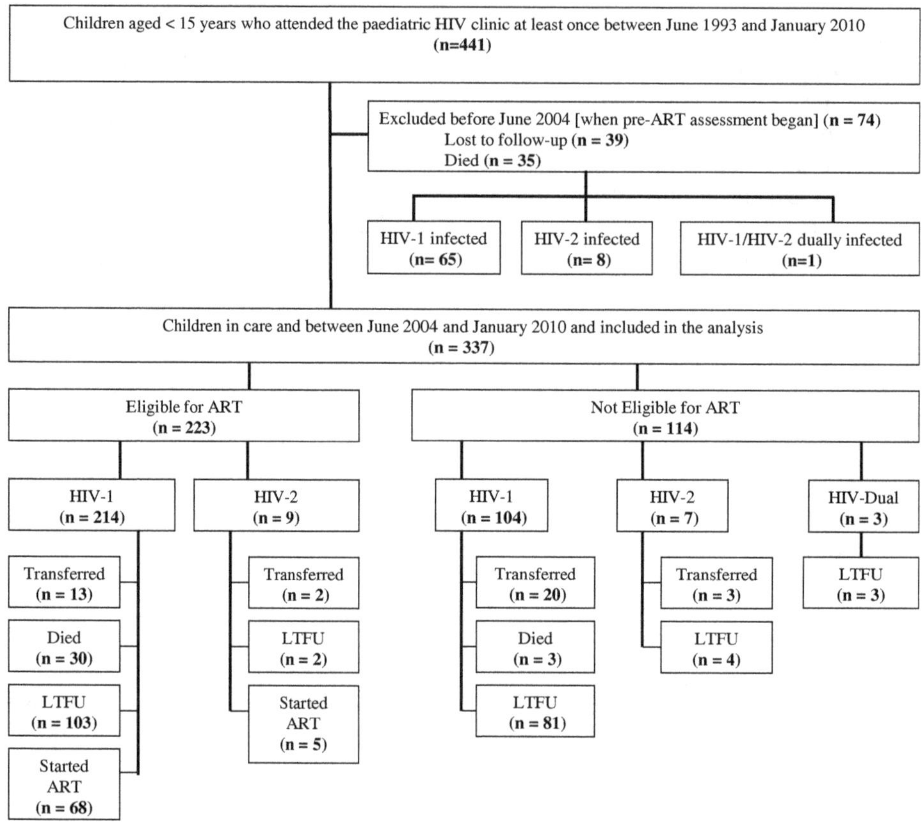

Figure 1 Flow chart of the cohort of HIV-infected children < 15 years of age enrolled in the Paediatric HIV programme, MRC Unit, The Gambia, 1993–2010.

Survival and retention in care among ART-eligible patients

Among the 73 children who commenced cART; the median time from eligibility to ART initiation and median age at initiation were 5.1 months (IQR: 2.8 – 11.2) and 4.9 years (IQR: 2.6 – 9.9) respectively.

Thirty (13.3%) ART-eligible children died without staring treatment giving a pre-treatment mortality rate of 25.7 per 100 child-years of follow-up (95% CI 19.9 – 36.8). The median survival following ART eligibility for children who died without starting treatment was 2.8 months (IQR: 0.9 – 5.8) with over half (60%) of all deaths occurring at home (Table 3).

One hundred and five (47%) treatment-eligible children who remained in the cohort for a median of 4.2 months (IQR: 3.4 – 5.3) were eventually LTFU before starting treatment. Nineteen (18%) of these children were last seen on the date that that they were diagnosed HIV-positive and/or assessed to be eligible for ART and of these, 14 were less than 2 years of age. WHO clinical stage at eligibility was documented in 75 of those lost to follow-up and 25 (33%) and 34 (45.3%) had a stage 3 and stage 4 condition respectively. Twenty-two (21%) of the children LTFU had one or both parents in HIV care whilst 35 (33%) were either single or double orphans.

A total of 135 ART-eligible children were lost to the programme before ART initiation giving an incidence rate for the composite endpoint of death or LTFU of 115.7 per 100 child-years of follow-up (95% CI 98.8 – 137). In both univariate and multivariable analyses of risk factors for death, no significant risk factors were identified (Table 4); however being less than 2 years of age at eligibility, having advanced clinical HIV disease (i.e. WHO stage 3 or 4) and having been assessed as eligible for ART between January 2006 and January 2010 were all significantly associated with loss to programme. Figure 2 shows the cumulative incidence of loss to programme overall, by age category, eligibility period and WHO clinical stage at ART eligibility. The graphs show significant unadjusted associations between age category (log rank test, p = 0.0001), eligibility period (log rank test, p = 0.0062), WHO clinical stage (log rank test, p = 0.0001) and loss to programme risk from the time of being assessed as ART-eligible. The unadjusted Hazard Ratio for loss to programme was 2.41 (95% CI 1.61 – 3.61) for children less than 2 years of age at the time of eligibility compared with children 5 years of age or older; 2.43 (95% CI 1.51 – 3.90) for being in WHO stage 3 or 4 relative to WHO stage 1 or 2 and 1.86 (95% CI 1.18 – 2.93)

Table 1 Clinical and socio-demographic characteristics of 223 ART-eligible HIV-infected children enrolled in the Paediatric HIV programme, MRC Unit, The Gambia, 2004–2010

Characteristics	n (%)
Sex: (n=223)	
Female	101 (45.3%)
Male	122 (54.7%)
Eligibility period [a] : (n= 223)	
June 2004 - December 2005	42 (18.8%)
January 2006 - January 2010	181 (81.2%)
Age at eligibility: (n=223)	
Median in years (IQR)	2.9 (1.4 - 7.4)
< 2 years	89 (40%)
2 - 4 years	49 (22%)
≥ 5 years	85 (38%)
HIV type: (n=223)	
HIV-1	214 (95.9%)
HIV-2	9 (4.0%)
HIV-Dual	0
WHO clinical stage at eligibility: (n=178)	
1 or 2	63 (35.4%)
3 or 4	115 (64.6%)
CD4% at eligibility: (n=196)	
Median (IQR)	11 (7 - 14)
<15%	151 (77.0%)
≥15%	45 (23.0%)
Haemoglobin at eligibility (n=192)	
Median (IQR)	9.3 (7.9 - 10.3)
Haemoglobin < 8 g/dl	50 (26%)
Vital status of parents: (n=173)	
One parent died	70 (40.5%)
Both died	16 (9.2%)
Both alive	87 (50.3%)

[a] Defined by age according to the WHO treatment guidelines in effect at the time of eligibility.

for being assessed as eligible for ART between January 2006 and January 2010 compared to the period between June 2004 and December 2005 (Table 4). In the multivariable Cox proportional hazard model, significant independent predictors of loss to programme were being less than 2 years of age and WHO stage 3 or 4. Being less than 2 years of age is the strongest independent predictor of loss to programme among ART-eligible patients - the Adjusted Hazard Ratio (AHR) for loss to programme was 2.06 (95% CI 1.12 – 3.83) for being aged less than 2 years relative to being 5 years of age or older and 1.92 (95% CI 1.05 – 3.53) for being in WHO stage 3 or 4 relative to WHO stage 1 or 2. The Proportional hazards assumption was met for all Cox proportional hazard models.

Outcomes among HIV-infected children ineligible for ART at enrollment

The 114 children who did not meet ART initiation criteria over the study period were followed up for a median of 1.7 months (IQR: 0.2 – 16.9) from enrolment. Twenty-three (20.2%) children were transferred to another clinic, 88 (77.2%) were LTFU and 3 (2.6%) died; all deaths occurred within three months of enrolment. All these children had been given follow-up appointments no later than 3 months after their last appointment, and were explicitly given permission to return earlier to the clinic in case of illness.

Discussion

Our study reports pre-treatment mortality and losses to follow-up among ART-eligible children from a cohort who were yet to initiate treatment at a West-African clinic. The majority of deaths in our cohort occurred in the first three months after eligibility and during the period of preparation for ART. The pre-treatment mortality rate observed in our setting is relatively higher than reports from other sites; a study in rural Zambia reported 10% mortality among ART-eligible children with a mortality rate of 2.73 (95% CI: 1.7 – 4.18) per 100 child-years [14] while another study reported that 1% of treatment-eligible children receiving care at an urban ART program in Zambia died prior to ART initiation [18]. In a large cohort of 1766 children in Cote d'Ivoire, the reported loss-to-programme rate of 50.3/100 child-years of follow up was also much lower than that reported in this study though, it was not clear if the children in that cohort were eligible for ART. One possible reason for the relatively higher pre-treatment mortality and loss-to-programme rates among ART-eligible children in our setting is the advanced stage of clinical disease and immunosuppression at diagnosis. Many children in resource limited settings are only tested for HIV as part of workup for recurrent or severe ill health; we reported that 80% of the treatment-eligible children attending our clinic were assessed as eligible for ART either at or within 6 months of their being diagnosed with HIV infection. The inclusion of home visits as part of our patient follow-up protocol provides a more accurate and complete ascertainment of survival status that could have contributed to the higher mortality rates observed in our cohort.

The proportion of children who initiated ART in our clinic is comparable to that reported in a study in South Africa where 39.5% (96/243) of ART-eligible children started treatment [19] but considerably lower than figures reported from Cote d'Ivoire [15] and Zambia [14] where 86% and 70% of ART-eligible children respectively started therapy. The median time of 5.1 months from eligibility to ART initiation in our cohort was comparable

Table 2 Association of baseline characteristics with outcomes among ART-eligible HIV-infected children enrolled in the Paediatric HIV programme, MRC Unit, The Gambia, 2004–2010

Variable	Started ART	Died	LTFU	Transferred	p-value
Total (n=223)	**73 (32.7%)**	**30 (13.5%)**	**105 (47.1%)**	**15 (6.7%)**	
Sex: (n=223)					
Female	35 (34.7%)	12 (11.8%)	48 (47.5%)	6 (5.9%)	0.868‡
Male	38 (31.2%)	9 (7.4%)	57 (46.7%)	18 (14.7%)	
Age at eligibility: (n=222)					
Median in years (IQR)	4.7 (1.9 – 8.4)	5.1 (1.6 – 10.0)	1.9 (1.2 – 4.7)	7.4 (3.2 – 8.7)	**0.0001ψ**
< 2 years	19 (21.4%)	10 (11.2%)	57 (64.0%)	3 (3.4%)	
2 – 4 years	21 (42.9%)	5 (10.2%)	22 (44.9%)	1 (2.0%)	
≥ 5 years	33 (38.8%)	15 (17.7%)	26 (30.6%)	11 (12.9%)	**<0.001 Ω**
HIV type: (n=223)					
HIV-1	68 (31.8%)	30 (14%)	103 (48.1%)	13 (6.1%)	0.065 Ω
HIV-2	5 (55.6%)	0	2 (22.2%)	2 (22.2%)	
WHO stage: (n=178)					
1 or 2	34 (54%)	8 (12.7%)	16 (25.4%)	5 (7.9%)	
3 or 4	33 (28.7%)	16 (13.9%)	59 (51.3%)	7 (6.1%)	**0.003 Ω**
CD4% at eligibility: (n=196)					
Median (IQR)	11% (8 – 14)	8% (4 – 11)	11% (8 – 15.0)	13% (8 – 14)	**0.039ψ**
<15%	55 (36.4%)	25 (16.6%)	60 (39.7%)	11 (7.3%)	0.574 Ω
≥15%	18 (40.0%)	4 (8.9%)	21 (46.7%)	2 (4.4%)	
Haemoglobin: (n=192)					
Median (IQR)	9.6 (7.9 – 10.6)	9.5 (7 – 11.4)	9.1 (8.1 – 9.9)	10 (8.6 – 10.5)	0.262ψ
< 8 g/dl	20 (40%)	9 (18%)	20 (40%)	1 (2%)	0.245 Ω
Vital status of parent: (n=173)					
Single orphan	25 (35.7%)	6 (8.6%)	31 (44.3%)	8 (11.4%)	
Double orphan	6 (37.5%)	3 (18.7%)	4 (25%)	3 (18.8%)	
Both alive	37 (42.5%)	9 (10.4%)	39 (44.8%)	2 (2.3%)	0.073 Ω

‡ Chi-square test.
Ω Fishers exact test.
ψ Kruskall-Wallis test.

to that reported from Cambodia where ART was initiated after a median of 4.7 months [13], but more than twice as long as the 2.1 months reported from rural Zambia [14]. Another study from Zambia reported that children eligible for ART at presentation in rural areas took longer time to initiate treatment than children in urban areas (3.6 vs. 0.9 months) [18].

Delays in treatment initiation among eligible children are reported to be due to several factors [12-14,19,20] some of which were observed in our cohort. Firstly, the long process of pre-treatment counselling required repeated clinic visits to ensure that care-givers are both willing and capable of taking the responsibility of supporting the child to take life-long medications with a high level of adherence. Lack of caregiver readiness as assessed during counselling sessions could prolong the process further. This often proved difficult for patients from rural areas and those with working parents though parents/caregivers who were in HIV care, specifically those already ART and with good adherence, underwent 'accelerated' counselling with emphasis on the challenges of administering drugs to children, drug-storage and side-effects. We however did not collect information on the number of parents/caregivers who completed the 4 pre-ART counselling sessions among children who died or were LTFU.

A second factor for treatment delay was the time required to obtain approval to start ART from the national ART eligibility committee. The fortnightly occurrence of the meeting frequently resulted in eligible children, whose caregivers had completed pre-ART counselling, waiting for days (sometimes as long as one month if the meeting date fell on a public holiday) to receive approval to start treatment. The concept of the national eligibility committee arose in the early days of ART availability in The Gambia when ART supplies were limited, providers inexperienced and practical application of eligibility criteria was still being debated. Though the committee now meets weekly, the inconvenience of travel

Table 3 Characteristics of 30 treatment eligible children who died prior to the initiation of ART

Cause of death	Age at eligibility	Sex	WHO clinical stage at eligibility	CD4% or absolute CD4 count at eligibility	Place of death
Disseminated Tuberculosis, Sepsis	13 years	M	1	140 cells/mm^3	Hospital
Disseminated Tuberculosis, Sepsis	8 years	M	3	10 cells/mm^3	Hospital
Kaposi Sarcoma	7 years	M	4	-	Hospital
Severe Malnutrition	8 months	M	4	22%	Hospital
Severe Malnutrition, Sepsis	19 months	M	4	27%	Hospital
Severe Malnutrition, Sepsis	8 years	F	4	120 cells/mm^3	Hospital
Tuberculosis	19 months	F	3	13%	Hospital
Tuberculosis	2 years	M	3	9%	Hospital
Tuberculosis	7 months	M	3	10%	Hospital
Tuberculosis	6 years	M	3	30 cells/mm^3	Hospital
Tuberculosis, Meningitis	11 years	M	4	10 cells/mm^3	Hospital
Very Severe Pneumonia	8 months	M	3	8%	Hospital
Unknown	2 years	F	2	3%	Home
Unknown	4 years	F	-	3%	Home
Unknown	20 months	M	4	9%	Home
Unknown	1 month	F	1	10%	Home
Unknown	13 months	F	3	19%	Home
Unknown	23 months	F	-	7%	Home
Unknown	2 years	F	4	16%	Home
Unknown	3 years	M	2	13%	Home
Unknown	19 months	F	-	8%	Home
Unknown	13 years	M	-	20 cells/mm^3	Home
Unknown	14 years	M	2	320 cells/mm^3 (8%)	Home
Unknown	10 years	F	1	20 cells/mm^3	Home
Unknown	6 years	M	1	160 cells/mm^3	Home
Unknown	10 years	M	1	10 cells/mm^3	Home
Unknown	12 years	M	-	380 cells/mm^3 (11%)	Home
Unknown	12 years	F	3	60 cells/mm^3	Home
Unknown	6 years	M	4	540 cells/mm^3	Home
Unknown	9 years	F	-	90 cells/mm^3	Home

to attend the meeting, increased uptake of HCT services nationwide and the widespread availability of ART favour decentralization of the committee to centres involved in provision of ART and may help shorten the time patients have to wait in order to initiate life-saving treatment.

Thirdly, caregivers failed to attend follow-up appointments; almost 20% of treatment eligible children attended only one clinic visit before being lost to follow-up. Poor uptake of paediatric HIV services is multifactorial and reasons include facility-related factors such as long queues, overcrowding, negative staff attitudes; unemployment, lack of money for food and transport, difficulty getting time off work, absenteeism from school and fear of social rejection from disclosure to family and neighbours [21]. While the cost of transport was not a hindrance to clinic attendance in our setting due to the practice of reimbursement of transport costs for all patients, disclosure of HIV-status to a family member or friend was a major factor for loss to follow-up among our adult cohort [12] and suggests that unwillingness to disclose the child's status to another caregiver may have contributed significantly to failure to keep clinic appointments as well as delays in initiation of ART among eligible children. Disclosure of paediatric infection is multifaceted being dependent on caregiver and family characteristics such as biologic relationship, caregiver permanence, caregiver beliefs and psychosocial function, as well as child-specific factors such as age, developmental stage, cognitive abilities and psychosocial function [22]. A child's positive status usually indicates maternal infection and the resultant anxiety, fear of blame, social and healthcare discrimination as well as marital abandonment may negatively influence the mother's acceptance of the HIV status of the

Table 4 Risk factors associated with death and loss to programme before initiation of ART among HIV-infected children eligible for ART in the Paediatric HIV programme, MRC Unit, The Gambia, 2004–2010

Patient Characteristics [b]		Death				Loss to programme			
		Crude HR 95% (CI)	P	Adjusted HR 95% (CI)	P	Crude HR 95% (CI)	P	Adjusted HR 95% (CI)	P
Sex: (n=219)									
Female	99 (45.2%)	1.0		1.0		1.0		1.0	
Male	120 (54.8%)	1.16 (0.56 – 2.41)	0.686	1.23 (0.43 – 3.51)	0.700	0.94 (0.67 – 1.32)	0.731	1.15 (0.68 – 1.95)	0.600
Age category: (n=219)									
< 2 years	88 (40.2%)	0.86 (0.38 – 1.94)	0.712	1.64 (0.50 – 5.38)	0.415	2.41 (1.61 – 3.61)	**<0.0001**	2.06 (1.12 – 3.83)	**0.023**
2 – 4 years	49 (22.4%)	0.66 (0.24 – 1.83)	0.429	0.50 (0.09 – 2.64)	0.410	1.58 (0.97 – 2.58)	0.069	0.95 (0.43 – 2.10)	0.896
≥ 5 years	82 (37.4%)	1.0		1.0		1.0		1.0	
WHO clinical stage: (n=174)									
1 or 2	60 (34.5%)	1.0		1.0		1.0		1.0	
3 or 4	114 (65.5%)	1.49 (0.63 – 3.55)	0.367	2.98 (0.78 – 11.31)	0.109	2.43 (1.51 – 3.90)	**<0.0001**	1.92 (1.05 – 3.53)	**0.035**
CD4%: (n=193)									
<15%	148 (76.7%)	1.69 (0.59 – 4.86)	0.330	1.26 (0.39 – 4.09)	0.700	0.90 (0.58 – 1.42)	0.662	1.23 (0.67 – 2.26)	0.499
≥15%	45 (23.3%)	1.0		1.0		1.0		1.0	
Vital status of parent: (n=169)									
Single orphan	68 (40.2%)	0.75 (026 – 2.11)	0.582	0.71 (0.23 – 2.20)	0.548	0.89 (0.58 – 1.38)	0.612	0.90 (0.52 – 1.57)	0.720
Double orphan	16 (9.5%)	1.93 (0.52 – 7.17)	0.323	1.32 (0.30 – 5.82)	0.711	0.95 (0.43 – 2.10)	0.903	1.12 (0.46 – 2.70)	0.800
Both alive	85 (50.3%)	1.0		1.0		1.0		1.0	
Eligibility period: (n= 219)									
Jun 2004 – Dec 2005	42 (19.2%)	1.0		1.0		1.0		1.0	
Jan 2006 – Jan 2010	177 (80.8%)	1.19 (0.50 – 2.83)	0.690	3.59 (0.40 – 32.4)	0.254	1.86 (1.18 – 2.93)	**0.007**	2.06 (0.86 – 4.96)	0.106

[a] Children were lost to the programme if they died or were lost to follow-up.
[b] 4 children excluded from the analysis: 1child had an of incorrect date of HIV eligibility while 3 children had incorrect date of exit.
Proportional hazards assumption was met for all Cox proportional hazard models as assessed by the global test based on the Schoenfeld residuals.
Φ Adjusted for Sex, Age, WHO stage, CD4% and eligibility period.

child [21,23]. Denial of results, despair or depression hinder health-care seeking and social support, and may lead to difficulties in reacting to the options and advice given by health workers [23-25]. Maternal depression (in cases of vertical transmission) and concurrent HIV or other comorbidities may also affect the mother's ability to care for the child; the belief that the child might die any moment may cause her not to take proper care of the child anymore. In circumstances where the biologic parents may have died or may be too ill to care for the child, responsibility for care is shifted to one or more relatives or family friends; poor coordination amongst multiple caregivers may also compromise the quality of care especially where secondary caregivers have not been disclosed to and therefore do not understand the importance of regular clinic visits or adherence to prescribed medications [21]. Studies from sub-Saharan Africa suggest that whilst many caregivers appreciate shared childcare, sustained adherence and community support as benefits of disclosing a child's HIV status to others, many still believe that disclosure to others could have negative effects [21,23,26]. Community-based support groups have been shown to play a major role in providing continuous support to caregivers of HIV-infected children [27] and though several support groups were linked to our clinic, we did not routinely collect data of patient/caregiver membership with such groups or assess what impact this had on their quality of life. Disclosing a diagnosis of HIV infection to a child has been suggested to have direct benefits for adherence to ART and among adolescents is associated with higher retention in care [26,28,29]. The average age of disclosure reported among children in sub-Saharan Africa is 8 years [30,31]; 75% of those LTFU in our cohort (data not shown) were less than 5 years of age at eligibility and therefore too young for a disclosure their HIV status.

Lastly, we report that tuberculosis was the most common cause of death among treatment-eligible children and may have also been an underlying cause of death among those who reportedly died at home. This is

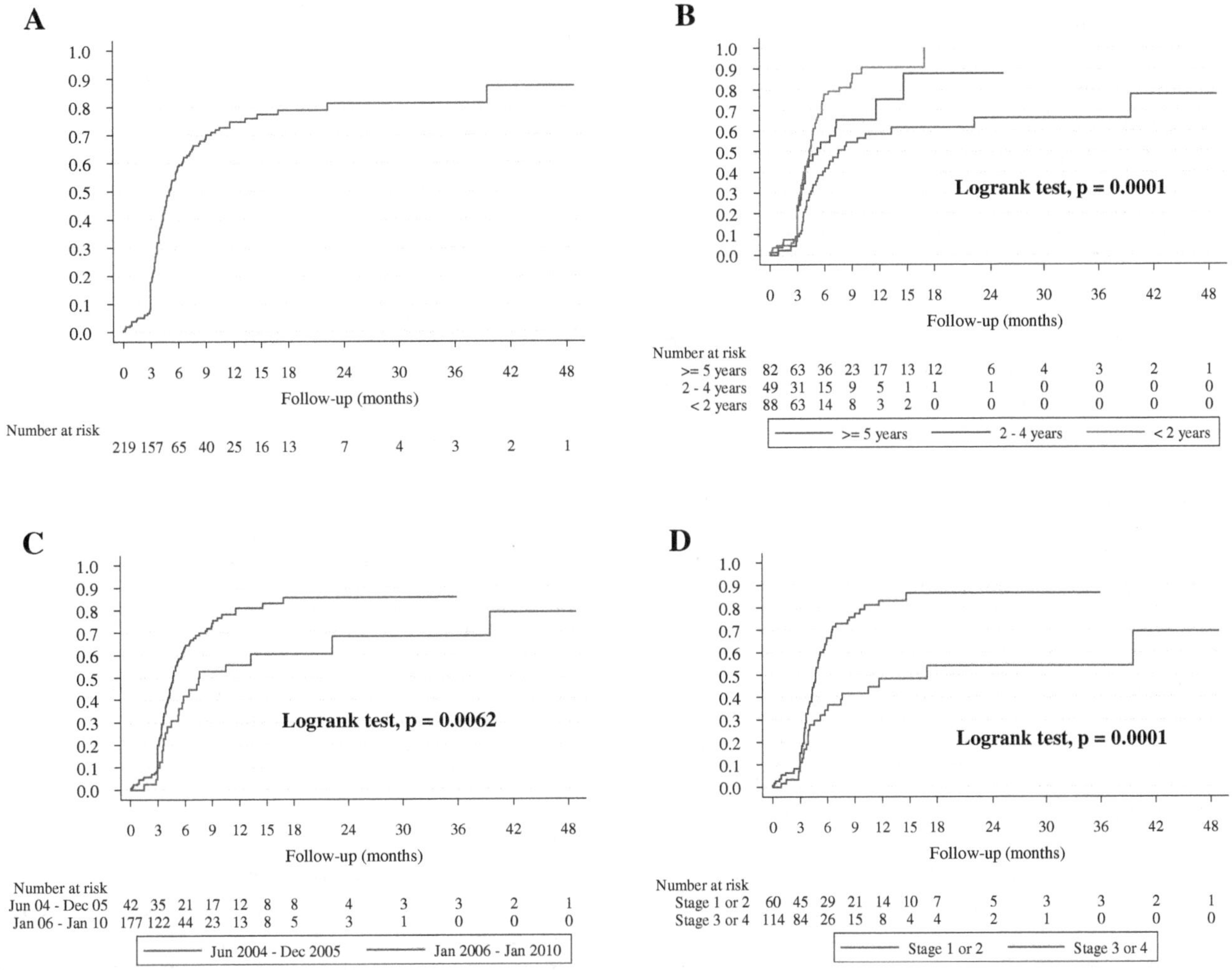

Figure 2 Cumulative incidence of loss to programme following eligibility for cART among HIV-infected children enrolled in the Paediatric HIV programme, MRC Unit, The Gambia, 2004 – 2010. Plot **A** shows the cumulative incidence of loss to programme before starting treatment for all ART-eligible patients; Plots **B**, **C**, and **D** show significant unadjusted associations between age category, WHO clinical stage and eligibility period respectively, and the risk of becoming lost to the programme.

consistent with data from paediatric cohorts in resource limited settings in which tuberculosis has been cited as a major reason for delayed treatment initiation [19,20] as well as the most common co-morbidity associated with early deaths among both ART naïve and experienced children [13,14,32]. As such, treatment for concurrent tuberculosis could also have contributed to the delay in initiation of ART.

Overall, 60% of ART-eligible children in our programme died or were lost to follow-up without starting treatment giving a loss-to-care incidence rate of 128 per 100 child-years of follow-up. We observed that the children who were lost to care were significantly more likely to be less than 2 years of age at ART eligibility or to have advanced clinical disease (predominantly tuberculosis and severe malnutrition - data not shown). Children aged less than 2 years or in WHO stage 3 or 4 had almost twice the risk of being lost to the programme before starting treatment respectively compared with those 5 years of age or older and those in WHO stage 1 or 2. The observation that just over half of children LTFU were in WHO stage 3 or 4 coupled with the relatively shorter median time to LTFU from eligibility compared with the time to initiation of ART (4.2 vs 5.1 months), suggests that many of those LTFU may have died as a result of rapid disease progression and advanced HIV disease during the time of preparation for ART and may have not even completed the process. This observation supports the 2010 WHO recommendation that ART be initiated for all HIV-infected infants and children between 12 and 24 months of age irrespective of their immunological threshold or clinical stage [5]. In our study the vital status of the parent was not related to death or loss to care, which was surprising as HIV-infected orphans in sub-Saharan have been shown to have delayed access to HIV care and treatment as well as reduced clinic attendance [33,34] .

Children assessed as eligible for ART between January 2006 and January 2010 using the revised 2006 guidelines were observed to have had a significantly higher risk of being lost to programme compared with those assessed as eligible between June 2004 and December 2005 based on the 2003 WHO treatment guidelines. As the paediatric cohort was a sub-cohort of a much larger adult cohort, this may be attributable to the increase in clinic enrolment over time and the reduced ability of clinic staff to effectively manage the patient load. This risk remained albeit insignificantly after adjusting for the effect of age, clinical stage and other variables.

As the only centre in the country performing virological tests for the diagnosis of HIV infection in children <18 months of age and the major paediatric HIV referral clinic in The Gambia, we experienced a good uptake of paediatric HIV services at our HIV clinic, which however, is not representative of paediatric HIV care in West Africa as patients had the advantage of reimbursement of all transport costs incurred in clinic visits, free treatment, nutritional support and provision and school fees for all children enrolled in school up till the age of 18 years. This coupled with the small size of our paediatric cohort, limit the generalizability of findings. There were however several limitations to this study; data were incomplete for many key variables such as WHO stage or CD4 T-cell percentage at eligibility and these children were classified based on immunologic or clinical criteria alone. Secondly, children with moderate or severe malnutrition in our setting were initially classified as WHO stage 3 or 4 respectively without assessing their response to nutritional support and treatment and thus may have been misclassified as eligible for treatment. Unreported deaths among ART-eligible children LTFU in our cohort suggest that the reported mortality rate may be underestimated; in addition, a good proportion of the children ineligible for ART and also LTFU may have progressed to an advanced stage of HIV-disease and died as they became eligible.

Conclusion

The results of our study have shown that HIV-infected children in The Gambia are enrolled into care at an advanced stage of disease with severe immunosuppression and a significant number of these treatment-eligible children die before initiating therapy. Only one-third of ART-eligible children go on to initiate ART but face a number of out-of-program and in-program delays before treatment is eventually commenced. Developing strategies to ensure early identification of HIV-infected children before they become eligible for ART, elimination of obstacles to prompt initiation of therapy as well as instituting measures to reduce losses to follow-up, will improve the overall outcomes of HIV-infected children.

Methods

Study setting and participants

This study was conducted in MRC HIV research clinic located in the urban area of Greater Banjul, the Gambia. The clinic established an adult cohort in 1986 with approval from the Joint Gambian Government/MRC Ethics Committee and started enrolment of children in 1993 based on written informed consent by the parent or legal guardian, with the adoption of a family-centred model of HIV-care. Paediatric patients consist of exposed or infected infants and children of adults enrolled in the MRC cohort, children with a positive HIV serologic test referred to the clinic from the MRC Clinical services or other health-care services in the country. HIV-exposed infants referred from other PMTCT programmes were also enrolled in the paediatric clinic. Provision of ART in The Gambia began in October 2004 through the support of the Global Fund. Nutritional support is provided and school fees for all children enrolled in school up till the age of 18 years are paid. All treatments, including cART, and treatment monitoring are provided free of charge and the parents/guardians of enrolled children also receive reimbursement of transport costs incurred in clinic visits.

Acquisition of clinical data in an electronic system includes capture of demographic characteristics, social history, basic anthropometric measurements, complete blood count, serum biochemistry, CD4 T-cell profile, chest radiograph, opportunistic/concomitant infections and clinical stage. Patients are required to be seen in clinic at least once every 3 months for follow-up clinical assessment, and CD4 T-cell monitoring is performed every 6 months or earlier if clinically indicated. All children receive daily cotrimoxazole prophylaxis [35,36].

Selection for ART

Eligibility for ART was determined using immunological and/or clinical criteria based on the Gambian National ART guideline [37] and WHO paediatric ART guidelines that were in place at the time of enrolment; for children enrolled on or before December 31 2005, eligibility was based on the 3-stage 2003 guidelines while for those enrolled from January 2006 eligibility was based on the 4-stage 2006 revision of the guidelines [38,39]. Following a further revision of the treatment guidelines in June 2008 [WHO 2008], ART was recommended for all children <12 months of age with confirmed HIV infection. In addition, all children were required to have at least one identifiable caregiver who would serve as a 'treatment supporter' and take responsibility for the administration of the child's medications. Pre-ART counselling was conducted twice a week and caregivers underwent a minimum of four one-on-one counselling sessions over a period of three to six weeks before selection was processed and confirmed by the national eligibility committee.

Patients who did not come to the clinic for at least 90 days beyond their last scheduled visit were considered LTFU and visited at home by trained field workers to ascertain survival status or change of address. For children who died at home, deaths were verified by close family members and cause of death ascertained by verbal autopsy. Recruitment of children into the programme ended in January 2010 as part of the transition process to transfer patient care from the MRC to the Gambian national health care system.

Laboratory methods

HIV diagnosis and CD4 measurement

Screening for HIV-1 and HIV-2 infection was done using a protocol described in detail elsewhere [40]. In children <18 months of age, HIV infection was diagnosed by two polymerase chain reaction (PCR) tests. Percentages and absolute counts of CD4 T lymphocytes were determined on a FACS Calibur (Becton Dickinson, US) using BD MultiTest reagents and MultiSet software (BD Immunocytometry Systems).

Statistical analysis

For the purpose of this analysis, eligibility for ART was determined from June 2004 when sensitization of patients began in preparation for the roll-out of ART, to January 2010 when patient recruitment ended. Children already in the paediatric cohort and eligible for treatment but who died or were lost to follow-up before June 2004 were excluded from the analyses. Severe anaemia was defined as haemoglobin <8 g/dl [41]. Distributions of categorical variables were compared between the four possible outcomes: [a] initiation of ART; [b] death; [c] loss to follow-up or [d] transfer by chi square statistics or Fisher exact test as appropriate. Continuous variables were compared using Kruskall-Wallis non-parametric test.

Follow-up duration in person-time was calculated from the date the children were assessed as eligible for ART; children who started ART were right-censored on the date treatment started; those who requested transfer were followed through to the date of transfer. Patients who died were followed to their date of death if known or date last seen alive. To avoid immortal person-time bias, patients LTFU were right-censored 90 days after the date of their last clinic visit (as loss to follow-up was not possible before this time). The probability of loss to programme following ART-eligibility was described using cumulative incidence curves and summarised by mortality rate and loss to programme rate (incident rate for the composite endpoint of death and LTFU) reported per 100 child-years of follow-up respectively. Cox proportional hazards regression models were used to identify baseline characteristics associated with death or a loss to programme. The proportional hazards assumption was assessed for all models by the global test based on the Schoenfeld residuals. All statistical analyses were performed with STATA release 11.1 software (Stata Corp., College Station, TX, USA) and statistical significance defined as $p < 0.05$ (two-sided).

Abbreviations

AHR: Adjusted Hazard Ratio; AIDS: Acquired Immune Deficiency Syndrome; cART: Combination Antiretroviral Therapy; CHR: Crude Hazard Ratio; CI: Confidence Interval; HCT: HIV Counselling and Testing; HIV: Human Immunodeficiency virus; IQR: Inter-quartile Range; LTFU: Loss to follow up; MRC: Medical Research Council; PCR: Polymerase chain reaction; PMTCT: Prevention of mother-to-child transmission; WHO: World Health Organization.

Competing interests

The authors declare that they have no competing interests.

Authors' contributions

UO coordinated the pediatric HIV clinical activities, performed the statistical analysis and drafted the manuscript. TT contributed to the study design, participated in the statistical analysis and helped to draft the manuscript. TT, FO and KP participated in the clinical care of the patients. AJ conceived the idea, edited the manuscript and gave overall support. All authors read and approved the final manuscript.

Acknowledgements

The authors thank the physicians, field workers and nurses of the MRC HIV Clinic, with special thanks to Mr. Saydiba Tamba. We also acknowledge and appreciate the efforts of Gilleh Thomas and Mehedi Shams-Rony in acquisition of the data; Ramu Sarge-Njie, Samuel Nyamweya and Sheikh Jarju for their assistance with HIV diagnostics and CD4 measurements.
UO work was supported by the Elizabeth Glaser Pediatric AIDS Foundation [grant number: ILA # 01-15 awarded to AJ]. Support for antiretroviral drugs and MRC HIV Clinic Staff was provided by the Global Fund for AIDS, TB and Malaria (GFATM).

Author details

[1]Medical Research Council (UK) Laboratories, Atlantic Road, Fajara, P.O. Box 273, Banjul, The Gambia. [2]Institute of Tropical Medicine, Nationalestraat 155, 2000, Antwerp, Belgium. [3]WAPHIR Network, Universite Cheikh Anta Diop Laboratoire de Bacteriologie Virologie, Hopital A. le Dantec, 30 Avenue Pasteur, Dakar, Senegal.

References

1. Ciaranello AL, Chang Y, Margulis AV, Bernstein A, Bassett IV, Losina E, Walensky RP: **Effectiveness of pediatric antiretroviral therapy in resource-limited settings: a systematic review and meta-analysis.** *Clin Infect Dis* 2009, **49**(12):1915–1927.
2. KIDS-ART-LINC Collaboration: **Low risk of death, but substantial program attrition, in pediatric HIV treatment cohorts in Sub-Saharan Africa.** *J Acquir Immune Defic Syndr* 2008, **49**(5):523–531.
3. Sauvageot D, Schaefer M, Olson D, Pujades-Rodriguez M, O'Brien DP: **Antiretroviral therapy outcomes in resource-limited settings for HIV-infected children <5 years of age.** *Pediatrics* 2010, **125**(5):e1039–e1047.
4. Sutcliffe CG, van Dijk JH, Bolton C, Persaud D, Moss WJ: **Effectiveness of antiretroviral therapy among HIV-infected children in sub-Saharan Africa.** *Lancet Infect Dis* 2008, **8**(8):477–489.
5. World Health Organization (WHO): *Antiretroviral therapy for HIV infection in infants and children: Towards universal access. Recommendations for a public health approach - 2010 revision.* Geneva: World Health Organization; 2010.

6. Newell ML, Coovadia H, Cortina-Borja M, Rollins N, Gaillard P, Dabis F: **Mortality of infected and uninfected infants born to HIV-infected mothers in Africa: a pooled analysis.** *Lancet* 2004, **364**(9441):1236–1243.
7. Little K, Thorne C, Luo C, Bunders M, Ngongo N, McDermott P, Newell ML: **Disease progression in children with vertically-acquired HIV infection in sub-Saharan Africa: reviewing the need for HIV treatment.** *Curr HIV Res* 2007, **5**(2):139–153.
8. Little K, Newell ML, Luo C, Ngongo N, Borja MC, McDermott P: **Estimating the number of vertically HIV-infected children eligible for antiretroviral treatment in resource-limited settings.** *Int J Epidemiol* 2007, **36**(3):679–687.
9. Rosen S, Fox MP: **Retention in HIV care between testing and treatment in Sub-Saharan Africa: a systematic review.** *PLoS Med* 2011, **8**(7):e1001056.
10. Fox MP, Larson B, Rosen S: **Defining retention and attrition in pre-antiretroviral HIV care: proposals based on experience in Africa.** *Trop Med Int Health* 2012, **17**:1235–1244.
11. Rosen S, Fox MP, Gill CJ: **Patient retention in antiretroviral therapy programs in sub-Saharan Africa: a systematic review.** *PLoS Med* 2007, **4**(10):e298.
12. Togun T, Peterson I, Jaffar S, Oko F, Okomo U, Peterson K, Jaye A: **Pre-treatment mortality and loss-to-follow-up in HIV-1, HIV-2 and HIV-1/HIV-2 dually infected patients eligible for antiretroviral therapy in The Gambia, West Africa.** *AIDS Res Ther* 2011, **8**(1):24.
13. Raguenaud ME, Isaakidis P, Zachariah R, Te V, Soeung S, Akao K, Kumar V: **Excellent outcomes among HIV+ children on ART, but unacceptably high pre-ART mortality and losses to follow-up: a cohort study from Cambodia.** *BMC Pediatr* 2009, **9**:54.
14. Sutcliffe CG, van Dijk JH, Munsanje B, Hamangaba F, Siniwymaanzi P, Thuma PE, Moss WJ: **Risk factors for pre-treatment mortality among HIV-infected children in rural Zambia: a cohort study.** *PLoS One* 2011, **6**(12):e29294.
15. Anaky MF, Duvignac J, Wemin L, Kouakoussui A, Karcher S, Toure S, Seyler C, Fassinou P, Dabis F, N'Dri-Yoman T, *et al*: **Scaling up antiretroviral therapy for HIV-infected children in Cote d'Ivoire: determinants of survival and loss to programme.** *Bull World Health Organ* 2010, **88**(7):490–499.
16. National Sentinel Surveillance Working Group: *National Sentinel Surveillance Bulletin 2008*. Banjul: Department of State for Health (DoSH); 2008.
17. UNICEF: *Unite for Children, Unite Against AIDS. Children and AIDS: The Fourth Stocktaking Report*. Geneva: UNICEF; 2009.
18. Sutcliffe CG, van Dijk JH, Bolton-Moore C, Cotham M, Tambatamba B, Moss WJ: **Differences in presentation, treatment initiation, and response among children infected with human immunodeficiency virus in urban and rural Zambia.** *Pediatr Infect Dis J* 2010, **29**(9):849–854.
19. Feucht UD, Kinzer M, Kruger M: **Reasons for delay in initiation of antiretroviral therapy in a population of HIV-infected South African children.** *J Trop Pediatr* 2007, **53**(6):398–402.
20. van Dijk JH, Sutcliffe CG, Munsanje B, Hamangaba F, Thuma PE, Moss WJ: **Barriers to the care of HIV-infected children in rural Zambia: a cross-sectional analysis.** *BMC Infect Dis* 2009, **9**:169.
21. Yeap AD, Hamilton R, Charalambous S, Dwadwa T, Churchyard GJ, Geissler PW, Grant AD: **Factors influencing uptake of HIV care and treatment among children in South Africa - a qualitative study of caregivers and clinic staff.** *AIDS Care* 2010, **22**(9):1101–1107.
22. Haberer J, Mellins C: **Pediatric adherence to HIV antiretroviral therapy.** *Curr HIV/AIDS Rep* 2009, **6**(4):194–200.
23. Kimani-Murage EW, Manderson L, Norris SA, Kahn K: **'You opened our eyes': care-giving after learning a child's positive HIV status in rural South Africa.** *Health Soc Care Community* 2010, **18**(3):264–271.
24. Brouwer CN, Lok CL, Wolffers I, Sebagalls S: **Psychosocial and economic aspects of HIV/AIDS and counselling of caretakers of HIV-infected children in Uganda.** *AIDS Care* 2000, **12**(5):535–540.
25. Meursing K, Sibindi F: **HIV counselling–a luxury or necessity?** *Health Policy Plan* 2000, **15**(1):17–23.
26. Vreeman RC, Nyandiko WM, Ayaya SO, Walumbe EG, Marrero DG, Inui TS: **The perceived impact of disclosure of pediatric HIV status on pediatric antiretroviral therapy adherence, child well-being, and social relationships in a resource-limited setting.** *AIDS Patient Care STDS* 2010, **24**(10):639–649.
27. Krabbendam AA, Kuijper B, Wolffers IN, Drew R: **The impact of counselling on HIV-infected women in Zimbabwe.** *AIDS Care* 1998, **10**(Suppl 1): S25–S37.
28. Arrive E, Dicko F, Amghar H, Aka AE, Dior H, Bouah B, Traore M, Ogbo P, Dago-Akribi HA, Eboua TK, *et al*: **HIV status disclosure and retention in care in HIV-infected adolescents on antiretroviral therapy (ART) in West Africa.** *PLoS One* 2012, **7**(3):e33690.
29. Fetzer BC, Mupenda B, Lusiama J, Kitetele F, Golin C, Behets F: **Barriers to and facilitators of adherence to pediatric antiretroviral therapy in a sub-Saharan setting: insights from a qualitative study.** *AIDS Patient Care STDS* 2011, **25**(10):611–621.
30. Brown BJ, Oladokun RE, Osinusi K, Ochigbo S, Adewole IF, Kanki P: **Disclosure of HIV status to infected children in a Nigerian HIV Care Programme.** *AIDS Care* 2011, **23**(9):1053–1058.
31. Moodley K, Myer L, Michaels D, Cotton M: **Paediatric HIV disclosure in South Africa – caregivers' perspectives on discussing HIV with infected children.** *S Afr Med J* 2006, **96**(3):201–204.
32. Reddi A, Leeper SC, Grobler AC, Geddes R, France KH, Dorse GL, Vlok WJ, Mntambo M, Thomas M, Nixon K, *et al*: **Preliminary outcomes of a paediatric highly active antiretroviral therapy cohort from KwaZulu-Natal, South Africa.** *BMC Pediatr* 2007, **7**(13):13.
33. Ntanda H, Olupot-Olupot P, Mugyenyi P, Kityo C, Lowes R, Cooper C, Lima V, Mills E: **Orphanhood predicts delayed access to care in Ugandan children.** *Pediatr Infect Dis J* 2009, **28**(2):153–155.
34. Vreeman RC, Wiehe SE, Ayaya SO, Musick BS, Nyandiko WM: **Association of antiretroviral and clinic adherence with orphan status among HIV-infected children in Western Kenya.** *J Acquir Immune Defic Syndr* 2008, **49**(2):163–170.
35. UNAIDS, WHO: *Provisional WHO/UNAIDS Secretariat recommendations on the use of cotrimoxazole prophylaxis in adults and children living with HIV/AIDS in Africa*. Geneva: Joint United Nations Program on HIV/AIDS and World Health Organization; 2000.
36. World Health Organization (WHO): *Guidelines on co-trimoxazole prophylaxis for HIV-related infections among children, adolescents and adults: Recommendations for a public health approach*. Geneva: World Health Organization; 2006.
37. Department of State for Health: *The Gambia: **Antiretroviral Therapy: A manual for health service providers***. Banjul: New Type Press; 2004.
38. World Health Organization (WHO): *Scaling up antitertiviral therapy in resource limited settings: Treatment guidelines for a public health approach (2003 Revision)*. Geneva: World Health Organization; 2004.
39. World Health Organization (WHO): *Antiretroviral therapy for HIV infection in infants and children: Towards universal access. Recommendations for a public health approach*. Geneva: World Health Organization; 2006.
40. van der Loeff MF S, Jaffar S, Aveika AA, Sabally S, Corrah T, Harding E, Alabi A, Bayang A, Ariyoshi K, Whittle HC: **Mortality of HIV-1, HIV-2 and HIV-1/HIV-2 dually infected patients in a clinic-based cohort in The Gambia.** *AIDS* 2002, **16**(13):1775–1783.
41. **Haemoglobin concentrations for the diagnosis of anaemia and assessment of severity. Vitamin and Mineral Nutrition Information System.** http://www.who.int/vmnis/indicators/haemoglobin.pdf, accessed January 27, 2012.

15

Coregulation of HIV-1 dependency factors in individuals heterozygous to the CCR5-delta32 deletion

Gero Hütter[1,2*], Christian Blüthgen[1], Martin Neumann[3], Mark Reinwald[4], Daniel Nowak[4] and Harald Klüter[1]

Abstract

Background: CCR5-delta32 heterozygous individuals are susceptible to HIV-1. However, it is not clear if there is a relevant protective effect against transmission and a beneficial effect in terms of HIV progression which cannot be attributed to CCR5 surface density alone. Therefore we investigated HIV-1 dependency factors (HDF) which might be differently regulated in CCR5 wild type (WT) and CCR5-delta32 heterozygous individuals.

Methods: We examined CD34+ hematopoietic progenitor cells derived from bone marrow samples from 19 healthy volunteers, 12 individuals with CCR5 WT and 7 with heterozygous CCR5-delta32 deletion. Samples were analyzed using a global gene expression oligonucleotide microarray (HG-U133plus 2.0, Affymetrix Inc.).

Results: A total of 205 genes were found with altered expression (3fold difference, present call rate of 75%, $p < 0.05$) and 7 of these had a connection to HIV-1 pathogenesis. In 4 genes: TOP1, CXCR2, SREBF2, and TAP we found a different regulation which was consistent with a supposed beneficial effect for CCR5-delta32 heterozygotes.

Conclusion: The CCR5-delta32 deletion is associated with other HDFs in HIV-1 pathogenesis as a possible explanation for beneficial effects regarding the deletion leading to a variant expression profile in heterozygous carriers of this mutation.

Keywords: CCR5-delta32, HIV-1, Coexpression, TOP1, CXCR2, SREBF2, TAP

Background

The human immunodeficiency virus type 1 (HIV-1) genome encodes a rather small number of 15 proteins. However, during infection and interaction with the target cells, the virus exploits multiple proteins of the host for its replication. Alterations of expression or functional changes based on genetic variances of critical genes are called HIV-dependency factors (HDFs). They are required for infection or disease progression, influencing the efficacy of HIV-1 transmission, viral load, and collapse of the immune system. Understanding these HDFs might play a key role in identifying new therapeutics strategies against the infection [1].

One of the most prominent HDF is the association of HIV-1 and the chemokine receptor CCR5. In combination with CD4, CCR5 is required for internalization of the viral genome. Up to date, over 70 mutations have been described in the CCR5 gene including the intensively studied 32 base pair deletion (CCR5-delta32) that introduces a premature stop-codon into the CCR5 locus [2,3].

Interestingly, CCR5 is highly preferred from the virus and people with a homozygous CCR5-delta32 deletion gain a nearly complete protection from HIV-1 transmission. This is remarkable as CXCR4 is always expressed as an alternative coreceptor in CCR5-deficient individuals and most HIV positive patients harbor a small fraction of CXCR4 using strains (X4 type) [4]. Therefore, CCR5 deficient individuals are frequently exposed against X4 but hardly ever get infected. It is still not clear whether this observation could only be explained by a presumed selective disadvantage of X4 in the absence of CCR5 or

* Correspondence: gero.huetter@medma.uni-heidelberg.de
[1]Institute of Transfusion Medicine and Immunology, Medical Faculty Mannheim, Heidelberg University; German Red Cross Blood Service Baden-Württemberg- Hessen, Mannheim, Germany
[2]Cellex GmbH, Dresden, Germany

Table 1 A selection of published surveys concerning possible clinical benefits (transmission or progression) of the CCR5-delta32 heterozygous genotype

N=	Study population	Benefit tested	Significance	Reference
1427	HIV + vs. sero-negative control group	Transmission	P = 0.012	[8]
30	ESN	Transmission	P = 0.04	[9]
54	ESN	Transmission	P = 0.05*	[10]
2605	Woman	Transmission	OR: 0.63 (95% CI 0.44-0.90)	[11]
2996	High risk groups	Transmission	Risk = 0.30 (95% CI: 0.08-0.97)	[12]
1252	MSM	Transmission	NS	[13]
1200	HIV + vs control	Transmission, progression to AIDS	Both significant	[14]
108	IDU	Progression to AIDS	NS	[15]
127	Children	Progression to AIDS	Significant (p = 0.008) Effect is abrogated in case of a SDF1-3'A genotype	[16]
1955	Hemophilia patients	Progression to AIDS	Significant	[17]
512	Mother-child	Transmission, progression to AIDS	NS, significant	[18]

These controversial data suggest that there might be additional factors beside the CCR5-delta32 genotype like SDF 1-3' which contribute to the clinical outcome of transmission and infection. (ESN = exposed seronegative, MSM = men having sex with men, IDU = injecting drug users, CI = confidence interval, OR = odds ratio, NS = not significant) *only significant in heterosexuals.

whether there are additional effects of the CCR5 deletion causing the protection from X4 transmission.

In addition, a certain protective effect in heterozygous CCR5-delta32 carriers is also controversially discussed (Table 1). It is well known that CCR5 receptor density on the target cells determines the susceptibility against transmission and that CCR5-delta32 heterozygotes have a reduced receptor expression on the surface [5]. However, CCR5 is a dynamic receptor and several studies have shown that CCR5 density in delta32 heterozygotes could be similar to wild type individuals and therefore the CCR5 surface expression might not be the single protective factor [6,7].

Taken together, the mechanism of a near-perfect protection of complete CCR5 deficiency as well as the observation that HIV-infected CCR5-delta32 heterozygotes may have a slower progression to AIDS has to be more elucidated and might help identifying other key players contributing to HIV pathogenesis [13,17].

Therefore, in this work we analyzed the gene expression patterns of CCR5-delta32 deletion in comparison to wild type carriers, further, how the alteration change in expression might contribute to the reduced clinical susceptibility and progression of HIV disease observed in carriers of this mutation. This might improve the understanding of the connection between HIV pathogenesis and immune system interaction of the underlying host.

Results and discussion

We screened CD34+ cells of 19 specimen contained within a blood donor bank and identified 12 healthy donors carrying wild type (WT) CCR5 while the remaining seven carried the CCR5-delta32 deletion allele heterozygously (Table 2). Gene expression analysis revealed 205 genes differentially expressed between WT and heterozygous carriers of CCR5-delta32 mutation. 96 were found to be overexpressed in heterozygotes (Additional file 1: Table S1) whereas the remaining 109

Table 2 Results and characteristics of analyzed specimen

	Specimen	Gender	Age	CCR5 WT	CCR5-delta32 heterozygous
1	N0014/05	m	19	+	
2	N0015/05	f	53	+	
3	N0023/05	m	24	+	
4	N0024/05	f	21	+	
5	N0031/05	m	25	+	
6	N0035/05	m	21		+
7	N0091/06	m	30	+	
8	N0094/06	m	20	+	
9	N0103/06	m	32	+	
10	N0106/06	m	23	+	
11	N0118/07	f	28		+
12	N0136/07	f	29		+
13	N0153/07	f	29		+
14	N0158/07	m	25		+
15	N0163/07	f	23		+
16	N0200/08	f	74	+	
17	N0204/08	f	85	+	
18	N0305/09	f	28		+
19	N0312/09	f	34	+	

CD34+ hematopoeitic progenitor cells for genotyping were obtained by bone marrow aspiration.

genes were found to be overexpressed in WT samples, respectively.

Further review of gene databases concerning the known or proposed function of these genes regarding HIV-1 infection revealed three genes in the WT group and four genes in the CCR5-delta32 group with significantly different overexpression profiles (Figures 1 and 2).

The theory that human host genes or polymorphic variants of genes may influence transmission or the outcome of HIV-1 infection goes back to the early 1980's [19]. Improved techniques using high throughput assays provide insight into a detailed view in the pathogenesis of HIV-1 and possible host or HIV-dependency factors (HDF) [1]. Besides the well-characterized chemokine entry mechanism there are several other allelic mutations described in HDF genes such as IL10, IFNG, or KIR3DS1 (together with HLA-Bw4). In addition, several HLA subtypes have been found to be associated either with delayed or accelerated progression to AIDS [20].

However, some phenomena remain unsolved. Especially the role of the CCR5-delta32 deletion in transmission and maintaining the infection is under investigation and there are currently more open questions than answers. Recent progress in HIV gene therapy revealed new insights of the CCR5-delta32 deletion [21,22]. In the SB-728-T Sangamo trial with anti CCR5 zinc-finger nuclease (ZFN) treated lymphocytes in HIV patients, only one candidate with a CCR5-delta32 heterozygous genotype in this group achieved spontaneous virus control during HAART discontinuation. Taken into account that the CCR5 density in heterozygotes does not substantially differ from the density in wild types, it is astonishing that an additional knock down of less than a few percent of CCR5 expression by ZFNs has subsequently such a deep impact on viral replication. Consequently it was not surprising that Sangamo initiated a follow up trial especially for carriers of the CCR5-delta32 genotype (SB-728-902-Cohort 5) [23].

Most recently, the report of a long term control of HIV in two patients receiving an allogeneic stem cell transplantation (SCT) with a CCR5 wild type allo-graft ("Boston patients") has brought up new questions. These patients showed a profound reduction of the viral reservoir, and declining HIV antibody levels with ongoing engraftment during the follow-up period of several years similar to the "Berlin patient" [24]. Finally, in 2013 antiretroviral medication was discontinued in these patients and none of them developed a rebound of HIV infection. Transplantation has led to a replacement of the old immune system, antiretroviral therapy has protected the new engrafting cells from re-infection, and probably GvHD has cleared residual viral reservoirs in the host. Interestingly, both patients were heterozygous for the CCR5-delta32 deletion [25].

Genes with higher expression in the wild type group

From 109 genes significantly overexpressed in the wild type group, three were recognized to have an association with HIV-1 (Table 3). Of these three, CXCR2 is expressed in higher quantities in the wild type group. Like CXCR1, CXCR2 acts as a receptor for interleukin 8

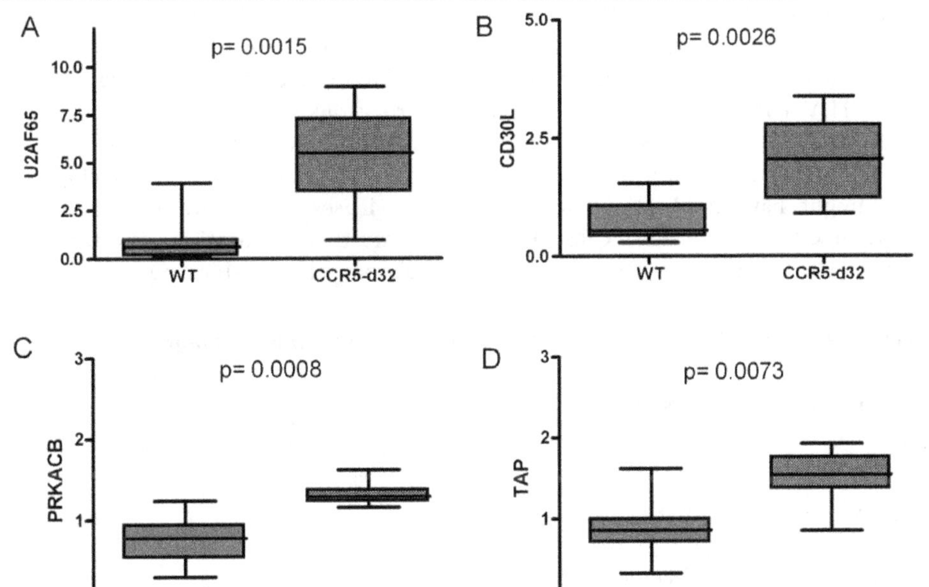

Figure 1 Results of the micro array gene expression analysis of 19 specimens. In the group of heterozygous CCR5-delta32 carriers 4 genes associated with HIV-1 pathogenesis have been found to be overexpressed: **A.** U2AF65, **B.** CD30L, **C.** PRKACB, and **D.** TAP. Normalized arbitrary expression levels.

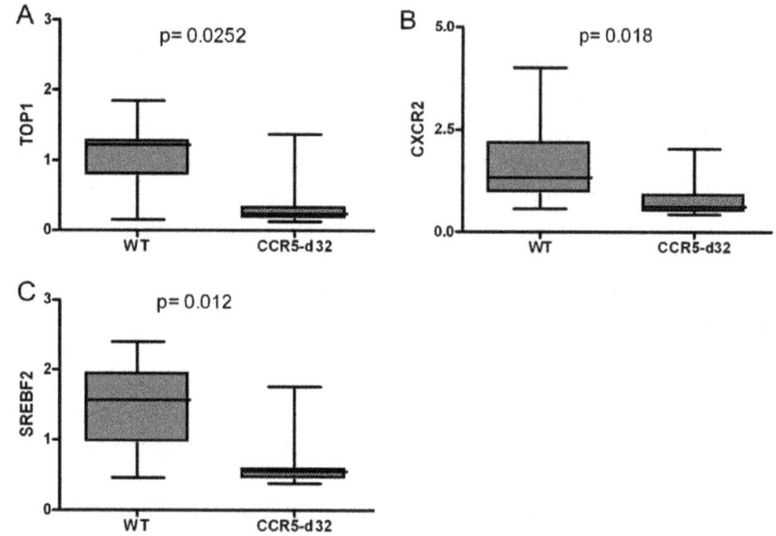

Figure 2 Results of the micro array gene expression analysis of 19 specimens. In wild type sample there were 3 genes associated with HIV-1 significantly overexpressed compared to heterozygous CCR5-delta32 carriers: **A.** TOP1, **B.** CXCR2, and **C.** SREBF2. Normalized arbitrary expression levels.

(IL-8) and is differentially expressed in subsets of lymphocytes like CD56+/CD16+ NK-cells [26]. Both receptors share intracellular cross-talk and in cells expressing either CXCR1 or CXCR2, exposure to IL-8 leads to an internalization of these receptors. This effect is significant lower in cells expressing both of the receptors like the CD56+/CD16+ NK-cells [27]. Additionally, binding of IL-8 on the CXCR1 receptors causes an additional cross-phosphorylation of both, CCR5 and CXCR4, resulting in a decreased susceptibility against HIV-1. Only the association of IL-8/CXCR1 and not IL-8/CXCR2 inherits this protective effect [28]. Most surprisingly in this context is that the HIV-1 matrix protein p17 binds to both, CXCR1 and CXCR2 in an IL-8-like manner [29]. Taken together, the higher expression of CXCR2 in the wild type group might have implications for the $p17_{HIV-1}$/IL-8 pathway of CXCR1 induced CCR5 internalization resulting in an altered susceptibility.

Topoisomerase 1 (TOP1) is a 91 kDa enzyme that critically regulates the topological state of DNA during transcription. TOP1 in association with reverse transcriptase is most relevant for HIV cDNA synthesis [32]. Moreover, TOP1 is essential to directly interact with HIV-1 nucleocapsid protein [33] In vitro assays with overexpression of TOP1 led to an 5fold increase of infective virions derived from these manipulated cells [34]. Our finding that TOP1 was significantly underexpressed in CCR5-delta32 samples than in wild type samples could contribute to the clinical observation of decreased rate of progression to AIDS in HIV-1-infected heterozygous carriers.

Finally, cholesterol is known to play an essential role in the life cycle of several enveloped viruses. Many of these viruses manipulate host cholesterol metabolism to facilitate their replication. The target gene of the sterol regulatory element-binding protein 2 (SREBP2) which

Table 3 Three genes with a link to HIV-1 pathogenesis were found to be significant higher expressed in the CCR5 wild type group

Significant higher Expression in CCR5 wild type samples				
Gene	Function *(link to HIV-1)*	Beneficial effect for CCR5-delta32 carriers		Reference
		Transm.	Repli.	
TOP1	Synthesis of cDNA *(in combination with RT transcription of viral RNA to DNA)*		Possible	[30]
CXCR2	Receptor for IL-8. Mediates neutrophil migration to sites of inflammation. *(binding side of $p17_{HIV-1}$, cross-linked to CXCR1 and indirectly cross-linked to CXCR1 mediated CCR5 internalisation)*	Possible		[29]
SREBF2	Cholesterol metabolism *(enhancing viral replication)*		Possible	[31]

For TOP1 and SREBF2 there are reports that overexpression of these genes might have a beneficial effect on HIV-1 infection. For CXCR2 overexpression this beneficial effect was described in case of HIV-1 transmission. (transm. = transmission, repli. = replication).

was found to be downregulated in the heterozygous CCR5-delta32 group is TFII-I, a gene critical for HIV-1 transcription in activated T cells [31]. Experimental knockdown of SREBP2 expression by small interfering RNA (siRNA) resulted in a significant reduced viral replication. Consecutively, decreased expression of SREBP2 in CCR5-delta32 heterozygotes may contribute to benefits of viral replication and progression to AIDS.

Genes with higher expression in the CCR5-delta32 group

In the CCR5-del32 group, 96 genes have been found to be overexpressed and four of them had a link to HIV-1 infection (Table 4).

PRKACB was significantly higher expressed in the CCR5-delta32 group. PRKACB is one of five human C subunits of the PKA group which acts as a serine/threonine kinase but only PRKACB together with PRKACA and PRKX do act as functional protein kinases [39]. Concerning HIV-1 pathogenesis this kinase has been described to be involved in infection such as activating viral transcription of monocytes/macrophages in vitro, or activation of T-cells in HIV-patients with ongoing HAART [40,41]. Most interestingly is the transcriptional regulation of CCR5 expression through a cAMP/PKA/CREB dependent pathway. [42] The CCR5 promoter region contains an cyclic AMP responsive element which could be critical for the regulation of gene expression [43]. Although authors could show that a temporal increase of CCR5 expression could be mediated by PKA, the role of differentially regulated PRKACB in HIV-1 pathogenesis still needs to be further determined.

One possible mechanism of HIV-1 escape from immune recognition and consecutive cytolysis is downregulation of the MHC I expression. TAP as a transporter for antigen presentation was overexpressed in the CCR5-delta32 carrier group. It is known that HIV-1 infection abolishes the ability of cells to translocate antigenic peptides via TAP to the endoplasmatic reticulum and thus indirectly abrogates peptides from MHC I presentation [38]. Overexpression of TAP in heterozygotes might partially compensate this HIV-induced inhibition leading to an enhanced clearance of infected cells and indirectly to a decreased susceptibility in this group.

U2AF^{65} is a 65 kDa auxiliary factor of pre-mRNA splicing and contains a sequence-specific RNA-binding region with 3′ RNA recognition motifs and an Arg/Ser-rich domain necessary for splicing. The spliced mRNA species in HIV-1 infected cells are *env/vpu*, *nef*, *rev*, *vpr*, and *vif*. The binding of a 35 kDa subunit stabilizes the binding of U2AF^{65} with the polypyrimidine tract (PPT) of introns during spliceosome assembly [35,44]. However, there are no reports that altered expression of U2AF^{65} contributes to HIV-1 viral progression or susceptibility of transmission.

CD30L is mainly expressed in high levels on activated T cells interacting either with membrane bound CD30 from B or T lymphocytes or soluble CD30. Soluble CD30 has been described to be expressed in high amounts during acute HIV-1 infection [36]. Recently, it has been reported that specified CD4 and CD8 T cell clones are capable of producing T helper (Th)2-type cytokines, which release soluble CD30 into the circulation [45]. The general function of the CD30/CD30L interaction is still unsolved. It has been suggested that this interaction promotes secondary humoral immune responses. However, an in vivo test system with CD30−/− knockout mice or anti CD30L antibodies have led to conflicting results [46]. Taken together, there is no convincing explanation whether the CD30L overexpression in CCR5-delta32 heterozygotes may contribute to a potential benefit in these patients or not.

Conclusions

We identified 7 genes previously found to be associated with HIV-1 pathogenesis and furthermore were differentially expressed in CCR5 wild type and CCR5-delta32 heterozygous individuals. Out of these two, CXCR2 and

Table 4 Four genes were found with link to HIV-1 in the CCR5-delta32 heterozygous group

Significant higher Expression in CCR5-delta32 samples				
Gene	Function *(link to HIV-1)*	Beneficial effect for CCR5-delta32 carriers		Reference
		Transm.	Repli.	
U2AF65	Splicing factor *(enhances with the polypyrimidine tract of the splicosome of several HIV-1 genes)*	Unknown		[35]
CD30L	Regulation immune response *(elevated CD30 levels during acute HIV-1 infection)*	Unknown		[36]
PRKACB	Catalytic subunit of camp-dependent protein kinase *(coexpression with the HDF GliPR)*	Unknown		[37]
TAP	Antigen presentation *(HIV-1 abrogates TAP mediated peptide transport to MHC I presentation)*	Possible		[38]

Only for TAP there was a beneficial effect pre-described in terms of viral transmission. For the other three genes there are currently no data concerning a beneficial effect available. (transm. = transmission, repli. = replication).

TAP may have a beneficial effect concerning HIV-1 transmission, and two genes, TOP1 and SREBF2, may be favorable in terms of replication and disease progression in heterozygous CCR5-delta32 carriers. Concerning the other three genes, there was no evidence of a beneficial effect described so far. The clinical relevance of these findings should be further tested in prospective studies.

Methods

Specimen

Input material for this analysis were immunomagnetically purified CD34+ cells from bone marrow aspiration of 19 healthy volunteers, 9 male 10 female, aged 19–85 (median 25) years. All donors gave written informed consent before investigation. Prior to CD34+ selection, mononuclear cells were isolated by density gradient centrifugation through Ficoll-Hypaque (Biochrom, Berlin, Germany). The study protocol was approved by the Ethical committee II, Medical Faculty Mannheim, Heidelberg University Institutional Review Board.

CCR5 genotyping analysis

Genomic DNA was extracted from heparinised peripheral blood monocytes (PBMC) of the donors with the QIAGEN-Blood-Midi-Kit (Qiagen, Germany). Screening of the donors for the CCR5-delta32-allele was performed with a genomic PCR using primers flanking the site of the deletion (forward: 5′-CTCCCAGGAATCAT CTTTACC-3′, reverse: 5′-TCATTTCGACACCGAAG CAG-3′) leading to a PCR fragment of 200 base pairs (bp) for the CCR5-allele and of 168 bp in case of a delta32 deletion. Results were confirmed by allele specific PCR and by direct sequencing using the BigDye®-Terminator-1.1.-Cycle-Sequencing-Kit (Applied Biosystems, Germany). Sequences were analyzed using the Vector-NTI-Contig-Express-software (Invitrogen, Germany).

RNA preparation and array based gene expression analysis

Total RNA was extracted from purified CD34+ hematopoietic progenitor cells using TRIzol (Invitrogen, Karlsruhe, Germany) according to the manufacturer's protocol. The quality of RNA was determined by the 2100 Bioanalyzer system (Agilent Technologies, Waldbronn, Germany) and only samples showing no RNA-degradation were included into the analysis. Oligonucleotide microarrays (HG-U133plus 2.0, Affymetrix Inc., Santa Clara, CA) were hybridized as described previously [47]. Data analysis was performed by the Microarray Suite 5.0 (Affymetrix), and the Genespring software 4.2 (Silicon Genetics, Redwood City, CA). The quality control parameters were in accordance to the MIAME consensus criteria for micro array data with a present call rate of at least 25% [48]. Previously, our group has shown a close correlation of micro-array data compared to quantitative PCR methods in the same sample [49].

Statistics

All samples were normalized with expression values raised to an arbitrary value of 1. Only expression values which reach a present call rate of 75% have been used. Only genes with a significant three-fold difference of expression ($p < 0.05$) between the CCR5 wild type and the CCR5-delta32 group were eligible for further statistical analysis. Expression analysis of the different groups was performed by using the Mann Whitney test.

Competing interests

The authors confirm that this article content has no conflicts of interest.

Authors' contributions

GH designed to study and wrote the manuscript, CB performed CCR5 genotyping, MN analyzed micro array data, DN performed the micro array, MR and HK Contributed to conception and design of the study and interpretation of the data. Revised the manuscript critically for important intellectual content. All authors read and approved the final manuscript.

Acknowledgements

This work was supported by the Bill & Melinda Gates Foundation (Grand Challenges Explorations Grant Number: OPP1033364). We thank Susanne Ganepola for proofreading the manuscript.

Author details

[1]Institute of Transfusion Medicine and Immunology, Medical Faculty Mannheim, Heidelberg University; German Red Cross Blood Service Baden-Württemberg- Hessen, Mannheim, Germany. [2]Cellex GmbH, Dresden, Germany. [3]Medical Department III (Hematology, Oncology), Charité Campus Benjamin Franklin, Berlin, Germany. [4]Medical Department III (Hematology, Oncology), University Medical Centre Mannheim, Heidelberg University, Heidelberg, Germany.

References

1. Brass AL, Dykxhoorn DM, Benita Y, Yan N, Engelman A, Xavier RJ, Lieberman J, Elledge SJ: **Identification of host proteins required for HIV infection through a functional genomic screen.** *Science* 2008, **319**:921–926.
2. Bream JH, Young HA, Rice N, Martin MP, Smith MW, Carrington M, O'Brien SJ: **CCR5 promoter alleles and specific DNA binding factors.** *Science* 1999, **284**:223.
3. Carrington M, Dean M, Martin MP, O'Brien SJ: **Genetics of HIV-1 infection: chemokine receptor CCR5 polymorphism and its consequences.** *Hum Mol Genet* 1999, **8**:1939–1945.
4. Delobel P, Sandres-Saune K, Cazabat M, Pasquier C, Marchou B, Massip P, Izopet J: **R5 to X4 switch of the predominant HIV-1 population in cellular reservoirs during effective highly active antiretroviral therapy.** *J Acquir Immune Defic Syndr* 2005, **38**:382–392.
5. Lin YL, Mettling C, Portales P, Reynes J, Clot J, Corbeau P: **Cell surface CCR5 density determines the postentry efficiency of R5 HIV-1 infection.** *Proc Natl Acad Sci USA* 2002, **99**:15590–15595.
6. Reynes J, Portales P, Segondy M, Baillat V, Andre P, Avinens O, Picot MC, Clot J, Eliaou JF, Corbeau P: **CD4 T cell surface CCR5 density as a host factor in HIV-1 disease progression.** *Aids* 2001, **15**:1627–1634.

7. Venkatesan S, Petrovic A, Van Ryk DI, Locati M, Weissman D, Murphy PM: **Reduced cell surface expression of CCR5 in CCR5Delta 32 heterozygotes is mediated by gene dosage, rather than by receptor sequestration.** *J Biol Chem* 2002, **277**:2287–2301.
8. Samson M, Libert F, Doranz BJ, Rucker J, Liesnard C, Farber CM, Saragosti S, Lapoumeroulie C, Cognaux J, Forceille C, Muyldermans G, Verhofstede C, Burtonboy G, Georges M, Imai T, Rana S, Yi Y, Smyth RJ, Collman RG, Doms RW, Vassart G, Parmentier M: **Resistance to HIV-1 infection in caucasian individuals bearing mutant alleles of the CCR-5 chemokine receptor gene.** *Nature* 1996, **382**:722–725.
9. Trecarichi EM, Tumbarello M, De Gaetano DK, Tamburrini E, Cauda R, Brahe C, Tiziano FD: **Partial protective effect of CCR5-Delta 32 heterozygosity in a cohort of heterosexual Italian HIV-1 exposed uninfected individuals.** *AIDS Res Ther* 2006, **3**:22.
10. Hoffman TL, MacGregor RR, Burger H, Mick R, Doms RW, Collman RG: **CCR5 genotypes in sexually active couples discordant for human immunodeficiency virus type 1 infection status.** *J Infect Dis* 1997, **176**:1093–1096.
11. Philpott S, Weiser B, Tarwater P, Vermund SH, Kleeberger CA, Gange SJ, Anastos K, Cohen M, Greenblatt RM, Kovacs A, Minkoff H, Young MA, Miotti P, Dupuis M, Chen CH, Burger H: **CC chemokine receptor 5 genotype and susceptibility to transmission of human immunodeficiency virus type 1 in women.** *J Infect Dis* 2003, **187**:569–575.
12. Marmor M, Sheppard HW, Donnell D, Bozeman S, Celum C, Buchbinder S, Koblin B, Seage GR III: **Homozygous and heterozygous CCR5-Delta32 genotypes are associated with resistance to HIV infection.** *J Acquir Immune Defic Syndr* 2001, **27**:472–481.
13. Huang Y, Paxton WA, Wolinsky SM, Neumann AU, Zhang L, He T, Kang S, Ceradini D, Jin Z, Yazdanbakhsh K, Kunstman K, Erickson D, Dragon E, Landau NR, Phair J, Ho DD, Koup RA: **The role of a mutant CCR5 allele in HIV-1 transmission and disease progression.** *Nat Med* 1996, **2**:1240–1243.
14. Oh DY, Jessen H, Kucherer C, Neumann K, Oh N, Poggensee G, Bartmeyer B, Jessen A, Pruss A, Schumann RR, Hamouda O: **CCR5Delta32 genotypes in a German HIV-1 seroconverter cohort and report of HIV-1 infection in a CCR5Delta32 homozygous individual.** *PLoS One* 2008, **3**:e2747.
15. Schinkel J, Langendam MW, Coutinho RA, Krol A, Brouwer M, Schuitemaker H: **No evidence for an effect of the CCR5 delta32/+ and CCR2b 64I/+ mutations on human immunodeficiency virus (HIV)-1 disease progression among HIV-1-infected injecting drug users.** *J Infect Dis* 1999, **179**:825–831.
16. Sei S, Boler AM, Nguyen GT, Stewart SK, Yang QE, Edgerly M, Wood LV, Brouwers P, Venzon DJ: **Protective effect of CCR5 delta 32 heterozygosity is restricted by SDF-1 genotype in children with HIV-1 infection.** *Aids* 2001, **15**:1343–1352.
17. Dean M, Carrington M, Winkler C, Huttley GA, Smith MW, Allikmets R, Goedert JJ, Buchbinder SP, Vittinghoff E, Gomperts E, Donfield S, Vlahov D, Kaslow R, Saah A, Rinaldo C, Detels R, O'Brien SJ: **Genetic restriction of HIV-1 infection and progression to AIDS by a deletion allele of the CKR5 structural gene: hemophilia growth and development study, multicenter AIDS cohort study, multicenter hemophilia cohort study, San Francisco City cohort, ALIVE study.** *Science* 1996, **273**:1856–1862.
18. Misrahi M, Teglas JP, N'Go N, Burgard M, Mayaux MJ, Rouzioux C, Delfraissy JF, Blanche S: **CCR5 chemokine receptor variant in HIV-1 mother-to-child transmission and disease progression in children: French pediatric HIV infection study group.** *Jama* 1998, **279**:277–280.
19. O'Brien SJ, Dean M: **In search of AIDS-resistance genes.** *Sci Am* 1997, **277**:44–51.
20. O'Brien SJ, Nelson GW: **Human genes that limit AIDS.** *Nat Genet* 2004, **36**:565–574.
21. Hütter G, Schneider T, Thiel E: **Transplantation of selected or transgenic blood stem cells - a future treatment for HIV/AIDS?** *J Int AIDS Soc* 2009, **12**:10.
22. Hütter G, Symond G: **Progress in HIV gene therapy.** In *Treatment strategies: AIDS.* 2nd edition. Edited by Hajba L. London: The Cambridge Research Centre; 2011:44–46.
23. Ando D, Tang WW, Stein D, Wang S, Lee G, Holmes M, Giedlin M, Gregory P, Tabas P, June C: *HAART Treatment Interruption following Adoptive Transfer of Zinc Finger Nuclease (ZFN) Modified Autologous CD4 T-cells (SB-728-T) to HIV-infected Subjects Demonstrates Durable Engraftment and Suppression of Viral Load [abstract].* Chicago: Interscience Conference on Antimicrobial Agents and Chemotherapy (ICAAC); 2011. 17–20 September.
24. Henrich TJ, Hu Z, Li JZ, Sciaranghella G, Busch MP, Keating SM, Gallien S, Lin NH, Giguel FF, Lavoie L, Ho VT, Armand P, Soiffer RJ, Sagar M, Lacasce AS, Kuritzkes DR: **Long-term reduction in peripheral blood HIV type 1 reservoirs following reduced-intensity conditioning allogeneic stem cell transplantation.** *J Infect Dis* 2013, **207**:1694–1702.
25. Henrich T, Hanhauser E, Sirignano M, Davis B, Lee TH, Keating S, Busch M, Marty F, LaCasce A, Armand P, Soiffer R, Altfeld M, Kuritzkes D: *In depth investigation of peripheral and gut HIV-1 reservoirs, HIV-specific cellular immunity, and host microchimerism following allogeneic hematopoetic stem cell transplantation.* Kuala Lumpur: 7th International AIDS Society Conference on HIV Pathogenesis, Treatment and Prevention; 2013.
26. Robertson MJ: **Role of chemokines in the biology of natural killer cells.** *J Leukoc Biol* 2002, **71**:173–183.
27. Attal H, Cohen-Hillel E, Meshel T, Wang JM, Gong W, Ben-Baruch A: **Intracellular cross-talk between the GPCR CXCR1 and CXCR2: role of carboxyl terminus phosphorylation sites.** *Exp Cell Res* 2008, **314**:352–365.
28. Richardson RM, Tokunaga K, Marjoram R, Sata T, Snyderman R: **Interleukin-8-mediated heterologous receptor internalization provides resistance to HIV-1 infectivity: role of signal strength and receptor desensitization.** *J Biol Chem* 2003, **278**:15867–15873.
29. Caccuri F, Giagulli C, Bugatti A, Benetti A, Alessandri G, Ribatti D, Marsico S, Apostoli P, Slevin MA, Rusnati M, Guzman CA, Fiorentini S, Caruso A: **HIV-1 matrix protein p17 promotes angiogenesis via chemokine receptors CXCR1 and CXCR2.** *Proc Natl Acad Sci USA* 2012, **109**:14580–14585.
30. Khurana B, Zhuang L, Moitra PK, Stantchev TS, Broder CC, Cutler ML, D'Arpa P: **Human TOP1 residues implicated in species specificity of HIV-1 infection are required for interaction with BTBD2, and RNAi of BTBD2 in old world monkey and human cells increases permissiveness to HIV-1 infection.** *Virol J* 2010, **7**:332.
31. Taylor HE, Linde ME, Khatua AK, Popik W, Hildreth JE: **Sterol regulatory element-binding protein 2 couples HIV-1 transcription to cholesterol homeostasis and T cell activation.** *J Virol* 2011, **85**:7699–7709.
32. Shoya Y, Tokunaga K, Sawa H, Maeda M, Ueno T, Yoshikawa T, Hasegawa H, Sata T, Kurata T, Hall WW, Cullen BR, Takahashi H: **Human topoisomerase I promotes HIV-1 proviral DNA synthesis: implications for the species specificity and cellular tropism of HIV-1 infection.** *Proc Natl Acad Sci USA* 2003, **100**:8442–8447.
33. Takahashi H, Matsuda M, Kojima A, Sata T, Andoh T, Kurata T, Nagashima K, Hall WW: **Human immunodeficiency virus type 1 reverse transcriptase: enhancement of activity by interaction with cellular topoisomerase I.** *Proc Natl Acad Sci USA* 1995, **92**:5694–5698.
34. Folks T, Kelly J, Benn S, Kinter A, Justement J, Gold J, Redfield R, Sell KW, Fauci AS: **Susceptibility of normal human lymphocytes to infection with HTLV-III/LAV.** *J Immunol* 1986, **136**:4049–4053.
35. Domsic JK, Wang Y, Mayeda A, Krainer AR, Stoltzfus CM: **Human immunodeficiency virus type 1 hnRNP A/B-dependent exonic splicing silencer ESSV antagonizes binding of U2AF65 to viral polypyrimidine tracts.** *Mol Cell Biol* 2003, **23**:8762–8772.
36. Pizzolo G, Vinante F, Nadali G, Krampera M, Morosato L, Chilosi M, Raiteri R, Sinicco A: **High serum level of soluble CD30 in acute primary HIV-1 infection.** *Clin Explmmunol* 1997, **108**:251–253.
37. Capalbo G, Muller-Kuller T, Dietrich U, Hoelzer D, Ottmann OG, Scheuring UJ: **Inhibition of HIV-1 replication by small interfering RNAs directed against glioma pathogenesis related protein (GliPR) expression.** *Retrovirology* 2010, **7**:26.
38. Kutsch O, Vey T, Kerkau T, Hunig T, Schimpl A: **HIV type 1 abrogates TAP-mediated transport of antigenic peptides presented by MHC class I: transporter associated with antigen presentation.** *AIDS Res Hum Retroviruses* 2002, **18**:1319–1325.
39. Soberg K, Jahnsen T, Rognes T, Skalhegg BS, Laerdahl JK: **Evolutionary paths of the cAMP-dependent protein kinase (PKA) catalytic subunits.** *PLoS One* 2013, **8**:e60935.
40. Johansson CC, Bryn T, Yndestad A, Eiken HG, Bjerkeli V, Froland SS, Aukrust P, Tasken K: **Cytokine networks are pre-activated in T cells from HIV-infected patients on HAART and are under the control of cAMP.** *Aids* 2004, **18**:171–179.
41. Rabbi MF, Al-Harthi L, Saifuddin M, Roebuck KA: **The cAMP-dependent protein kinase A and protein kinase C-beta pathways synergistically interact to activate HIV-1 transcription in latently infected cells of monocyte/macrophage lineage.** *Virology* 1998, **245**:257–269.

42. Banerjee A, Pirrone V, Wigdahl B, Nonnemacher MR: **Transcriptional regulation of the chemokine co-receptor CCR5 by the cAMP/PKA/CREB pathway.** *Biomed Pharmacother* 2011, **65:**293–297.
43. Kuipers HF, Biesta PJ, Montagne LJ, Van Haastert ES, Van Der Valk P, Van Den Elsen PJ: **CC chemokine receptor 5 gene promoter activation by the cyclic AMP response element binding transcription factor.** *Blood* 2008, **112:**1610–1619.
44. Jenkins JL, Agrawal AA, Gupta A, Green MR, Kielkopf CL: **U2AF65 adapts to diverse pre-mRNA splice sites through conformational selection of specific and promiscuous RNA recognition motifs.** *Nucleic Acids Res* 2013, **41:**3859–3873.
45. Romagnani S, Del Prete G, Maggi E, Chilosi M, Caligaris-Cappio F, Pizzolo G: **CD30 and type 2 T helper (Th2) responses.** *J Leukoc Biol* 1995, **57:**726–730.
46. Kennedy MK, Willis CR, Armitage RJ: **Deciphering CD30 ligand biology and its role in humoral immunity.** *Immunology* 2006, **118:**143–152.
47. Hofmann WK, De Vos S, Komor M, Hoelzer D, Wachsman W, Koeffler HP: **Characterization of gene expression of CD34+ cells from normal and myelodysplastic bone marrow.** *Blood* 2002, **100:**3553–3560.
48. Brazma A: **Minimum information about a microarray experiment (MIAME)–successes, failures, challenges.** *Scientific World J* 2009, **9:**420–423.
49. Gueller S, Komor M, Nowak D, Baldus CD, De Vos S, Hoelzer D, Ottmann OG, Hofmann WK: **Identification of defects in the transcriptional program during lineage-specific in vitro differentiation of CD34(+) cells selected from patients with both low- and high-risk myelodysplastic syndrome.** *Exp Hematol* 2010, **38:**718–732. 732 e711-716.

16

Trends and determining factors associated with adherence to antiretroviral therapy (ART) in Cameroon

Lawrence Mbuagbaw[1,2*], Lehana Thabane[2,3], Pierre Ongolo-Zogo[1], David Yondo[1], Stephen Noorduyn[2], Marek Smieja[2,4] and Lisa Dolovich[5]

Abstract

Background: The benefits of antiretroviral therapy (ART) cannot be experienced if they are not taken as prescribed. Yet, not all causes of non-adherence are dependent on the patient. Having to pay for medication reduces adherence rates. Non- adherence has severe public health implications which must be addressed locally and globally. This paper seeks to describe the trends in adherence rates reported in Cameroon and to investigate the determinants of adherence to ART in the Cameroon Mobile Phone SMS (CAMPS) trial.

Methods: We conducted a systematic review of electronic databases (PubMed, Google Scholar, Web of Science, CINAHL, EMBASE and PSYCINFO) for publications on adherence to ART in Cameroon (from January 1999 to May 2012) and described the trend in reported adherence rates and the factors associated with adherence. Data were extracted in duplicate. We used multivariable analyses on the baseline data for 200 participants in the CAMPS trial to determine the factors associated with adherence in four models using different measures of adherence (more than 90% or 95% on the visual analogue scale, no missed doses and a composite measure: 100% on the visual analogue scale, no missed doses and all pills taken on time).

Results: We identified nine studies meeting our inclusion criteria. Adherence to ART in Cameroon has risen steadily between 2000 and 2010, corresponding to reductions in the cost of medication. The factors associated with adherence to ART in Cameroon are grouped into patient, medication and disease related factors. We also identified factors related to the health system and the patient-provider relationship. In the CAMPS trial, education, side effects experienced and number of reminder methods were found to improve adherence, but only using multiple reminder methods was associated with better adherence in all the regression models (Adjusted Odds Ratio [AOR] 4.11, 95% Confidence Interval [CI] 1.89, 8.93; p<0.001; model IV).

Conclusions: Reducing the cost of ART is an important aspect of ensuring adequate adherence rates. Using multiple reminder methods may have a cumulative effect on adherence to ART, but should be investigated further.

Keywords: Adherence, Antiretroviral therapy, Cameroon, Reminder methods, CAMPS

* Correspondence: mbuagblc@mcmaster.ca
[1]Centre for Development of Best Practices in Health (CDBPH), Yaoundé Central Hospital, Avenue Henri Dunant, Messa, PO Box 87, Yaoundé, Cameroon
[2]Department of Clinical Epidemiology and Biostatistics, McMaster University, Hamilton, ON, Canada
Full list of author information is available at the end of the article

Background

The advent of antiretroviral medication as a treatment for HIV is one of the most celebrated advances in medicine [1]. Antiretroviral therapy (ART) reduces viral loads to undetectable levels, and dramatically decreases morbidity and mortality. Decreasing serum viral load with antiretroviral medication also reduces mother to child transmission rates [2,3]. However, viral replication still occurs in reservoirs like lymph node or gastrointestinal T-cells even when viral loads are undetectable [4,5]. As such, good adherence is necessary to maintain prolonged viral suppression [5]. Non-adherence to HIV medication is a major reason for treatment failure, the development of resistant strains, and increased costs [6]. It is also one of the key predictors or determinants of success in the management of HIV/AIDS and the progression to AIDS and death [7,8]. Non-adherence reduces the immunologic potential of ART and is associated with drops in CD4-positive-T-lymphocyte counts [9-11]. Non-adherence has also been found to be associated with increased hospitalisations and longer hospital stays [10,12]. Initial worries in the scientific community about non-adherence in sub-Saharan Africa were dispelled when research findings demonstrated similar or higher rates of adherence than in the developed world [13]. However, only a third of people living with HIV (PLHIV) take their medication as prescribed [1]. Non-adherence leads to increased viremia which might lead to increased transmissibility and consequently a higher incidence of HIV. High risk activity may also lead to the transmission of resistant strains to newly infected individuals, thereby reducing their therapeutic options [14,15]. Adherence to ART has clinical and public health implications, and should therefore be addressed on global and local levels.

Defining adherence

Adherence can be narrowly defined as the "extent to which patients take medications as prescribed by their health care providers" [16], or more broadly as the "the extent to which a person's behaviour—taking medication, following a diet, or executing lifestyle changes, corresponds with agreed recommendations from a health care provider" [1]. The former definition refers to compliance with medication as prescribed by the provider while the latter goes beyond medication to include all the recommendations jointly agreed upon by both provider and client to improve health care. The latter definition also highlights or acknowledges additional factors such as diet or lifestyle which may affect adherence. It also recognises that the client may not agree with the recommendations of the health care provider. Such factors are even more relevant in HIV where dietary restrictions are required for the uptake of certain medications [17,18] and that certain lifestyles (e.g. substance abuse) can lead to non- adherence to ART [19]. In this paper, all degrees of adherence which are not optimal are referred to as non-adherence.

The factors associated with adherence to ART exist in many categories, defined in literature [1,16,19]:

Patient factors such as substance abuse, being male (i.e. gender), depression, lower levels of education, lack of self efficacy, extreme anxiety, extreme pain, no change in health status despite ART and non-white race are significantly associated with non-adherence [1,19].
Medication factors like dose frequency, pill burden, type of drug, inability to take medication when away from home, food requirements, side effects are also responsible for less than optimal adherence [1,19]. In other words the complexity of the regimen and its side-effects are associated with non-adherence.
Provider-related factors such as a poor patient-health care provider relationship can affect the patient's overall satisfaction and trust in the provider. The quality of these relationships is significantly associated with better adherence [1,20,21].
Disease characteristics, notably stage and duration of HIV infection, symptoms experienced and the presence of opportunistic infections play a role in adherence to ART. HIV related symptoms like nausea may impede a patient from swallowing pills. Some studies report that patients who have experienced an opportunistic infection tend to be more adherent than those who have not [1,22,23].
Clinical setting and health system factors may influence use of services and adherence [19].

Adherence to ART in Cameroon

Cameroon has one of the highest rates of HIV in west and central Africa, with 5.3% of the adult population living with HIV. Of these, only 30% are receiving ART [24]. Adherence to ART in Cameroon has changed over the years for a multitude of reasons. Health system changes like the decentralization of HIV treatment centres and the subsidy of costs of medication and testing over the years have contributed to the variations in the reported adherence rates. A substantial reduction in costs occurred in 2004 [25] and ART has been provided for free since 2007 [26]. As a result, the designs and the contexts of the studies reporting rates of adherence to ART in Cameroon also vary. The set of similar and varying contextual factors in Cameroon make it a worthwhile case study to examine adherence to ART and learn lessons that could be applied across the country. Adherence rates in Cameroon have been measured using patient reports, pharmacy refill data, attendance at scheduled visits and blood testing [25-35]. These different methods have spawned adherence rates varying from 10.1% to 97.5%, between 2000 and 2010. Faced with these enormous discrepancies, we sought to use data from a recent trial [36] to describe adherence to ART and the associated determining factors. Adherence rates are not only a predictor of treatment success, but also an indication of how many resources should be invested in adherence enhancement research and practice. This cannot be done without stable estimates for adherence or a comprehensive list of locally relevant determinants.

Additionally, in a changing world where new methods and technologies arise to improve adherence rates, and levels of stigma are declining, there may be a shift in patients' attitudes and practices related to adherence.

The objectives of this paper are:

- to review the literature on adherence in Cameroon with specific emphasis on ART adherence rates and its correlates or determinants, and
- to report the factors associated with adherence to ART at baseline in the Cameroon Mobile Phone SMS trial (CAMPS;36).

Methodology

Literature review of ART adherence rates in Cameroon

We searched electronic databases (PubMed, Google Scholar, Web of Science, CINAHL, EMBASE and PSYCINFO) for publications on adherence to ART in Cameroon (from January 1999 to May 2012) using appropriate combinations of keywords such as *Cameroon, Cameroun (French), adherence, compliance, antiretroviral therapy, antiretroviral treatment* and *HIV*. ART was introduced in Cameroon in 1999 [37]. No language restrictions were set. Citations were screened and full text obtained if they reported any measure of adherence to ART in Cameroonian subjects. Completeness and adequacy of reporting in the selected studies were assessed in duplicate by noting their compliance to the 22-item Strengthening the Reporting of Observational Studies in Epidemiology (STROBE) checklist [38]. Data were also extracted in duplicate: citation details; year study was conducted, city in which study was conducted, adherence rate, method of measure of adherence, study design, sample size and the cost of ART at the time. Discrepancies were resolved by discussion. We examined the evolution of adherence rates taking into account the above characteristics. We also identified the reported factors associated with adherence and classified them as patient variables, medication variables, patient-provider relationship and health system characteristics. These categories have previously been identified in literature [16,19]. No statistical pooling was performed. The factors associated with adherence were extracted only if they resulted from multivariable analyses. The reported odds ratios and p-values were used to confirm the associations reported.

Adherence to ART in CAMPS

We conducted a cross-sectional analytical study based on the baseline data for the Cameroon Mobile Phone SMS (CAMPS) trial [36]. Data were collected from a subset of patients (eligible for the trial) aged 21 or older, who owned mobile phones and who agreed to take part in the trial. The independent variables included socio-demographics like age (in years), gender (male or female), level of education (none and primary or secondary and university), disclosure of status to family members (family aware or not aware of HIV status); clinical features like presence or absence of an opportunistic infection, Centers for Disease Control and Prevention (CDC; [39]) classification (categorised as AIDS defining condition or not), regimen (first line or second line), duration on treatment (in months); the number of drug side-effects experienced and the number of recall methods used. All the independent variables were those reported in literature and collected for the CAMPS trial [36]. The dependent variables were adherence measured using a visual analogue scale (0–100), self report on the number of missed doses and whether the doses were taken on time in the week preceding the interview. We also designed a composite measure of adherence based on all three measures, which we dichotomized as adherent (VAS=100; number of missed doses=0; all doses taken on time=yes) and non-adherent (VAS<100; missed doses >0; all doses taken on time=no).

We performed multivariable logistic regression with adherence (dependent variable) dichotomized at the VAS cut-offs of 90 and 95% (Model I and II). These cut-off points represent the levels of adherence at which sustained viral suppression can occur [5], and those often used in literature [40,41]. We also analyzed the data using the self reports of adherence as the dependent variable, in which case one or more missed doses was considered as non-adherence and no missed dose was considered as good adherence (Model III). We repeated these analyses using the composite measure of adherence (Model IV). The interaction between independent variables was investigated based on associations reported in the general literature and specifically for Cameroon. Variables were introduced into the model in blocks defined by the following categories: socio-demographic, disease-related and medication-related. Model fit was assessed using the Hosmer and Lemeshow goodness of fit statistic [42].

Data were analysed using Predictive Analytic Software (PASW) Version 17.0 (SPSS, Inc., 2009, Chicago, IL, USA). Statistical significance was set at alpha= 0.05. Adjusted odds ratios (AOR), 95% confidence intervals (CI) and p-values are presented. The forest plot was drawn using Stata Statistical Software (STATA) Release 12 (StataCorp LP, 2011, College Station, TX, USA).

Results

Literature review

We identified 9 studies conducted between 2000 and 2010 which reported adherence rates in Cameroon. The mean number of reported items on the STROBE checklist was 19.7 (standard deviation [SD] 1.38). Data from the CAMPS trial was included in the analysis [36]. Five of them were conducted in Yaoundé, the capital city of Cameroon. The characteristics of these studies are reported in Table 1. We observed an increasing trend in adherence rates over time, which corresponds to the reductions in cost of ART (Figure 1). Two studies were outliers to this quasi-linear relationship. The first was Kouanfack *et al.* [27], which reported high adherence rates (88.7% and 97.5%, using biological markers and self report respectively). This study was a drug trial and participants received medication free of charge at a time when medication costed 51.2 USD/month. The second, Mosoko *et al.* [25], reported very low adherence rates (10.1% using hospital records of the number of scheduled clinic visits attended). These data may be affected by inaccuracies in hospital records (incompleteness was handled using imputation techniques); participants who lived far away were sometimes given medication for more than one month; patients who lived in the nearby city of Douala had other ART opportunities and this measure (scheduled visits) considers all deaths and lost to follow-up as non-adherent. Ideally, the cases of death should be excluded from the denominator. The other study using attendance of scheduled visits [29] also reported low adherence rates (<50%).

Determinants of, and factors associated with ART adherence

In addition to the nine papers that reported adherence rates, we identified two papers which reported on the determinants of adherence to ART. These studies were conducted in cross-national cohorts of patients from Cameroon, the Democratic Republic of Congo and Burundi (Table 2). These papers were provided additional information on factors associated with adherence [34,35]. They were not used in the trend analysis.

These factors were found to reduce adherence to ART: binge drinking, drug use, tobacco use, lack of family support, experience of stigma, switching regimen, advanced stage of disease, cost of care, distance from clinic, large hospital size and no task shifting from physician to other staff [25,28,30-35].

These factors increased adherence to ART: Female gender, age greater than 49 years, higher levels of education, positive perceptions of treatment, high motivation, using reminder methods, satisfaction with information provided by physician, higher CD4 count at initiation of ART, and being transferred-in from another clinic [30,31,33-35].

High monthly income [31,32] and increased duration on medication [30,33,35] were both reported to either increase or reduce adherence.

Table 1 Characteristics of studies reporting adherence to ART in Cameroon

Reference	Year	City	Study design (sample size)	Adherence rate	Method	Cost of ART/month for that year in USD*
Laurent et al.	2000-2003	Douala	Cross-sectional retrospective (788)	<50% [µ]	Scheduled visits attended	128
Kouanfack et al.	2002-2003	Yaoundé	Prospective cohort (60)	88.7%, (97.5%)	Biological markers, (Self Report)	51.2 (free for participants)
Mosoko et al.	2002-2005	Limbe	Cross-sectional retrospective [α] (2920)	10.1%	Scheduled visits attended	51.2
Boyer et al. [28]	2006	Yaoundé	Cross-sectional (532)	56.6%	Self Report [β]	12.8
Rougemont et al.	2006	Yaoundé	Prospective cohort (312)	64% (78%)	Pharmacy data (Self report)	12.8
Boyer et al. [32]	2006-2007	Multiple locations	Cross-sectional (3151)	53.9%	Self report [β]	12.8
Roux et al.	2006-2008	Yaoundé	Prospective cohort (401)	61-73%	Self report [β]	12.8
Mahy et al.	2007-2008	Tokombere	Cross-sectional (56)	95% (80%)	self report [β] (Pharmacy data)	0
Mbopi-Keou et al.	2010	Dschang	Cross-sectional (356)	80.2% (48.7)	Self report [β] (Pharmacy data)	0
CAMPS	2010	Yaoundé	Cross-sectional (200)	90.5%	Self report [β]	0

*Costs vary per regimen, the highest costs are reported.
[α] Cross- sectional analysis of previously collected data without planning for needs of an investigation.
[β] All methods in which all information used to measure adherence was obtained by interviewing the participant with either one question or a series of questions.
[µ] 50% was imputed to represent the trend graphically.

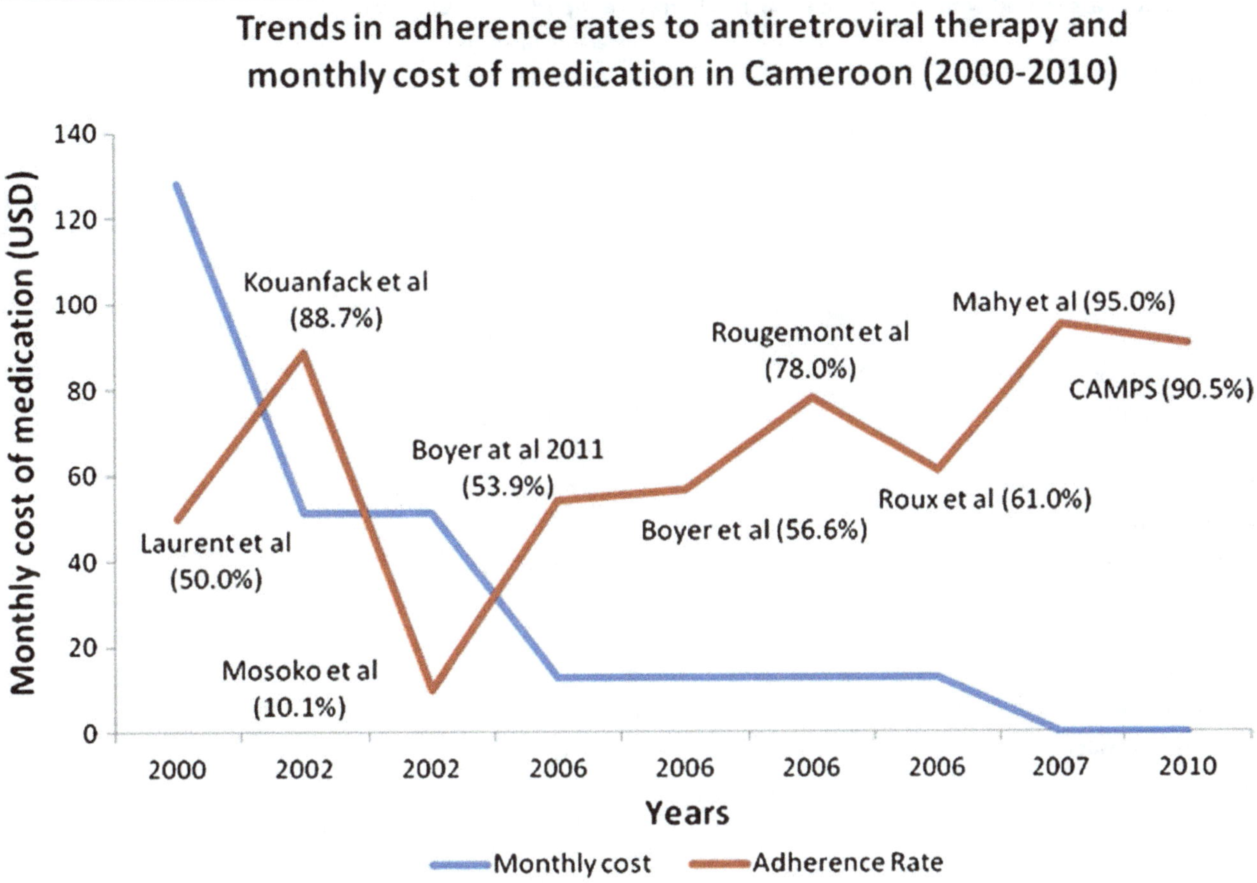

Figure 1 Trends in adherence rates to antiretroviral therapy and monthly cost of medication.

Factors associated with adherence to ART at baseline in the CAMPS Trial

In this sample of 200 adults, one fifth was older than 50 years, three-quarters were female, 98% had at least primary education, and 90% reported that their families were aware of their HIV status. The rest of their characteristics are reported in Table 3. All the factors associated with adherence that were collected in this data set were used in the regression analysis. The baseline data for participants in the CAMPS trial are reported in Table 3.

In the first model, we dichotomized adherence using the VAS at 95%. Using multiple recall methods was significantly associated with adherence >95% (AOR 6.7, 95% CI 2.69, 16.56; p<0.001). In our second model, adherence was dichotomized at 90%. Female gender was associated with adherence >90% (AOR 0.28, 95% CI 0.09, 0.90; p=0.032), while secondary education (AOR, 4.4 95% CI 1.64, 11.92; p= 0.003) and multiple recall methods (AOR, 7.89 95% CI 3.22, 19.33; p<0.001) were associated with adherence >90%. In the third model we used the number of missed doses as our measure of adherence. Experiencing more side effects (AOR 2.25, 95% CI 1.13, 4.50; p= 0.021) and using multiple recall methods increased the odds for not missing doses (AOR 7.28, 95% CI 3.06, 17.32; p<0.001). In our last model we used a composite measure of adherence that incorporated the VAS, number of missed doses and timing of doses. Only the use of multiple recall methods was associated with adherence (AOR 4.11, 95% CI 1.89, 8.91; p<0.001). The Hosmer and Lemeshow goodness-of-fit statistic for all the four models had p-values greater than 0.05 implying a good fit [42]. These models are displayed in Figure 2.

Discussion

By reviewing the literature on adherence rates in Cameroon, and analysing a new data set we have produced an explanatory account of the trends in adherence observed and the reported determinants. We also identified another plausible means of enhancing adherence to ART: using multiple reminder methods.

Despite the different study designs, locations and sample sizes there is a clear improvement in adherence rates over time irrespective of how it is measured. This finding confirms and supports health policies that reduce

Table 2 Factors associated with adherence to ART in literature reports from Cameroon

Factors	Reference (findings)
Patient variables	
Female gender	Rougemont et al. (↑)
Age>49 years	Newman et al.* (↑); Freeman et al.**(↑)
High monthly income	Rougemont et al. (↓); Boyer et al. ([28] ; ↑)
Education	Freeman et al. (↑)*
Binge drinking	Boyer et al. ([32] ; ↓); Roux et al. (↓); Newman et al.(↓)*
Drug use	Freeman et al.(↓)*
Tobacco use	Freeman et al.(↓)*
Lack of family support for adherence	Boyer et al. ([32]; ↓);
Experiencing discrimination and stigma	Boyer et al. ([32]; ↓);
Positive perception of treatment	Roux et al. (↑)
Being transferred-in to HIV clinic	Mbopi-Keou (↑)
Medication variables	
Switching regimen	Boyer et al. ([32]; ↓);
High motivation	Roux et al.(↑)
Using a reminder method	Roux et al.(↑)
Patient Provider Relationship	
Satisfaction with information provided by physician	Roux et al.(↑)
Disease characteristics	
Advanced stage of disease	Rougemont et al. (↓); Roux et al.(↑)
Increased duration on medication	Roux et al.(↓); Freeman et al.(↑)*Mbopi-Keou (↑)
Higher CD4[¥] count at initiation of ART [β]	Mbopi-Keou (↑)
Health System/clinic Characteristics	
Cost of care/Having to pay for care	Mosoko et al.(↓), Boyer et al. ([32] ; ↓) ; Boyer et al. ([28] ; ↓) Laurent et al. (↓)
Increased distance from clinic	Mosoko et al. (↓)
Large hospital size	Boyer et al. ([32]; ↓);
No task shifting from physician to other staff	Boyer et al. ([32]; ↓);

↓Reduces adherence; ↑increases adherence; * Cohort included participants from Cameroon, Burundi and the Democratic Republic of Congo; ** Cohort included females from Cameroon, Burundi and the Democratic Republic of Congo; [¥] CD4-positive-T-lymphocyte; [β] Antiretroviral therapy.

the cost of care to improve access and use. This is also in line with studies reporting that the main hindrances to adherence in Africa are related to health system weaknesses such as inadequate supply, human resource shortages and poor infrastructure [29,32].

The determinants of adherence to ART identified in the Cameroonian literature are a subset of factors identified elsewhere [19]. However, there are discrepancies as to the role of monthly income and duration on ART on adherence. Boyer *et al.* [32] reported better adherence with a higher monthly income, while Rougemont *et al.* [31] reported the contrary. Both studies were initiated in the same period (2006) and therefore the cost of medication is unlikely to be the reason for this discrepancy. On the other hand Boyer *et al.* conducted a multisite (27 sites) study with a larger sample size (n=3151) compared to Rougemont *et al.* (n=312) in a single site. The results from Boyer *et al.* may be more plausible in the Cameroonian context where, apart from free ART, other related services are still funded by out-of-pocket payments and having to pay for care has been identified as a cause of non-adherence [25,28,29,32]. The larger sample is also more likely to have more accurate and generalizable data, especially since one of the sites included in Boyer *et al.* is the same site where the Rougemont study was conducted.

Roux *et al.* [30] noted a drop in adherence rates with increased duration on ART while Freeman *et al.* and Mbopi-Keou *et al.* [33,35] noted the contrary. However, these two samples differ greatly. Roux *et al.* describe a multisite study in the Centre region of Cameroon, in 401 PLHIV over two years. Freeman *et al.* describe a cross-national cohort of 8419 women from Cameroon, Burundi and the Democratic Republic of Congo followed up for two years. Female gender has been reported as a factor for better adherence [31] and this discrepancy may explain the interaction between gender and duration on

Table 3 Baseline characteristics of participants in the CAMPS trial

Variable	Statistic
Age (years) : mean (SD) $^{\alpha}$	40.1 (10.10)
21-49	157 (79.3)
50+	41 (20.7)
Gender: n (%)	
Female	147 (73.5)
Level of education: n (%)	
None or primary	78 (39.0)
Secondary or university	122 (61.0)
Family aware of HIV status: n (%)	180 (90.0)
Presence of an opportunistic infection: n(%)	62 (31.0)
BMI : mean (SD) $^{\beta}$	25.2 (4.00)
Underweight	4 (2.2)
Normal	90 (48.6)
Overweight	91 (49.2)
CDC* classification - AIDS defining illness§:n (%)	146 (73.0)
Regimen: n (%)$^{\delta}$	
First line	179 (90.9)
Second line	18 (9.1)
Duration on ART (months): median (Q1, Q3) $^{\alpha}$	28.5 (9.0, 48.0)
CD4 (cells per mm^3): median (Q1, Q3)	336.0 (200.5,487.7)
Adherence	
Visual Analogue Scale: mean (SD) $^{\varepsilon}$	90.5 (12.76)
Number of missed doses: mean (SD) $^{\mu}$	1.0 (0.00)
No missed doses: n (%)	127 (65.1)
Treatment taken on time: n (%)	108 (54.0)
Reasons for missing doses: n (%)	
Forgot	54 (27.0)
Out of home	23 (11.5)
Out of tablets	7 (3.5)
Too busy	8 (4.0)
Side effects	2 (1.0)
Other reason	5 (2.5)
Medication side effects experienced: n (%)	
None	127 (63.5)
One	43 (21.5)
Two	30 (15.0)
Reminder methods: n (%)$^{¥}$	
None	49 (25.7)
One	125 (65.4)
Multiple	17 (8.5)

SD: standard deviation; BMI: body mass index; *Centres for Disease Control, § =CDC classifications: A3, B3, C1, C1, C3 [39]; α= 2missing; δ=3 missing; β=15 missing; ε= 10 missing ¥= 9missing; μ= 5 missing.
The reminder methods reported were: personal verbal reminders by individuals, phone alarms, meal times, timing with TV shows and watches.

medication. Mbopi-Keou *et al.* suggest that this trend might be the effect of continuous psycho-social support [33].

One study reported higher levels of adherence for patients who initiated ART with high levels of CD4-positive-T-lymphocytes [33]. This finding is in favor of earlier initiation of ART. Why patients who were transferred to the clinic would have better adherence rates is unclear. However, if they left their previous clinics due to service provision issues or unsatisfactory interactions with clinic staff, the latter clinic may provide a more favorable environment for adherence.

Using multivariable analysis we identified gender, education, side effects experienced, and number of reminder methods as factors that affect adherence rates.

The male gender has often been reported as the most likely to be non-adherent, maybe because males are more likely to engage in other behaviours that influence adherence such as binge drinking, tobacco use and drug use [19]. This effect was not found in all models and is not consistent across studies [19].

Level of education seems to play a role in adherence behaviour. A significant difference in adherence exists between people with secondary and those with no education. Further increments in educational level show no effect. This may imply that as concerns adherence to ART there are no benefits to be gained from very high levels of education. The benefits of education on adherence to ART can be obtained from secondary education. This effect was not consistent across all models.

Our findings regarding side effects are contrary to what is reported in literature. People who experienced more side-effects were more likely to be adherent. No other Cameroonian studies have identified side effects as a determinant for adherence to ART. In the CAMPS trial only 1% of those who missed doses reported side effects to be the reason for not taking medication (Table 3).

Only the number of reminder methods was associated with adherence in all the models. Another Cameroonian study reported the use of reminder methods to be associated with better adherence [30]. This is the first study to show that multiple reminders may have a cumulative effect. A randomized clinical trial in Kenya found alarms to have no effect on virological outcomes [43]. Simple electronic alarms are not as complex as the reminder methods described in this population (personal verbal reminders by individuals, phone alarms, meal times, timing with TV shows and watches). Other studies have reported the use of mobile phone beeps and prayer times by Muslims to remind them of when to take their medication [44]. The use of multiple and varied reminder methods may address other causes of non-adherence like forgetfulness and lack of social support.

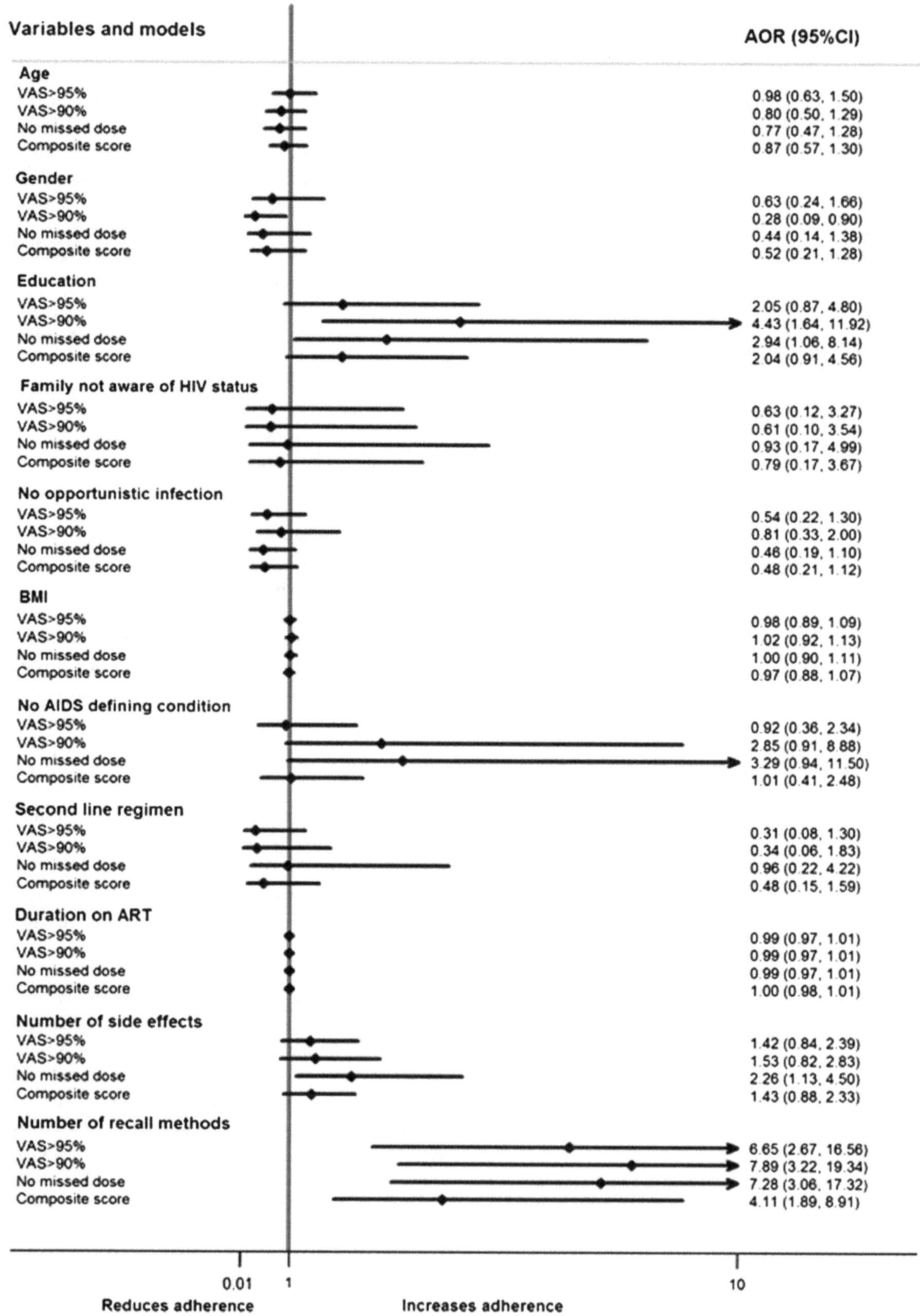

Figure 2 Multivariable analysis using different measures of adherence.

The difference in the four models suggests that the factors associated with adherence depend somewhat on how adherence is defined and the thresholds for acceptable adherence. Different levels of adherence are associated with different factors. It is unclear how this issue can be resolved without a uniform and validated tool for measuring adherence rates in clinical practice or research, as all methods have their advantages and flaws [16,45]. Self reported adherence is by far the most popular method used, but how it is used varies greatly [16,46]. On the one hand, a simple visual analogue scale can be used to situate a patient's adherence; and on the other a series of questions related to number of pills, timing, missed doses and identification of pills, all fall under the canopy of self report.

In low resource settings, self report, attendance-based and dispensing-based adherence measuring methods can predict important clinical outcomes [46] and should be collected routinely. Some measure of drug availability or the occurrence of drug stock-outs should be documented to explain trends in adherence behaviours.

Both sections of this paper may have limitations. Even though we observed an increasing trend in adherence as the cost of ART reduces, other temporal factors may contribute to this trend, notably health system improvements over the years and reductions in stigma and discrimination. These factors are reported as potential threats to optimal adherence and are very likely to change over time. The availability and use of reminder methods like mobile phones may also enhance adherence over time [25,32]. Participants in this study (CAMPS) may not adequately represent all the people living with HIV, but a subgroup who are already on ART, and who own mobile phones. Even though mobile phone ownership is widespread in Cameroon, those who own them may differ significantly from those who don't.

Conclusions

A prerequisite to optimal adherence is the availability of free or cheap medication. Irrespective of how it is measured, adherence rates tend to improve as the cost of medication is reduced. Improved financing mechanisms for ART are an important way of ensuring adequate adherence and improving outcomes for people living with HIV. Multiple and varied reminder methods are more likely to improve adherence than any single method alone. Further research is required to elucidate what combinations of reminder methods can produce the most desirable effects.

Competing interests

The authors declare that they have no competing interests.

Authors' contributions

LM and LT conceived of the study; LM and SN performed the searches and extracted the data; LM, LT, SN, POZ, DY, LD and MS provided intellectual content and revised several versions of the manuscript. All authors read and approved the final manuscript.

Funding

This study was funded in part by the CIHR Canadian HIV Trials Network (CTN).

Author details

[1]Centre for Development of Best Practices in Health (CDBPH), Yaoundé Central Hospital, Avenue Henri Dunant, Messa, PO Box 87, Yaoundé, Cameroon. [2]Department of Clinical Epidemiology and Biostatistics, McMaster University, Hamilton, ON, Canada. [3]Biostatistics Unit, Father Sean O'Sullivan Research Centre, St Joseph's Healthcare, Hamilton, ON, Canada. [4]St. Joseph's Healthcare Hamilton, Hamilton, ON, Canada. [5]Department of Family Medicine, McMaster University, McMaster Innovation Park, Hamilton, ON, Canada.

References

1. WHO: *Adherence to long-term therapies: Evidence for action*; 2003. Available from: http://www.who.int/chp/knowledge/publications/adherence_report/en/ (Accessed 27 May 2012).
2. Vernazza PL, Troiani L, Flepp MJ, Cone RW, Schock J, Roth F, Boggian K, Cohen MS, Fiscus SA, Eron JJ: **Potent antiretroviral treatment of HIV-infection results in suppression of the seminal shedding of HIV. The Swiss HIV Cohort Study.** *AIDS* 2000, **14:**117–121.
3. Sperling RS, Shapiro DE, Coombs RW, Todd JA, Herman SA, McSherry GD, O'Sullivan MJ, Van Dyke RB, Jimenez E, Rouzioux C, Flynn PM, Sullivan JL, Pediatric AIDS Clinical Trials Group Protocol076 Study Group: **Maternal viral load, zidovudine treatment, and the risk of transmission of human immunodeficiency virus type 1 from mother to infant.** *N Engl J Med* 1996, **335:**1621–1629.
4. Montaner JS, Reiss P, Cooper D, Vella S, Harris M, Conway B, Wainberg MA, Smith D, Robinson P, Hall D, *et al*: **A randomized, double-blind trial comparing combinations of nevirapine, didanosine, and zidovudine for HIV-infected patients: the INCAS Trial. Italy, The Netherlands, Canada and Australia Study.** *JAMA* 1998, **279:**930–937.
5. Paterson DL, Swindells S, Mohr J: **Adherence to protease inhibitor therapy and outcomes in patients with HIV infection.** *Ann Intern Med* 2000, **133:**21–30.
6. Gill CJ, Hamer DH, Simon JL, Thea DM, Sabin LL: **No room for complacency about adherence to antiretroviral therapy in sub-Saharan Africa.** *AIDS* 2005, **19:**1243–1249.
7. de Olalla Garcia P, Knobel H, Carmona A, Guelar A, Lopez-Colomes JL, Cayla JA: **Impact of adherence and highly active antiretroviral therapy on survival in HIV-infected patients.** *J Acquir Immune Defic Syndr* 2002, **30:**105–110.
8. Bangsberg DR, Perry S, Charlebois ED, Clark RA, Roberston M, Zolopa AR, Moss A: **Non-adherence to highly active antiretroviral therapy predicts progression to AIDS.** *AIDS* 2001, **15:**1181–1183.
9. Mannheimer S, Friedland G, Matts J, Child C, Chesney M: **The consistency of adherence to antiretroviral therapy predicts biologic outcomes for human immunodeficiency virus-infected persons in clinical trials.** *Clin Infect Dis* 2002, **34:**1115–1121.
10. Paterson DL, Swindells S, Mohr J, Brester M, Vergis EN, Squier C, Wagener MM, Singh N: **Adherence to protease inhibitor therapy and outcomes in patients with HIV infection.** *Ann Intern Med* 2000, **133:**21–30.
11. Haubrich RH, Little SJ, Currier JS, Forthal DN, Kemper CA, Beall GN, Johnson D, Dube MP, Hwang JY, McCutchan JA, California Collaborative Treatment Group: **The value of patient-reported adherence to antiretroviral therapy in predicting virologic and immunologic response.** *AIDS* 1999, **13:**1099–1107.
12. Knobel H, Codina C, Miro JM, Carmona A, Garcia B, Antela A, Gomez-Domingo MR, Arrizabalaga J, Iruin A, Laguna F, *et al*: **The recommendations of GESIDA/SEFH/PNS for improving adherence to antiretroviral treatment. AIDS Study Group of the Spanish Society of Hospital Pharmacy and the National Plan on AIDS of the Minister of Health and Consumers.** *Enferm Infecc Microbiol Clin* 2000, **18:**27–39.
13. Mills EJ, Nachega JB, Buchan I, Orbinski J, Attaran A, Singh S, Rachlis B, Wu P, Cooper C, Thabane L, *et al*: **Adherence to antiretroviral therapy in sub-Saharan Africa and North America: a meta-analysis.** *JAMA* 2006, **296:**679–690.

14. Boden D, Hurley A, Zhang L, Cao Y, Guo Y, Jones E, Tsay J, Ip J, Farthing C, Limoli K, *et al*: **HIV-1 drug resistance in newly infected individuals.** *JAMA* 1999, **282:**1135–1141.
15. Hecht FM, Grant RM, Petropoulos CJ, Dillon B, Chesney MA, Tian H, Hellmann NS, Bandrapalli NI, Digilio L, Branson B, Kahn JO: **Sexual transmission of an HIV-1 variant resistant to multiple reverse-transcriptase and protease inhibitors.** *N Engl J Med* 1998, **339:**307–311.
16. Osterberg L, Blaschke T: **Adherence to medication.** *N Engl J Med* 2005, **353:**487–497.
17. Stone VE, Hogan JW, Schuman P, Rompalo AM, Howard AA, Korkontzelou C, Smith DK: **Antiretroviral regimen complexity, self-reported adherence, and HIV patients' understanding of their regimens: survey of women in the her study.** *J Acquir Immune Defic Syndr* 2001, **28:**124–131.
18. Sax PE, Gathe JC Jr: **Beyond efficacy: the impact of combination antiretroviral therapy on quality of life.** *AIDS Patient Care STDS* 2005, **19:**563–576.
19. Chesney MA: **Factors affecting adherence to antiretroviral therapy.** *Clin Inf Dis* 2000, **30**(S2):S171–S176.
20. Beach MC, Keruly J, Moore RD: **Is the quality of the patient-provider relationship associated with better adherence and health outcomes for patients with HIV?** *J Gen Intern Med* 2006, **21:**661–665.
21. Roberts KJ: **Physician-patient relationships, patient satisfaction, and antiretroviral medication adherence among HIV-infected adults attending a public health clinic.** *AIDS Patient Care STDS* 2002, **16**(1):43–50.
22. Singh N, Squier C, Sivek C, Wagener M, Nguyen MH, Yu VL: **Determinants of compliance with antiretroviral therapy in patients with human immunodeficiency virus: prospective assessment with implications for enhancing compliance.** *AIDS Care* 1996, **8:**261–269.
23. Gao X, Nau DP, Rosenbluth SA, Scott V, Woodward C: **The relationship of disease severity, health beliefs and medication adherence among HIV patients.** *AIDS Care* 2000, **12:**387–398.
24. UNAIDS: *UNAIDS report on the global AIDS epidemic*. 2010. Available from: http://www.unaids.org/globalreport/Global_report.htm. (Accessed 29 December 2011).
25. Mosoko JJ, Akam W, Weidle PJ, Brooks JT, Aweh AJ, Kinge TN, Pals S, Raghunathan PL: **Retention in an antiretroviral therapy programme during an era of decreasing drug cost in Limbe, Cameroon.** *J Int AIDS Soc* 2011, **14:**32.
26. Mahy S, Duong M, Huraux JM, Aurenche C, Ndong JG, Birguel J, Piroth L, Chavanet P: **Measure of effectiveness and adherence to antiretroviral therapy in HIV-infected patients in Cameroon.** *Med Mal Infect* 2011, **41:**176–180.
27. Kouanfack C, Laurent C, Peytavin G, Mawamba Nkene Y, Essomba C, Ciaf L, Ngolle M, Delaporte E, Calmy A, Mpoudi-Ngole' E, *et al*: **Adherence to antiretroviral therapy assessed by drug level monitoring and self-report in Cameroon.** *J Acquir Immune Defic Syndr* 2008, **48:**216–219.
28. Boyer S, Marcellin F, Ongolo-Zogo P, Abega SC, Nantchouang R, Spire B, Moatti JP: **Financial barriers to HIV treatment in Yaoundé, Cameroon: first results of a national cross-sectional survey.** *Bull World Health Organ* 2009, **87:**279–287.
29. Laurent C, Meilo H, Guiard-Schmid JB, Mapoure Y, Noel JM, M'Bangue M, Joko A, Rozenbaum W, Ntone FN, Delaporte E: **Antiretroviral therapy in public and private routine health care clinics in Cameroon: lessons from the Douala antiretroviral (DARVIR) initiative.** *Clin Infect Dis* 2005, **41:**108–111.
30. Roux P, Kouanfack C, Cohen J, Marcellin F, Boyer S, Delaporte E, Carrieri P, Laurent C, Spire B: **Adherence to antiretroviral treatment in HIV-positive patients in the Cameroon context: promoting the use of medication reminder methods.** *J Acquir Immune Defic Syndr* 2011, **57**(Suppl 1):S40–S43.
31. Rougemont M, Stoll BE, Elia N, Ngang P: **Antiretroviral treatment adherence and its determinants in Sub-Saharan Africa: a prospective study at Yaounde Central Hospital, Cameroon.** *AIDS Res Ther* 2009, **6:**21.
32. Boyer S, Clerc I, Bonono CR, Marcellin F, Bile PC, Ventelou B: **Non-adherence to antiretroviral treatment and unplanned treatment interruption among people living with HIV/AIDS in Cameroon: individual and healthcare supply-related factors.** *Soc Sci Med* 2011, **72:**1383–1392.
33. Mbopi-Keou FX, Dempouo Djomassi L, Monebenimp F: **Etude des facteurs liés à l'observance au traitement antirétroviral chez les patients suivis à l'Unité de Prise En Charge du VIH/SIDA de l'Hôpital de District de Dschang, Cameroun.** *PAMJ* 2012, **12:**55.
34. Newman J, Iriondo-Perez J, Hemingway-Foday J, Freeman A, Akam W, Balimba A, Kalenga L, Mbaya M, Mfangam Molu B, Mukumbi H, *et al*: **Older adults accessing HIV care and treatment and adherence in the IeDEA Central Africa cohort.** *AIDS Res Treat* 2012, **2012:**725713.
35. Freeman A, Newman J, Hemingway-Foday J, Iriondo-Perez J, Stolka K, Akam W, Balimba A, Kalenga L, Mbaya M, Mfangam Molu B, *et al*: **Comparison of HIV-positive women with children and without children accessing HIV care and treatment in the IeDEA Central Africa cohort.** *AIDS Care* 2012, **24:**673–679.
36. Mbuagbaw L, Thabane L, Ongolo-Zogo P, Lester R, Mills E, Volmink J, Yondo D, Essi M-J, Bonono-Momnougui R-C, Mba R, *et al*: **The Cameroon Mobile Phone SMS (CAMPS) trial: a protocol for a randomized controlled trial of mobile phone text messaging versus usual care for improving adherence to highly active anti-retroviral therapy.** *Trials* 2011, **12:**5.
37. Boyer S, Protopopescu C, Marcellin F, Carrieri MP, Koulla-Shiro S, Moatti J-P, Spire B, Group tES: **Performance of HIV care decentralization from the patient's perspective: health-related quality of life and perceived quality of services in Cameroon.** *Health Policy Plan* 2011, **27:**301–315.
38. von Elm E, Altman DG, Egger M, Pocock SJ, Gotzsche PC, Vandenbroucke JP: **The Strengthening the Reporting of Observational Studies in Epidemiology (STROBE) statement: guidelines for reporting observational studies.** *J Clin Epidemiol* 2008, **61:**344–349.
39. Centers for Disease Control and Prevention: **1993 revised classification system for HIV infection and expanded surveillance case definition for AIDS among adolescents and adults.** *MMWR Recomm Rep* 1992, **18:**41(RR-17):1–19.
40. Lester RT, Ritvo P, Mills EJ, Kariri A, Karanja S, Chung MH, Jack W, Habyarimana J, Sadatsafavi M, Najafzadeh M, *et al*: **Effects of a mobile phone short message service on antiretroviral treatment adherence in Kenya (WelTel Kenya1): a randomised trial.** *Lancet* 2010, **376:**1838–1845.
41. Pop-Eleches C, Thirumurthy H, Habyarimana JP, Zivin JG, Goldstein MP, de Walque D, MacKeen L, Haberer J, Kimaiyo S, Sidle J, *et al*: **Mobile phone technologies improve adherence to antiretroviral treatment in a resource-limited setting: a randomized controlled trial of text message reminders.** *AIDS* 2011, **25:**825–834.
42. Hosmer DW, Lemeshow S: *Applied logistic regression*. New York: Wiley; 2000.
43. Chung MH, Richardson BA, Tapia K, Benki-Nugent S, Kiarie JN, Simoni JM, Overbaugh J, Attwa M, John-Stewart GC: **A randomized controlled trial comparing the effects of counseling and alarm device on HAART adherence and virologic outcomes.** *PLoS Med* 2011, **8:**e1000422.
44. Mbuagbaw L, Bonono-Momnougui RC, Thabane L: **Considerations in using text messages to improve adherence to highly active antiretroviral therapy: a qualitative study among clients in Yaounde, Cameroon.** *HIV AIDS* 2012, **4:**45–50.
45. Farmer KC: **Methods for measuring and monitoring medication regimen adherence in clinical trials and clinical practice.** *Clin Ther* 1999, **21:**1074–1090.
46. Ross-Degnan D, Pierre-Jacques M, Zhang F, Tadeg H, Gitau L, Ntaganira J, Balikuddembe R, Chalker J, Wagner AK: **Measuring adherence to antiretroviral treatment in resource-poor settings: the clinical validity of key indicators.** *BMC Health Serv Res* 2010, **10:**42.

17

The development of simple anthropometric measures to diagnose antiretroviral therapy-associated lipodystrophy in resource limited settings

Zulfa Abrahams[1], Joel A Dave[1], Gary Maartens[2], Maia Lesosky[3] and Naomi S Levitt[1*]

Abstract

Background: Lipohypertrophy does not appear to be an adverse ART reaction while lipoatrophy is clearly associated with the use of stavudine (d4T) and zidovudine (AZT). In low and middle income countries d4T has only recently been phased out and AZT is still widely being used. Several case definitions have been developed to diagnose lipodystrophy, but none of them are generalizable to sub-Saharan Africa where black women have less visceral adipose tissue and more subcutaneous adipose tissue than white women. We aimed to develop a simple, objective measure to define lipoatrophy and lipohypertrophy by comparing patient report to anthropometric and dual-energy X-ray absorptiometry (DXA) -derived variables.

Methods: DXA and anthropometric measures were obtained in a cross sectional sample of black HIV-infected South African men (n = 116) and women (n = 434) on ART. Self-reported information on fat gain or fat loss was collected using a standard questionnaire. Receiver operating characteristic (ROC) curves were used to describe the performance of anthropometric and DXA-derived variables using patient reported lipoatrophy and lipohypertrophy as the reference standard.

Results: Lipoatrophy and lipohypertrophy were more common in women (25% and 33% respectively) than in men (10% and 13% respectively). There were insufficient numbers of men with DXA scans for meaningful analysis. The best predictors of lipoatrophy in women were the anthropometric variables tricep (AUC = 0.725) and thigh skinfold (AUC =0.720) thicknesses; and the DXA-derived variables percentage lower limb fat (AUC = 0.705) and percentage lower limb fat/height (AUC = 0.713). The best predictors of lipohypertrophy in women were the anthropometric variable waist/hip ratio (AUC = 0.645) and the DXA-derived variable percentage trunk fat/percentage limb fat (AUC = 0.647).

Conclusions: We were able to develop simple, anthropometric measures for defining lipoatrophy and lipohypertrophy, using a sample of black HIV-infected South African women with DXA scans. This is of particular relevance in resource limited settings, where health professionals need simple and inexpensive methods of diagnosing patients with lipoatrophy and lipohypertrophy.

Keywords: HIV, Lipoatrophy, Lipohypertrophy, Lipodystrophy, DXA, Anthropometry, Sub-Saharan africa, Antiretroviral therapy

* Correspondence: Naomi.levitt@uct.ac.za
[1]Division of Diabetic Medicine and Endocrinology, Department of Medicine, University of Cape Town, Cape Town, South Africa
Full list of author information is available at the end of the article

Background

Antiretroviral therapy (ART) has significantly reduced the morbidity and mortality of people infected with HIV [1], however, long-term use of ART has been associated with a number of metabolic complications such as dysglycaemia, insulin resistance, dyslipidaemia and lipodystrophy [2]. Lipodystrophy is characterized by either subcutaneous fat loss (lipoatrophy), which is most noticeable in the face, limbs, and buttocks, or fat accumulation (lipohypertrophy) seen in the abdomen, breast or posterior neck, or a combination of both [3,4].

Both subjective and objective methods have been used to diagnose lipodystrophy, resulting in a number of case definitions. The most widely used subjective methods of diagnosis are patient perception and report [5,6], physician examination and report [7], and physician confirmation of patient report [8-11]. Objective measures include imaging by dual-energy X-ray absorptiometry (DXA) [6,12,13] and computed tomography (CT) scans [12,14]. These imaging measures are expensive and not widely available in resource limited settings. Anthropometric and DXA-derived variables have also been developed, in an attempt to provide standard measures of defining lipodystrophy [15-17]. Furthermore, criteria established to define lipodystrophy did not include data from any African country. These diagnostic criteria may not be generalizable to sub-Saharan Africans, as there are important ethnic differences in fat distribution, especially in black women who have less visceral adipose tissue and more subcutaneous adipose tissue than white women [18-20].

Lipohypertrophy does not appear to be an adverse ART reaction as participants on different ART drug regimens gained similar amounts of trunk fat over time [21]. Lipoatrophy, in contrast is clearly an adverse ART reaction. The use of stavudine (d4T) and zidovudine (AZT) is associated with subcutaneous fat loss and is partially reversed after changing to abacavir or tenofovir [21,22]. Lipoatrophy remains common in low and middle income countries where d4T has only recently been phased out and AZT is still widely used [23]. However, even if lipohypertrophy is not associated with ART, lipodystrophy, and lipoatrophy in particular, is independently associated with an increased risk of vascular disease [24,25]. Therefore recognising lipodystrophy is important to identify patients at risk for vascular disease so that screening can be targeted for other vascular risk factors, while recognising lipoatrophy is important so that d4T or AZT can be substituted.

The aim of our study was to develop a simple, objective measure to define lipoatrophy and lipohypertrophy by comparing patient report to anthropometric and DXA-derived variables in a sample of black South Africans on ART.

Results

Participant characteristics are presented in Table 1. The study sample consisted of 550 participants on ART. Based on patient report, 121 (22%) had lipoatrophy and 157 (29%) had lipohypertrophy. Both lipoatrophy and lipohypertrophy were significantly more common in females than in males ($p \le 0.001$). Participants with lipoatrophy had spent a significantly longer period of time on ART (25 vs. 17 months) and a longer time on d4T (15.5 vs. 13 months).

Anthropometric variables are shown separately for women and men (Tables 2 and 3 respectively). In women, all median skinfold measurements, with the exception of sub-scapular skinfold thickness, were significantly lower in participants with lipoatrophy compared with those without lipoatrophy. Measurements for waist circumference, waist/hip ratio and supra-iliac skinfold thickness were significantly higher in women with lipohypertrophy compared with those without lipohypertrophy. There were no statistically significant differences in anthropometric variables in males with and without lipoatrophy (Table 3). Males with lipohypertrophy had a significantly ($P = 0.008$) greater thigh circumference than those without (13.5 mm vs. 8.1 mm).

DXA-derived measures are shown for women only (Table 4), as there were insufficient numbers of men with DXA scans for meaningful analysis. Women with lipoatrophy as well as those with lipohypertrophy, had significantly higher percentage trunk fat/lower limb fat and percentage trunk fat/total limb fat and significantly lower percentage lower limb fat/BMI. Women with lipoatrophy had significantly less percentage limb fat while women with lipohypertrophy had significantly more percentage trunk fat.

ROC curves for lipoatrophy and lipohypertrophy were generated and reported in female participants for anthropometric and DXA-derived variables with the highest AUC's (Figure 1). For lipoatrophy, the two anthropometric variables with the highest AUC were tricep skinfold thickness (AUC = 0.725) and thigh skinfold thickness (AUC = 0.720) and for lipohypertrophy they were waist/hip ratio (AUC = 0.645) and waist circumference (AUC = 0.589). For lipoatrophy, the two DXA-derived variables with the highest AUC were the percentage of lower limb fat standardised to height (AUC = 0.713) and percentage lower limb fat (AUC = 0.705) and for lipohypertrophy they were percentage trunk fat/percentage total limb fat (AUC = 0.647) and percentage trunk fat/ percentage lower limb fat (AUC = 0.646). An illustration of anthropometric and DXA-derived variables in females is shown in Figure 2.

Optimum cut-points for lipoatrophy and lipohypertrophy variables, based on likelihood ratios, were selected. Table 5 shows the sensitivity, specificity, likelihood ratios and predictive values for the two anthropometric and

Table 1 Characteristics of participants on ART

Variable	Lipoatrophy* With n = 121 Median [IQR]	Lipoatrophy* Without n = 429 Median [IQR]	P-value**	Lipohypertrophy*** With n = 157 Median [IQR]	Lipohypertrophy*** Without n = 393 Median [IQR]	P-value**
Age	34 [30–42]	35 [30–41]	0.256	34 [29–41]	35 [30–41]	0.198
Current CD4 count	397 [249–539]	315 [218–481]	0.023	389 [248–548]	314 [220–481]	0.015
Time on ART (months)	25 [14–32]	17 [10–27]	0.001	20 [12–31]	17 [11–28]	0.080
Time on Stavudine (months)	15.5 [10–26]	13 [8–19]	0.004	13 [8–21]	13 [9–20]	0.961
	n [%]	n [%]		n [%]	n [%]	
Sex						
Males	12 [10.34]	104 [89.66]	0.001	15 [12.93]	101 [87.07]	<0.001
Females	109 [25.12]	325 [74.88]		142 [32.72]	292 [67.28]	
Highest standard passed						
No schooling	6 [18.8]	26 [81.3]	0.289	9 [28.13]	23 [71.88]	0.272
Primary school	14 [15.4]	77 [84.6]		20 [21.98]	71 [78.02]	
Secondary school	96 [23.4]	315 [76.6]		121 [29.44]	290 [70.56]	
Tertiary	5 [31.3]	11 [68.8]		7 [43.75]	9 [56.25]	
ART Regimen						
First-line	99 [22.30]	345 [77.70]	0.730	130 [29.28]	314 [70.72]	0.608
Second-line	22 [20.75]	84 [79.25]		27 [25.47]	79 [74.53]	

*based on patient report, those with moderate or severe fat loss in 2 or more regions.
**Wilcoxon Rank-sum (Mann-Whitney) tests for continuous variables and chi-square tests for binary variables.
***based on patient report, those with moderate or severe fat gain in 2 or more regions.

DXA-derived variables with the highest AUC for lipoatrophy and lipohypertrophy at the optimum cut-points.

Discussion

We showed that simple anthropometric measures were at least as good as DXA-derived measures to diagnose lipoatrophy and lipohypertrophy in African women on ART. The best predictors of lipoatrophy in women were the anthropometric variables tricep and thigh skinfold thicknesses; and the DXA-derived variables percentage lower limb fat and percentage lower limb fat/height. The best predictors of lipohypertrophy in women were the anthropometric variable waist/hip ratio and the DXA-derived variable percentage trunk fat/percentage limb fat. Women with lipoatrophy had considerably smaller limb circumferences, limb skinfold thicknesses and lower percentages of limb fat than women without lipoatrophy, despite similar BMIs. Lipoatrophy and lipohypertrophy were both more common in women than in the small sample of men.

Previous studies, conducted in high-income countries, developed objective measures for lipodystrophy, thus combining lipoatrophic and lipohypertrophic individuals [15-17]. They proposed the use of fat mass ratio (FMR), defined as the ratio between the percentage of trunk fat mass and the percentage of lower-limb fat mass. We however sought to investigate lipoatrophy and lipohypertrophy as separate entities. Identification of lipoatrophy is important as it is an adverse antiretroviral drug reaction, which improves on switching antiretroviral drugs [21]. Although lipohypertrophy is thought to be a consequence of treating HIV infection rather than an adverse antiretroviral drug reaction [21], like lipoatrophy, it is associated with an increased risk of vascular disease [26] therefore it is worth identifying so that appropriate screening and prevention interventions can be implemented.

Despite the subjective nature of assessing lipoatrophy and lipohypertrophy by using patient self-report, previous studies have shown a strong correlation between patient and physician reported lipodystrophy scores [27-29]. In South Africa, as well as in many other African countries, nurses, rather than physicians, prescribe antiretroviral therapy and follow up patients. For these reasons we used patient self-report [5,6] as the reference measure to define lipoatrophy and lipohypertrophy.

Our study, like several others [11,21], showed a significant association between lipoatrophy and time on ART, and time on d4T in particular. As South Africa has only recently phased out d4T, and AZT is still being used, it is not unexpected that a quarter of the women and a tenth of the men, had lipoatrophy. The prevalence of lipoatrophy found in this study is not easy to compare with other studies as studies from high-income countries

Table 2 Anthropometric measurements of female participants on ART

Variable	Lipoatrophy* With n = 106 Median [IQR]	Lipoatrophy* Without n = 312 Median [IQR]	P-value**	Lipohypertrophy*** With n = 142 Median [IQR]	Lipohypertrophy*** Without n = 292 Median [IQR]	P-value**
Height (m)	1.6 [1.5-1.6]	1.6 [1.5-1.6]	0.603	1.6 [1.6-1.6]	1.6 [1.5-1.6]	0.112
Weight (kg)	65.4 [56.0-74.5]	68.1 [58.9-80.9]	0.019	69.5 [60.7-80.4]	67.1 [57.6-79.3]	0.127
BMI	26.2 [23.8-29.3]	27.1 [24.1-31.6]	0.036	27.4 [24.6-31.3]	26.65 [23.9-31.2]	0.187
Sagittal Abdominal Diameter (cm)	20.5 [19.0-23.0]	20.0 [18.5-23.0]	0.552	21 [19–24]	20 [18–23]	0.004
Circumferences						
Waist (cm)	86.3 [79.5-96.3]	87.0 [78.5-97.0]	0.704	90.7 [80.3-98.5]	86 [78.4-95]	0.003
Hip (cm)	98.0 [92.0-104.0]	102.0 [95.0-112.0]	<0.001	100 [95–110]	101 [94–110]	0.824
Waist/hip ratio	0.90 [0.83-0.94]	0.85 [0.80-0.90]	<0.001	0.89 [0.83-0.93]	0.84 [0.79-0.90]	<0.001
Mid-upper arm (cm)	27.0 [25.0-29.0]	29.0 [26.5-32.0]	<0.001	28 [26–32]	28 [26–32]	0.789
Mid-thigh (cm)	54.5 [51.0-59.0]	57.0 [53.0-63.0]	<0.001	56 [52–61]	57[52–63]	0.589
Skinfolds						
Bicep (mm)	6.0 [4.4-8.4]	8.1 [5.7-11.7]	<0.001	7.1 [5.2-10.7]	8 [5.4-11.45]	0.189
Tricep (mm)	13.3 [9.5-17.4]	18.4 [13.6-26.0]	<0.001	16.2 [12–22]	18.3 [13–25.15]	0.059
Abdomen (mm)	20.4 [11.9-30.0]	24.4 [16.8-35.3]	0.001	24.1 [15.9-35.8]	23.6 [15.0-31.2]	0.210
Thigh (mm)	23.8 [15.4-32.8]	34.7 [24.2-44.7]	<0.001	29.8 [20.5-42.5]	32.0 [22.5-43.5]	0.359
Sub-Scapular (mm)	16.9 [12.5-23.0]	19.2 [12.2-28.8]	0.058	20 [14.8-29.4]	18.5 [11.7-27.1]	0.050
Supra-iliac (mm)	13.2 [7.7-18.7]	15.1 [8.8-22.8]	0.033	16.6 [9.9-24.0]	13.9 [8.2-21.7]	0.022
Calf (mm)	10.8 [8.0-17.5]	17.5 [12.2-24.2]	<0.001	15.6 [9.2-21.3]	17.3 [11.4-23.6]	0.061

*based on patient report, those with moderate or severe fat loss in 2 or more regions.
**Wilcoxon Rank-sum (Mann–Whitney) tests for continuous variables and chi-square tests for binary variables.
***based on patient report, those with moderate or severe fat gain in 2 or more regions.

focussed on men [12,24], while most studies from Africa looked at the prevalence of lipodystrophy [30-32] rather than studying the two entities of lipoatrophy and lipodystrophy separately. Our finding that tricep skinfold thickness was a predictor of lipoatrophy is supported by other studies. George et al. [33], using a small sample of HIV-infected South Africans, found that after 2 years of exposure to ART, patients had significantly decreased tricep skinfold thicknesses. Similarly, a Ugandan study using a sample of HIV-infected men and women [32], found that decreased tricep skinfold thicknesses was associated with the use of AZT.

There were some limitations to our study. The cross sectional design, while allowing us to make associations, does not allow us to infer causality. With changes in fat distribution, repeated objective measures would have given us a better reference standard than patient report, even though patient report is commonly used [5,6]. We did not have enough men with lipoatrophy or lipohypertrophy, to explore predictive anthropometric and DXA-derived variables. Finally, the likelihood ratios for the most predictive anthropometric and DXA-derived variables were only weakly diagnostic of self-report lipoatrophy and lipohypertrophy. Future research of longitudinal studies in African cohorts, using changes in DXA-derived variables as the reference standard, is needed to confirm the value of anthropometric measures for the diagnosis of lipoatrophy and lipohypertrophy.

Conclusion

Using a large sample of black HIV-infected South African women who had DXA scans performed, we were able to develop anthropometric measures for defining lipoatrophy and lipohypertrophy. The development of anthropometric measures which admittedly needs training and well maintained skinfold callipers to ensure their accuracy, are of particular relevance in resource limited settings, where health professionals need simple and inexpensive methods of diagnosing patients with lipoatrophy and lipohypertrophy.

Methods

Participants

A convenience sample of HIV-infected black men and women presenting to ART clinics in Cape Town were selected. The recruitment procedure is described elsewhere [34]. The study sample comprised 116 male and 434 female participants on ART. At the time of the study

Table 3 Anthropometric measurements of male participants on ART

Variable	Lipoatrophy*		P-value**	Lipohypertrophy***		P-value**
	With n = 12 Median [IQR]	Without n = 104 Median [IQR]		With n = 15 Median [IQR]	Without n = 101 Median [IQR]	
Height (m)	1.7 [1.6-1.7]	1.7 [1.6-1.7]	0.942	1.7 [1.6-1.8]	1.7 [1.7-1.7]	0.954
Weight (kg)	65.5 [59.7-68.6]	63.5 [57.0-74.4]	0.895	67.4 [57.8-78.3]	62.7 [57.3-73.4]	0.408
BMI	23.3 [20.2-23.9]	22.4 [20.6-25.2]	0.772	23.6 [21.1-25.5]	22.3 [20.5-24.8]	0.324
Sagittal Abdominal Diameter (cm)	17.0 [16.0-19.5]	18.0 [17.0-20.0]	0.384	17.0 [16.0-22.0]	18.0 [17.0-20.0]	0.967
Circumferences						
Waist (cm)	81.75 [77–84.9]	80.4 [75.0-90.2]	0.953	83.8 [75.0-97.0]	79.8 [75.8-89.5]	0.338
Hip (cm)	90 [87–93.5]	90.0 [85.0-97.0]	0.768	91.0 [85.0-97.0]	90.0 [85.0-96.0]	0.556
Waist/hip ratio	0.89 [0.85-0.95]	0.91 [0.87-0.94]	0.740	0.93 [0.86-0.97]	0.90 [0.86-0.94]	0.325
Mid-upper arm (cm)	27.0 [24–28.5]	26.0 [24.0-29.0]	0.877	27.0 [25.0-29.0]	26.0 [24.0-29.0]	0.817
Mid-thigh (cm)	50.5 [43.5-52.5]	49.0 [46.0-54.0]	0.401	49.0 [46.0-56.0]	49.0 [46.0-54.0]	0.567
Skinfolds						
Bicep (mm)	3.9 [3.4-4.2]	3.5 [3.0-4.5]	0.329	4.1 [3.2-4.8]	3.5 [3.0-4.3]	0.180
Tricep (mm)	6.8 [5.6-8.2]	6.4 [5.1-9.3]	0.921	8.4 [5.0-11.4]	6.4 [5.1-8.7]	0.444
Abdomen (mm)	13.5 [10.5-16.9]	12.3 [8.5-30.1]	1.00	15.8 [9.3-28.2]	12.3 [8.5 -18.1]	0.309
Thigh (mm)	8.4 [7.2-14.8]	8.5 [6.0-12.4]	0.490	13.5 [8.4-21.1]	8.1 [6.0-11.3]	0.008
Sub-Scapular (mm)	9.4 [6.5-13.2]	8.3 [6.3-13.4]	0.605	10.5 [5.7-18.0]	8.2 [6.5-11.1]	0.770
Supra-iliac (mm)	6.3 [4.4-6.8]	6.2 [4.9-9.4]	0.196	6.4 [4.7-12.1]	6.2 [4.9-8.5]	0.934
Calf (mm)	5.5 [4.8-9.0]	5.8 [4.4-8.2]	0.739	6.8 [5.4-10.5]	5.5 [4.4-7.7]	0.094

*based on patient report, those with moderate or severe fat loss in 2 or more regions.
**Wilcoxon Rank-sum (Mann–Whitney) tests for continuous variables and chi-square tests for binary variables.
***based on patient report, those with moderate or severe fat gain in 2 or more regions.

Table 4 DXA-derived measurements of female participants on ART

Variable	Lipoatrophy*		P-value**	Lipohypertrophy***		P-value**
	With n = 29 Median [IQR]	Without n = 143 Median [IQR]		With n = 46 Median [IQR]	Without n = 126 Median [IQR]	
DXA-derived measures						
Arm fat (%)	37.4 [30.8-44.1]	38.3 [31.8-47.1]	0.380	39.8 [31.5-48.3]	38.1 [31.7-45.1]	0.319
Lower limb fat (%)	37.6 [31.5-40.6]	43.4 [36.6-49.7]	0.001	39.2 [33.3-49.7]	41.8 [36.3-48.8]	0.761
Trunk fat (%)	34.7 [29.9-38.0]	35.1 [27.9-43.1]	0.719	37.9 [30.7-45.3]	34.4 [26.6-40.4]	0.019
Lower limb fat/ht (%)	23.6 [19.7-25.4]	27.4 [23.4-31.5]	0.001	25.4 [21.9-31.1]	26.5 [23.2-29.7]	0.631
Total limb fat/ht (%)	22.7 [20.8-27.0]	25.4 [22.0-29.9]	0.015	25.4 [20.8-31.1]	25.2 [21.8-29.1]	0.825
Lower limb fat/BMI (%)	1.3 [1.2-1.7]	1.6 [1.3-1.8]	0.049	1.4 [1.2-1.6]	1.6 [1.3-1.8]	0.019
Total limb fat/BMI (%)	1.3 [1.3-1.6]	1.5 [1.3-1.6]	0.193	1.3 [1.2-1.5]	1.5 [1.3-1.7]	0.006
Trunk fat/lower limb fat (%)	0.94 [0.76-1.15]	0.83 [0.66-0.96]	0.017	0.93 [0.80-1.10]	0.81 [0.66-0.94]	0.003
Trunk fat/ total limb fat (%)	1.0 [0.8-1.0]	0.9 [0.7-1.0]	0.045	0.93 [0.85-1.03]	0.85 [0.72-0.97]	0.003

*based on patient report, those with moderate or severe fat loss in 2 or more regions.
**Wilcoxon Rank-sum (Mann–Whitney) tests for continuous variables and chi-square tests for binary variables.
***based on patient report, those with moderate or severe fat gain in 2 or more regions.

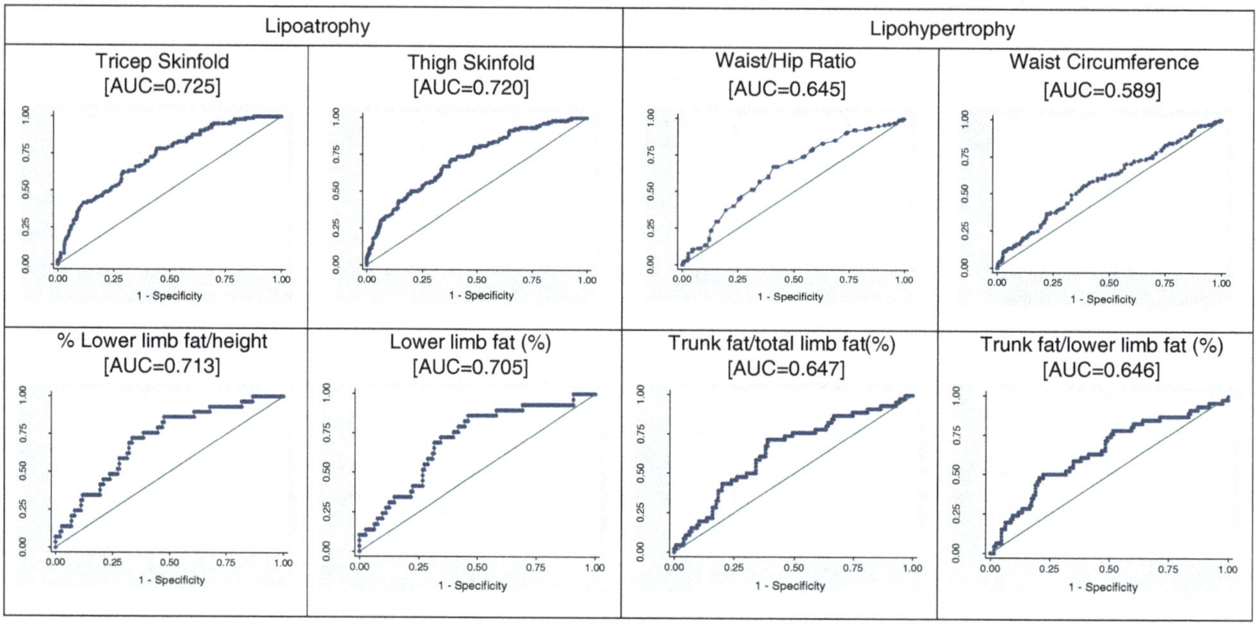

Figure 1 ROC curves for the 2 anthropometric and DXA-derived variables with the highest AUC for lipoatrophy and lipohypertrophy in female participants on ART.

two ART regimens were available to South Africans accessing primary health care facilities. The first-line regimen consisted of d4T, lamivudine (3TC) and efavirenz (EFV) or nevirapine, and a second-line regimen consisting of AZT with 3TC and lopinavir/ritonavir (LPV/r) [35].

Testing procedures

Questionnaires were used to collect socio-demographic information from participants. Their clinical records at the health facilities were reviewed to obtain data on ART regimen, time on ART, and CD4 count. Self-reported information on fat gain or fat loss was collected using a standard questionnaire [8]. Lipoatrophy was defined as moderate or severe fat loss in 2 or more regions and lipohypertrophy defined as moderate or severe fat gain in two or more areas [36].

Anthropometric measurements: [weight, height, circumferences (waist, hip, mid-upper arm, and mid-thigh),

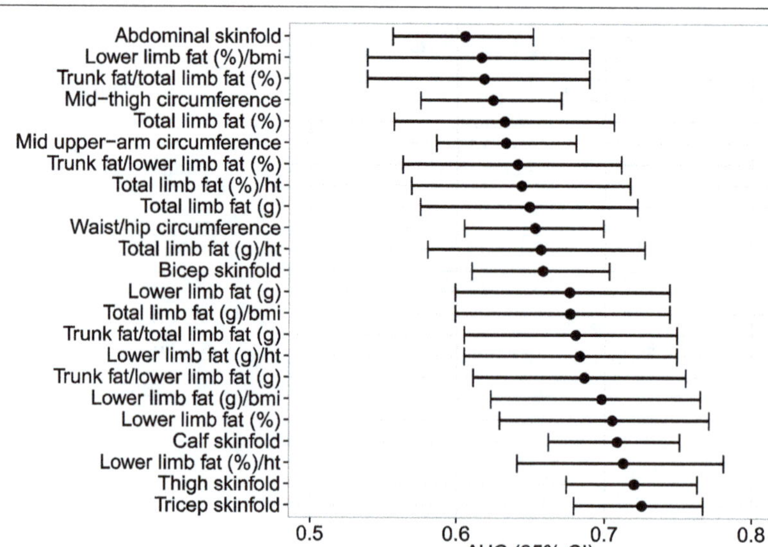

Figure 2 Lipoatrophy variables for female participants on ART with ROC AUCs of ≥0.6 and their 95% confidence intervals in descending order of AUC.

Table 5 Variables for prediction and classification used to identify lipoatrophy and lipohypertrophy cut-points

Lipoatrophy variable cut-point	N	Sensitivity	Specificity	Likelihood ratio positive test	Likelihood ratio negative test	Positive predictive value	Negative predictive value	% correctly classified
Tricep skinfold ≤14.5 mm	418	0.62	0.71	2.13	0.53	0.42	0.85	68.66*
Thigh skinfold ≤28.0 mm	417	0.67	0.65	1.93	0.51	0.39	0.85	65.70*
% Lower limb fat/height ≤ 24.7	418	0.19	0.85	1.28	0.95	0.30	0.76	68.42*
Lower limb fat (%) ≤ 39.1	418	0.19	0.84	1.20	0.96	0.29	0.75	67.70*
Lipohypertrophy variable cut-point								
Waist/Hip Ratio ≥ 0.899	434	0.44	0.75	1.75	0.75	0.46	0.73	64.75**
Waist Circumference ≥ 88.5 cm	434	0.57	0.59	1.40	0.73	0.41	0.73	58.53**
Trunk fat/total limb fat (%) ≥0.8895	172	0.50	0.70	1.66	0.72	0.38	0.79	64.5**
Trunk fat/leg fat (%) ≥ 0.8816	172	0.72	0.61	1.84	0.46	0.40	0.86	64.0**

*percentage of those classified with and without lipoatrophy using the new cut-point compared to those defined by subject-report.
**percentage of those classified with and without lipohypertrophy using the new cut-point compared to those defined by subject-report.

skinfold thickness (bicep, tricep, subscapular, abdomen, suprailiac, thigh and calf) and sagittal abdominal diameter (SAD)] taken have previously been described [37]. DXA (Hologic Discovery-W, software version 12.7; scan region 195 × 65 cm^2 and weight limit 160 kg) was used to measure fat mass and fat free soft tissue mass in a subsample of participants (females: n = 172; males: n = 53). DXA cut off lines positioned at anatomical markers were used to obtain fat mass for the whole body as well as for the various regions of interest. A more detailed description has been previously described [34].

Ethical approval

The study proposal was submitted and approved by the Research Ethics Committee of the Faculty of Health Sciences at the University of Cape Town. Written informed consent was obtained from all participants prior to participation in the study.

Data analyses

Data analysis was carried out using the STATA/SE statistical software package version 12.0 (StataCorp., College Station, TX, USA). Data were collected between February 2007 and June 2009. Participants were categorised into those with and those without lipoatrophy. Continuous variables were described as medians and inter-quartile ranges (IQR), and were compared using Wilcoxon Rank Sum tests. Binary variables were described using chi-square tests.

Receiver operating characteristic (ROC) curves were used to describe the performance of a number of anthropometric and DXA-derived variables using patient reported lipoatrophy and lipohypertrophy as the reference standard. The area under the curve (AUC) was used to assess the diagnostic performance of each variable. In addition, sensitivity, specificity, likelihood ratios and predictive values were calculated for variables with the highest AUC at the optimum cut-points. Cut-point selection was based on positive likelihood ratios.

Competing interests

Supported by grants from the World Diabetes Foundation and the South African Department of Health. GM was supported in part by the National Research Foundation (NRF) of South Africa (grant specific unique reference number (UID) 85810). The Grant holder acknowledges that opinions, findings and conclusions or recommendations expressed in any publication generated by the NRF supported research are that of the author(s), and that the NRF accepts no liability whatsoever in this regard.

Authors' contributions

ZA conducted all statistical analyses, interpreted the findings and drafted the manuscript; JD, NL and GM designed and conducted the study; ML assisted with study design and data interpretation; NL, GM, JD and ML edited the manuscript and drafted revisions. All authors read and approved the manuscript.

Acknowledgements

We thank Linda Bewerunge for doing the DXA scans, Sasha West for anthropometric measurements, and Carmen Delport for co-ordinating the study.

Author details

[1]Division of Diabetic Medicine and Endocrinology, Department of Medicine, University of Cape Town, Cape Town, South Africa. [2]Division of Clinical Pharmacology, Department of Medicine, University of Cape Town, Cape Town, South Africa. [3]Department of Medicine, University of Cape Town, Cape Town, South Africa.

References

1. Johnson LF: **Access to antiretroviral treatment in South Africa, 2004-2011.** *SA J HIV Med* 2012, **13**(1):22–27.
2. Schambelan M, Benson CA, Carr A, Currier JS, Dubé MP, Gerber JG, Grinspoon SK, Grunfeld C, Kotler DP, Mulligan K: **Management of metabolic complications associated with antiretroviral therapy for HIV-1 infection: recommendations of an International AIDS Society-USA panel.** *J Acquir Immune Defic Syndr* 2002, **31**(3):257–275.
3. Grinspoon S, Carr A: **Cardiovascular risk and body-fat abnormalities in HIV-infected adults.** *N Engl J Med* 2005, **352**(1):48–62.
4. Carr A: **HIV protease inhibitor-induced lipodystrophy syndrome.** *AIDS Rev* 1999, **1**:29–36.
5. Carter V, Hoy J, Bailey M, Colman P, Nyulasi I, Mijch A: **The prevalence of lipodystrophy in an ambulant HIV-infected population: it all depends on the definition.** *HIV Med* 2001, **2**(3):174–180.
6. Casado JL, Iglesias V, Del Palacio M, Marín A, Perez-Elías MJ, Moreno A, Moreno S: **Social isolation in HIV-infected patients according to subjective patient assessment and DEXA-confirmed severity of lipodystrophy.** *AIDS Care* 2013, **25**(12):1599–1603.
7. Savès M, François R, Jacqueline C, Rozenbaum W, Ragnaud J, Perronne C, Basdevant A, Leport C, Geneviève C: **Factors related to lipodystrophy and metabolic alterations in patients with human immunodeficiency virus infection receiving highly active antiretroviral therapy.** *Clin Infect Dis* 2002, **34**(10):1396–1405.
8. Carr A: **An objective case definition of lipodystrophy in HIV-infected adults: a case–control study.** *Lancet* 2003, **361**(9359):726–735.
9. Worm D, Kirk O, Andersen O, Vinten J, Gerstoft J, Katzenstein T, Nielsen H, Pedersen C: **Clinical lipoatrophy in HIV-1 patients on HAART is not associated with increased abdominal girth, hyperlipidaemia or glucose intolerance.** *HIV Med* 2002, **3**(4):239–246.
10. Sievers M, Walker U, Sevastianova K, Setzer B, Wågsäter D, Eriksson P, Yki-Järvinen H, Sutinen J: **Gene expression and immunohistochemistry in adipose tissue of HIV type 1–infected patients with nucleoside analogue reverse-transcriptase inhibitor–associated lipoatrophy.** *J Infect Dis* 2009, **200**(2):252–262.
11. Menezes C, Maskew M, Sanne I, Crowther N, Raal F: **A longitudinal study of stavudine-associated toxicities in a large cohort of South African HIV infected subjects.** *BMC Infect Dis* 2011, **11**(1):244.
12. McComsey GA, Kitch D, Sax PE, Tebas P, Tierney C, Jahed NC, Myers L, Melbourne K, Ha B, Daar ES: **Peripheral and central fat changes in subjects randomized to abacavir-lamivudine or tenofovir-emtricitabine with atazanavir-ritonavir or efavirenz: ACTG Study A5224s.** *Clin Infect Dis* 2011, **53**(2):185–196.
13. Haubrich RH, Riddler SA, DiRienzo AG, Komarow L, Powderly WG, Klingman K, Garren KW, Butcher DL, Rooney JF, Haas DW: **Metabolic outcomes in a randomized trial of nucleoside, nonnucleoside and protease inhibitor-sparing regimens for initial HIV treatment.** *AIDS* 2009, **23**(9):1109.
14. Valantin M, Lanoy E, Bentata M, Kalmykova O, Boutekadjirt A, Allavena C, Rozenbaum W, Peytavin G, Amellal B, Calvez V: **Recovery of fat following a switch to nucleoside reverse transcriptase inhibitor-sparing therapy in patients with lipoatrophy: results from the 96-week randomized ANRS 108 NoNuke Trial.** *HIV Med* 2008, **9**(8):625–635.
15. Asha HS, Seshadri MS, Paul TV, Abraham OC, Rupali P, Thomas N: **Human immunodeficiency virus-associated lipodystrophy: an objective definition based on dual-energy x-ray absorptiometry-derived regional fat ratios in a South Asian population.** *Endocr Pract* 2012, **18**(2):158–169.
16. Bonnet E, Delpierre C, Sommet A, Marion-Latard F, Herve R, Aquilina C, Labau E, Obadia M, Marchou B, Massip P: **Total body composition by DXA of 241 HIV-negative men and 162 HIV-infected men: proposal of reference values for defining lipodystrophy.** *J Clin Densitom* 2005, **8**(3):287–292.

17. Freitas P, Santos AC, Carvalho D, Pereira J, Marques R, Martinez E, Sarmento A, Medina JL: **Fat mass ratio: an objective tool to define lipodystrophy in hiv-infected patients under antiretroviral therapy.** *J Clin Densitom* 2010, **13**(2):197–203.
18. Goedecke JH, Levitt NS, Lambert EV, Utzschneider KM, Faulenbach MV, Dave JA, West S, Victor H, Evans J, Olsson T: **Differential effects of abdominal adipose tissue distribution on insulin sensitivity in black and white South African women.** *Obesity* 2009, **17**(8):1506–1512.
19. Kanaley J, Giannopoulou I, Tillapaugh-Fay G, Nappi J, Ploutz-Snyder L: **Racial differences in subcutaneous and visceral fat distribution in postmenopausal black and white women.** *Metab Clin Exp* 2003, **52**(2):186–191.
20. Carroll JF, Chiapa AL, Rodriquez M, Phelps DR, Cardarelli KM, Vishwanatha JK, Bae S, Cardarelli R: **Visceral fat, waist circumference, and BMI: impact of race/ethnicity.** *Obesity* 2008, **16**(3):600–607.
21. De Waal R, Cohen K, Maartens G: **Systematic review of antiretroviral-associated lipodystrophy: lipoatrophy, but not central fat gain, is an antiretroviral adverse drug reaction.** *PLoS One* 2013, **8**(5):e63623.
22. Feleke Y, Fekade D, Mezegebu Y: **Prevalence of highly active antiretroviral therapy associated metabolic abnormalities and lipodystrophy in HIV infected patients.** *Ethiop Med J* 2012, **50**(3):221–230.
23. World Health Organization: **Global update on HIV treatment 2013: results, impact and opportunities.** [http://www.who.int/hiv/pub/progressreports/update2013/en/]
24. Freitas P, Carvalho D, Souto S, Santos AC, Xerinda S, Marques R, Martinez E, Sarmento A, Medina JL: **Impact of Lipodystrophy on the prevalence and components of metabolic syndrome in HIV-infected patients.** *BMC Infect Dis* 2011, **11**(1):246.
25. Masiá M, Padilla S, García N, Jarrin I, Bernal E, López N, Hernández I, Gutiérrez F: **Endothelial function is impaired in HIV-infected patients with lipodystrophy.** *Antivir Ther* 2010, **15**(1):101–110.
26. Lake JE, Wohl D, Scherzer R, Grunfeld C, Tien PC, Sidney S, Currier JS: **Regional fat deposition and cardiovascular risk in HIV infection: the FRAM study.** *AIDS Care* 2011, **23**(8):929–938.
27. Guaraldi G, Murri R, Orlando G, Giovanardi C, Squillace N, Vandelli M, Beghetto B, Nardini G, De Paola M, Esposito R: **Severity of lipodystrophy is associated with decreased health-related quality of life.** *AIDS Patient Care STDS* 2008, **22**(7):577–585.
28. Huang JS, Harrity S, Lee D, Becerra K, Santos R, Mathews WC: **Body image in women with HIV: a cross-sectional evaluation.** *AIDS Res Ther* 2006, **3**(17):1–7.
29. Tungsiripat M, O'Riordan MA, Storer N, Harrill D, Ganz J, Libutti D, Gerschenson M, McComsey GA: **Subjective clinical lipoatrophy assessment correlates with DEXA-measured limb fat.** *HIV Clin Trials* 2009, **10**(5):314–319.
30. Van Oosterhout JJ, Mallewa J, Kaunda S, Chagoma N, Njalale Y, Kampira E, Mukaka M, Heyderman RS: **Stavudine toxicity in adult longer-term ART patients in Blantyre.** *Malawi PLos One* 2012, **7**(7):e42029.
31. Bussmann H, Wester CW, Thomas A, Novitsky V, Okezie R, Muzenda T, Gaolathe T, Ndwapi N, Mawoko N, Widenfelt E, Moyo S, Musonda R, Mine M, Makhema J, Moffat H, Essex M, Degruttola V, Marlink RG: **Response to zidovudine/didanosine-containing combination antiretroviral therapy among HIV-1 subtype C-infected adults in Botswana: two-year outcomes from a randomized clinical trial.** *J Acquir Immune Defic Syndr* 2009, **51**(1):37–46.
32. Thompson V, Medard B, Taseera K, Chakera AJ, Andia I, Emenyonu N, Hunt PW, Martin J, Scherzer R, Weiser SD: **Regional anthropometry changes in antiretroviral-naive persons initiating a Zidovudine-containing regimen in Mbarara.** *Uganda AIDS Res Hum Retroviruses* 2011, **27**(7):785–791.
33. George JA, Venter WD, Van Deventer HE, Crowther NJ: **A longitudinal study of the changes in body fat and metabolic parameters in a South African population of HIV-positive patients receiving an antiretroviral therapeutic regimen containing stavudine.** *AIDS Res Hum Retroviruses* 2009, **25**(8):771–781.
34. Goedecke JH, Micklesfield LK, Levitt NS, Lambert EV, West S, Maartens G, Dave JA: **Effect of different antiretroviral drug regimens on body fat distribution of HIV-infected South African women.** *AIDS Res Hum Retroviruses* 2013, **29**(3):557–563.
35. Department of Health: **The South African antiretroviral treatment guidelines.** [http://www.auruminstitute.org/phocadownload/guidelines-short.pdf]
36. Lichtenstein KA, Ward DJ, Moorman AC, Delaney KM, Young B, Palella FJ Jr, Rhodes PH, Wood KC, Holmberg SD: **Clinical assessment of HIV-associated lipodystrophy in an ambulatory population.** *AIDS* 2001, **15**(11):1389–1398.
37. Dave JA, Lambert EV, Badri M, West S, Maartens G, Levitt NS: **Effect of nonnucleoside reverse transcriptase inhibitor-based antiretroviral therapy on dysglycemia and insulin sensitivity in South African HIV-infected patients.** *J Acquir Immune Defic Syndr* 2011, **57**(4):284–289.

Lipodystrophy among HIV-infected patients: a cross-sectional study on impact on quality of life and mental health disorders

Charlotte M Verolet[1*], Cécile Delhumeau-Cartier[2], Marlène Sartori[2,4], Simona Toma[4], Sophie Zawadynski[5], Minerva Becker[6], Enos Bernasconi[7], Laurence Toutous Trellu[3], Alexandra Calmy[2] and The LIPO Group Metabolism

Abstract

Background: Lipodystrophy (LD) is a frequent adverse event of combination antiretroviral therapy (ART) and occurs mainly in patients exposed to first-generation antiretroviral drugs. The aim of this study was to explore and measure the interaction between LD, mental health, and quality of life of human immunodeficiency virus (HIV) positive individuals seen in a metabolic clinic.

Methods: We conducted a single-site cross-sectional study including all HIV-infected patients attending the *LIPO group and metabolism* day clinic at the University Hospitals of Geneva, Switzerland between January 31, 2008 and November 28, 2013. Data on LD were prospectively collected using the HIV Outpatient Study (HOPS) score, the Lipodystrophy Case Definition (LDCD), ART regimens, anthropometric measures, imaging, and standardized questionnaires. Quality of life was evaluated using a visual analog scale of 0–100. Depression and anxiety were assessed using the Beck Depression Inventory and the State Trait Anxiety Inventory scales, respectively.

Results: One hundred ninety-four patients (54.6% male; 45.4% female; median age, 50 years) on successful ART (median CD4 cell count, 569.0 cells/mm^3; median viral load, 20 copies/mL) were evaluated. Among these, 62.7, 63.5 and 35.5% of patients reported at least one body site affected by fat hypertrophy, atrophy or both, respectively. Using the LDCD score conservative definition, including imaging and biological values, 57.8% were diagnosed with LD. Of these, 39.7% suffered from severe/very severe LD. Depression was reported by 35.6% of individuals; 51.9% had anxiety symptoms and 49.5% reported poor quality of life (defined as being inferior to 50% on a scale from 0 to 100%). LD (odds ratio (OR = 5.22, 95% confidence interval (CI) 1.07–25.37, p-value: 0.040), depression (OR = 4.67, 95% CI 1.08–20.31, p-value 0.040), and anxiety (OR = 7.83, 95% CI 1.91–32.03, p-value 0.004) all affected significantly the quality of life.

Conclusions: LD, depression and anxiety were frequent features among HIV-infected individuals seen in the metabolic clinic and significantly impacted on their quality of life.

Keywords: HIV infection, Lipodystrophy, Lipohypertrophy, Lipoatrophy, Quality of life, Mental health disorder, Depression, Anxiety

Background

Since the description of the first case of acquired immune deficiency syndrome (AIDS) in 1981, human immunodeficiency virus (HIV) infection has reached pandemic proportions and has continued to expand in worldwide; in 2012 an estimated of 35.3 million of peoples were infected by HIV [1]. Nucleoside reverse transcriptase inhibitors (NRTIs), followed by protease inhibitors (PIs), were the first antiretroviral (ARV) drugs used to treat HIV [2] and succeeded in decreasing

*Correspondence: Charlotte.Verolet@hcuge.ch
[1] Department of Pediatrics, Children's Hospital-University Hospitals of Geneva, 6 Rue Willy-Donzé, 1211 Geneva 14, Switzerland
Full list of author information is available at the end of the article

mortality by an estimated of 4.2 million of deaths during the previous decade [1, 3, 4]. However, this therapeutic revolution was not without complications as multiple side-effects were associated with these first-generation ARV drugs. Among these, lipodystrophy (LD) was highlighted in 1998 by Carr et al. [5]. This syndrome comprises three phenotypes: lipohypertrophy (LH); lipoatrophy (LA); or a mixed pattern of both [5, 6]. LD can be associated also with metabolic disorders, therefore increasing the risk of cardiovascular disease [7].

There is currently no universal definition of LD. This implies significant variation in the prevalence rate, incidence, severity, and risk factors, which makes difficult any comparison between studies and across countries and ethnicities [7]. Diagnosis is based mainly on clinical observations by the patients themselves and by the physicians. To help meeting this challenge, the HIV Outpatients Study (HOPS) scale provides a subjective, but standardized LD evaluation using specific questions related to the clinical signs of the disorder [8]. Carr et al. developed a score in order to offer a more objective definition of LD, the Lipodystrophy Case Definition (LDCD), with a reported 79% sensitivity and 80% specificity [9, 10]. Nevertheless, this score does not allow differentiating between disease phenotypes [6].

Systematic reviews have discussed the impact of ARV agents and regimens on LD, but with discordant conclusions. If a clear relationship between NRTIs (thymidine analogs) and LA has been demonstrated, the causal role of specific drugs in the development of fat accumulation remains to be clarified [11, 12]. With the advent of newer drugs and the earlier detection of HIV, the prevalence of LD is now decreasing [11], although 48 weeks after the tests of a novel, potent NRTI, BMS-986001 a peripheral and central fat accumulation was observed [13]. However, the overall prevalence of LD remains high as many patients were exposed to first-generation molecules and damage caused to adipose tissue has only limited reversibility [14].

Several research groups have focused on the impact of LD on quality of life [15–23]. In addition, these reports have described discrepant results and conclusions regarding the interplay with mental health disorders, such as depression or anxiety [24–28].

This study aimed to identify the complex relationships between LD, mental health disorders, and the quality of life in patients attending the *LIPO group and metabolism* day clinic at the University Hospitals of Geneva, Switzerland.

Methods

Patients

All patients participating to the metabolic clinic (*LIPO group and metabolism*) at the University Hospitals of Geneva between January 31, 2008 and November 28, 2013 were included in the study. This multidisciplinary consultation (day hospital) is held once monthly and patients are referred to the clinic by their treating physician for several reasons, such as the evaluation of HIV-related or unrelated multiple medical co-morbidities, or LD management. A complete medical check-up is coordinated by the infectious diseases team and includes blood analyses, imaging [body composition and bone dual-energy X-ray absorptiometry (DXA), and thoracic vertebral level (T12) as well as lumbar vertebral level (L5) computed tomography (CT) single slice scans], and psychological, plastic surgery, dermatology, endocrinology, bone diseases and dietary consultations. Physicians from other medical specialties are available upon request e.g., nephrologist, endocrinologist, bone specialist, cardiologist, hepatologist. All patients provided written informed consent and the study protocol was approved by the clinical ethics committee of the University Hospitals of Geneva (CER #09017).

Definitions

LD Patients and physicians both completed a questionnaire based on the HOPS scale [8]. Different parts of the patient body (arms, legs, cheeks and buttocks for signs of atrophy; abdomen, neck and breast for signs of hypertrophy) were evaluated and described as absent, subtle, moderate or severe. The different values were then stratified into five categories (none, all subtle, subtle/moderate, one severe, two or more severe). According to Lichtenstein et al. [8], this score was then classified in two strata; absent vs present and used like this in all the statistical analysis.

We used also the complete model of LDCD score, developed by Carr et al. and validated in a large cohort of patients [9], to determine the categories used to define the presence of LD [10]. LD was stratified in four classes, from very subtle/absent (<0 to 9.9 points) to severe/very severe (15 to >23 points). This score was then classified in two classes; absent (subtle/absent, subtle, moderate) versus present (severe/very severe) and used like this for all the statistical analysis. These definitions are presented in the Additional file 1: Table S1.

Quality of life Patients were asked by a trained psychologist to score their perceived quality of life on a 20 cm quantitative scale ranging from 0 to 100%. Zero corresponds to the "worst possible quality of life" and 100 to the "best possible quality of life". This measure is often used in cognitive behavioral therapy and is a part of a wider score validated in different studies [29]. In our study, we used the short version of the score. Patients were classified as having a low (0–50%) or high quality of life (51–100%).

Anxiety was evaluated by a trained psychologist using the State Trait Anxiety Inventory (STAI Y-B) grading by a questionnaire with 20 items regarding the trait anxiety developed by Spielberger in 1983 [30]. A score equal or greater than 46 indicated the presence of anxiety symptoms.

Depression was measured by a trained psychologist using the Beck Depression Inventory (BDI) score [31], including a questionnaire with 21 items. Patients were considered to have depression when the score was above 19.

The waist was measured halfway between the last rib and the iliac crest, and the hips by the maximal buttock circumference.

Imaging studies

A CT-scan consisting of two single slices of 6 mm thickness each obtained at the T12 and L5 level was performed in each patient in order to calculate the ratio between the visceral adipose tissue and the subcutaneous adipose tissue (VAT/SAT). Abdominal VAT and SAT were measures by contouring manually the areas with attenuation values of adipose tissue (range 190 Hounsfield Units to 30 Hounsfield Units) according to the literature [32]. Limb as well as leg fat measurement, both needed for LDCD score calculation, was obtained by Total Body Dual X Ray Absorbsometry (DXA) on a Discovery A Bone densitometer (Hologic Inc. Bedford, MA, USA). Total body scans were performed by DXA (Dual X Ray Absorbsometry) using the same Discovery A Bone densitometer all over the study period (Hologic Inc. Bedford, MA, USA). To assure reliability and stability of our device, Phantom was scanned daily; QC (quality control) data plot was verified online by a secured, centralized database program. ISCD (International Society of Clinical Densitometry) recommendations for precision assessment, scans acquisition and analysis are applied.

Statistical analyses

We used a kappa test with an alpha threshold of 5% to measure the level of agreement between patients and physicians regarding the presence of fat loss or accumulation by using the HOPS score. A Chi-square test with an alpha threshold of 5% was used to verify if gender had an impact on qualitative variables (depression, anxiety, quality of life, and LDCD). We conducted a multivariate logistic regression model to identify risk factors for a low quality of life, including the severe LD (LDCD) variable and all other variables with a p value lower than 0.2 in the univariate model, to assess the specific contribution of severe LD (LDCD). To identify specific, potential confounding risk factors of quality of life, such as depression and anxiety, we developed an additional model including clinical risk factors considered to have a potential impact on quality of life in HIV population: age; gender; severe LD (LDCD), atrophy and hypertrophy observed by patients and physicians (HOPS); body mass index (≥30 kg/m^2); HIV duration (≥10 years); United States Centers for Disease Control and Prevention HIV stage (B&C); CD4 count (≤300 cells/mm^3); and HIV viral load (≥40 copy/mL). Finally, we performed the Hosmer–Lemeshow test, as well as the area under the ROC curve, to evaluate the overall fit of our two logistic regression models. Statistical analyses were carried out with STATA software, version 13.0 (StataCorp, College Station, TX, USA).

Results

Characteristics of the study population

One hundred ninety-four HIV+ individuals were included in the analysis median time since HIV diagnosis was 17 years and a median age of 50 years old [interquartile range (IQR) 44.0–55.0]; 88 (45.4%) were female and 108 (72.5%) were Caucasians (Table 1). Twenty patients (10.4%) were obese with a body mass index ≥30 kg/m^2. Almost all patients (99.0%) were on antiretroviral therapy with a majority (88.5%) on nucleoside reverse transcriptase inhibitor (NRTI) treatment. Protease inhibitors (PIs) were used in 50.1% of the patients while 43.7% were taking non-nucleoside reverse transcriptase inhibitor (NNRTI). Among those, 36 (18.6%) were taking efavirenz (EFV), 34 (17.6%) on etravirine and 14 (7.2%) on nevirapine. Eighty-six percent had a viral load below the threshold of 40 copies/mL; median CD4 count was 569.0 cell/mm^3 (IQR: 403.0–710.0). Sixty-eight patients (35.6%) reported signs of depression (moderate 23.6%; severe 12.0%). Of them, a psychiatric intervention was indicated in 89.0%, including a psychiatric evaluation in 22.9%, a psychopharmacologic treatment in 33.3%, and a psychotherapeutic treatment in 65.6%. Ninety-nine patients (51.9%) were anxious (moderate 27.8%; severe 24.1%). A psychiatric intervention was indicated in 83.9% of those, including a psychiatric evaluation in 18.3%, a psychopharmacologic treatment in 29.6%, and a psychotherapeutic treatment in 72.3%. However, we do not have the information on whether the patient came or not to his or her appointment. Finally, 93 (49.5%) mentioned poor quality of life (≤50%) (Table 1).

Prevalence of LD

The prevalence of LD signs and symptoms were assessed using both the LDCD [10] and HOPS scores [8] (Additional file 1: Table S1). The LDCD score diagnosed LD among 57.8% individuals (from subtle to very severe LDCD score). Of these, 39.7% had imaging or biological features corresponding to severe/very severe LD

Table 1 Characteristics of the study population

	N missing	All patients	Quality of Life[a]		p-value
			Poor (≤50% visual score)	High (>50% visual score)	
		Median (IQR)	Median (IQR)	Median (IQR)	
		N = 194	N = 93	N = 95	
Patient characteristics					
Sex female, n (%)		88.0 (45.4)	50 (53.8)	34 (35.8)	0.013*
Age (years)		50.0 (44.0–55.0)	48.0 (43.0–52.0)	51.0 (45.0–59.0)	0.008*
Ethnicity	45				0.005*
Caucasians n (%)		108 (72.5)	42 (61.8)	62 (82.7)	
Africans n (%)		29 (19.5)	21 (30.9)	7 (9.3)	
Others n (%)		12 (8.0)	5 (7.3)	6 (8.0)	
Waist/hip ratio	9	0.9 (0.9–1.0)	0.9 (0.8–1.0)	0.9 (0.9–1.0)	0.105
VAT/SAT ratio[b,c]	9	0.5 (0.3–1.0)	0.4 (0.2–0.7)	0.5 (0.3–1.1)	0.009*
Body mass index (kg/m^2)[d]	1	24.0 (22.0–27.0)	24.0 (22.0–27.0)	24.0 (22.0–26.0)	0.547
Triglycerides (mmol/l)		1.3 (0.9–2.2)	1.2 (0.8–1.9)	1.4 (1.0–2.4)	0.252
Total cholesterol (mmol/l)		5.1 (4.4–5.7)	5.0 (4.3–5.7)	5.1 (4.7–5.9)	0.105
HDL cholesterol (mmol/l)		1.2 (0.9–1.4)	1.1 (0.9–1.4)	1.2 (0.9–1.4)	0.795
HIV characteristics					
HIV duration (years)	20	17.0 (11.0–22.0)	15.5 (10.0–21.0)	18.5 (12.0–22.0)	0.099
CDC HIV stage[e]	14				0.362
A, n (%)		85.0 (47.2)	36.0 (41.9)	46.0 (52.3)	
B, n (%)		33.0 (18.3)	16.0 (18.6)	15.0 (17.0)	
C, n (%)		62.0 (34.4)	34.0 (39.5)	27.0 (30.7)	
CD4 (cells/mm^3)	4	569.0 (403.0–710.0)	612.0 (411.5–752.0)	533.5 (394.0–700.0)	0.116
HIV viral load (copy/ml)	2	20.0 (20.0–40.0)	20.0 (20.0–40.0)	20 (20.0–40.0)	0.495
Antiretroviral therapy, n (%)		192.0 (99.0)	92.0 (98.9)	94.0 (98.9)	0.988
Protease inhibitors containing, n (%)	1	97.0 (50.5)	42.0 (46.1)	51.0 (54.3)	0.271
Integrase inhibitor containing, n (%)	1	41.0 (21.3)	17.0 (18.7)	24.0 (25.5)	0.262
NRTI[e] containing, n (%)	1	170.0 (88.5)	83.0 (91.2)	81.0 (86.2)	0.280
NNRTI[f] containing, n (%)	1	84.0 (43.7)	42.0 (46.1)	41.0 (43.6)	0.729
Efavirenz, n (%)	1	36.0 (18.6)	20.0 (22.0)	15.0 (16.0)	0.296
Etravirine, n (%)	1	34.0 (17.6)	16.0 (17.6)	18.0 (19.1)	0.783
Nevirapine, n (%)	1	14.0 (7.2)	6.0 (6.6)	8.0 (8.5)	0.622
Other regimens, n (%)	1	7.0 (3.6)	2.0 (2.1)	5.0 (5.5)	0.230
Questionnaire assessments					
Depression (BDI score)[g]	3				0.001*
Absent/very subtle (≤10 points), n (%)		61 (31.9)	11.0 (11.8)	50.0 (52.6)	
Subtle (11–18 points), n (%)		62 (32.5)	30.0 (32.3)	31.0 (32.6)	
Moderate (19–29 points), n (%)		45 (23.6)	31.0 (33.3)	12.0 (12.6)	
Severe/very severe (≥30 points), n (%)		23 (12.0)	21.0 (22.6)	2.0 (2.1)	
Anxiety (STAI-Y-B score)[g]	3				0.001*
Absent/very subtle (≤35 points), n (%)		35.0 (18.3)	3.0 (3.2)	32.0 (34.0)	
Subtle (36–45 points), n (%)		57.0 (29.8)	19.0 (20.4)	36.0 (38.3)	
Moderate (46–55 points), n (%)		53.0 (27.8)	34.0 (36.6)	19.0 (20.2)	
Severe/very severe (≥56 points), n (%)		46.0 (24.1)	31.0 (33.3)	6.0 (6.4)	
Lipodystrophy (LDCD score)[i]	59				
Absent/very subtle (≤9.9 points), n (%)		57.0 (42.2)	28.0 (46.7)	27.0 (38.6)	0.581
Subtle (10–14.9 points), n (%)		35.0 (25.9)	12.0 (20.0)	22.0 (31.4)	

Table 1 continued

	N missing	All patients	Quality of Life[a]		p-value
			Poor (≤50% visual score)	High (>50% visual score)	
		Median (IQR)	Median (IQR)	Median (IQR)	
		N = 194	N = 93	N = 95	
Moderate (15–22.9 points), n (%)		12.0 (8.9)	6.0 (10.0)	5.0 (7.1)	
Severe/very severe (≥23 points), n (%)		31.0 (23.0)	14.0 (23.3)	16.0 (22.8)	

[a] Quality of Life Quantitative scale numbered 0%–100 according to the short version of EQ-5D-3L score.
[b] VAT: by CT-scan cross-section of 6 mm, level of L5: intra-abdominal adipose tissue.
[c] SAT: by CT-scan cross-section of 6 mm, level of L5: extra-abdominal adipose tissue.
[d] CDC HIV stage: according to CDC Classification System for HIV Infection by the United States Center for Disease Control and Prevention.
[e] NRTI: Nucleoside reverse transcriptase inhibitors.
[f] NNRTI: Non-nucleoside reverse transcriptase inhibitors.
[g] Depression: according to Beck Depression Inventory score by *Beck definition* (BDI).
[h] Anxiety: according to State Trait Anxiety Inventory by *Spielberger definition* (STAI-Y-B).
[i] LDCD: Lipodystrophy Case Definition by Carr et al.
* Significant *p*-value <0.05.

(Table 1). According to the HOPS score, 62.7, 63.5 and 35.5% of patients subjectively reported at least one site affected by fat hypertrophy or atrophy or both, respectively. Patients and physicians were agree on 80.3% (substantial agreement, kappa 0.61; p-value 0.001) regarding the atrophy and on 79.1% (substantial agreement, kappa 0.57; p-value 0.001) regarding the hypertrophy (Table 2). The agreement regarding the atrophy between the two LD tests (HOPS score and LDCD score) was moderate (patients and physicians observations; 55.9 and 48.1% respectively, p-values <0.001 for both). Regarding hypertrophy, the results were not significant (patients and physicians observations (data not shown).

Mental health, quality of life, and LD stratified by gender

Women were more likely to present signs of depression or anxiety compared to men (46.0 versus 26.9%; p-value = 0.006; and 62.5 versus 42.7%; p-value = 0.006 for depression and anxiety, respectively) (Table 3). Although there was no gender difference in severe LD according to the LDCD score (p-value = 0.082). Men seem to be more affected by LA, while women suffered mainly from LH according to the HOPS score (Table 3). Moreover, women were more likely to score lower on quality of life than men (59.5 versus 41.4%, respectively; p-value = 0.013).

Factors associated with poor quality of life (QoL)

Among the 188 patients who completed the questionnaire, 93 (49.5%) described a poor quality of life (median (IQR): 40.0 (30.0–50.0) with a visual score of <50% [29]. Although none of the demographic variables was found to be associated with poor quality of life in the multivariate models (M1, M2, Table 4), HIV-related variables, such as duration of HIV diagnosis (categorized by ≥10 years) and the presence of a detectable viral load (categorized by ≥40 copy/mL) both were associated with a poor quality of life; the shorter the time after HIV diagnosis, the worse the quality life (Table 4). Fat atrophy observed by patients and physicians was associated with a poor quality of life in the univariate model, but was no longer statistically significant in the adjusted analyses. Symptoms of depression [M1: OR = 3.62 (95% CI 0.99–13.27); M2: OR = 4.67 (95% CI 1.08–20.31), anxiety features (M1: OR = 7.10 (95% CI 1.99–25.30); M2: OR = 7.83 (95% CI 1.91–32.03)), and severe LD (LDCD) (M1: OR = 6.25

Table 2 Level of agreement between patients and physicians; HIV Outpatient Study (HOPS) score

	Patients observation N (%)	Physicians observation N (%)	Agreements (%)	Kappa	p-value	Interpretation
	N = 167	N = 144				
Atrophy	106 (63.5)	71 (49.3)	80.3	0.61	0.001*	Substantial
Hypertrophy	106 (62.7)	79 (54.9)	79.1	0.57	0.001*	Substantial

Atrophy/hypertrophy observed by patients/physicians: according to HOPS score by Lichtenchtein et al.
* Significant *p*-value <0.05.

Table 3 Prevalence of mental health alterations and lipodystrophy symptoms by gender

	Male N (%)	Female N (%)	p value
Presence of depression (BDI score ≥19)[a]	28 (26.9)	40 (46.0)	0.006*
Presence of anxiety (STAI-Y-B score ≥46)[b]	44 (42.7)	55 (62.5)	0.006*
Poor QoL (≤50% visual score)[c]	43 (41.4)	50 (59.5)	0.013*
Severe LD (LDCD score ≥23 points)[d]	21 (28.8)	10 (16.1)	0.082
HOPS score:[e]			
Atrophy observed by patients	66 (72.5)	40 (52.6)	0.008*
Atrophy observed by physicians	46 (60.0)	25 (37.3)	0.007*
Hypertrophy observed by patients	47 (51.1)	59 (76.6)	0.001*
Hypertrophy observed by physicians	35 (46.7)	44 (63.8)	0.039*

[a] Presence of depression: according to Beck Depression Inventory score by *Beck definition* (BDI).

[b] Presence of anxiety: according to State Trait Anxiety Inventory by *Spielberger definition* (STAI-Y-B).

[c] Quality of Life Quantitative scale numbered 0%–100 according to the short version of EQ-5D-3L score.

[d] Severe LD: according to LDCD score Lipodystrophy Case Definition by *Carr* et al.

[e] Atrophy/Hypertrophy observed by patients/physicians: according to HOPS score by *Lichtenchtein* et al.

* Significant *p*-value <0.05.

(95% CI:1.33–29.40); M2: OR = 5.22 (95% CI: 1.07–25.37)] were all associated with a poor quality of life in the univariate model (Table 4). They remained statistically significant in both multivariate analyses, apart from depression, which was significantly associated in the second model only (Table 4). No interaction between mental health disorders (depression or anxiety) and LD has been highlighted within the multivariate logistic regression model M2 (data not shown). Finally, we have assumed that the two models are correctly specified with no statistical difference and are in concordance (for M1 and M2, respectively: Hosmer–Lemeshow test: p-value: 0.521 and 0.286; area under the ROC curve 0.847 and 0.863; p-value: 0.338).

Discussion

Results of our study indicate a high frequency of LD and mental health disorders among HIV-infected men and women on successful ART presenting at the *LIPO group and metabolism* day clinic. Almost half of all patients considered themselves as suffering from a poor quality of life. Severe LD, depression, and anxiety were all associated with poor quality of life. This high level of LD frequency is partly due because the patients are referred to the day clinic by their treating physician.

Through these findings, we demonstrate that the objective signs of LD, based on a validated score (LDCD) and including morphologic data and metabolic values, are associated with a decreased quality of life and with the presence of mental health disorders. Fat loss observed by the patient and the physician (HOPS score) was also associated with a poor quality of life, but only in the univariate analysis.

Our results are consistent with several previous studies. First, some authors have highlighted a poor quality of life, severe stigma, and lower values in social and psychological scores regarding HIV-infected patients with or without reported LD [33, 34]. Of note, treatment of mental health disorders improved quality of life [33]. Secondly, other studies emphasized an association between LD and a negative effect on body image [18, 28, 34]. Indeed, because of body changes, stigma remains, leading to poor self esteem [20]. This leads to social isolation [24], decrease of sexual activity [26], and mental health disorders, such as anxiety and depression [35], which contribute to poor quality of life [21]. Guaraldi et al. evaluated LD by three scores, i.e., the Multicenter AIDS Cohort Study score (MACS)-HOPS-LDCD. The results of their study is consistent with our finding that LD is related to a poor quality of life [19]. Similar to other reports, they observed that the presence of LD can lead to ART discontinuation [19, 36, 37]. By contrast, a large study showed that individuals suffering from morphological alterations, such as LD, maintain a good adherence regarding ART [38].

Other studies show discordant results. Quality of life scales and psychological questionnaire often change from one study to another (i.e.: Health Related QoL (HRQoL) [13, 16, 18]; Profil der Lebensqualität Chronischkranker (PLC) [19], HIVspecific QoL [32]) and thus complicates comparison between the targeted population. In addition, study objectives vary (i.e.: cosmetic result, antiretroviral tolerance, global wellbeing, social isolation) and may influence the results. Barata et al. assessed a psychological questionnaire in outpatients with and without LD and found no difference in mental health disorders between the two groups [25]. Rajagopalan et al. found similar results regarding quality of life; however, a subgroup analysis showed that patients with LD, particularly homosexual men and patients undergoing psychiatric treatment, suffered from a low QoL [22].

LD remains a prevalent adverse event, despite the advent of new generation ARV drugs [18]. A recent French observational multicenter study showed that more than half of all patients on long-term effective ART suffer from disturbing and stigmatizing facial lipoatrophy. Congruent with reports from other groups, its prevalence is around 30% in patients who recently started

Table 4 Risk factors for poor quality of life

	Poor quality of life[a] (≤50% visual score)					
	Univariate regression		M1: p-value ≤0.2 in univariate model regression		M2: Clinical risk factors	
	OR (95%IC)	p-values	OR (95%IC)	p-values	OR (95%IC)	p-values
Patient characteristics						
Age (≥50 years)	0.62 (0.35–1.11)	0.109*	1.16 (0.38–3.54)	0.794	1.73 (0.52–5.68)	0.365
Gender (F)	2.09 (1.16–3.74)	0.014*	1.05 (0.35–3.10)	0.930	1.49 (0.46–4.78)	0.502
BMI (≥30 kg/m^2)[b]	0.90 (0.53–2.33)	0.828	–	–	1.01 (0.14–7.18)	0.988
Triglycerides (≥2.0 mmol/L)	0.62 (0.33–1.16)	0.135*	0.60 (0.19–1.94)	0.397		
HIV characteristics						
HIV duration (≥ 10 years)	0.43 (0.21–0.92)	0.030*	0.14 (0.03–0.79)	0.026**	0.10 (0.01–0.63)	0.014**
CDC HIV stage (B&C)[c]	1.52 (0.84-–2.77)	0.170*	0.81 (0.27–2.39)	0.697	0.95 (0.30–3.00)	0.936
CD4 (≤300 $cells/mm^3$)	0.57 (0.20–1.64)	0.300	–	–	0.09 (0.01–1.04)	0.054
HIV viral load (≥40 copy/mL)	2.55 (1.04–6.2)	0.039*	10.4 (1.73–2.55)	0.011**	10.39 (1.79–60.16)	0.009**
Current use of efavirenz	1.46 (0.69–3.06)	0.316	–	–		
Questionnaire assessments						
Severe LD (LDCD score ≥23 points)[d]	1.02 (0.45–2.33)	0.949	6.25 (1.33–29.40)	0.020**	5.22 (1.07–25.37)	0.040**
HOPS score:[e]						
Atrophy observed by patients	0.51 (0.27–0.99)	0.047*	0.49 (0.12–2.07)	0.334	0.27 (0.05–1.40)	0.120
Atrophy observed by physicians	0.51 (0.26–1.00)	0.051*	1.13 (0.30–4.26)	0.860	1.47 (0.37–5.84)	0.580
Hypertrophy observed by patients	1.37 (0.73–2.58)	0.325	–	–	0.50 (0.10–2.49)	0.396
Hypertrophy observed by physicians	0.75 (0.38–1.47)	0.400	–	–	0.56 (0.13–2.39)	0.438
Presence of depression (BDI score ≥19)[f]	7.33 (3.64–14.77)	0.001*	3.62 (0.99–13.27)	0.053	4.67 (1.08–20.31)	0.040**
Presence of anxiety (STAI-Y-B score ≥46)[g]	8.44 (4.37–16.30)	0.001*	7.10 (1.99–25.30)	0.003**	7.83 (1.91–32.03)	0.004**

[a] Quality of Life Quantitative scale numbered 0%–100 according to the short version of EQ-5D-3L score.

[b] BMI: body mass index (bodyweight in kilogram/(height in meter).

[c] CDC HIV stage: according to CDC Classification System for HIV Infection used by the United States Center for Disease Control and Prevention.

[d] Severe LD: according to LDCD score Lipodystrophy Case Definition by Carr et al.

[e] Atrophy/Hypertrophy observed by patients/physicians: according to HOPS score by Lichtenchtein et al.

[f] Presence of depression: according to Beck Depression Inventory score by *Beck definition* (BDI).

[g] Presence of anxiety: according to State Trait Anxiety Inventory by *Spielberger definition* (STAI-Y-B).

* Significant *p*-value in univariate model <0.2.

** Significant *p*-value <0.05.

their ARV treatment (1–5 years) [39]; the extent to which signs of LH reflect the physiological aging process is debated [40]. In our cohort, no difference was observed in the prevalence of LA and LH among individuals aged 50 or more and younger patients.

In a recent analysis of 15,275 participants to the Swiss HIV Cohort Study, Keiser et al. describe the suicide rate in HIV patients from 1998 to 2008. Despite a significant decrease rate of suicide between the pre era ARV drugs and the late era, suicides are more frequent in HIV population compared to general population [41]. In 62% of them, mental health disorders, as depression and anxiety, have been highlighted after the HIV diagnosis [41]. HIV infection and its possible impact on mental health can be compared to other chronic diseases, such as diabetes, asthma, or chronic kidney disease [42–47]. Indeed, a similar relationship has been highlighted in a recent study showing a major increase of anxiety symptoms as well as depression in patients with chronic obstructive pulmonary syndrome disease [48]. Interestingly, although the symptoms related to pulmonary disease could not be improved, recognition of psychological distress by the physician led to an enhancement of quality of life [48].

This study shows a complex interplay between quality of life, mental health disorders, and signs of LD. Severe LD and mental health disorders were all associated with a subjective impairment of quality of life. Moreover, individuals with a more recent diagnosis (<10 years) or those with a detectable viral load (≥40 copy/mL), more likely due to insufficient adherence to treatment, had also a poor quality of life. Therefore, psychological issues in HIV chronic infection is of major importance for daily constraints associated with the disease, adherence to therapy, and quality of life.

Women were more likely to express signs of depression and anxiety as found in other studies [49, 50]. Depressive symptoms are more than two-fold than those reported in the general population, while the number of men and women patients with anxiety symptoms is multiplied by 2.5 [51]. Men were more likely addressed to our group for LA and women for LH. We may speculate that the acceptability of LA and LH phenotype is gender-influenced.

Our study has some limitations. First, we used a modified quality of life score. This scale registers the self-estimation of the patient within a very specific timeframe. For this reason, a various number of independent variables can interfere with this estimate. We arbitrarily defined poor quality of life as between 0–50 and good quality of life between 51–100 and these thresholds could be challenged. However, this measure is simple to evaluate, and easily repeatable. Moreover, the QoL score that we used in our study has the advantage to be used directly during the clinical interview and measure synthetically the psychic pain in a biopsychosocial situation. As the validated Visual Analog Scale (VAS) largely used for pain appreciation, our QoL scale measure a subjective definition. Secondly, LD assessment remains difficult because of the lack of a gold standard definition. However, we consider that the use of two different scores, one based on the physician and patient perceptions and the other based on objective features, allowed us to capture with sufficient precision the prevalence and the severity of LD in this population. We were able to assess LD with great precision, using multiple and routinely-performed tools during the patient one-day visits to the day hospital. These included 191 of validated questionnaires, representing 98.5% of the patients included in the cohort, and 135 imaging (69.6%) (CT and DXA scans), as well as biological values, which are all features related to the LD. Regarding the HOPS score, there was good concordance between physician and patient assessments for fat atrophy and hypertrophy. Moreover, although the study population represented selected individuals referred by their practicing physician, it included both men and women of diverse ethnicity, thus making our results more consistent.

Conclusions

The majority of the HIV-infected patients seen in the metabolic clinic in Geneva describe, at least, one body site affected by LA or LH and are diagnosed with LD regarding the LDCD score. Depression as well as anxiety feature are also very frequent in our studied population, and, with the presence of LD, are related to a poor quality of life, leading to psycho-social consequences. Mental health and a simple score for quality of life should be routinely assessed among HIV-infected individuals, including those on effective ART, in order to recognize early signs and symptoms of psychological distress and to help patients have better outcomes in their daily life.

Abbreviations

AIDS: acquired immune deficiency syndrome; HIV: human immunodeficiency virus; NRTIs: nucleoside reverse transcriptase inhibitors; NNRTIs: non-nucleoside reverse transcriptase inhibitors; PIs: protease inhibitors; ARV: antiretroviral; ART: antiretroviral therapy; LD: lipodystrophy; LH: lipohypertrophy; LA: lipoatrophy; HOPS: HIV outpatients study; LDCD: lipodystrophy case definition; QoL: quality of life; CDC HIV stage: CDC Classification System for HIV Infection used by the United States Center for Disease Control and Prevention; DXA: bone dual-energy X-ray absorptiometry; CT: computed tomography; STAI Y-B: state trait anxiety inventory; BDI: beck depression inventory; VAT: visceral adipose tissue; SAT: subcutaneous adipose tissue; CI: confidence interval; OR: odds ratio.

Authors' contributions

AC and CV participated in the project study design. SZ, MB, EB, LTT, MS and ST were involved in data acquisition. CV and CD conducted statistical analysis. All authors read and approved the final manuscript.

Author details

[1] Department of Pediatrics, Children's Hospital-University Hospitals of Geneva, 6 Rue Willy-Donzé, 1211 Geneva 14, Switzerland. [2] HIV Unit, Department of Infectious Diseases, University Hospitals of Geneva, 4, Rue Gabrielle-Perret-Gentil, 1211 Geneva 4, Switzerland. [3] Department of Dermatology and Venerology, University Hospitals of Geneva, 4, Rue Gabrielle-Perret-Gentil, 1211 Geneva 4, Switzerland. [4] Department of Psychiatric Diseases, University Hospitals of Geneva, 4, Rue Gabrielle-Perret-Gentil, 1211 Geneva 4, Switzerland. [5] Department of Nuclear Medicine, University Hospitals of Geneva, 4, Rue Gabrielle-Perret-Gentil, 1211 Geneva 4, Switzerland. [6] Department of Radiology, University Hospitals of Geneva, 4, Rue Gabrielle-Perret-Gentil, 1211 Geneva 4, Switzerland. [7] Department of Infectious Diseases, Hospital of Lugano, Via Tesserete 46, 6900 Lugano, Switzerland.

Acknowledgements

The authors would like to acknowledge the support of this work by the members of the day clinic *LIPO group and metabolism* day clinic at the University Hospitals of Geneva. http://www.lipodystrophy-hug-ge.ch. We thank Rosemary Sudan for editorial assistance.

Funding sources

LIPO Group and Metabolism is sponsored by the Center for Research, University Hospitals of Geneva, SIDAIDE Foundation, AbbVie, Gilead, ViiV Healthcare, Merck Sharpe & Dohme AG, and Janssen-Cilag.

Competing interest

AC received travel grants from Gilead, Boehringer-Ingelheim, Janssen-Cilag.

References

1. UNAIDS/WHO (2013) AIDS epidemic update: November 2013; http://www.unaids.org/sites/default/files/media_asset/UNAIDS_Global_Report_2013_en_1.pdf. Accessed 15 Jan 2014
2. H-C Collaboration, Ray M, Logan R, Sterne JA, Hernandez-Diaz S, Robins JM et al (2010) The effect of combined antiretroviral therapy on the overall mortality of HIV-infected individuals. AIDS 24(1):123–137. doi:10.1097/QAD.0b013e3283324283
3. Fauci AS, Marston HD (2013) Achieving an AIDS-free world: science and implementation. Lancet 382(9903):1461–1462. doi:10.1016/S0140-6736(13)62042-5
4. Palella FJ Jr, Delaney KM, Moorman AC, Loveless MO, Fuhrer J, Satten GA et al (1998) Declining morbidity and mortality among patients with advanced human immunodeficiency virus infection. HIV Outpatient Study Investigators. N Engl J Med 338(13):853–860. doi:10.1056/NEJM199803263381301
5. Carr A, Samaras K, Burton S, Law M, Freund J, Chisholm DJ et al (1998) A syndrome of peripheral lipodystrophy, hyperlipidaemia and insulin resistance in patients receiving HIV protease inhibitors. AIDS 12(7):F51–F58
6. Rakotoambinina B, Medioni J, Rabian C, Jubault V, Jais JP, Viard JP (2001) Lipodystrophic syndromes and hyperlipidemia in a cohort of HIV-1-infected patients receiving triple combination antiretroviral therapy with a protease inhibitor. J Acquir Immune Defic Syndr 27(5):443–449
7. Calmy A (2003) La lipodystrophie. Rev Med Suisse 2453
8. Lichtenstein KA, Ward DJ, Moorman AC, Delaney KM, Young B, Palella FJ Jr et al (2001) Clinical assessment of HIV-associated lipodystrophy in an ambulatory population. AIDS 15(11):1389–1398
9. Carr A, Emery S, Law M, Puls R, Lundgren JD, Powderly WG et al (2003) An objective case definition of lipodystrophy in HIV-infected adults: a case–control study. Lancet 361(9359):726–735
10. Carr A, Law M, Group HIVLCDS (2003) An objective lipodystrophy severity grading scale derived from the lipodystrophy case definition score. J Acquir Immune Defic Syndr 33(5):571–576
11. Guaraldi G, Stentarelli C, Zona S, Santoro A (2013) HIV-associated lipodystrophy: impact of antiretroviral therapy. Drugs 73(13):1431–1450. doi:10.1007/s40265-013-0108-1
12. de Waal R, Cohen K, Maartens G (2013) Systematic review of antiretroviral-associated lipodystrophy: lipoatrophy, but not central fat gain, is an antiretroviral adverse drug reaction. PLoS One 8(5):e63623. doi:10.1371/journal.pone.0063623
13. McComsey GA (2014) H-1644-HIV NRTI BMS-986001 in Antiretroviral-naïve subjects: evaluation of bone and metabolic safety data through week 48. Abstract ICAAC 2014; http://www.abstractsonline.com/Plan/ViewAbstract.aspx?sKey=36303ae1-2a15-4dd2-a960-f370b3647859&cKey=7f87a869-d8a9-44f4-912d-b46b7c65c5de&mKey=5d6b1802-e453-486b-bcbb-b11d1182d8bb. Accessed 8 Nov 2015
14. Martinez E (2011) Disorders of fat partitioning in treated HIV-infection. Best Pract Res Clin Endocrinol Metab 25(3):415–427. doi:10.1016/j.beem.2010.10.019
15. Guaraldi G, Murri R, Orlando G, Squillace N, Stentarelli C, Zona S et al (2008) Lipodystrophy and quality of life of HIV-infected persons. AIDS Rev 10(3):152–161
16. Guaraldi G, Orlando G, Murri R, Vandelli M, De Paola M, Beghetto B et al (2006) Quality of life and body image in the assessment of psychological impact of lipodystrophy: validation of the Italian version of assessment of body change and distress questionnaire. Qual Life Res 15(1):173–178. doi:10.1007/s11136-005-8342-y
17. Shenoy A, Ramapuram JT, Unnikrishan B, Achappa B, Madi D, Rao S et al (2013) Effect of lipodystrophy on the quality of life among people living with HIV/AIDS (PLHIV) on highly active antiretroviral therapy. J Int Assoc Provid AIDS Care. doi:10.1177/2325957413488205
18. Leclercq P, Goujard C, Duracinsky M, Allaert F, L'Henaff M, Hellet M et al (2013) High prevalence and impact on the quality of life of facial lipoatrophy and other abnormalities in fat tissue distribution in HIV-infected patients treated with antiretroviral therapy. AIDS Res Hum Retroviruses 29(5):761–768. doi:10.1089/AID.2012.0214
19. Guaraldi G, Murri R, Orlando G, Giovanardi C, Squillace N, Vandelli M et al (2008) Severity of lipodystrophy is associated with decreased health-related quality of life. AIDS Patient Care STDS 22(7):577–585. doi:10.1089/apc.2007.0173
20. Power R, Tate HL, McGill SM, Taylor C (2003) A qualitative study of the psychosocial implications of lipodystrophy syndrome on HIV positive individuals. Sex Transm Infect 79(2):137–141
21. Rajagopalan R, Laitinen D, Dietz B (2008) Impact of lipoatrophy on quality of life in HIV patients receiving anti-retroviral therapy. AIDS Care 20(10):1197–1201. doi:10.1080/09540120801926993
22. Blanch J, Rousaud A, Martinez E, De Lazzari E, Peri JM, Milinkovic A et al (2002) Impact of lipodystrophy on the quality of life of HIV-1-infected patients. J Acquir Immune Defic Syndr 31(4):404–407
23. Santos CP, Felipe YX, Braga PE, Ramos D, Lima RO, Segurado AC (2005) Self-perception of body changes in persons living with HIV/AIDS: prevalence and associated factors. AIDS 19(Suppl 4):S14–S21
24. Casado JL, Iglesias V, del Palacio M, Marin A, Perez-Elias MJ, Moreno A et al (2013) Social isolation in HIV-infected patients according to subjective patient assessment and DEXA-confirmed severity of lipodystrophy. AIDS Care 25(12):1599–1603. doi:10.1080/09540121.2013.793275
25. Barata A, Malouf J, Gutierrez M, Mateo GM, Sambeat MA, Gich I et al (2013) Psychopathology and psychosocial adjustment in patients with HIV-associated lipodystrophy. Braz J Infect Dis 17(4):444–449. doi:10.1016/j.bjid.2012.11.011
26. Guaraldi G, Luzi K, Murri R, Granata A, De Paola M, Orlando G et al (2007) Sexual dysfunction in HIV-infected men: role of antiretroviral therapy, hypogonadism and lipodystrophy. Antivir Ther 12(7):1059–1065
27. Crane HM, Grunfeld C, Harrington RD, Uldall KK, Ciechanowski PS, Kitahata MM (2008) Lipoatrophy among HIV-infected patients is associated with higher levels of depression than lipohypertrophy. HIV Med 9(9):780–786. doi:10.1111/j.1468-1293.2008.00631.x
28. Marin A, Casado JL, Aranzabal L, Moya J, Antela A, Dronda F et al (2006) Validation of a specific questionnaire on psychological and social repercussions of the lipodystrophy syndrome in HIV-infected patients. Qual Life Res 15(5):767–775. doi:10.1007/s11136-005-5001-2
29. http://www.euroqol.org/fileadmin/user_upload/Documenten/PDF/Folders_Flyers/UserGuide_EQ-5D-5L_v2.0_October_2013.pdf. Accessed 15 Jan 2014
30. Spielberger CD, Gorusch RL, Lushene R, Vagg PR, Jacobs GA (1983) Manual for State-Trait Anxiety Inventory. Consulting Psychologist Press, Palo Alto, CA
31. Beck ATSR (1988) Carbin MG psychometric properties of the Beck Depression Inventory: twenty-five years of evaluation. Clin Psychol Rev 8(1):77–100
32. Ferland M, Despres JP, Tremblay A, Pinault S, Nadeau A, Moorjani S et al (1989) Assessment of adipose tissue distribution by computed axial tomography in obese women: association with body density and anthropometric measurements. Br J Nutr 61(2):139–148
33. Arseniou S, Arvaniti A, Samakouri M (2014) HIV infection and depression. Psychiatry Clin Neurosci 68(2):96–109. doi:10.1111/pcn.12097
34. Burgoyne R, Collins E, Wagner C, Abbey S, Halman M, Nur M et al (2005) The relationship between lipodystrophy-associated body changes and measures of quality of life and mental health for HIV-positive adults. Qual Life Res 14(4):981–990
35. Tien PC, Barron Y, Justman JE, Hyman C, Cohen MH, Young M et al (2007) Antiretroviral therapies associated with lipoatrophy in HIV-infected women. AIDS Patient Care STDS 21(5):297–305. doi:10.1089/apc.2006.128
36. Ammassari A, Murri R, Pezzotti P, Trotta MP, Ravasio L, De Longis P et al (2001) Self-reported symptoms and medication side effects influence adherence to highly active antiretroviral therapy in persons with HIV infection. J Acquir Immune Defic Syndr 28(5):445–449
37. Duran S, Saves M, Spire B, Cailleton V, Sobel A, Carrieri P et al (2001) Failure to maintain long-term adherence to highly active antiretroviral therapy: the role of lipodystrophy. AIDS 15(18):2441–2444
38. Guaraldi G, Murri R, Orlando G, Orlandi E, Sterrantino G, Borderi M et al (2003) Morphologic alterations in HIV-infected people with lipodystrophy are associated with good adherence to HAART. HIV Clin Trials 4(2):99–106
39. Cabrero E, Griffa L, Burgos A, Group HIVBPCS (2010) Prevalence and impact of body physical changes in HIV patients treated with highly active antiretroviral therapy: results from a study on patient and physician perceptions. AIDS Patient Care STDS 24(1):5–13. doi:10.1089/apc.2009.0191
40. Guaraldi G, Stentarelli C, Zona S, Santoro A, Beghetto B, Carli F et al (2014) The natural history of HIV-associated lipodystrophy in the changing scenario of HIV infection. HIV Med. doi:10.1111/hiv.12159

41. Keiser O, Spoerri A, Brinkhof MW, Hasse B, Gayet-Ageron A, Tissot F et al (2010) Suicide in HIV-infected individuals and the general population in Switzerland, 1988–2008. Am J Psychiatry 167(2):143–150. doi:10.1176/appi.ajp.2009.09050651
42. Wand H, Calmy A, Carey DL, Samaras K, Carr A, Law MG et al (2007) Metabolic syndrome, cardiovascular disease and type 2 diabetes mellitus after initiation of antiretroviral therapy in HIV infection. AIDS 21(18):2445–2453. doi:10.1097/QAD.0b013e3282efad32
43. Jurisic-Erzen D, Benko K, Ljubic S, Jerkovic R (2011) The prevalence of depression and anxiety in seafarers type 2 diabetic patients. Coll Antropol 35(4):1067–1070
44. Cinar N, Kizilarslanoglu MC, Harmanci A, Aksoy DY, Bozdag G, Demir B et al (2011) Depression, anxiety and cardiometabolic risk in polycystic ovary syndrome. Hum Reprod 26(12):3339–3345. doi:10.1093/humrep/der338
45. Takeuchi T, Nakao M, Nomura K, Inoue M, Tsurugano S, Shinozaki Y et al (2009) Association of the metabolic syndrome with depression and anxiety in Japanese men: a 1-year cohort study. Diabetes Metab Res Rev 25(8):762–767. doi:10.1002/dmrr.1041
46. Trzcinska H, Przybylski G, Kozlowski B, Derdowski S (2012) Analysis of the relation between level of asthma control and depression and anxiety. Med Sci Monit 18(3):CR190–CR194
47. Lee YJ, Kim MS, Cho S, Kim SR (2013) Association of depression and anxiety with reduced quality of life in patients with predialysis chronic kidney disease. Int J Clin Pract 67(4):363–368. doi:10.1111/ijcp.12020
48. Yildirim A, Asilar RH, Bakar N, Demir N (2013) Effect of anxiety and depression on self-care agency and quality of life in hospitalized patients with chronic obstructive pulmonary disease: a questionnaire survey. Int J Nurs Pract 19(1):14–22. doi:10.1111/ijn.12031
49. Dumont IP, Olson AL (2012) Primary care, depression, and anxiety: exploring somatic and emotional predictors of mental health status in adolescents. J Am Board Fam Med 25(3):291–299. doi:10.3122/jabfm.2012.03.110056
50. Schandl A, Bottai M, Hellgren E, Sundin O, Sackey P (2012) Gender differences in psychological morbidity and treatment in intensive care survivors—a cohort study. Crit Care 16(3):R80. doi:10.1186/cc11338
51. Kessler RC, Berglund P, Demler O, Jin R, Merikangas KR, Walters EE (2005) Lifetime prevalence and age-of-onset distributions of DSM-IV disorders in the National Comorbidity Survey Replication. Arch Gen Psychiatry 62(6):593–602. doi:10.1001/archpsyc.62.6.593

19

HIV-1 transmitted drug resistance mutations among antiretroviral therapy-Naïve individuals in Surabaya, Indonesia

Tomohiro Kotaki[1,2], Siti Qamariyah Khairunisa[1], Adiana Mutamsari Witaningrum[1], Muhammad Qushai Yunifiar M[1], Septhia Dwi Sukartiningrum[1], Muhammad Noor Diansyah[4], Retno Pudji Rahayu[1], Nasronudin[1,3] and Masanori Kameoka[2,5*]

Abstract

Background: The emergence of transmitted drug resistance (TDR) compromises the effect of antiretroviral therapy (ART), resulting in treatment failure of human immunodeficiency virus (HIV) disease. Although more than a decade has passed since ART was introduced into Indonesia, information on TDR is limited. Here, a genotypic study of TDR among ART-naïve individuals was conducted in Surabaya, Indonesia.

Method: HIV-1 seropositive participants were recruited from the communities of commercial sex workers and intravenous drug users as well as from the university teaching hospital in Surabaya. Protease (PR) and reverse transcriptase (RT) genes were sequenced in order to conduct HIV-1 subtyping and phylogenetic analysis and to detect TDR. TDR was defined as the presence of at least one surveillance drug resistance mutation on the WHO list or major drug resistance mutations in the International AIDS Society-USA panel.

Result: Fifty two and 47 of the PR and RT genes, respectively, were successfully sequenced in the 58 samples. HIV-1 subtyping revealed that 86.3% (50/58) of the sequenced samples were classified as CRF01_AE, 8.6% as subtype B, 3.4% as B/CRF01_AE, and 1.7% as A/G/CRF01_AE. TDR of PR inhibitors was not detected in this study. In contrast, TDR of RT inhibitors was detected in 4.3% (2/47) of samples. In addition, minor drug resistance mutations were detected in 98.1% (51/52) and 12.8% (6/47) of PR and RT genes, respectively.

Conclusion: This study clarified the predominance of the CRF01_AE strain in Surabaya, Indonesia. The prevalence of TDR was below 5%, indicating that the currently available first-line regimen is still effective in Surabaya. However, the prevalence might be underestimated since we detected only major population of HIV-1 in individuals. Therefore, continuous surveillance is required in order to detect the emergence of TDR in the early phase.

Keywords: HIV-1, Antiretroviral therapy, Transmitted drug resistance, Indonesia

Backgrounds

Antiretroviral therapy (ART) achieved the reduction of viral transmission, morbidity and mortality associated with human immunodeficiency virus (HIV) disease. However, the emergence of transmitted drug resistance (TDR) as a consequence of ART expansion represents a serious public health problem because TDR affects the treatment efficacy and clinical outcome [1,2]. Although the prevalence of TDR in resource-limited countries is currently <5% [3], it is expected to increase with ART expansion. TDR is a permanent challenge for HIV disease control.

HIV-1 is subdivided into four groups, M (major), O (outlying), N (new or non-M, non-O), and P. Group M accounts for the majority of HIV-1 infections. The viruses in group M are further classified into subtypes, circulating recombinant forms (CRFs) and unique recombinant forms (URFs), which are prevalent in specific geographic regions. While subtype B of HIV-1 is the predominant subtype in the Americas, Europe, and Australia,

* Correspondence: mkameoka@port.kobe-u.ac.jp
[2]Center for Infectious Diseases, Kobe University Graduate School of Medicine, Hyogo, Japan
[5]Department of International Health, Kobe University Graduate School of Health Sciences, Hyogo, Japan
Full list of author information is available at the end of the article

there is a growing epidemic of non-B subtypes and CRFs in Africa and Asia [4]. CRF01_AE is the major CRF prevalent throughout Southeast Asian countries including Indonesia [4]. Although surveillance studies on TDR have been conducted in Southeast Asian countries where CRF01_AE is prevalent, information on TDR as well as on CRF01_AE viruses is still limited [3,5].

In Indonesia, the estimated number of people living with HIV has been increasing and reached 610,000 in 2012, even though that of other Southeast Asian countries is stable or in decline [6]. Accordingly, it was estimated that the number of people eligible for ART, whose CD4+ T-cell count was below 500 cells/mm^3 (WHO criteria), would reach 510,000 in 2013 [6]. Even though the Indonesian government launched an ART expansion program in 2004 [7], the coverage rate among patients in need of ART was less than 18% until 2010 [6]. However, it increased markedly to 40% in 2011 according to the Ministry of Health, Mathematic Model of HIV Epidemic in Indonesia [8]. The number of patients with access to ART is therefore increasing in Indonesia.

The first-line regimen of ART recommended in Indonesia is a combination of two nucleoside reverse-transcriptase inhibitors (NRTIs) and a non-nucleoside reverse-transcriptase inhibitor (NNRTI) [5]. Lamivudine (3TC), zidovudine (AZT), tenofovir (TDF), nevirapine (NVP) and efavirenz (EFV) are commonly used. For patients with virological failure or adverse effects, ritonavir-boosted protease inhibitors (PIs) in combination with two NRTIs are recommended as the second-line regimen [5]. Other drugs, including didanosine (ddI), etravirine (ETR) and rilpivirine (RPV), are uncommon in Indonesia.

Although ART is successful in Indonesia, the emergence of drug resistance has been reported among treatment-failure patients [9]. After a decade of ART expansion in Indonesia, the emergence of TDR is inevitable. However, there are limited data on TDR among ART-naïve patients in Indonesia. It is important to monitor the prevalence of TDR in countries where the drug options are limited. In this report, a genotypic study of TDR among ART-naïve patients was conducted in Surabaya, Indonesia.

Results

Demographic data of the study subjects

Peripheral blood samples were collected from the participants from the communities of commercial sex workers (CSWs) and intravenous drug users (IDUs) as well as from the university teaching hospital in Surabaya. All participants were confirmed to be ART naïve at interview and/or from medical records. RNA and DNA were extracted from plasma and peripheral blood mononuclear cells (PBMC), respectively, isolated from peripheral blood samples. If a viral gene fragment failed to be amplified from the cDNA even after multiple attempts, it was amplified instead from DNA. In order to examine the genomic fragment of the major viral population in a sample, PCR products amplified at the end-point dilution of DNA templates were subjected to sequencing analysis.

As a result, 52 and 47 of the protease (PR) and reverse transcriptase (RT) genes, respectively, were successfully sequenced in the 58 samples. Of these, 13 and 22 of the PR and RT genes, respectively, were derived from DNA. The demographic data of the 58 individuals are shown in Table 1, along with the results of viral subtyping described below. Mean age was 33.2 years old (range 17–51). There was no significant difference in age and subtype among study participants. Detailed patient information including age, sample collection date and transmission route is shown in Additional file 1.

HIV-1 subtyping and phylogenetic analysis

HIV-1 subtyping was carried out for PR and RT gene sequences separately using recombinant identification program (RIP). Most PR and RT gene sequences were classified as CRF01_AE or subtype B. However, two RT gene sequences derived from SM11 and IDU11 were classified as B/CRF01_AE, and PR and RT gene sequences derived from PJ121 were G/CRF01_AE and A/G/CRF01_AE, respectively (Additional file 1). Phylogenetic trees of PR and RT gene sequences are shown in Figure 1. HIV-1 subtyping by phylogenetic analysis was consistent with RIP results, except for PJ121. With regard to the samples from PJ121, for the PR gene, phylogenetic analysis showed that it was clustered with subtype G and CRF02_AG, while RIP showed that it was G/CRF01_AE. For the RT gene, phylogenetic analysis showed its relevance to CRF01_AE, whereas RIP showed that it was A/G/CRF01_AE. Taken together, 50 samples (86.3%) were classified as CRF01_AE, 5 samples (8.6%) as subtype B, 2 samples (3.4%) as B/CRF01_AE and a sample (1.7%) derived from PJ121 as A/G/CRF01. In addition, jumping profile Hidden Markov Models (jpHMM) analysis revealed that viral gene fragments derived from SM11 and IDU11 (B/CRF01_AE) had their breakpoints at 2884–2883 and 2889–2909 (HXB2 position), respectively, which were similar to that of CRF33_01B reference strains (2847–2884) (Additional file 2). The breakpoint of the viral gene fragment from PJ121 was not similar to that of the CRFs registered in the Los Alamos HIV sequence database (http://www.hiv.lanl.gov/content/sequence/HIV/CRFs/CRFs.html).

Genotypic analysis of drug resistance for PR gene

In this study, TDR was defined as the presence of at least one major drug resistance mutation listed in the international AIDS Society (IAS)-USA panel or surveillance drug resistance mutation in world health organization

Table 1 Demographic characteristics, viral subtypes and time after infection of study subjects*

	All (n = 58)	CSW community (n = 22)	IDU community (n = 16)	Hospital (n = 20)
Mean age (years old)	32.2	30.3	33.9	33.0
Gender				
Male	26 (44.8%)**	0 (0%)	15 (93.8%)	11 (55.0%)
Female	32 (55.2%)	22 (100%)	1 (6.2%)	9 (45.0%)
Viral subtype				
CRF01_AE	50 (86.3%)	20 (91.0%)	12 (75.0%)	18 (90.0%)
Subtype B	5 (8.6%)	0 (0%)	3 (18.8%)	2 (10.0%)
B/CRF01_AE recombinant	2 (3.4%)	1 (4.5%)	1 (6.2%)	0 (0%)
A/G/CRF01_AE recombinant	1 (1.7%)	1 (4.5%)	0 (0%)	0 (0%)

*There was no significant difference among study participants from the communities of CSWs and IDUs, and from Airlangga University Teaching Hospital in terms of mean age and viral subtype. Gender was statistically different because we aimed to recruit female CSW.
**The proportion (%) of the number of individuals in a question item is shown in parentheses.

(WHO) surveillance list [10,11]. According to the lists, TDR was not detected in PR gene sequences. However, minor drug resistance mutations listed in the IAS-USA panel were detected in 98.1% (51/52) of the study subjects, shown in Table 2 [10]: L10I/V, G16E, K20R, L33F, M36I/L, I62V, L63P, I64V, H69K/R, V77I, V82I, L89M/I and I93L. Each CRF01_AE strain possessed at least 3 and up to 8 mutations. M36I/L, H69K/R and L89M/I were highly conserved in the CRF01_AE strain, at rates of 95.7% (45/47), 100% and 100%, respectively (Table 2). These mutations were known as natural polymorphism among CRF01_AE [12].

Genotypic analysis of drug resistance for RT gene

Two of 47 samples (4.3%) possessed TDR in RT gene sequences. The RT gene fragment from SM18 contained a K101E mutation, which is a major drug resistance mutation to NNRTI; ETR and RPV [10]. Interestingly, the sample from UA6 contained 6 major drug resistance mutations: D67N, K70R, M184V, T215F, K219Q, conferring resistant to almost all NRTI (except ddI), and K103N conferring resistance to NNRTI; NVP and EFV [10]. RT gene fragment of UA6 was amplified from undiluted DNA (because of the failure of PCR from diluted DNA), indicating that minor population of HIV also possessed multiple TDR. The failure of PCR using RNA might be due to poor sample storage condition. Other than TDR, four minor drug resistance mutations (A98G, E138G/A, V179D), which confer resistance to ETR and/or RPV, were detected among 6 samples of CRF01_AE (12.8%: 6/47) [10]. The data are summarized in Table 3.

Discussion

Here we report the circulating HIV-1 subtype and the prevalence of TDR among 58 HIV-1-infected drug-naïve individuals in Surabaya, Indonesia. Of 58 sequenced samples, 50 (86.3%) were classified as CRF01_AE, 5 (8.6%) as subtype B, 2 (3.4%) as B/CRF01_AE, and 1 (1.7%) as A/G/CRF01_AE. These results are consistent with a previous report on the predominance of CRF01_AE in Southeast Asian countries [4]. According to the phylogenetic tree of RT gene and jpHMM analysis, B/CRF01_AE recombinants in Surabaya were closely related to CRF33_01B, which was currently reported in Indonesia [13]. The viral gene derived from PJ121, an A/G/CRF01_AE recombinant, seems a URF because its breakpoint and recombination pattern had not been reported as of December 2014, in the Los Alamos HIV sequence database. The HIV gene fragment analyzed in the present study was not informative enough to determine actual CRFs. Further sequence analysis of different regions must therefore be carried out.

Genotypic analysis of drug resistance revealed no evidence of the circulation of TDR against PIs in Surabaya. This was not surprising because access to PIs is limited in Surabaya, even though PI is recommended as the second-line regimen. Interestingly, each CRF01_AE strain possessed 3 to 8 minor drug resistance mutations based on the IAS-USA panel [10]. Although these mutations were considered natural polymorphisms of CRF01_AE, the accumulation of minor mutations may affect the efficacy of PIs. Further studies are necessary to clarify their impact on the susceptibility of PIs.

In contrast, the prevalence of TDR against RT inhibitors was 4.3% (2/47). This was consistent with a previous report that TDR in Asian countries was <5%, but is gradually increasing [3]. The sample from SM18 contained a K101E mutation conferring resistance to ETR and RPV [10]. However, the emergence of K101E is probably not associated with ART expansion in Indonesia because ETR and RPV are not commonly used. It is considered that K101E appeared as a natural polymorphism in Indonesian CRF01_AE. In contrast, the RT gene fragment derived from UA6 possessed 6 major mutations and 1 minor mutation. The virus in UA6 is considered to be resistant to the common first-line regimen in Indonesia

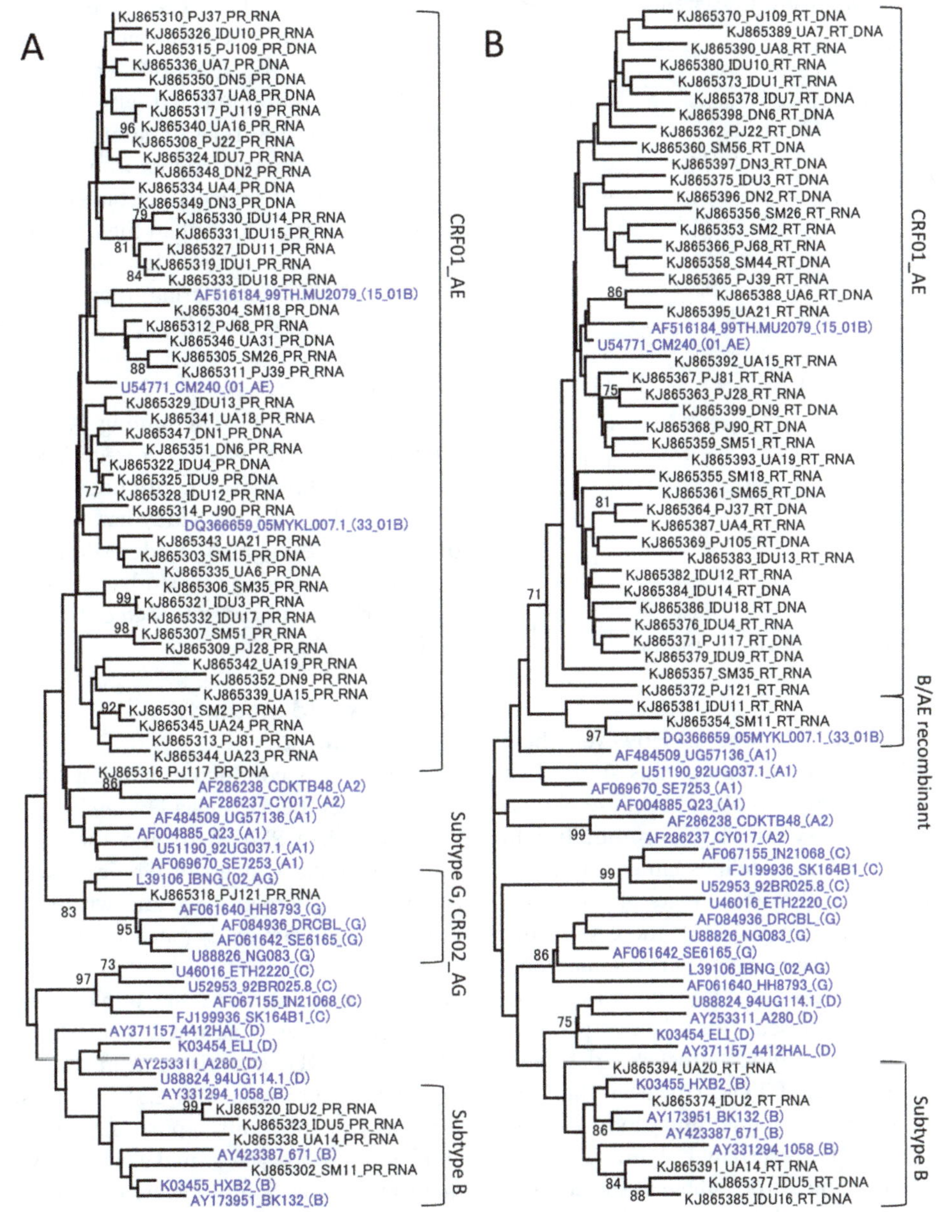

Figure 1 Neighbor-joining phylogenetic trees of PR and RT gene sequences. Phylogenetic trees were constructed for newly sequenced HIV-1 PR **(A)** and RT **(B)** genes along with the corresponding viral gene of reference HIV-1 strains, representing subtype A1, subtype A2, subtype B, subtype C, subtype D, subtype G, CRF01_AE, CRF02_AG, CRF15_01B and CRF33_01B. The reference strains of the HIV-1 subtype were shown in blue and bold. The sequence codes are presented as the GenBank accession number, patient ID or name of reference strain, and the subtype or CRF of reference strain (shown in parentheses) in order. DNA or RNA following the patient ID indicates the origin of the viral sequence, i.e., DNA extracted from PBMC or RNA extracted from a plasma sample, respectively. Bootstrap values are shown when the values are >70.

(3TC, AZT, TDF, NVP and EFV). The patient UA6 was probably infected with HIV-1 by heterosexual intercourse (Additional file 1), indicating that the HIV-1 with multiple TDR had enough growth fitness for sexual transmission. A multiple drug resistant HIV was confirmed among drug-naïve HIV patient in Surabaya.

Four minor mutations (A98G, E138G/A, V179D) conferring resistance to ETR and/or RPV were detected among 6 samples. However, they are considered natural polymorphisms because these mutations are excluded from the WHO list [11], and ETR and RPV are not commonly used in Indonesia.

In the WHO TDR surveillance guideline, the prevalence of TDR is categorized into three groups: <5% (low level), 5–15% (medium level) and >15% (high level) [14,15]. The <5% level is the desired threshold for any country scaling up ART. According to this guideline, the currently recommended first- and second-line regimens

Table 2 Appearance of minor drug resistance mutations in PR gene*

Mutation	Frequency (%)			
	All (n = 52)	CRF01_AE (n = 47)	Subtype B (n = 4)	G/CRF01_AE (n = 1)
L10I/V	11 (21.2)	10 (21.3)	1 (25.0)	0 (0)
G16E	16 (30.8)	15 (31.9)	1 (25.0)	0 (0)
K20R	19 (36.5)	19 (40.4)	0 (0)	0 (0)
L33F	7 (13.5)	7 (14.9)	0 (0)	0 (0)
M36I/L	46 (88.5)	45 (95.7)	0 (0)	1 (100)
I62V	6 (11.5)	6 (12.8)	0 (0)	0 (0)
L63P	5 (9.6)	4 (8.5)	0 (0)	1 (100)
I64V	3 (5.8)	2 (4.3)	1 (25.0)	0 (0)
H69K/R	48 (92.3)	47 (100)	0 (0)	1 (100)
V77I	12 (23.1)	10 (21.3)	2 (50.0)	0 (0)
V82I	3 (5.8)	3 (6.4)	0 (0)	0 (0)
L89M/I	48 (92.3)	47 (100)	0 (0)	1 (100)
I93L	15 (28.8)	12 (25.5)	3 (75.0)	0 (0)

*Mutations were detected manually according to the International AIDS Society-USA panel.

are appropriate in Surabaya, Indonesia. However, there were several limitations in the design of this study. Our sample collection might have been biased because participants were recruited from CSW and IDU communities. In addition, although the WHO guidelines aimed to recruit recently infected individuals (below 25 years of age, CD4$^+$ T-cell counts above 500 cells/mm^3) [15], these were not used in this study for practical reasons. A previous report indicated that certain drug resistance mutations would revert to the wild type in the absence of selective pressure by ART [16]. Therefore, it is probable that our data may underestimate the prevalence of TDR. However, the TDR including most thymidine analogue mutations (M41L, D67N, K70R, L210W, T215 revertant but not T215Y/F and K219Q) and K103N, which were stable in the absence of ART, were rarely detected in our study subjects even though they have been frequently detected among treatment-failure patients in Indonesia [9,16]. Therefore, it was estimated that the prevalence of TDR among the population recently infected with HIV-1 is not high. It is helpful for the future ART strategy to clarify the prevalence of TDR among patients who are about to start ART, even if the study subjects are biased and may not reflect recent infections. Other than the quality of samples, direct sequencing might cause underestimation, as previously reported [17,18]. Considering these limitations, the data must be evaluated carefully.

Conclusion

The prevalence of TDR among ART-naïve patients in Surabaya was <5%, which is categorized as low by WHO. However, additional or continuous surveillance must be conducted because this study had several limitations, and the prevalence might be underestimated and biased. The low TDR observed in this study calls for continuous monitoring of TDR in order to detect the emergence of TDR in the early phase.

Materials and methods

Ethics statement

This study was conducted with approval from the ethics committee of the Airlangga University (permission number: 25-995/UN3.14/PPd/2013) and the medical ethics committee at Kobe University Graduate School of Medicine (permission number: 784), and written informed consent was obtained from study participants.

Participant recruitment and sample collection

Participants were recruited from the communities of CSWs and IDUs as well as from the university teaching hospital in Surabaya. The CSW study subjects were the same as in a previous report [19]. All participants were confirmed to be ART naïve at interview and/or from medical records. Samples were collected between October 2012 and April 2014. Ten milliliters of

Table 3 Demographic characteristics of 6 individuals infected with HIV-1 with drug resistance mutation to RT inhibitors*

ID	Group	Subtype	Drug resistance mutation		
			NNRTI	NRTI	Resistance
SM18	CSW	CRF01_AE	**K101E****E138G		**RPV***** ETR
UA6	Hospital	CRF01_AE	**K103N** A98G	**D67N K70R, M184V T215F K219Q**	**3TC, AZT, TDF, NVP, EFV, ABC, d4T, FTC,** ETR, RPV
IDU9	IDU	CRF01_AE	E138A		RPV, ETR
UA7	Hospital	CRF01_AE	E138A		RPV, ETR
UA15	Hospital	CRF01_AE	V179D		RPV, ETR
DN6	Hospital	CRF01_AE	E138G		RPV, ETR

*HIV-1 drug resistance mutations were detected according to the International AIDS Society-USA panel and WHO surveillance list.
**Major drug resistance mutations are shown in bold.
***Highly resistant drugs are shown in bold.

ethylenediaminetetraacetic acid anti-coagulated peripheral blood was collected from each participant. Plasma was then isolated from peripheral blood samples. In addition, peripheral blood mononuclear cells (PBMC) were isolated by density gradient centrifugation using Histopaque 1077 (Sigma-Aldrich, St. Louis, MO, USA). RNA and DNA were extracted from plasma and PBMC using the QIAamp Viral RNA Mini kit (Qiagen, Hilden, Germany) and the GenElute Mammalian Genomic DNA Miniprep kit (Sigma-Aldrich), respectively.

Amplification of HIV-1 genomic fragment and sequence analysis

Viral RNA was reverse transcribed to cDNA using the SuperScript III First-Stand Synthesis kit (Invitrogen, Carlsbad, CA, USA). Generated cDNA was subjected to amplification of the viral gene for both the PR and RT encoding regions in a separate reaction by nested PCR using Ex Taq (Takara Bio, Shiga, Japan). Primer information is shown in Additional file 3. If a viral gene fragment failed to be amplified from the cDNA even after multiple attempts, it was amplified instead from DNA extracted from PBMC. In order to examine the genomic fragment of the major viral population in a sample, PCR products amplified at the end-point dilution of DNA templates were subjected to sequencing analysis.

Sequencing analysis of the amplified fragment was performed using the BigDye Terminator v3.1 Cycle Sequencing kit with an ABI PRISM 3500 × 1 genetic analyzer (Applied Biosystems, Foster City, CA, USA). Data were assembled and aligned using Genetyx ver. 10 software (Genetyx, Tokyo, Japan). Nearly the full length of the PR gene [(280 bp; corresponding to nucleotides 2262 to 2541 of a HIV-1 reference strain, HXB2 (GenBank accession no. K03455)] and part of the RT gene (762 bp; nucleotides 2550 to 3311) were sequenced and subjected to subsequent analysis.

HIV-1 subtyping and phylogenetic analysis

Obtained sequence data were subjected to HIV-1 subtyping using the RIP, available at the website of the HIV sequence database (www.hiv.lanl.gov/). In addition, neighbor-joining (NJ) trees with a Kimura two-parameter model were constructed using MEGA5.2 software [20–22]. Bootstrap values (1,000 replicates) for relevant nodes were reported on a representative tree [23]. If one of the PR and RT genes are failed to be sequenced, the subtype was assigned based on the other gene. In addition, breakpoints of the recombinant forms were determined by using the jpHMM (http://jphmm.gobics.de/) [24]. The nucleotide sequences of these PR and RT genes have been deposited in the GenBank database under accession numbers KJ865301-KJ865352 and KJ865353-KJ865399.

Detection of drug resistance mutations

HIV-1 TDRs were detected manually according to the IAS-USA panel and WHO surveillance list [10,11]. In this study, TDR in a patient was defined as the presence of at least one major drug resistance mutation listed in the IAS-USA panel or surveillance drug resistance mutation in WHO surveillance list. In addition to TDR, minor drug resistance mutations in the IAS-USA panel were detected as well [10].

Statistical analysis

Statistical analysis was performed using Fisher's exact test for categorical variables. The P value was calculated using the program available at the web site, http://aoki2.-si.gunma-u.ac.jp/exact/fisher/getpar.html. P values ≤0.05 were considered to be significant.

Abbreviations

ART: Antiretroviral therapy; HIV: Human immunodeficiency virus; TDR: Transmitted drug resistance; CRF: Circulating recombinant form; URF: Unique recombinant form; NRTI: Nucleoside reverse-transcriptase inhibitor; NNRTI: Non-nucleoside reverse-transcriptase inhibitor; 3TC: Lamivudine; AZT: Zidovudine; TDF: Tenofovir; NVP: Nevirapine; EFV: Efavirenz; PI: Protease inhibitor; ddI: Didanosine; ETR: Etravirine; RPV: Rilpivirine; CSW: Commercial sex worker; IDU: Intravenous drug user; PBMC: Peripheral blood mononuclear cells; PR: Protease; RT: Reverse transcriptase; RIP: Recombinant Identification Program; jpHMM: Jumping profile Hidden Markov Models; IAS: International AIDS Society; WHO: World Health Organization; NJ: Neighbor-joining.

Competing interests

The authors declare that they have no competing interest.

Authors' contributions

TK carried out the molecular genetic studies, the sequence alignment and drafted the manuscript. SQK, AMW, MQYM and SDS carried out the molecular genetic studies. MN, RPR and N participated in the design and coordination of this study. MK conceived of the study, and participated in its design and coordination, and helped to draft the manuscript. All authors read and approved the final manuscript.

Acknowledgement

This work was supported by the program of the Japan Initiative for Global Research Network on Infectious Diseases (J-GRID); by the Ministry of Education, Culture, Sports, Science and Technology of Japan; and the Center of Excellence (COE) program by the Ministry for Research and Technology (RISTEK) of Indonesia. The funders had no role in the study design, data collection and analysis, decision to publish, or preparation of the manuscript. The manuscript was proofread by Medical English Service, Kyoto, Japan.

Author details

[1]Institute of Tropical Disease, Indonesia-Japan Collaborative Research Center for Emerging and Re-emerging Infectious Diseases, Airlangga University, Surabaya, Indonesia. [2]Center for Infectious Diseases, Kobe University Graduate School of Medicine, Hyogo, Japan. [3]Faculty of Medicine, Airlangga University, Surabaya, Indonesia. [4]Airlangga University Teaching Hospital, Surabaya, Indonesia. [5]Department of International Health, Kobe University Graduate School of Health Sciences, Hyogo, Japan.

References

1. Popp D, Fisher JD. First, do no harm: a call for emphasizing adherence and HIV prevention interventions in active antiretroviral therapy programs in the developing world. AIDS. 2002;16:676–8.
2. Pillay D, Bhaskaran K, Jurriaans S, Prins M, Masquelier B, Dabis F, et al. The impact of transmitted drug resistance on the natural history of HIV infection and response to first-line therapy. AIDS. 2006;20:21–8.
3. Sohn AH, Srikantiah P, Sungkanuparph S, Zhang F. Transmitted HIV drug resistance in Asia. Curr Opin HIV AIDS. 2013;8:27–33.
4. Hemelaar J, Gouws E, Ghys PD, Osmanov S. Global trends in molecular epidemiology of HIV-1 during 2000–2007. AIDS. 2011;25:679–89.
5. Trotter AB, Hong SY, Srikantiah P, Abeyewickreme I, Bertagnolio S, Jordan MR. Systematic review of HIV drug resistance in Southeast Asia. AIDS Rev. 2011;15:162–70.
6. UNAIDS. UNAIDS report on the global AIDS epidemic 2013. [www.unaids.org/en/resources/campaigns/globalreport2013/globalreport/]
7. WHO. Summary country profile for HIV/AIDS treatment scale up Indonesia. [www.who.int/3by5/support/june2005_idn.pdf]
8. Indonesian National AIDS Commission. Republic of Indonesia country report on the follow up to the Declaration of Commitment on HIV/AIDS (UNGASS) reporting period 2010–2011. [www.unaids.org/en/dataanalysis/knowyourresponse/countryprogressreports/2012countries/ce_ID_Narrative_Report.pdf]
9. Fibriani A, Wisaksana R, Indrati A, Hartantri Y, van de Vijver D, Schutten M, et al. Virological failure and drug resistance during first line anti-retroviral treatment in Indonesia. J Med Virol. 2013;85:1394–401.
10. Johnson VA, Calvez V, Gunthard HF, Paredes R, Pillay D, Shafer RW, et al. Update of the drug resistance mutations in HIV-1: March 2013. Top Antivir Med. 2013;21:6–14.
11. Bennett DE, Camacho RJ, Otelea D, Kuritzkes DR, Fleury H, Kiuchi M, et al. Drug resistance mutations for surveillance of transmitted HIV-1 drug-resistance: 2009 update. PLoS One. 2009;4:e4724.
12. Auwanit W, Isarangkura-Na-Ayuthaya P, Kasornpikul D, Ikuta K, Sawanpanyalert P, Kameoka M. Detection of drug resistance-associated and background mutations in human immunodeficiency virus type 1 CRF01_AE protease and reverse transcriptase derived from drug treatment-naive patients residing in central Thailand. AIDS Res Hum Retroviruses. 2009;25:625–31.
13. SahBandar IN, Takahashi K, Motomura K, Djoerban Z, Firmansyah I, Kitamura K, et al. The Indonesian variants of CRF33_01B: near-full length sequence analysis. AIDS Res Hum Retroviruses. 2010;27:97–102.
14. Bennett DE, Bertagnolio S, Sutherland D, Gilks CF. The world health organization's global strategy for prevention and assessment of HIV drug resistance. Antivir Ther. 2008;2(13):1–13.
15. Bennett DE, Myatt M, Bertagnolio S, Sutherland D, Gilks CF. Recommendations for surveillance of transmitted HIV drug resistance in countries scaling up antiretroviral treatment. Antivir Ther. 2008;2(13):25–36.
16. Castro H, Pillay D, Cane P, Asboe D, Cambiano V, Phillips A. Dunn DT; UK collaborative group on HIV drug resistance: persistence of HIV-1 transmitted drug resistance mutations. J Infect Dis. 2013;208:1459–63.
17. Simen BB, Simons JF, Hullsiek KH, Novak RM, MacArthur RD, Baxter JD, et al. Low-abundance drug-resistant viral variants in chronically HIV-infected, antiretroviral treatment-naïve patients significantly impact treatment outcomes. J Infect Dis. 2009;199:693–701.
18. Lataillade M, Chiarella J, Yang R, Schnittman S, Wirtz V, Uy J, et al. Prevalence and clinical significance of HIV drug resistance mutations by ultra-deep sequencing in antiretroviral-naïve subjects in the CASTLE study. PLoS One. 2010;5:e10952.
19. Kotaki T, Khairunisa SQ, Sukartiningrum SD, Arfijanto MV, Utsumi T, Normalina I, et al. High prevalence of HIV-1 CRF01_AE viruses among female commercial sex workers residing in Surabaya. Indonesia PLoS One. 2013;8:e82645.
20. Tamura K, Peterson D, Peterson N, Stecher G, Nei M, Kumar S, et al. Molecular evolutionary genetics analysis using maximum likelihood, evolutionary distance, and maximum parsimony methods. Mol Biol Evol. 2011;28:2731–9.
21. Kimura M. A simple method for estimating evolutionary rates of base substitutions through comparative studies of nucleotide sequences. J Mol Evol. 1980;16:111–20.
22. Saitou N, Nei M. The neighbor-joining method: a new method forreconstructing phylogenetic trees. Mol Biol Evol. 1987;4:406–25.
23. Felsenstein J. Confidence limits on phylogenies: an approach using the bootstrap. Evolution. 1985;39:783–91.
24. Bulla I, Schultz AK, Meinicke P. Improving hidden markov models for classification of human immunodeficiency virus-1 subtypes through linear classifier learning. Stat Appl Genet Mol Biol. 2012. 11: doi:10.2202/1544-6115.1680

20

Nutritional status and its association with quality of life among people living with HIV attending public anti-retroviral therapy sites of Kathmandu Valley, Nepal

Rajshree Thapa[1*], Archana Amatya[1], Durga Prasad Pahari[1], Kiran Bam[2] and M Sophia Newman[3]

Abstract

Background: Little evidence exists on the connections between nutrition, diet intake, and quality of life (QoL) among people living with HIV (PLHIV). The study aimed to estimate the prevalence of under-nutrition among PLHIV in Nepal, and identify risk factors and assess correlations with PLHIVs' QoL and nutritional status.

Methods: This quantitative cross-sectional study used Body Mass Index (BMI) as an indicator for nutritional status, and additional information on opportunistic infections (OIs), CD4 count, and World Health Organization (WHO) clinical staging was collected from medical records. Participants were asked to complete surveys on food security and QoL. Descriptive analysis was used to estimate the prevalence of under nutrition. To assess associations between nutrition status and independent variables, bivariate and multivariate analysis was completed. Spearman's rank correlation test was used to assess the association between nutritional status and QoL.

Results: One in five PLHIVs was found to be under nourished (BMI <18.5 kg/m^2). Illiteracy, residence in care homes, CD4 cells count <350 cells/mm^3, OIs, and illness at WHO clinical stages III and IV were found to be significant predictors of under nutrition. BMI was significantly correlated with three domains of QoL (psychological, social and environmental).

Conclusion: Nutrition interventions should form an integral part of HIV care programs. Understanding the presence of OI, decline in CD4 count, and advancing WHO clinical stages as risk factors can be helpful in preventing under nutrition from developing. Longitudinal research is necessary to further explicate associations between nutritional status and QoL.

Keywords: Nutritional status, Quality of life (QoL), People living with HIV (PLHIV), Nepal, Food security

Introduction

Per Joint United Nations Programme on HIV and AIDS (UNAIDS), the number of people newly infected with Human Immunodeficiency Virus (HIV) each year is continuing to decline in most parts of the world. The new infections declined by 38 percent from 3.4 million in 2001 to 2.1 million in 2013 [1]. Meanwhile, care is increasing. The percentage of people living with HIV (PLHIV) who are receiving antiretroviral therapy (ART) have increased from around 10 percent in 2006 to around 37 percent in 2013, with 12.9 million people receiving ART worldwide by the end of 2013 [1]. As a result, Acquired Immune Deficiency Syndrome (AIDS)-related deaths have fallen by 35% since 2005, when the highest number of deaths was recorded [2]. As a result of life-saving treatment, the number of PLHIV is rising in spite of falling rates of new infection. At the end of 2013, there were approximately 35 million PLHIV [2].

The role of HIV infection on nutrition was identified early in the epidemic [3]. Wasting is one of the most visible signs of malnutrition as patients progress from HIV to AIDS [3]. HIV was found to affect nutritional status by increasing energy requirements, reducing food intake, and adversely affecting nutrient absorption and metabolism

* Correspondence: raazshree.thapa@gmail.com
[1]Institute of Medicine, Maharajgunj Medical Campus, Tribhuwan University, Kathmandu, Nepal
Full list of author information is available at the end of the article

[4]. Failing to meet nutritional needs may lead to decreased immunity and increased susceptibility to opportunistic infections (OIs), which can lead to further malnutrition. Additionally, nutrient intake can improve antiretroviral absorption and tolerance [5]. Receiving appropriate nutrition can help improve PLHIV's quality of life (QoL) [6]. Poor nutritional status in PLHIV speeds the disease progression, increases morbidity, and reduces survival time [7]. For these reasons, nutritional support should be a fundamental part of a comprehensive response to HIV and AIDS [8]. The World Health Organization (WHO) recommends ensuring micronutrient needs are met by increasing access to a diversified diet, fortified foods, and micronutrient supplements, particularly in areas where micronutrient deficiencies are endemic [8]. However, these clinical issues remain common, despite improvements in the treatment and survival of PLHIV [7].

Similarly, food insecurity and HIV and AIDS are intertwined in a vicious cycle [9]. Food insecurity is the condition of not having physical or economic access to enough food to be productive and healthy. Each condition increases the vulnerability to and worsen the severity of the other [9]. Among PLHIV, food insecurity is associated with incomplete HIV-1 RNA suppression, CD4 decline, increased opportunistic infections, hospitalizations, and HIV-related mortality [10]. Good nutrition for PLHIV has been proven to increase resistance to infection, help PLHIV maintain weight, and improve QoL, drug compliance, and drug efficacy [10,11].

In a chronic disease like HIV and AIDS the QoL of the patients is also important [12]. The WHO defines QoL as "an individuals' perception of their position in life in the context of their culture and value systems in which they live and in relation to their goals, standards, expectations and concerns" [13]. Health Related QoL (HRQoL) comprises the components of QoL that are directly related to health status. Studies have reported a strong association between HRQoL and socioeconomic characteristics [14,15] and health related indicators [16] in resource-poor settings. Various symptoms, including wasting, are known to potentially reduce QoL among PLHIV [17]. But the relationship between nutritional status and QoL are not yet clearly defined [10], and the investigation of the relationship between food security and HRQoL among PLHIV is just beginning to emerge [10,11,18]. In particular, there is a lack of clarity on the dimensions of food security critical for improving HRQoL for PLHIV. By the latest estimate (2013), the current prevalence of HIV is 0.23 percent among adults (aged 15-49 years) in Nepal [19]. A total of 40,720 people are estimated to be living with HIV [19]. There has been a large decline in new infections annually, from 8,039 in 2000 to 1,408 in 2013 [19]. Per the country's Millennium Development Goal 2013 progress report, around 28.7 percent of PLHIV with advanced HIV infection are now receiving antiretroviral combination therapy, a figure that increased from 21 percent in 2010 [20].

A recent study from the Food and Agricultural Organization (FAO) shows that in Nepal, around 3.7 million people, representing 16.4 percent of the rural population of Nepal, are food insecure [21]. The number of these who are PLHIV is difficult to ascertain. In a food insecure area, assessing food security during clinical care for the PLHIV population is important. This study aims to identify nutritional status of PLHIV in Nepal, to identify how food security may impact nutritional status, and to clarify the relationship between nutritional status and HRQoL and PLHIV in Nepal.

Methods

Study design

This is a cross-sectional study using quantitative domain to assess the relationship between nutrition status and other variables.

Study location and timeframe

We conducted this study at two public ART sites, Tribhuvan University Teaching Hospital (TUTH) and Sukraraj Tropical and Infectious Disease Control Hospital (STIDH). These were selected out of four public ART sites in Kathmandu Valley, Nepal, that provide ART. TUTH and STIDH were taken purposively based on the high number of PLHIVs registered at these two sites. Data was collected for six months, from July to December 2013.

Study population and sampling technique

The study population was PLHIV who are accessing services from these health institutions. Inclusion criteria were a diagnosis of HIV at least six months prior to the study period, age 18 years or more, and ability to consent to the study. Both ART and pre-ART clients were included, and for those participants on ART, only those clients who have been taking ART for at least six months prior to the study period were included. As per the national ART guideline [22], those PLHIV in WHO stages III and IV or with CD4 cells count less than 350 cells/mm^3 are enrolled on ART.

The exclusion criteria were PLHIV who are severely sick or unable to respond. In addition, pregnant women were excluded and those clients who had started ART within six months of the study were excluded. This last exclusion was to allow for accurate comparison of ART and pre-ART clients.

Other studies have established estimated malnutrition prevalence among PLHIV of 30% [23,24]. With a confidence interval of 95%, an allowable error of 5% and a 5% non-response rate, the total calculated sample size was 340. The sample was determined using formula by Kothari [25].

Clients on ART were identified via the ART and pre-ART registers maintained at the sites, and a random sampling technique was employed to select 340 prospective research participants. These 340 people were contacted for study recruitment. As PLHIV is recommended for the regular CD4 cells count monitoring, prospective participants were approached during their visit at health facility for ART or pre-ART services. At first contact, researchers briefly screened prospective participants to ensure that participants enrolled in the study were those who had been diagnosed with HIV for at least six months, and that those who were on ART, had been on the regimen for a minimum duration of six months.

Ethics and consent

To accommodate the sensitivity of the issue and maintain participant confidentiality, verbal informed consent was taken from each participant before data collection. The informed consent process included a verbal explanation describing the purpose of the study, potential risks and benefits of participating, procedures for maintaining confidentiality, and the participants' right to refuse to participate. Each participant was then given an opportunity to provide verbal consent, and this was recorded by the research team.

Acknowledging the sensitivity of the issue, researcher behavior that reinforced prevailing stigma and discrimination against PLHIVs was strictly prohibited. Sensitivity and appropriate language were included as topics in researcher preparation prior to data collection.

This informed consent followed the ethical norms and values stated in the National Ethical Guidelines for Health Research in Nepal (2001) [26]. Ethical approval was obtained from the Institutional Ethical Review Board (ERB) of the Institute of Medicine, Tribhuvan University.

Data collection instruments

The study collected anthropometric data: a reference weight and height measured by standard methods, and a body mass index (BMI) calculated as a basic indicator of nutritional status. CD4 cell counts and WHO HIV and AIDS clinical staging data were taken from the health records of each participant. Each participant's ART use status was also taken from client's personal ART and pre-ART records and was confirmed at the time of recruitment. Clinical information such as the enrollment in ART, time since diagnosis, WHO clinical staging, and TB co-infection at any time after the diagnosis of HIV were recorded from individual clients records and triangulated with the ART and pre-ART registers maintained at the service facility.

Following this, each participant completed a questionnaire. The participant's demographic information (age, literacy, educational level, marital status, caste, religion, and household status) and health behaviors (tobacco use and alcohol consumption) were included as self-report items on the first part of the questionnaire. To assess the QoL of the patients, the 26-item WHOQOL-HIV BREF [27] was used. This instrument has been utilized in many studies to determine the health related quality of life among PLHIV [28,29]. The instrument uses 26 items and measures QoL across four domains: physical well-being, psychological well-being, level of independence, and environment. The participant ranked their QoL on each item on a scale of one to five, where higher scores indicated greater QoL.

Household food insecurity was measured using Household Food Insecurity Access Scale (HFIAS) [30], a well-validated instrument used to measure household food insecurity in many countries [31-33]. It consists of nine questions on experiences of food insecurity, with possible responses of never, rarely, sometimes, or often. The highest score for HFIAS is 27; the higher the score, the greater the food insecurity.

The data collection tools were translated into the Nepali language and pre-tested with 10% of the sample size in the ART center at TUTH in Kathmandu. These samples were not included in the final analysis. Factual information obtained from these samples was cross-checked with ART and Pre-ART registers at the study sites. After the pretesting, various questions relating to co-infections were omitted, as only TB was found to have been recorded accurately. Similarly questions pertaining to fortified food supply from the ART center was also omitted as the supply of the fortified food was interrupted for more than six months during the time of study and very few study participants could actually recall of the receipt. Additionally, face validity was checked during the pretest and modifications were made to increase cultural competency in the question phrasing. Finally, the pre-testing process included discussion of stigma and discrimination with pre-testing participants, and their feedback was integrated into ensuring sensitive language and behavior was maintained in the data collection processes.

Statistical analysis

Every completed questionnaire was reviewed at the end of each day to ensure its consistency and completeness. After data collection, 10 percent of the sample was randomly cross-checked for accuracy, and where errors were found, these were corrected. All recorded data was coded to facilitate data entry process. BMI was calculated from the height and weight using the standard formula: BMI = Weight (kg)/ Height^2 (m). The WHOQOL- HIV BREF [27] was used to produce a QoL profile derived from four domain scores denoting facets of an individual's perceived QoL. The mean score of items within each domain is used to calculate the domain score. Mean scores are then multiplied by four in order to make domain scores comparable with the scores used in the WHOQOL-100, a commonly used scale. The instruments' guidelines for checking and cleaning data and computing domain scores were rigorously followed.

Where more than 20% of data is missing from a questionnaire, the questionnaire was discarded. Where an item is missing, the mean of other items in the domain was substituted. Where more than two items are missing from the domain, the domain score was not calculated (with the exception of domain 3, where the domain could only be calculated if <1 item is missing). Finally, two items were examined separately: a question about an individual's overall perception of QoL and a question about an individual's overall perception of their health.

The calculation of the household food security score was based on the HFIAS version 3 [30]. The instrument had a top score of 27 points, where greater scores indicate more severe food insecurity. Four strata of food security were created based on the guideline (secure, mildly insecure, moderately insecure, and severely insecure). For the analysis purpose HFIA category 1 is termed as food secure and HFIA category 2 to 4 are categorized as food insecure. To assess associations between nutrition status and independent variables, bivariate and multivariate analysis was completed. Spearman's rank correlation test was used to assess the association between nutritional status and QoL.

Results

Total participants

A total of 340 PLHIV were contacted for interviews in the two public ART sites in Kathmandu Valley; 120 were approached in TUTH and 220 were approached in STIDH. Of these, 15 people declined to participate. The response rate was therefore 95.58% (325/340). The major reasons for non- participation in TUTH was fear of breach of confidentiality (n = 6). Many of the clients who declined said they had not disclosed their status to anyone. In STIDH the major reason for non-participation was inability to commit the necessary amount of time (n =5), although other feared disclosure of their status or were disinterested in the study (n = 4).

Among the 325 interviews taken, 24 were not complete. Thus, 301 samples were taken for final analysis, for a final response rate of 88.56%. Of these, 101 participants from TUTH and 200 participants from STIDH completed the study.

Population characteristics

The mean age of the population was 36.2 years with the standard deviation of 8.2 years. The majority of respondents (61.1%) were male. About one-third (30.2%) had completed primary level education or less, and around 77 percent were able to read and write. The majority were married (70.7%). A considerable percent were widows or widowers (8.6%). With respect to caste (the local equivalent of socioeconomic class); Janajatis (around 41%) accounted for the highest proportion of the PLHIVs seeking treatment at these sites, followed by Brahmins/Chettri (33%) and Dalits (18.6%). The majority were Hindus (70.8%), followed by Buddhists (15.9%), Christians (7%), and other faiths, mainly Kirat (3%) and Muslim (1.3%). Most resided with their family (87%), although 9% were living in group homes run by charitable organizations or in prison, and another 4% were living alone in rented homes. Background characteristics of the study participants are given in Table 1.

Nutritional status of PLHIV

To determine nutritional status, BMI was calculated. The standard cut-offs were used: <18.5 kg/m^2 is underweight, 18.5-24.9 kg/m^2 is normal, and greater than or equals to 25.0 kg/m^2 is considered overweight. Out of the 301 samples analyzed, 60 participants had BMI less than 18.5 kg/m^2. Thus 19.93% of the PLHIVs visiting the ART centers in Kathmandu valley were undernourished. Females were found to be more undernourished than the males; 17.4 percent of males and 23 percent of females had BMI less than 18.5 kg/m^2. On the other hand, 29 PLHIV (9.7%) were found to be overweight. Details are presented in Table 2.

Socioeconomic, behavioral factors, HIV related factors and nutrition status

The association between the various socioeconomic and HIV related variables and nutritional status was assessed through binary logistic regression. The statistical significance was tested at 95% confidence interval or p-value <0.05.

Among the demographic variables, age, gender, ethnicity, religion and occupation were found to have no significant association with nutritional status of the PLHIV. The mean age of the study participants was 36.2 ± 8.2, and the age of the study participants was not significantly associated with the nutritional status of the PLHIV.

Education status was found to be significantly associated with the nutritional status of PLHIV. Those PLHIV who were illiterate were almost 2.5 times more likely to be undernourished than those who were literate (Crude OR = 2.45; 95% C.I, 1.32-4.54).

During bivariate analysis, marital status was a significant factor for under-nutrition. Those who are unmarried were 2.7 times more likely to be undernourished than those who were married. Similarly, those PLHIV living single or at care homes were around three times more likely to be undernourished than those who resided with their families (Crude OR =3.45; 95% C.I, 1.68-7.05).

Household access to food is a key indicator for predicting under-nutrition. Of the 301 clients, 71 participants (23.6 percent) were found to have some food insecurity (denoted as levels 2, 3, or 4 on a scale of one to four). Households with food insecurity were more than twice as likely to be

Table 1 Socio demographic characteristics of study participants

Variables	N (%)
Treatment sites	
TUTH	101(33.6%)
STIDH	200(66.4%)
Age (Mean ± SD)	36.2 ± 8.2
≤36 years	159(52.8%)
>36 years	142(47.2%)
Gender	
Male	184(61.1%)
Female	117(38.9%)
Literacy status	
Yes	233(77.4%)
No	68(22.6%)
Educational level	
Illiterate	68(22.6%)
Primary	91(30.2%)
Secondary	68(22.6%)
Higher secondary and above	74(24.6%)
Marital status	
Married	213(70.7%)
Unmarried	38(12.6%)
Divorced	12(4.0%)
Separated	12(4.0%)
Widower/Widowed	26(8.6%)
Caste	
Dalit	57(18.6%)
Terai Janajati	12(4.0%)
Janajati	123(40.9%)
Brahmin/Chettri	100(33.2%)
Other	9(3.0%)
Place of residence	
Residing with family	262(87.0%)
Residing with a care organization	27(9.0%)
Residing alone	12(4.0%)
Religion	
Hindu	219(70.8%)
Muslim	4(1.3%)
Buddhists	48(15.9%)
Christian	21(7.0%)
Others	9(3.0%)
Occupation	
Agriculture	54(17.9%)
Labor	23(7.6%)
Service	61(20.3%)
Self-business	46(15.3%)
Household work	61(20.3%)
No work	35(11.6%)
Others	21(7.0%)
Smoking habits	
Regular smokers	111(36.9%)
Non smokers	190(63.1%)
Alcohol use	
Regular alcohol user	98(22.6%)
Non alcoholic	203(67.4%)

undernourished as those PLHIV with adequate access to food (Crude OR = 2.75; 95% C.I, 1.50-5.04).

Behavioral factors such as smoking and alcohol use were not found to be significantly associated with nutrition status. The association between various socio-demographic and behavioral factors and nutrition status is presented in Table 3.

HIV-related variables and nutritional status

Various factors related to the HIV infection such as the duration from diagnosis, ART status, and duration on ART, presence of any OIs and WHO stage was integrated into study analyses. During bivariate analysis, no significant association was found between the time since diagnosis and nutritional status.

Differences between nutritional status and enrollment in the ART were assessed. A higher proportion of pre-ART PLHIV were undernourished than those on ART. Out of 40 PLHIV on pre-ART, ten were undernourished (25%). In comparison, out of 261 PLHIV on ART, 50 were undernourished (19.2.%). This association, however, was not statistically significant (Crude OR = 0.71; 95% C.I, 0.31-1.02) (Table 3).

Multivariate analysis of associated factors

Those variables significantly related with under-nutrition (p-value <0.05) in bivariate analysis were further subjected into multivariate analysis using a logistic regression model. Only the variables found significant at 95% confidence interval in bivariate analysis were used for multivariate analysis. Binary logistic regression using the

Table 2 Nutritional status of PLHIV

BMI	N (%)
BMI < 18.5 kg/m^2 (underweight)	60 (19.9%)
BMI (18.5-24.4 kg/m^2) (Normal weight)	212 (70.4%)
BMI (>24.4 kg/m^2 (overweight)	29 (9.7%)
Total	301 (100%)

Table 3 Socioeconomic factors associated with the nutritional status

Variables	Categories	Underweight n(%) n = 60	Well-nourished n (%) n = 241	Crude OR (95% C.I.)	P-value	Adjusted OR (95% C.I.)	P-Value
Age	≤36 years*	41 (25.8)	118 (74.2)	0.55 (0.28-1.09)	0.088		
	>36 years	19 (13.4)	123 (86.6)	1			
Educational status	Illiterate	22 (32.4)	46 (67.6)	**2.45 (1.33-4.54)**	**0.004**	**2.31 (1.10-4.82)**	**0.027**
	Literate	38 (16.3)	195 (83.7)	**1**			
Gender	Female	28 (23.9)	89 (76.1)	1.49 (0.85-2.64)	0.235		
	Male	32 (17.4)	152 (82.6)	1			
Marital status	Unmarried	13 (34.2)	25 (65.8)	**2.76 (1.36-5.59)**	0.005	2.14 (0.94-4.88)	0.701
	Separated/widowed/ divorced	16 (32.0)	34 (68.0)	0.91 (0.31-2.22)	0.827	0.74 (0.24-2.29)	0.603
	Married	31 (14.6)	182 (85.4)	1			
Ethnicity	Dalits	6 (10.5)	51 (89.5)	2.42 (0.98-5.98)	0.054		
	Non- Dalits	54 (24.1)	190 (75.9)	1			
Wealth quintile	Middle class	20 (19.6)	82 (80.4)	1.30 (0.65-2.61)	0.458		
	Lower class	22 (22.2)	77 (77.8)	1.17 (0.54-2.31)	0.649		
	Upper class	18 (18.0)	82 (82.0)	1			
Religion	Hindu	44 (20.1)	175 (79.9)	0.76 (0.41-1.41)	0.391		
	Other than Hindu#	16 (19.5)	66 (79.1)	1			
Residence	Care homes/Single	16 (41.0)	23 (59.0)	**3.45 (1.69-7.05)**	**0.009**	**4.47 (1.79-11.15)**	**0.001**
	Family	44 (16.8)	218 (83.2)	**1**			
Alcohol use	No	44 (21.7)	159 (78.3)	0.71 (0.38-1.33)	0.278		
	Yes	16 (16.3)	82 (83.7)	1			
Associated with PLHIV network	No	43 (28.6)	150 (71.4)	1.54 (0.83-2.85)	0.175		
	Yes	17 (15.7)	91 (84.3)	1			
Household food security	Food insecure	24 (33.8)	47 (66.1)	**2.75 (1.50-5.05)**	**0.001**	**2.89 (1.39-5.95)**	**0.004**
	Food secure	36 (15.6)	194 (84.3)	1			
Smoking habits	No	41 (21.6)	149 (78.4)	0.75 (0.41-1.37)			
	Yes	19 (17.1)	92 (82.9)	1			
HIV related factors							
Duration from diagnosis	≤12 months	47 (24.7)	143 (75.3)	0.57 (0.32-1.03)	0.062		
	>12 months	13 (11.7)	98 (88.3)	1			
ART	Yes	50 (19.2)	211 (80.8)	0.71 (0.33-1.55)	0.391		
	No	10 (25.0)	30 (75.0)	1			
CD4 count	>350 cells/mm^3	17 (10.4)	146 (89.6)	**0.26 (0.14-0.48)**	**0.000**	**0.26 (0.13-0.56)**	**0.000**
	≤350 cells/mm^3	43 (31.2)	95 (68.8)	**1**			
ART duration	≤12 months	16 (21.1)	60 (78.9)	0.914 (0.46-1.81)	0.797		
	>12 months	44 (19.6)	181 (80.4)	1			
TB infection	Yes	17 (40.4)	25 (59.6)	**3.42 (1.70-6.86)**	**0.001**	**3.16 (1.43-7.01)**	**0.005**
	No	43 (16.6)	216 (83.4)	**1**			
WHO clinical stage	III/IV	41 (29.1)	100 (70.9)	**3.04 (1.67-5.55)**	**0.000**	**2.09 (1.04-4.21)**	**0.038**
	I/II	19 (11.9)	141 (88.1)	1			

1 = Reference Category.
*Mean value was used.
#Others include Muslim, Christian, Buddhist and Kirat.
Variables (education, age, gender, marital status, residence, OIs, WHO clinical stage, household food security and CD4 cell counts) are adjusted to minimize the effect of possible confounders in multivariate analysis.

enter method was applied to get the final model, and the Hosmer and Lemeshow test was done to test goodness of fit. The model was found to be fit ($p = 0.153 > 0.05$). Multivariate analysis was performed to examine the independent effect of each of the significant independent variables in bivariate analysis with the effect of other variables remaining constant. In the multivariate analysis, the coefficient of determination (R^2) was 0.67.

In bivariate analysis, marital status was found to be significantly associated with under-nutrition. However, this relation was not significant when subjected to multivariate analysis.

The association of literacy status with under-nutrition was found to be significant. Illiterate people were 2.3 times as likely to be undernourished as people who could read and write (Adjusted OR = 2.31; 95% C.I, 1.10-4.82).

PLHIVs' residence with their family members, alone, or at care homes also determines their nutritional status. Residing with family members provides a protective effect against under-nutrition. Those participants who resided alone or in care homes were more than four times as likely to be undernourished than those living with their family members (Adjusted OR = 4.47; 95% C.I,1.79-11.14). Food security remains the prominent factor affecting nutritional status even when subjected to multivariate analysis (Adjusted OR = 2.88; 95% C.I, 1.39-5.95).

CD4 count was a significant factor associated with under-nutrition. PLHIVs with CD4 counts of 350cells/mm^3 or more were 74% less likely to be undernourished than their counter parts (Adjusted OR = 0.26; 95% C.I, 0.12-0.55). Similarly, WHO clinical stages III and IV were found to be significant factors associated with under nutrition. PLHIVs in stage III and IV were more than twice as likely to be under-nourished than WHO stage I and II (adjusted OR - 2.09, 95% C.I, 1.04-4.21). Previous OIs with tuberculosis was also found to be the prominent risk factor for under nutrition (Adjusted OR = 3.16, 95% C.I, 1.42-7.0). The multivariate analysis is presented in Table 3.

Health-related QoL of PLHIV

QoL descriptive statistics

QoL was measured using the WHOQolBREF [27]. Four domains capture different aspects of health-related QoL: physical health (including medical issues, pain, work capacity, and other aspects), psychological health (including negative and positive feelings, self-esteem, spirituality, and cognitive functions), social relationships (including social support and intimate relationships), and environment (including financial resources, safety, physical surroundings, and more).

Socio demographic factors and QoL

In the bivariate analysis of demographic variables and QoL scores, a significant difference in the QoL mean scores of male and female participants was noted. Males reported higher mean scores than females. Literate participants were also found to have higher QoL scores. Other demographic characteristics, such as marital status, religion and occupation, showed no significant differences in QoL scores.

Mean QoL scores were also found to be significantly higher among PLHIV with higher CD4 counts and those who were at WHO clinical stage I and II. The association, however, was not significant in the physical health and social domains.

The mean scores for all four different domains were found to be lower among the undernourished than those PLHIV having a BMI >18.5 kg/m^2 and this difference was significant for psychological, social and environmental domains (Table 4).

Correlation between QoL and nutritional status

A Spearmen Rank correlation test was carried out to observe if there was any correlation between nutritional status and QoL. A positive correlation was seen between weight and all four domains, as well as between BMI and all four domains. However, the correlation is weak (<0.3) throughout. Notably, height is also found to be significantly correlated with three domains (psychological, level of independence and environment) of QoL (Table 5).

Discussion

Nutritional status of PLHIV

The study estimates the rate of under-nutrition among PLHIVs and assesses correlations to other elements of their lives. The role of HIV infection on nutrition has been well-documented. Wasting is one of the most visible signs of malnutrition in patients who progress to AIDS [34]. Food insecurity, the condition of not having physical or economic access to sufficient food to meet dietary needs for a productive and healthy life [35], remains a common problem among PLHIV despite advances in their treatment and survival. However, the complex interactions of under-nutrition, food insecurity, QoL, and health status are not well-documented.

HIV affects the proportion of population already struggling with malnutrition and food security. In 2011, the Nepal Demographic and Health Survey (NDHS) reported that 18% of all adult females in Nepal were malnourished. The study suggests that HIV-infected women are more vulnerable to malnutrition, with 23 percent of female participants having BMI less than 18.5 kg/m^2 [36].

According to the WHO, nutritional support should be fundamental to a comprehensive response to HIV and AIDS [37]. Poor nutritional status in PLHIV is associated with disease progression, increased morbidity, and reduced survival, even when ART is available [38]. A study in the United States found that micronutrient

Table 4 Mean scores of different domains of the QoL

Variables	Categories	Physical domain ± SD	Psychological domain ± SD	Social domain ± SD	Environmental domain ± SD
Gender	Male	48.8 ± 9.8	46.5 ± 10.8	43.8 ± 13.	44.5 ± 10.9
	Female	45.3 ± 8.3	41.7 ± 10.2	38.5 ± 12.3	40.2 ± 9.5
Education	Illiterate	45.8 ± 9.6	45.8 ± 10.6	43.0 ± 13.4	44.5 ± 10.7
	Some education	40.6 ± 7.8	40.6 ± 10.6	36.6 ± 11.3	37.3 ± 8.2
CD4 count (cells/mm^3)	<350	46.4 ± 10.10	43.3 ± 11.4	41.0 ± 12.9	41.6 ± 11.0
	≥350	48.6 ± 8.5	46.2 ± 9.8	42.6 ± 13.4	44.3 ± 9.8
WHO stage	I/II	46.2 ± 8.0	41 ± 8.9	39 ± 9.3	40 ± 8.2
	III/IV	48.38 ± 8.4	46 ± 10.6	43 ± 14.5	44.9 ± 11.2
BMI (Kg/m^2)	<18.5	45.41 ± 9.4	41.5 ± 11.7	36.06 ± 12.3	38.4 ± 9.4
	≥18.5	47.9 ± 10.6	45.4 ± 10.4	43.1 ± 13.0	43.9 ± 10.6

supplements significantly increased CD4 count among PLHIV [39], and studies among HIV-infected adults in Haiti, Kenya, Malawi and Zambia have demonstrated significant positive effects of macronutrient supplementation on adherence to antiretroviral medication, weight gain and CD4 counts [38-42]. Similarly, in food-insecure settings, food support programs (increasing total calories) are often required in addition to nutrition support (increasing specific micronutrients) to optimize health outcomes in PLHIV [38]. This supports the idea of nutritional support to PLHIVs in countries (like Nepal) where food insecurity is endemic.

Factors associated with under nutrition among PLHIV

Various socio-demographic and HIV-related factors determine the nutritional status of PLHIVs. Education status was significantly associated with nutritional status, in that illiterate people were more likely to be undernourished. Previous studies of underlying factors in under-nutrition among the illiterate demonstrate that differences may include their dietary pattern, their understanding on the disease processes, and ART adherence [43]. A study carried out in Ethiopia in 2013 indicates that occupation and economic status might account for the vulnerability of illiterate people to under nutrition [44]. In this study, no significant association was seen between under-nutrition and socioeconomic status.

Table 5 Correlation between the nutritional status and QoL

Domains/ Nutritional status	Physical	Psychological	Level of independence	Environment
Weight	0.124*	0.236*	0.272*	0.262*
Height	0.059	0.148*	0.207*	0.164*
BMI	0.136*	0.154*	0.208*	0.215*

*Significant at 95% CI, P value <0.05.

Independent of all other variables, WHO clinical stages III and IV have significant effects on the likelihood of malnutrition development. Malnutrition is usually encountered at the advanced phase of HIV infection. An anthropometric measurement like BMI is lower in symptomatic patients as classified by WHO HIV disease stages [45]. Since disease status could modulate the immunological responses to HIV infection over time [44], further research with longitudinal design can be helpful in assessing the effect of malnutrition on HIV infection progression.

It was found that an OIs (tuberculosis) was an independent risk factor for under nutrition. Similar other studies support the findings that TB is associated with under nutrition [46-49]. The HIV-induced immune impairment and heightened subsequent risk of OIs can worsen nutritional status [50]. This exemplifies the importance of managing patients with OIs promptly.

Regarding CD4 count, we found that PLHIV with more than 350 cells/mm^3 were more well-nourished than PLHIV with less than or equal to 350 cells/mm^3. Since this is a cross-sectional study, some longitudinal study can better explain the relationship between CD4 count and nutritional status. The same is true for understanding the relationship between OIs and under nutrition.

Correlation between nutritional status and health related QoL

There are very little evidence linking nutritional status and health related QoL. In our study all three parameters (height, weight, and BMI) were found to be significantly associated with the domains of QoL. A cross-sectional study carried out at West Bengal, India, among HIV-positive women in 2012 similarly showed that QoL scores were correlated positively with all the parameters of nutritional status [12]. The correlation of height and QoL may indicate that lifelong undernourishment resulting in stunting, rather than current HIV status, may correlate with lower levels of QoL. However, further investigation is necessary to determine this.

Limitations

The cross-sectional nature of the study limits the investigation into causal relationship between determinants and outcomes of interest (malnutrition). Likewise, further comparative study between HIV-infected and non-HIV infected persons could explore additional nutrition and food security risk factors. The study, like others, is subject to some systematic errors, including measurement error, recall bias for self-reported components, and incomplete medical records. These are the key limitations. Additionally, self-reported HRQoL measures may feature important confounds, in that some aspects of HRQoL may also be affected by factors in a study participants life unrelated to nutrition status or HIV and AIDS that nevertheless affect their answers.

Conclusions

In our findings, one in every five PLHIV is undernourished. Nutritional status was found to be positively correlated with QoL. Although further longitudinal research will be helpful in determining the role of nutritional status in QoL, the results of this study suggest that the existing care options for PLHIV do not appear to fully address this issue. Nutritional support should form a fundamental part of the response to HIV and AIDS in Nepal, including more efforts toward providing nutritional counseling, support, and encouragement to clients. Our results also make a case for a PLHIV-specific food security program, additional to ones targeting HIV-negative food-insecure populations, to ensure this especially vulnerable population receives adequate support.

Competing interests

The authors declare that they have no competing interests.

Authors' contributions

RT, DPP and KB designed, implemented and drafted the manuscript. MSN analyzed the data and revised the paper. AA is responsible for overall supervision of the research process and reviewed the article. All the authors have read and approved the final manuscript.

Acknowledgements

We would like to acknowledge the support of Prof. Dr. Prem Krishna Khadga, TUTH, Dr. Anup Bastola, Dermatologist, STIDH, Mr. Madhav Pant, ART counselor, TUTH, Ms. Uma Chitrakar, TUTH, for their support in carrying out and successfully complete this study. We are grateful to all the participants. We also offer sincere and earnest thankfulness to Prof. Dr. Amod Poudel, who helped us with the analysis, and the entire team of TUTH, Department of Community Medicine and Public Health for their support and help which made this study possible and feasible. Our sincere thanks goes to Ms. Barsha Thapa, Mr. Deepak Jha and Ms. Anita Shrestha for their active help and assistance during data collection and analysis. RT adds special thanks to all her friends in the MPH program 15th Batch for their kind assistance.

Funding of the Project

This is a self-funded project with the technical support from the Institute of Medicine, Maharajgunj, Kathmandu.

Author details

[1]Institute of Medicine, Maharajgunj Medical Campus, Tribhuwan University, Kathmandu, Nepal. [2]James P Grant School of Public Health, BRAC University, Dhaka, Bangladesh. [3]Independent Scholar, Chicago, IL, USA.

References

1. Joint United Nations Programme on HIV/AIDS (UNAIDS). The Gap Report. Geneva: UNAIDS. 2014. Available at: http://www.unaids.org/sites/default/files/en/media/unaids/contentassets/documents/unaidspublication/2014/UNAIDS_Gap_report_en.pdf.
2. Joint United Nations Programme on HIV/AIDS (UNAIDS). Fast-track: ending the AIDS epidemic by 2030. Geneva: UNAIDS; 2014. Available at: http://www.unaids.org/sites/default/files/media_asset/JC2686_WAD2014report_en.pdf.
3. Trujillo EB, Borlase BC, Bell SJ, Guenther KJ, Swails W, Queen PM, et al. Assessment of nutritional status, nutrient intake, and nutrition support in AIDS patients. J Am Diet Assoc. 1992;92(4):477–8.
4. World Health Organization: Nutrient requirements for people living with HIV/AIDS: report of a technical consultation. Geneva, Switzerland 2003. Available at: http://www.who.int/nutrition/publications/hivaids/9241591196/en/.
5. Maertens, JA. Barriers to Nutrition management among people living with HIV on Antiretroviral Therapy. Dissertation for Doctor for philosophy. 2011. Available at: http://digitool.library.colostate.edu/exlibris/dtl/d3_1/apache_media/L2V4bGlicmlzL2R0bC9kM18xL2FwYWNoZV9tZWRpYS8xMTc0ODA=.pdf.
6. Anand D, Puri S, Mathew M. Assessment of Quality of Life of HIV-Positive People Receiving ART: An Indian Perspective. Indian J Community Med. 2012;37(3):165.
7. Hsu JW, Pencharz PB, Macallan D, Tomkins A. Macronutrients and HIV/AIDS: A Review of Current Evidence in Consultation on Nutrition and HIV/AIDS in Africa: Evidence, Lessons and Recommendations for Action. Durban, South Africa: WHO, Department of Nutrition for Health and Development; 2005.
8. PEPFAR. Report on Food and Nutrition for People Living with HIV/AIDS. 2006.
9. Anema A, Vogenthaler N, Frongillo EA, Kadiyala S, Weiser SD. Food insecurity and HIV/AIDS: current knowledge, gaps, and research priorities. Curr HIV/AIDS Rep. 2009;6(4):224-31.
10. Palermo T, Rawat R, Weiser SD, Kadiyala S. Food Access and Diet Quality Are Associated with Quality of Life Outcomes among HIV-Infected Individuals in Uganda. PLoS One. 2013;8(4):e62353. doi:10.1371/journal.pone.0062353.
11. Food and Nutrition technical Assistance (FANTA) and World Food Program (WFP). Food Assistance Programming in context of HIV. Washington, DC: FANTA Project, Academy for Educational Development; 2007.
12. Bhowmik A, Ghugre P, Udipi S, Guha SK. Nutritional Status and Quality of Life of Women with HIV/AIDS. Am J Infect Dis. 2012;8(1):13–8.
13. World Health Organization. Division of mental health and prevention of substance abuse. WHOQOL and spirituality, religiousness and personal beliefs (SRPB). WHO;1998.
14. Ruutel K, Pisarev H, Loit HM, Uuskula A. Factors influencing quality of life of people living with HIV in Estonia: A cross-sectional survey. J Int AIDS Soc. 2009;12:13.
15. Louwagie G, Bachmann M, Meyer K, Booysen FIR, Fairall L, Heunis JC. Highly active antiretroviral treatment and health related quality of life in South African adults with human immunodeficiency virus infection: a cross-sectional analytical study. BMC Public Health. 2007;7(244):1-33.
16. Folasire OF, Irabor AE, Folasire AM. Quality of life of People living with HIV and AIDS attending the Antiretroviral Clinic, University College Hospital, Nigeria. Afr J Prm Health Care Fam Med. 2012;4(1):294.
17. Testa MA, Lenderking WR. The impact of AIDS-associated wasting on quality of life: qualitative issues of measurement and evaluation. J Nutr. 1999;129:282-9.
18. Venter E, Gericke GJ, Bekker PJ. Nutritional status, quality of life and CD4 cell count of adults living with HIV/AIDS in the Ga-Rankuwa area (South Africa). S Afr J Clin Nutr. 2009;22:124–129.
19. NCASC: Nepal Country Progress Report. Kathmandu: National Centre for AIDS and STD Control; 2014.
20. United Nations Development Programme(UNDP).Millennium Development Goals (MDG) Progress Report 2013. Available at: http://www.np.undp.org/content/nepal/en/home/library/mdg/mdg-progress-report-2013.html.
21. Food and Agricultural Organization (FAO). Assessment of Food Security and Nutrition Situation in Nepal 2010. Available at: ftp://ftp.fao.org/TC/CPF/Country%20NMTPF/Nepal/thematic%20studies/Food%20Security%20_Final_.pdf.

22. National Centre for AIDS and STD Control (NCASC). National Guidelines for Antiretroviral Therapy. Kathmandu: National Centre for AIDS and STD Control, Apr; 2012. Available at: http://www.who.int/hiv/pub/guidelines/nepal_art.pdf.
23. Nti A, Hayford J, Obisaw, CP. Nutrition Knowledge, Diet Quality and Nutritional Status of People Living with HIV (PLHIV) in Ghana. Food and Public Health 2012;2(6):219–227.
24. Daniel M, Mazengia F, Birhanu D. Nutritional Status and Associated Factors among Adult HIV/AIDS Clients in Felege Hiwot Referral Hospital, Bahir Dar. Ethiopia Science Journal of Public Health. 2013;1(1):24–31.
25. Kothari CR. Research Methodology Methods & Techniques. 2nd ed. New Delhi: New Age International publisher; 2004.
26. NHRC. National Ethical Guidelines for Health Research in Nepal And Standard Operating Procedures. 2011. Available at http://nhrc.org.np/guidelines.
27. WHO. WHO QoL HIVBREF. Department of Mental health and Substance Dependence. 2002.
28. Imam MH, Karim MR, Ferdous C, Akhter S. Health related quality of life among the people living with HIV. Bangladesh Med Res Counc Bull. 2011;37:1–6.
29. Giri S, Neupane M, Pant S, Timalsina U, Koirala S, Timalsina S, Sharma S. Quality of life among people living with acquired immune deficiency syndrome receiving anti-retroviral therapy: a study from Nepal. Dove Press. 2013;277–282.
30. Coates J, Swindale A, Bilinsky P. Household Food Insecurity Access Scale (HFIAS) for Measurement of Food Access: Indicator Guide. Washington, DC: Food and Nutrition Technical Assistance Project (FANTA), Academy for Educational Development. 2007. Available at: http://www.fao.org/fileadmin/user_upload/eufao-fsi4dm/doc-training/hfias.pdf.
31. Baiyegunhi LJS, Makwangudze KE. Home Gardening and Food Security Status of HIV/AIDS-Affected Households in Mpophomeni, KwaZulu-Natal Province. South Africa J Hum Ecol. 2013;44(1):1–8.
32. Weiser SD, Frongillo EA, Ragland K, Hogg RS, Riley ED, Bangsberg DR. Food Insecurity is Associated with Incomplete HIV RNA Suppression Among Homeless and Marginally Housed HIV-infected Individuals in San Francisco. J Gen Intern Med. 2009;24(1):14–20. doi:10.1007/s11606-008-0824-5.
33. Kadiyala S, Rawat R, Babirye F, Ochai R. Food security is strongly associated with nutritional status mong HIV-infected individuals in Uganda: AIDS 2010 - XVIII International. AIDS Conference: Abstract no. CDB0046.
34. Mangili A, Murman DH, Zampini AM, Wanke CA. Nutrition and HIV infection: review of weight loss and wasting in the era of highly active antiretroviral therapy from the nutrition for healthy living cohort. Clin Infect Dis. 2006;42(6):836–42.
35. Xiong K. Review of the Evidence: Linkages between Livelihood, Food Security, Economic Strengthening, and HIV Related Outcomes. Measure Evaluation, 2012. Available at: http://www.cpc.unc.edu/measure/publications/sr-12-71.
36. Ministry of Health and Population (MOHP) [Nepal], New ERA, & ICF International Inc. Nepal Demographic and Health Survey 2011. Kathmandu, Nepal : Ministry of Health and Population, New ERA, and ICF International, Calverton, Maryland. 2012.
37. WHO. Regional Consultation on Nutrition and HIV and AIDS: Evidence Lesson Learnt and recommendation for action in South East Asia. 2007. p. 8–11.
38. Houtzager, LM. Nutrition in HIV: A Review. Nutrition Development Division, Albion Street Centre, Sydney, Australia
39. Kaiser JD, Campa AM, Ondercin JP, Leoung GS, Pless RF, Baum MK. Micronutrient supplementation increases CD4 count in HIV-infected individuals on highly active antiretroviral therapy: a prospective, double-blinded, placebo-controlled trial. J Acquir Immune Defic Syndr. 2006;42:523-8.
40. Tirivayi N, Koethe J, Groot W. Clinic-Based Food Assistance is Associated with Increased Medication Adherence among HIV-Infected Adults on Long-Term Antiretroviral Therapy in Zambia. Journal of AIDS and Clinical Research. 2012;3:171.
41. Ndekha MJ, van Oosterhout JJ, Zijlstra EE, Manary M, Saloojee H, Manary MJ. Supplementary feeding with either ready-to-use fortified spread or corn-soy blend in wasted adults starting antiretroviral therapy in Malawi: randomised, investigator blinded, controlled trial. BMJ. 2009;338:b1867.
42. Gichunge CN, Hogan J, Sang E, Wafula S, Mwangi A, Petersen T et al. Role of food assistance in survival and adherence to clinic appointments and medication among HIV-infected patients on antiretroviral therapy (ART) in Western Kenya. Vienna: XVIII International AIDS Conference; 2010.
43. Unge C, Sodergard B, Marrone G, Thorson A, Lukhwaro A, Carter J, et al. Long-term adherence to antiretroviral treatment and program drop-out in a high-risk urban setting in sub-saharan Africa: a prospective cohort study. PLoS One. 2010;5(10):e13613.
44. Hailemariam S, Bune GT, Ayele HT. Malnutrition: Prevalence and its associated factors in People living with HIV/AIDS, in Dilla University Referral Hospital. Archives of Public Health. 2013;71(1):13. doi:10.1186/0778-7367-71-13.
45. Somarriba G, Neri D, Schaefer N, Miller LT. The effect of aging, nutrition, and exercise during HIV infection. HIV/AIDS. Research and Palliative Care. 2010;2:191–20.
46. Bhargava A, Chatterjee M, Jain Y, Chatterjee B, Kataria A, Bhargava, M, et al. Nutritional Status of Adult Patients with Pulmonary Tuberculosis in RuralCentral India and Its Association with Mortality. PLoS ONE 2013,. doi:10.1371/journal.pone.007797
47. Macallan DC. Malnutrition in tuberculosis. Diagn Microbiol Infect Dis. 1999;34:153–7. doi: 10.1016/S0732-8893(99)00007-3 PubMed:0354866.14.
48. Schaible UE, Kaufmann SH. Malnutrition and infection: complex mechanisms and global impacts. PLoS Med. 2007;4:e115. doi:10.1371/journal.pmed.0040115.
49. Nnyepi MS. The risk of developing malnutrition in people living with HIV/ AIDS: Observations from six support groups in Botswana. S Afr J Clin Nutr. 2009;22(2):89–93.
50. Paton NI, Sangeetha S, Earnest A, Bellamy R. The impact of malnutrition on survival and the CD4 count response in HIV-infected patients starting antiretroviral therapy. HIV Med. 2006;7:323–30. doi:10.1111/j.1468-1293.2006.00383.x.

21

Trends in prevalence of diarrhoea, Kaposi's sarcoma, bacterial pneumonia, malaria and geohelminths among HIV positive individuals in Uganda

John Rubaihayo[1,2*], Nazarius M Tumwesigye[1] and Joseph Konde-Lule[1]

Abstract

Background: Trends in prevalence of opportunistic infections (OIs) associated with the human immunodeficiency virus (HIV) in resource poor settings have previously not been well documented. The objective of this study was to describe the trends in prevalence of Diarrhoea, Bacterial pneumonia, Kaposi's sarcoma, Malaria and Geohelminths among HIV positive individuals over a 12 year period in Uganda.

Methods: Observation data for 5972 HIV positive individuals enrolled with the AIDS support organisation (TASO) in Uganda were analysed. Study participants were drawn from three HIV clinics located in different geographical areas of Uganda and followed from January 2002 to December 2013. The prevalence trends for the above OIs were plotted using the Box Jenkins moving average technique. X^2-test for trend was used to test for the significance of the trends and Pearson's correlation coefficient used to test for the strength of linear relationship between OI prevalence and calendar time. Mixed effect linear regression was used to estimate average monthly change in prevalence with monthly variation modelled as a random effect.

Results: A total of 204,871 monthly medical reports were retrieved and analysed. 73 % (4301/5972) were female with a median age of 32 years (inter-quartile range 26–39). Overall, significant decreasing mean annual prevalence trends ($p < 0.05$, X^2_{trend}) were observed for Diarrhoea (<1 month) with Pearson's correlation coefficient ($r = -0.89$), Malaria ($r = -0.75$), Bacterial Pneumonia ($r = -0.52$), and Geohelminth ($r = -0.32$). Non-significant increasing mean annual prevalence trend was observed for Kaposis sarcoma ($p = 0.20$, X^2_{trend}; $r = +0.26$). After adjusting for age, sex and clinic in a mixed effects linear regression model, average monthly prevalence declined significantly at a rate of 0.4 % for Kaposis sarcoma, 0.3 % for Geohelminths, 2 % for Malaria, 1 % for Bacterial Pneumonia and 3 % for Diarrhoea(<1 month). However, the rate of decline per month differed significantly ($p < 0.05$) by HIV clinic for Diarrhoea (<1 month), and age, sex and clinic for malaria.

Conclusions and recommendations: Overall, decreasing trends were observed in the above OIs. However the trends differed significantly by OI, geographical location and demographic characteristics. There is urgent need to integrate interventions targeting malaria and geohelminths in HIV programmes.

* Correspondence: rubaihayoj@yahoo.co.uk
[1]Department of Epidemiology and Biostatistics, School of Public Health, College of Health Sciences, Makerere University, Kampala, Uganda
[2]Department of Public Health, School of Health Sciences, Mountains of the Moon University, Fort Portal, Uganda

Background

Several African countries with a generalised HIV epidemic are struggling with availing lifelong ARVS to an increasing population of eligible HIV patients amidst scarce resources. According to the World health Organization [1], 9.7 million persons living with HIV in low and middle income countries had access to highly active antiretroviral therapy by the end of 2012, and AIDS-related deaths were reduced to about 1.6 million compared to 2 million deaths attributed to AIDS in 2002 [2]. Uganda is one of the few sub-Saharan countries in which the magnitude of the HIV epidemic has been substantially reduced and stabilized in the past decades; though recent reports show a slight increase in HIV prevalence among adults from a national average of 6.4 % in 2005 to 7.3 % by 2011 [3]. According to the Uganda AIDS indicator survey (2011), the burden of HIV differs by geographical area with central Uganda having the highest prevalence of HIV (10.6 %), followed by mid-northern (8.3 %) and then mid and south western (8–8.2 %) and lowest prevalence in mid-eastern(4.1 %) [3] but was not clear whether the burden of HIV related morbidity and mortality follows the same pattern.

Access to highly active antiretroviral therapy (HAART) in Uganda has been steadily increasing since HAART was introduced in 2004 and by the end of 2013, 69.4 % (570,373/821,721) of eligible adults and children had access to HAART; though this was still below the 80 % national target by 2015 [4]. Co-trimoxaxole (TMP-SMX) prophylaxis has also been shown to prevent or significantly reduce the incidence of opportunistic infections and related mortality in HIV-infected individuals [5–8] . In Sub-Saharan Africa where access to HAART is still limited, cotrimoxazole prophylaxis remains the most viable alternative and has greatly increased the chances of survival for HIV-infected individuals who are eligible but cannot access HAART [9]. UNAIDS recommends cotrimoxazole prophylaxis for life to all persons living with HIV/AIDS regardless of their immunological status and whether they are on HAART or not [10]. However, even with increasing availability of HAART and co-trimoxazole (TMP-SMX) prophylaxis, life threatening opportunistic infections remain the most important aspect of care for persons living with HIV associated with stigma, poor quality of life and high medical care costs. Opportunistic infections therefore have greatly contributed to poverty among those infected and affected by HIV hence an impediment to the attainment of the millennium development goals (MDGs) on health and poverty eradication particularly in resource poor countries [4]

In Uganda, universal cotrimoxazole prophylaxis was introduced in 2003 in all public and private health facilities providing care and treatment to persons infected with HIV/AIDS [11]. The AIDS support Organisation (TASO), one of the oldest and largest non-governmental organisation (NGO) providing treatment and care to persons living with HIV/AIDS in Uganda, rolled out universal co-trimoxazole prophylaxis in early 2003 and HAART in 2004. However, it was not known whether TASO HIV/AIDS care and treatment programme had any significant effect on trends of opportunistic infections or not. Trends of OIs in Uganda have previously not been fully examined due to lack of sufficient data. Trends of OIs provide invaluable information that can be used to evaluate the impact of treatment and preventive interventions over time and can also help to inform planning and policy on future preventive and treatment strategies in resource poor settings. We analysed trends in prevalence of diarrhoea, bacterial pneumonia, kaposi sarcoma, malaria and geohelminths among HIV positive individuals enrolled with TASO HIV/AIDS care and treatment programme from 2002 to 2013 inclusive. The trends of others OIs (TB, cryptococcosis, candidiasis, genital ulcer and herpes zoster) were also analysed but were considered elsewhere. These OIs were selected on the basis that they are the commonest OIs in Uganda and are easy to diagnose.

Methods

Study design

Observational data for 5972 HIV positive individuals enrolled with the AIDS support organisation (TASO) in Uganda were retrieved and analysed. The study period was from January 2002 to December 2013 and the opportunistic infections of interest were diarrhoea, bacterial pneumonia, kaposi sarcoma, malaria and geohelminths. Kaposis sarcoma though strictly speaking is not an opportunistic infection but was included because of being associated with opportunistic viral infections ((human herpes virus type 8) [12]. The 12 year review period was categorised into three time periods that signify important milestones in the prevention and treatment of opportunistic infections associated with HIV/AIDS in Uganda. First period covered 2 years immediately prior to HAART rollout in Uganda (2002–2003). Second period is from 2004 to 2008 denoted as "Early HAART" in which there was very limited access to HAART only available to a few severely ill HIV positive individuals (CD4 cell count $<$200cells/μl of blood). The third period is from 2009 to 2013 denoted as "Late HAART" in which HAART access was extended to include even HIV+ individuals with CD4 cell equal to 350cells/ μl to of blood. Data were analyzed using autoregressive moving average time series and multilevel mixed effects linear regression models adjusting for potential confounders whose data was available.

Study settings

Data for the study were obtained from TASO electronic data bases. TASO is one of the oldest and largest HIV/

AIDS care programme in Uganda and sub-Saharan Africa [13]. The organisation which was started in 1987 has 11 HIV clinics spread across Uganda and has accumulated data on HIV/AIDS for the last 3 decades and thus provided a good opportunity to examine trends of common and rare opportunistic infections associated with HIV/AIDS in Uganda. TASO HAART programme started as part of the National HAART roll-out programme in public health facilities in 2004. Being one of the largest HAART providers in the country, TASO attracted a lot of support from different funders supporting HAART programmes in sub-Saharan Africa including the President's Emergency Plan for AIDS Relief (PEPFAR) and the Global Fund to Fight AIDS, Tuberculosis and Malaria. Initially, HAART eligibility was based on WHO 2006 guidelines i.e. WHO stage 3 or 4 illness or a CD4 cell count < 200 cells/μl for adults and adolescents and WHO stage III, advanced stage II or stage I with CD4 cell percentage less than 20 % for children more than 18 months of age [14]. However, in 2010 new HAART guidelines [15] that raised the threshold for adults and adolescents to a CD4 cell count >200 cells/μl but ≤350 cells/μl or WHO clinical stage3 or 4 irrespective of CD4 cell count were adopted [16]. Those who were not eligible for HAART were offered cotrimoxazole prophylaxis. All HIV positive patients were usually screened for tuberculosis (TB) at admission and at HAART initiation. HIV-1 viral load monitoring was not used in theses settings. Given the resource constraints and pressing clinical needs, HIV positive patients could be initiated on HAART basing on clinical presentation without CD4 evaluations. The TASO HAART programme has a robust community counselling and social support component including provider initiated and voluntary HIV testing and counselling, monitoring adherence to ART, assessing general clinical conditions of their clients and reporting those severely ill or dead. All services are free of charge including anti-retroviral drugs (ARVs) for those who are eligible [17].

Sampling and sample size

Three TASO HIV clinics were purposively selected basing on volume, quality of data and geographical representation. The HIV clinics selected were TASO Mulago HIV clinic in central Uganda, TASO Mbarara HIV clinic in south-western Uganda and Tororo HIV clinic in Eastern Uganda. All HIV positive adults (15 years and above) who were in care at the three selected HIV clinics from 1st January 2002 were included in the study.

Data collection

The data were collected by TASO medical staff following an established protocol for all TASO HIV clinics. In brief, each client was expected to attend the clinic at least once a month. At each clinic visit, data per client was collected on a standardized medical form detailing the client's demographic information, clinical condition, medical history, OI diagnosis, ART use and level of adherence, prophylaxis use, any other treatment given and side effects/toxicities if any. Diagnosis of the different disease conditions was based on the Ugandan Ministry of Health and WHO case definition guidelines [18]. Bacterial pneumonia was clinically defined as acute onset of fever, cough, dyspnoea associated with chest pain and responsive to antibiotics; diarrhoea < 1 month was clinically defined as three or more loose or liquid bowel movements per day lasting for a period not exceeding 1 month; malaria was clinically defined as fever, body temperature >37 °C and with a laboratory confirmed positive malaria blood slide or a positive rapid diagnosis test (RDT); Kaposi's sarcoma was clinically defined as persistent skin lesions developing into plaques or nodules; geohelminthiasis was defined as laboratory confirmed positive stool slide for the eggs of any of the following: *Ascaris lumbricodes*, *Trichuris trichiura*, *Necator americanus*, *Strongyloides stercoralis* or *Ancylostoma duodenale*.

Both clinical and laboratory Data were then compiled and entered into the TASO electronic data base by TASO data administrator using EPIINFO vs3 in Access format. Monthly medical data for each participant covering the period January 2002 to December 2013 were extracted by the data administrator, delinked from overt identifiers and then handed over for analysis.

Data management and analysis

Data cleaning, validation and analysis were done using STATA 12(Stata Corp, Collage station, Texas). Baseline demographic data was summarised and presented by frequency distribution. To analyse trends, data on each OI was assembled and summarised by year and month. Monthly prevalence was calculated from the total number of clients recorded with an event in a month divided by the total number that attended the clinic in that particular month. Annual prevalence per OI was calculated from the mean of the monthly prevalences in a year. A time plot was generated using the Box Jenkins moving average smoothening technique [19]. The moving average smoothing technique achieves this by replacing each element of the time series by *n* neighbouring elements, where n is the width of the smoothening window. We used a centred moving average including 3 observations before and 2 observations after the current observation inclusive, and then computed the mean value as the centred moving average. Pearson's correlation coefficient was used to test for the strength of linear relationship between OI prevalence and calendar time.

To test for the significance of annualised trends, a X^2-test for trend [20, 21] was used. The trend was considered significant if X^2-trend < 0.05 [21]. To test for the significance of the difference between trends, we used kruskal wallis test [22]. To estimate average monthly change and the effect of covariates, we used mixed effect linear regression analysis with monthly variation modelled as a random effect adjusting for all available potential confounders.

Ethical considerations

The study obtained ethical clearance from Makerere University School of Public Health Higher Degrees Research and Ethics committee and the Uganda National Council for Science and Technology. Informed consent from study participants was not required as this was routinely collected operational data and the above ethical committees waived the need for consent. However, written consent was obtained from TASO for conducting study and publication of findings with any accompanying images.

Results

Baseline characteristics

A total of 204,871 monthly medical reports were analysed. 73 % (4301) were female with a median age of 32 years (inter-quartile range 26–39). More than half of the study participants were subsistence farmers (56 %) with majority having only primary level education (50 %) and 30 % were widowed (Table 1). By 2004, only 9 % of these had access to HAART compared to more than 90 % on HAART in 2013. The overall median age at HAART initiation was 44 years (inter-quartile range 37–50) but was significantly lower for women at 43 (inter-quartile range 37–49) than that of men at 45 (inter-quartile range 40–52) ($p = 0.001$) (Table 3). Baseline WHO clinical stage, CD4 count and HAART regimen were not significantly different by gender ($p > 0.05$) (Table 3). The median CD4 cell count at the start of HAART was 128 cells (inter-quartile range 55–190) and the commonly used HAART regimes were zidovudine plus lamivudine and nevirapine (ZDV + 3TC+ NVP) (44 %), followed by stavudine, lamivudine and nevirapine (d4T + 3TC + NVP) (40 %), and other regimen combinations that includes efavirenz (EFV), Tenofovir (TDF) and Lopinavir/ritonavir, etc. were rarely used in this cohort (20 %) (Table 2). Only 3 % of the study participants were on cotrimoxazole/dapson prophylaxis in 2002 compared to 98 % in 2013

Prevalence and trends of OIs

Overall monthly trends for each OI are shown in Fig. 1. Best-fit regression lines, R^2 and p-values for each OI are

Table 1 Baseline characteristics of the cohort at the start of the study period (2002), total and clinic-specific

Variable	Total cohort n(%)	Tororo HIV clinic n(%)	Mulago HIV clinic n(%)	Mbarara HIV Clinc n(%)
Sex (n = 5,972)				
Female	4,301(73)	1,071 (71)	1,368 (76)	1,862 (70)
Male	1,671 (27)	433 (29)	436 (24)	802 (30)
Median age (IQR) (n = 5964)	32 (26,39)	33 (28,40)	30(25,36)	32 (27,39)
Occupation (n = 5031)				
paid employee	627(12)	120(8)	232(18)	275(12)
self employed	1125(22)	271(18)	336(27)	518(23)
subsistence farmer	2808(56)	932(62)	563(45)	1313(58)
others	471(9)	196(13)	127(10)	148(7)
Education (n = 5,005)				
None	1199(23)	414(27)	135(11)	650(29)
Primary	2521(50)	789(52)	623(50)	1106(49)
Secondary	1063(21)	286(19)	415(33)	364(16)
Tertiary or above	220(4)	22(1)	82(6.5)	116(5)
Marital status (n = 5029)				
Single (never married)	195(4)	24(2)	98(8)	73(3)
Married	2074(21)	690(45)	441(35)	943(42)
Divorced	678(13)	152(10)	324(26)	202(9)
Widowed	1504(30)	462(30)	236(19)	806(36)
Others	578(11)	191(13)	159(13)	228(10)

Table 2 Mean number of study participants who were in care and those accessing HAART each year

Year	Total number in care	Number LFU/died(−) or returning for care(+) n(%)	Total on ART n(%)	Tororo HIV clinic n(%)		Mulago HIV clinic n(%)		Mbarara HIV clinic n(%)	
				In care	On ART	In care	On ART	In care	On ART
2002	5972	-	-	-	-	-	-	-	-
2003	4725	1247(−21)	-	-	-	-	-	-	-
2004	3896	829(−18)	371(9)	1181	-	1185	252(21)	1530	119(8)
2005	3551	345(−9)	837(23)	1261	61(5)	1157	343(30)	1133	433(38)
2006	2980	571(−16)	934(32)	972	71(7)	931	392(42)	1077	471(44)
2007	2401	579(−19)	1051(43)	863	84(10)	686	438(64)	852	529(62)
2008	2087	314(−13)	1135(54)	823	101(12)	581	466(80)	683	568(83)
2009	2127	42(+2)	1281(60)	887	176(20)	579	497(86)	661	608(92)
2010	2190	63(+3)	1693(77)	888	557(63)	570	514(90)	632	622(98)
2011	2002	188(−9)	1741(87)	689	577(84)	558	524(94)	655	640(98)
2012	1724	278(−14)	1724(100)	578	578(100)	515	515(100)	631	631(100)
2013	1772	48(+3)	1772(100)	592	592(100)	533	533(100)	647	647(100)

LFU = Lost to follow up

shown in Fig. 2. Demographic characteristics are shown in Table 1 while study participants accessing HAART over time are shown in Table 2. Background characteristics at the commencement of HAART are shown in Table 3. Average annual prevalence by each OI and statistical tests for trend are shown in Table 4. Average monthly changes in OI prevalence over time after controlling for age, sex and clinic as fixed effects and monthly clustering as a random effect are shown in Table 5.

Diarrhoea (<1 month) monthly prevalence trend exhibited a curvilinear decrease with time, declined rapidly in the first 12 months (45 %) and thereafter levelled off in the following months (Fig. 1). However, after log transformation, monthly prevalence decreased linearly

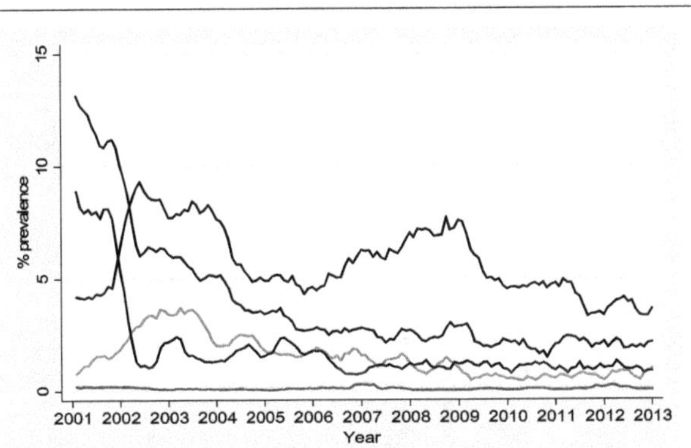

Fig. 1 Plot of monthly prevalence for bacterial pneumonia (green line), malaria (red line), diarrhea <1 month)(blue line), geohelminths(black line) and kaposi's sarcoma (maroon line) over a period of 12 years (2002–2013) expressed as a proportion of HIV-positive persons diagnosed with a particular OI out of the total number who turned up for care per month for the period January 2002 to December 2013

with time ($R^2 = 0.79$, $\beta = -0.02$, $p < 0.001$) and negative correlation coefficient of 0.89 was found in Pearson's correlation between calendar time and prevalence of diarrhoea (Fig. 2). Diarrhoea mean annual prevalence reduced by 83 % (12 % to 2 %) between 2002 and 2013 and the largest decline was in 2003 (45 %). The mean annual prevalence showed a signicant reducing trend ($X^2_{trend} = 177.6$, $P < 0.001$) (Table 4). After adjusting for age, sex and clinic as fixed effects and monthly clustering as a random effect in a mixed effects linear regression model, average monthly prevalence declined at a rate of 2 % per month ($p < 0.05$). The rate of decline per month did not differ significantly by age and sex ($p > 0.05$) but differed significantly by clinic ($p < 0.05$) (Table 5). The monthly rate for Mulago HIV clinic in central Uganda declined 9 % times more compared to that of Tororo HIV clinic in Eastern Uganda($p < 0.001$) whereas the monthly rate for Mbarara HIV clinic in western Uganda declined 0.03 times that of Tororo HIV clinic after adjusting for age and sex.

Bacterial pneumonia had an increasing monthly prevalence trend in the first 24 months (2002–2003) and thereafter monthly prevalence declined gradually (Fig. 1). A negative correlation coefficient of 0.52 was found in Pearson's correlation between calendar time and prevalence of bacterial pneumonia (Fig. 2). Bacterial pneumonia mean annual prevalence reduced by 56 % (3.2 % to 0.7 %) between 2002 and 2013 and the largest impact was in 2010 (41 %) The mean annual prevalence for bacterial pneumonia showed a signicant reducing trend ($X^2_{trend} = 21.7$, $P < 0.001$) (Table 4). The peak prevalence was in 2003 at (32/1000) but the largest reduction was between 2009 and 2010(41 %) (Table 4). Generally

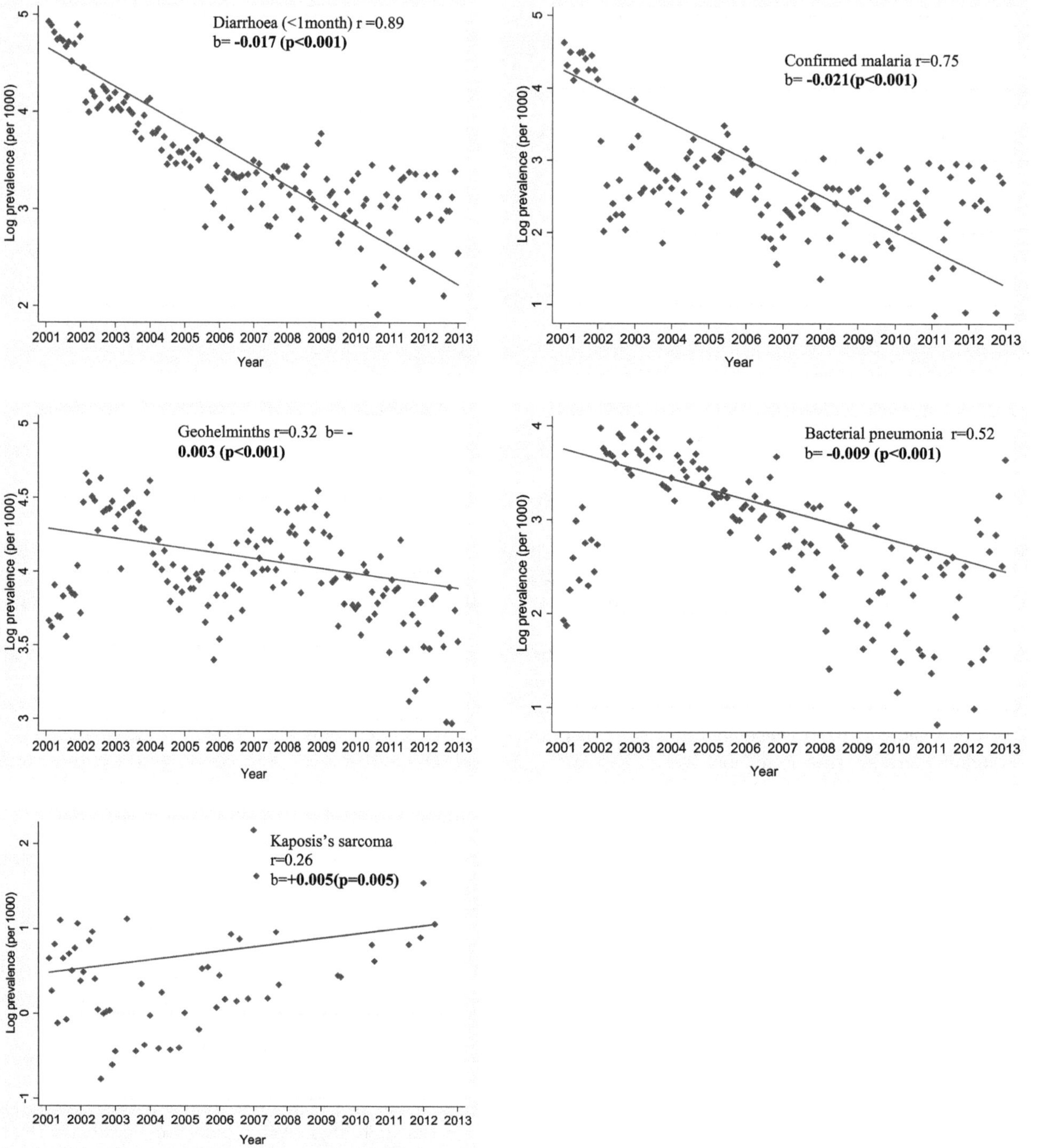

Fig. 2 Scatter plot and fitted regression line for monthly prevalence over time (in months) for each OI expressed as a proportion of HIV-positive persons diagnosed with a particular OI out of the total number who turned up for care per month for the period January 2002 to December 2013

monthly prevalence did not decrease consistently but was characterised by increasing and decreasing trends over time. Hence the net monthly decrease was small ($R^2 = 0.27$, $\beta = -0.01$, $p < 0.001$) (Fig. 2). After adjusting for age, sex and clinic as fixed effects and monthly clustering as a random effect in a mixed effects linear regression model, average monthly prevalence of bacterial pneumonia declined at a rate of 1 % per month ($p < 0.05$). The rate of change per month did not differ significantly by age, sex and clinic ($p > 0.05$) (Table 5).

Table 3 Baseline characteristics of the study participants at commencement of HAART, total and gender segregated

Characteristic	Total (N = 1741)	Female (N = 1413)	Male (N = 328)	p-value*
Age in years, median (IQR)	44(37,50)	43(37,49)	45(40,52)	0.001
WHO stage III & IV, n (%)	1113(63.9)	929(65.7)	184(56.1)	0.121
CD4 cells/μl, median (IQR) (2005–6)	128(55,190)	144(65,191)	49(49,92)	0.074
ART regime (2005–2013), n (%)				
d4T + 3TC+ NVP	693(40)	638(45)	136(41)	0.233
ZDV +3TC + NPV	774(44)	562(40)	131(40)	
Other**	274(16)	213(15)	61(19)	

*Chi^2-Test
**includes Tenofovir(TDF), Lopinavir/ritonavir, etc.

The sum of the mean number of reported malaria cases per year was 3471 of which 309 (8.9 %) were confirmed malaria cases and 3162 (91.1 %) were suspected cases treated for malaria. However only confirmed cases were considered for analysis. Malaria monthly prevalence trends exhibited a curvilinear decrease with time, decreased rapidly in the first 12 months from 8 % to 2 % (80 %) and thereafter levelled off in the following months (Fig. 1). A negative correlation coefficient of 0.75 was found in Pearson's correlation between calendar time and prevalence of malaria (Fig. 2). Malaria mean annual prevalence reduced by 87 % (8 % to 1 %) between 2002 and 2013 and the largest impact was in 2003 (80 %). The mean annual prevalence showed a signicant reducing trend ($X^2_{trend} = 102.6$, $P < 0.001$) (Table 4). After adjusting for age, sex and clinic as fixed effects and monthly clustering as a random effect in a mixed effects linear regression model, average monthly prevalence declined at a rate of 2 % per month ($p < 0.05$) (Table 5). The monthly rate differed significantly by age, sex and clinic ($p < 0.05$). Malaria prevalence declined by 6 % times more in men compared to women ($p = 0.01$) after adjusting for age and clinic. The monthly rate also declined 9 % more in those aged 30-39years and 10 % more in those aged 40 years and above as compared to those <30 years (<0.001) after adjusting for sex and clinic. However the monthly rate of decline for Mulago HIV clinic was not significantly different from that of Tororo HIV clinic ($p > 0.05$) but the monthly rate for Mbarara HIV clinic was significantly different from that of Tororo HIV clinic ($p < 0.05$) after adjusting for age and sex) (Table 5).

Geohelminths included *Ascaris lumbricodes, Trichuris trichiura, Necator americanus, Strongyloides stercoralis* and *Ancylostoma duodenale.* Overall the monthly prevalence was characterised by increasing and decreasing trends, first increased between 0–12 months, then declined between 12-60months, then increased again between 60-96months and thereafter declined for the rest of the remaining study period (Fig. 1). A negative correlation coefficient of 0.32 was found in Pearson's correlation between calendar time and prevalence of geohelminths (Fig. 2). Geohelminthic infection mean annual prevalence reduced by 56 % (9 % to 4 %) between 2002 and 2013 and the largest impact was in 2005 (34 %) The mean annual prevalence showed a signicant reducing trend ($X^2_{trend} = 6.2$, $P = 0.01$) (Table 4). The peak prevalence was in 2003 at (88/1000) but the largest reduction was between 2004 and 2005(34 %) (Table 4). Because monthly prevalence did not decrease consistently but was characterised by increasing and decreasing trends over time, the net monthly decrease was small ($R^2 = 0.10$, $\beta = -0.03$, $p < 0.001$) (Fig. 3). After adjusting for age, sex and clinic as fixed effects and monthly clustering as a random effect in a mixed effects linear regression model, average monthly prevalence declined at a rate of 0.3 % per month ($p < 0.05$) (Table 5). However, the rate of change per month did not differ significantly by age, sex and clinic ($p > 0.05$)

Kaposis sarcoma was found very rare (Fig. 1) and a showed non-significant mean annual increasing trend ($X^2_{trend} = 1.67$, $P = 0.20$) (Table 4). A positive correlation coefficient of 0.26 was found in Pearson's correlation between calendar time and prevalence of Kaposis sarcoma (Fig. 2). After adjusting for age, sex and clinic as fixed effects and monthly clustering as a random effect in a mixed effects linear regression model, average monthly prevalence increased at a rate of 0.4 % per month ($p < 0.05$). However, the rate of change per month did not differ significantly by age, sex and clinic ($p > 0.05$) (Table 5)

Discussion

Diarrhoea has for long been reported to be one of the commonest complication in HIV positive individuals associated with opportunistic enteric infections [23]. Previous studies show up to 60 % of people living with HIV experience diarrhoea, that negatively affects their quality of life and adherence to HAART [24]. Diarrhoea among HIV positive individuals may be due to multiple causes including infectious causes (bacterial, viral, protozoal,

Table 4 Test for trend of mean annual prevalence (per 1000) with calendar time (2002–2013)

	Before HAART		Early HAART					Late HAART					
OI	2002	2003	2004	2005	2006	2007	2008	2009	2010	2011	2012	2013	X^2_{trend} *(p-value)*
Diarrhoea (<1 month)	117.6	64.2	54.6	37.7	31.6	25.8	25.5	25.9	20.9	18.4	22.0	20.2	177.6 (<0.001)
% change	-	−45	−15	−31	−16	−18	−1	+1	−19	−12	+19	−1	
Kaposis sarcoma	2.1	1.5	1.5	1.0	1.5	4.5	3.5	-	1.5	2.1	3.1	2.7	1.67 (0.197)
% change	-	−29	0	−33	+50	+200	−22	-	-	+40	+48	−13	
Bacterial Pneumonia	13.2	32.3	30.1	22.4	15.9	16.7	13.3	9.8	5.8	5.4	5.8	7.7	21.7 (<0.001)
% change	-	+145	−7	−26	−29	+5	−20	−26	−41	−7	+7	+33	
Malaria	78.7	16.0	15.2	16.7	19.6	10.5	10.2	11.3	11.4	11.0	9.4	9.6	102.6 (<0.001)
% change	-	−80	−5	+10	+17	−46	−3	+11	+1	−3	−14	+1	
Geohelminths	43.9	87.9	81.8	54.3	47.3	54.4	62.5	71.6	54.9	45.8	40.9	36.6	6.2 (0.0124)
% change	-	+100	−7	−34	−13	+15	+15	+15	−23	−16	−11	−10	

heliminthic, etc.) or non-infectious causes(ARV drug effects e.g. ritonavir-boosted protease inhibitors such as Lopinavir/ritonavir or nelfinavir) [24–28]. Its prevalence is significantly higher among HIV-positive people when compared to matched controls [24]

A previous study in Uganda reported the commonest causes of diarrhoea to be helminthic infections(29.5 %), bacterial infections (19.2 %) and protozoal infections (9.2 %) [29]. Enteric viruses have also been reported associated with diarrhoea [23]. In the current study, diarrhoea prevalence declined from 12 % in the period before HAART to 2 % in 2013. In fact the biggest decline in diarrhea prevalence happened in 2003(45 %) before HAART was introduced. This was proabably due to the introduction of cotrimoxazole prophyalaxis in 2003. Our findings are consistent with other previous studies that examined the effect of cotrimoxazole prophylaxis on diarrhoea. A study in Eastern Uganda found a significant reduction in the incidence of diarrhoea after 18 months of cotrimoxazole prophylaxis(RR = 0.65; 95%CI = 0.53-0.81; p < 0.0001) [6]. Trends of bacterial diarrhoea in persons infected with HIV in the USA from 1992 to 2002 also showed a significant decrease in the period after HAART compared to the period before HAART (OR 0.4, 95%CI 0.2-0.6) [30]. The persitence of diarrhoea in spite of the increassing access to HAART and universal cotrimoxazole prophylaxis is most likely due to non-infectious causes as has previously been reported [24, 31]. A cohort study in Uganda that followed children and adolescents aged 6 weeks to 18 years who were ART for 5 years(2004–9) reported 13.% had diarrhoea attributed to ART use [31]. With global scale up of HAART access, the incidence of infectious diarrhoea has decreased but incidence of non-infectious diarrhoea has increased. More studies are urgently required to give more insight on how we can overcome this challenge and improve the quality of life for persons living with HIV/AIDS.

In Uganda, malaria is still the leading cause of illness and death particularly among the vulnerable groups including pregnant women, children under five years and people living with HIV/AIDS. In recent years, tremendous progress has been made in the fight against malaria through various interventions including increased public awareness about preventive measures; increased access to insecticide treated nets, introduction of rapid diagnostic tests (RDTs) and improved anti-malarial treatment. In this study we have observed a steep decline in malaria prevalence in 2003(80 %) which levelled off in the following years. This decline could partly be attributed to the introduction of universal cotrimoxazole prophylaxis for all HIV positive patients in Uganda in 2003 [32]. This finding is consistent with previous studies that reported a lower risk of malaria after cotrimoxazole prophylaxis compared to before (p = 0.02) [33]. A study in Eastern Uganda, showed 72 % decrease in the rate of malaria among HIV positive individuals attributed to cotrimoxazole prophylaxis[6]. Another study in Uganda showed that ART associated with daily cotrimoxazole was more protective against malaria compared to daily cotrimoxazole alone, when administered to HIV-infected adults [34]. Many studies have also reported antimalarial treatment effect of antiretroviral drugs [35–37]. This could perhaps explain the observed low malaria prevalence after the introduction HAART. However, our estimated prevalence could be an underestimate because of excluding clinically diagnosed cases that did not get a laboratory confirmation. Additionally, the decline in malaria prevalence over time could also have been caused by the other malaria interventions in Uganda including massive distribution of insecticide treated mosquito bed nets and introduction of indoor residual spraying especially in Northern Uganda [38].

Soil transmitted helminths are endemic in sub-Saharan Africa but very little has been written about their

Table 5 Mixed effects linear regression of monthly prevalence (per 1000) and calendar time (months) adjusted for fixed effects (age, sex and clinic) and random effects (monthly clustering)

	Diarrhoea < 1 month[1] β (95 % CI) [p-value]	Malaria[2] β (95 % CI) [p-value]	Geohelminths[3] β (95 % CI) [p-value]	Bacterial Pneumonia[4] β (95 % CI) [p-value]	Kaposis sarcoma[5] β (95 % CI) [p-value]
Time*	−0.017	−0.018	−0.003	−0.01	0.004
	(−0.0172 to −0.0168)	(−0.018 to −0.017)	(−0.003 to −0.002)	(−0.01 to −0.01)	(0.0006 to to.007
	[<0.001]	[<0.001]	[<0.001]	[<0.001]	[0.020]
Sex					
Female	1	1	1	1	1
Male	0 .0026	−0.061	−0.002	0.004	−0.08
	(−0.018 to 0.013) [0.743]	(−0.11 to −0.015) [,0.009]	(−0.019 to 0.014) [0.763]	(−0.039 to0.049) [0.845]	(−0.33 to 0.18) [0.544]
Age					
<30 yrs	1	1	1	1	1
30-39	−0.0019	0.09	0.015	0.03	−0.26
	(−0.017 to 0.014)	(0.05 to 0.13)	(−0.001 to 0.03)	(−0.012 to 0.072)	(−0.57 to .049)
	[0.809]	[0.001]	[0.071]	[0.168]	[0.100]
40+	−0.0047	0.096	0.011	−0.007	−0.30
	(−0.0134to 0.023)	(0.04to 0.15)	(−0.008 to 0.029)	(−0.06 to 0.045)	(−0.70 to 0.11)
	[0.612]	[<0.001]	[0.269]	[0.789]	[0.148]
HIV clinic					
Tororo	1	1	1	1	1
Mulago	−0.072	0.056	0.016	0.026	−0.014
	(−0.09 to −0.05)	(0.02to 0.13)	(−0.002 to 0.035)	(−0.024to 0.077)	(−0.29 to 0.26)
	[<0.001]	[0.129]	[0.083]	[0.306]	[0.920]
Mbarara	−0.033	0.43	0.022	0.018	0.12
	(−0.08 to −0.017)	(0.37 to 0.49)	(0.006 to 0.039)	(−0.037to 0.073)	(−0.17 to 0.42)
	[0.001]	[,0.001]	[0.009]	[0.518]	[0.404]
Constant (β_0)	4.7	3.8	4.3	3.4	0.64
	(4.6 to 4.8)	(3.7to 3.9)	(4.2 to 4.3)	(3.3 to 3.5)	(0.27 to 1.03)
	[<0.001]	[<0.001]	[<0.001]	[<0.001]	(0.001)
Month					
δ^2_μ	0.0063	0.007	0.0016	0.017	0.044
(95 % CI)	(0.0028 to 0.014)	(0.003 to 0.019	(0007to 0.004)	(0.007 to 0.040)	(0.008 to 0.22)
[SE]	[0.003]	[0.003]	[0.0007]	[0.007]	[0.036]
δ^2_ε	0.071	0.26	0.087	0.179	0.32
(95 % CI)	(0.069 to 0.074)	(0.25 to 0.28)	(0.084 to 0.09)	(0.17 to 0.19)	(0.23 to 0.42)
[SE]	[0.001]	[0.007]	[0.0014]	[0.006]	[0.048]

*Time =144 months, β = beta coefficient, SE = standard error, CI = confidence interval, δ^2_ε = Residual variance
δ^2_μ = random effect monthly variance
[1]Natural log monthly prevalence (per 1000) for Diarrhoea (<1 month)
[2]Natural log monthly prevalence (per 1000) for Malaria
[3]Natural log monthly prevalence (per 1000) for Geohelminths
[4]Natural log monthly prevalence (per 1000) for Bacterial Pneumonia
[5]Natural log monthly prevalence (per 1000) for Kaposis sarcoma

association of with HIV infection and let alone their trends. A few previous studies showed a significant association between HIV and geohelminthic infections though this association was not consistent for all helminths. A study in Honduras found a strong association between *Strongyloides stercoralis* and HIV infection but lower risk for infections of *Giardia lamblia*, *Ascaris lubricoides* and *Trichuris trichiurias* [39]. Another study found a high prevalence of *Giardiasis* and *Strongyloidiasis* among HIV-positive patients in Brazil [40]. A similar study in Ethiopia also found higher prevalence of *Strongyloides stercoralis* among HIV-positive patients with CD4 count <200 cells/µl [41]. All these point to the fact that a reduced immunity increases the risk of infection by helminthic infections and anything that improves this immunity would ideally reduce the risk of infection. In the current study prevalence of helminthic infections remained relatively higher compared to other opportunistic infections and was less affected by the expanded coverage of HAART with time. More studies are required to have more insight on the effect of HAART on severity of infection and risk of new geohelminthic infections.

Bacterial pneumonia is one of the commonest respiratory infections associated with HIV/AIDS in Africa [42]. Whereas pneumocystis pneumonia (PCP) is common in European countries and the United states but is uncommon in Africa [43]. Community-acquired bacterial pneumonia caused by *Streptococcus pneumoniae* is one of the commonest respiratory tract infections in persons living with HIV/AIDS [44]. Though preventable, bacterial pneumonia is one of the leading causes of morbidity and mortality among persons living with HIV/AIDS in many sub-Saharan Africa countries [45–48]. A review of studies on HIV/AIDS related opportunistic infections in sub-Saharan Africa show high prevalence of *S. pneumonia* infection ranging from 25 % in Cameroon to 31 % in Uganda [47]. In the current study, prevalence of bacterial pneumonia showed an increasing trend up to 2003, and thereafter reduced consistently with increasing access to HAART. This is probably due to universal cotrimoxazole prophylaxis introduced in 2003 and HAART in 2004. Some studies have shown HIV infection to be associated with a 10-fold increase in incidence of bacterial pneumonia [42]. However our findings are consistent with other previous studies which showed a significant reducing effect of cotrimoxazole prophylaxis and HAART. For instance a study Kohli et al. showed HAART and cotrimoxazole prophylaxis were associated with an 8 % monthly risk reduction of bacterial pneumonia [49]. However our findings differs from those obtained in a study in the USA that evaluated annual trends for 13 most common AIDS-defining opportunistic infections by examining medical records in more than 90 hospitals and clinics in 9 US cities before HAART (1991–96) that showed decreasing trend in all the OIs except pneumonia [50]. Another study in the USA reported high rates of bacterial pneumonia among HIV-positive women compared to HIV-negative women [49]. The rate of bacterial pneumonia among HIV-infected women was 8.5 cases per 100 person-years, compared with 0.7 cases per 100 person-years in HIV-uninfected women ($P < .001$). Relatively few studies have characterised the impact of HAART on bacterial pneumonia in resource poor settings and more studies are therefore recommended.

Kaposis's sarcoma which is an AIDS-related malgnancy had no evidence of a significant trend. Kaposi's sarcoma usually associated with advanced HIV disease was found rare in our study. Though strictly speaking, it's not an opportunistic infection but was studied because of its close association with viral infections (human herpes virus type 8) [12]. In developed countries, the introduction of highly active antiretroviral therapy (HAART) in 1996 led to a tremendous decrease in the incidence of Kaposi's sarcoma (KS) among people with HIV or AIDS (PWHA) [51]. Our findings are consistent with another study in Kenya in which medical records at Nairobi hospital were reviewed for Kaposis sarcoma covering the period 1968 to 1997 and was found to be very rare at only 2-5 % [52]. A retrospective review of clinical records in a teaching hospital in North-western Nigeria covering the period 1994–2004 also found the prevalence of Kaposis sarcoma to be very low (only 27cases in 11 years) [53]. Another study that examined trends of Kaposis sarcoma for the period 1982–2009 in Brazil found a prevalence of only 2.4 % among HIV+ individuals [54]. The study also showed a significant reduction in Kaposis sarcoma prevalence attributed to increased access to HAART over time [54]. Another study that evaluated time trends of AIDS-defining diseases diagnosed in Italy during the pre-HAART period (1982–1996) noted downward trends for mycoses, PCP, Karposis sarcoma and non-Hodgkin's lymphomas and upward trends for mycobacterioses, bacterial and protozoal infections [55]. However, more studies giving insight on the impact of HAART on Kaposis sarcoma and other HIV-related opportunistic cancers in resource poor settings are still required.

Limitations

This study had a number of limitations. First, data analysed was limited to what was available in the TASO electronic data base and so certain variables whose data was not captured could not be analysed. Being a retrospective cohort, there was no information available on the clients who never returned for care. So we did not have information on the connection to care or survival status of clients who were lost to follow up. However we assumed that these simply relocated to another clinic for care or died as had been reported in other previous studies [56–60]. Even from sensitivity analysis (results not shown), we established that cases who remained in care were not significantly different from those that were lost to follow up and so we conservatively assumed that cases who remained in care were a representative sample of all the cases in the original cohort and that missing clinic visits happened randomly. The TASO clients whose medical records were analysed may not represent all HIV positive individuals in Uganda which means generalisability could be limited but still this does not compromise the evidence we have adduced since most if not all beneficiaries of public health care programmes in Uganda are generally the same. There may also have been a possibility that some OIs went away undiagnosed or were not recorded during clinic visits as was reported in a previous study conducted in Uganda [61]. Though we believe this was minimized by selected OIs which were easy to diagnose and could have been a small number which may not have significantly influenced the overall trends. The decreasing trends of OIs could partially be related to immune recovery due to HAART. However CD4 monitoring data for most patients were not available probably because of being unaffordable in these resource poor settings. Additionally, trends in the reported disease conditions needs to be compared with trends in HIV-negative controls since these conditions are not exclusively limited to HIV-infected individuals. This would have helped to explain better whether the decline in trends could only be attributed to HAART and/or co-trimoxazole prophylaxis. Even with these limitations, there is sufficient evidence that increasing HAART availability in resource poor settings is having a meaningful impact on prevalence of opportunistic infections.

Conclusions and recommendations

Our findings show a declining trend in the prevalence of most OIs, though some like geohelminths remain an important public health problem even in the era of HAART. The differences in trends between clinics were likely to be due to differences to exposure to infectious agents and the rural/urban disparity. Tororo being most remote and rural had the highest prevalence of the OIs studied and needs special consideration for targeted interventions. With an increasing number of HAART eligible HIV-infected patients amidst limited resources to sustain lifelong access to treatment, more studies are needed to assess the effectiveness of current treatment strategies on the quality of life of persons living with HIV/AIDS to better inform policy and planning of HIV/AIDS health care service. Future studies should compare trends in HIV positive individuals with trends in HIV negative controls to better understand whether the declining trends are exclusively due to increasing access to HAART and co-trimoxazole prophylaxis. There is also urgent need to integrate interventions targeting malaria and geohelminths in HIV programmes.

Competing interests

The authors declare that they have no competing interests.

Authors contributions

JR: Conceived the study, participated in the study design, data collection, analysis and manuscript writing; NMT: Participated in study design, data analysis and manuscript writing; JKL: Participated in study design, data analysis and manuscript writing. All authors read and approved the final manuscript.

Acknowledgement

We are grateful to the AIDS Support Organisation (TASO) in Uganda for providing the data for the study. We would also like to extend our sincere appreciation to Mountains of the Moon University for the financial support.

References

1. UNAIDS. Access to Antiretroviral therapy in Africa: Satus report on progress towards 2015 targets. Geneva: UNAIDS; 2014.
2. UNAIDS. Global report. UNAIDS report on the global AIDS epidemic 2013. Geneva: WHO; 2013.
3. Uganda MOH. National AIDS Indicator Survey 2011. Uganda Ministry Of Health: Kampala; 2011.
4. Ministry of Finance, Planning and Economic development (MoFPED) Uganda. Millenium Development Goals Report for Uganda. Kampala; 2010.
5. Watera C, Todd J, Muwonge R, Whitworth J, Nakiyingi-Miiro J, Brink A, et al. Feasibility and effectiveness of cotrimoxazole prophylaxis for HIV-1-infected adults attending an HIV/AIDS clinic in Uganda. J Acquir Immune Defic Syndr. 2006;42(3):373–8.
6. Mermin J, Lule J, Ekwaru JP, Malamba S, Downing R, Ransoma R, et al. Effect of cotrimoxazole prophylaxis on morbidity, mortality, CD4 cell count, and viral load in HIV infection in rural Uganda. Lancet. 2004;364:1428–34.
7. Holmes BC, Wood R, Badri M, Margolin S, Wang B, Martens G. Incidence of primary opportunistic infections in Cape Town South Africa: Implications for prophylaxis. Denver, USA: 13th conference of Retroviruses and opportunistic infections: 2005; 2005.
8. Wiktor SZ, Sassan-Morokro M, Grant AD, Abouya L, Karon JM, Mourice C, et al. Efficacy of trimethoprim-sulphamethoxazole prophylaxis to decrease morbidity and mortality in HIV-1 infected patients with tuberculosis in Abidjan, Cote d'Ivoire: a randomised controlled trial. Lancet. 1999;353:1469–75.
9. Walker AS, Ford D, Gilks CF, Munderi P, Ssali F, Reid A, et al. Daily Cotrimoxazole prophylaxis in severely immune-suppressed HIV-infected adults in Africa started on combination antiretroviral therapy: an observational analysis of the DART cohort. Lancet. 2010;375:1278–86.
10. UNAIDS. Guidelines on Cotrimoxazole prophylaxis for HIV-related infections among children, adolescents and adults; Recommendations for a Public health approach. Geneva: WHO; 2006.
11. Ministry of Health Uganda. National policy guidelines for cotrimoxazole prophylaxis for people with HIV/AIDS. Kampala: Ministry of Health; 2005.
12. Paradžik M, Bučević-Popović V, Šitum M, Jaing C, Degoricija M, McLoughlin K, et al. Association of Kaposi's sarcoma-associated herpesvirus (KSHV) with bladder cancer in Croatian patients. Tumour Biol. 2014;35(1):567–72.
13. Calvarese M, Bame S, Bakanume B. Historical analysis of AIDS patients in Uganda using innovative community clinical service: The AIDS Support Organisation (TASO). Journal of Humanities and Social Sciences. 2007;1:1–13.
14. WHO. Antiretroviral therapy for HIV infection in adults and adolescents; recommendations for a public health approach. Geneva: WHO; 2006.
15. WHO. Antiretroviral therapy for HIV infection in adults and adolescents: recommendations for a public health approach 2010 revision. Geneva: WHO; 2010.
16. Ministry of Health Uganda. Antiretroviral treatment policy. Kampala: Uganda Ministry of Health; 2009.
17. TASO Services and Programmes [http://www.tasouganda.org/]
18. Ministry of Health Uganda. Uganda Clinical guidelines: National guidelines on management of common conditions. Kampala; 2010.
19. Box, Jenkins, Reinsel. Time Series Analysis, Forecasting and Control. 3rd ed. Englewood Clifs, NJ: Prentice Hall; 1994.
20. Cuzick J. A Wilcoxon-type test for trend. Stat Med. 1985;4:87–90.
21. Stata corp. Nonparametric analysis:trend test across ordered groups. 2012th ed. College station, Texas, USA: Stata Corp; 2012.
22. Stata corp. Nonparametric analysis: kruskal wallis rank test. 2012th ed. College statation, Texas, USA: Stata corp LP; 2012.
23. Grohmannp G, Glass R, Pereira H, Monroem S, Ainerweber AH, Bryan A. Enteric Viruses And Diarrhea In Hiv-Infected Patients. N Engl J Med. 1993;329(1):14–20.

24. MacArthur R, DuPont H. Etiology and Pharmacologic Management of Noninfectious Diarrhea in HIV-Infected Individuals in the Highly Active Antiretroviral Therapy Era. Clin Infect Dis. 2012;55(6):860–7.
25. Guest J, Ruffin C, Tschampa J, DeSilva K, Rimland D. Differences in Rates of Diarrhea in Patients with Human Immunodeficiency Virus Receiving Lopinavir-Ritonavir or Nelfinavir. Pharmacotherapy. 2004;24(6):727–35.
26. Johnson M, Grinsztejn B, Rodriguez C, Coco J, DeJesus E, Lazzarin A, et al. 96-week comparison of once-daily atazanavir/ritonavir and twice-daily lopinavir/ritonavir in patients with multiple virologic failures. AIDS. 2006;20(5):711–8.
27. Heiser C, Ernst J, Barrett J, French N, Schutz M, Dube M. Probiotics, soluble fiber and L-glutamine (GLN) reduce nelfinavir (NFV)- or lopinavir/ritonavir (LPV/r)- related diarrhea. J Int Assoc Physicians AIDS Care. 2004;3:121–9.
28. Molina J, Andrade-Villanueva J, Echevarria J, Chetchotisakd P, Corral J, David N, et al. Once-daily atazanavir/ritonavir versus twice-daily lopinavir/ritonavir, each in combination with tenofovir and emtricitabine, for management of antiretroviral-naive HIV-1-infected patients: 48 week efficacy and safety results of the CASTLE study. Lancet. 2008;372(9639):646–55.
29. Binka A, Mahe C, Watera C, Lugada E, Gilks CF, Whitworth JAG, et al. Diarrhoea, CD4 Counts and Enteric Infections in a Community-Based Cohort of HIV-Infected Adults in Uganda. J Infect. 2002;45(2):99–105.
30. Sanchez TH, Brooks J, Sullivan P, Juhasz M, Mintz E, Dworkin M, et al. Bacterial Diarrhea in Persons with HIV Infection, United States, 1992–2002. Clin Infect Dis. 2005;41:1621–7.
31. Tukei V, Asiimwe A, Maganda A, Atugonza R, Sebuliba I, Bakeera-Kitaka S, et al. Safety and tolerability of antiretroviral therapy among HIV-infected children and adolescents in Uganda. J Acquir Immun Defic Syndr. 2012;59(3):274–80.
32. Manyando C, Njunju E, D'Alessandro U, Van Geertruyden J. Safety and Efficacy of Co-Trimoxazole for Treatment and Prevention of Plasmodium falciparum Malaria: A Systematic Review. PLoS One. 2013;8(2):e56916.
33. Saracino A, Nacarapa EA, Massinga EC, Martinelli D, Scacchetti M, de Oliveira C, et al. Prevalence and clinical features of HIV and malaria co-infection in hospitalized adults in Beira, Mozambique. Malar J. 2012;11:241.
34. Mermin J, Ekwaru JP, Liechty CA, Were W, Downing R, Ransom R, et al. Effect of co-trimoxazole prophylaxis, antiretroviral therapy, and insecticide-treated bednets on the frequency of malaria in HIV-1-infected adults in Uganda: a prospective cohort study. Lancet. 2006;367:1256–61.
35. Skinner-Adams T, McCarthy J, Gardiner D, Hilton P, Andrews K. Antiretrovirals as Antimalarial Agents. J Infect Dis. 2004;190(11):1998–2000.
36. Greenhalgh S, Ndeffo M, Galvani A, Parikh S. The epidemiological impact of HIV antiretroviral therapy on malaria in children. AIDS. 2015;29(4):473–82.
37. Nakanjako D, Kiragga A, Castelnuovo B, Kyabayinze D, Kamya M. Low prevalence of Plasmodium falciparum antigenaemia among asymptomatic HAART-treated adults in an urban cohort in Uganda. BMC Malaria Journal. 2011;10:66.
38. Ministry of Health Uganda. Malaria Control Report 2011 Aide Memoire. Kampala: Ministry of Health, Uganda; 2011.
39. Lindo JF, Dubon JM, Age RA, De Gourville EM, Solo-Gabriele H, Klaskala WI, et al. Intestinal parasitic infections in human immunodeficiency virus (HIV)-positive and HIV-negative individuals in San Pedro Sula, Honduras. Am J Trop Med Hyg. 1998;58:431–5.
40. Feitosa G, Bandeira AC, Sampaio DP, Badaro R, Brites C. High prevalence of Giardiasis and strongyloidiasis among HIV- infected patients in Bahia, Brazil. Braz J Infect Dis. 2001;5:339–44.
41. Assefa S, Erko B, Medhin G, Assefa Z, Shimelis T. Intestinal parasitic infections in relation to HIV/AIDS status, diarrhea and CD4 T-cell count. BMC Infect Dis. 2009;9:155.
42. Benito N, Moreno A, Miro JM, Torres A. Pulmonary infections in HIV-infected patients: an update in the 21st century. Eur Respir J. 2012;39:730–45.
43. Kaplan JE, Hanson D, Dworkin MS, Frederick T, Bertolli J, Lindergren ML, et al. Epidemiology of human immunodeficiency virus-associated opportunistic infections in the united states in the era of highly active antiretroviral therapy. Clin Infect Dis. 2000;30 Suppl 1:S5–S14.
44. Staine JG. AIDS up date 2007: An overview of acquired immune deficiency syndrome. McGraw-Hill co.,Inc: New York; 2008.
45. French N, Nakiyingi J, Carpenter LM, Lugada E, Moi K, Watera C, et al. 23—valent pneumococcal polysaccharide vaccine in HIV-1-infected Ugandan adults: double-blind, randomised and placebo controlled trial. Lancet. 2000;355(9221):2106–11.
46. Gilks CF, Ojoo SA, Ojoo JC, Brindle RJ, Paul J, Batchelor BI, et al. Invasive pneumococcal disease in a cohort of predominantly HIV-1 infected female sex-workers in Nairobi, Kenya. Lancet. 1996;347(9003):718–23.
47. Holmes BC, Losina E, Walensky RP, Yazdanpanah Y, Freedberg KA. Review of Human Immunodeficiency Virus Type 1–Related Opportunistic Infections in Sub-Saharan Africa. Clin Infect Dis. 2003;36:652–62.
48. Miiro G, Kayhty H, Watera C, Tolmie H, Whitworth JA, Gilks CF, et al. Conjugate pneumococcal vaccine in HIV-infected Ugandans and the effect of past receipt of polysaccharide vaccine. J Infect Dis. 2005;192(10):1801–5.
49. Kohli R, Lo Y, Homel P, Flanigan TP, Gardner LI, Howard AA, et al. Bacterial Pneumonia, HIV Therapy, and Disease Progression among HIV-Infected Women in the HIV Epidemiologic Research (HER) Study. Clin Infect Dis. 2006;43:90–8.
50. Jones JL, Hanson DL, Dworkin MS, Kaplan JE, Ward JW. Trends in AIDS-Related Opportunistic Infections among Men Who Have Sex with Men and among Injecting Drug Users, 1991–1996. J Infect Dis. 1998;178:114–20.
51. Franceschi M, Lise M, Clifford GM, Rickenbach M, Levi F, Maspoli M, et al. Changing patterns of cancer incidence in the early- and late-HAART periods: the Swiss HIV Cohort Study. Br J Cancer. 2010;103:416–22.
52. Onyango JF, Njiru A. Kaposis sarcoma in a Nairobi hospital. East Afr Med J. 2004;81(3):120–3.
53. Mbah N, Abdulkareem IH, Panti A. AIDS-associated Kaposi's sarcoma in Sokoto, Nigeria. Niger J Clin Pract. 2008;11(3):181–4.
54. Saraceni V, Talhari CC, Pereira GF, Golub JE, Talhari S, Miranda AE. AIDS-related Kaposi's sarcoma in Brazil: trends and geopolitical distribution. Int J Dermatol. 2013;52(12):1525–9.
55. Pezzotti P, Serraino D, Rezza G, Maso LD, Vaccher E, Lepri AC, et al. The spectrum of AIDS-defining diseases:Temporal trends in Italy prior to the use of highly active antiretroviral therapies, 1982–1996. Internat J of Epid. 1999;28:975–81.
56. Braitstein P, Brinkhof MW, Dabis F, Schechter M, Boulle A, Miotti P, et al. Mortality of HIV-1-infected patients in the first year of antiretroviral therapy: comparison between low-income and high-income countries. Lancet. 2006;367(9526):817–24.
57. Brinkhof MW, Dabis F, Myer L, Bangsberg DR, Boulle A, Nash D, et al. Early loss of HIV-infected patients on potent antiretroviral therapy programmes in lower-income countries. Bull World Health Organ. 2008;86:559–67.
58. Egger M, Spycher BD, Sidle J, Weigel R, Geng EH, Fox MP, et al. Correcting mortality for loss to follow-up: a nomogram applied to antiretroviral treatment programmes in sub-Saharan Africa. PLoS Med. 2011;8(1):e1000390.
59. Geng EH, Glidden DV, Bwana MB, Musinguzi N, Emenyonu N, Muyindike W, et al. Retention in Care and Connection to Care among HIV-Infected Patients on Antiretroviral Therapy in Africa: Estimation via a Sampling-Based Approach. PLoS One. 2011;6(7):e21797.
60. Kiragga NA, Lok JJ, Musick SB, Bosch JR, Mwangi A, Wools-Kaloustian KK, et al. CD4 trajectory adjusting for dropout among HIV-positive patients receiving combination antiretroviral therapy in an East African HIV care centre. J Int AIDS Soc. 2014;17:18957.
61. Kiragga NA, Castelnuovo B, Schaefer P, Muwonge T, Easterbrook JP. Quality of data collection in a large HIVobservational clinic database in sub-Saharan Africa: implications for clinical research and audit of care. J Int AIDS Soc. 2011;14:3.

Effectiveness of first-line antiretroviral therapy in the IPEC cohort, Rio de Janeiro, Brazil

Sandra W Cardoso[1], Paula M Luz[1*], Luciane Velasque[1,2], Thiago Torres[1], Lara Coelho[1], Kenneth A Freedberg[3], Valdilea G Veloso[1], Rochelle P Walensky[3] and Beatriz Grinsztejn[1]

Abstract

Background: While Brazil has had a long-standing policy of free access to antiretroviral therapy (ART) for all in need, the epidemiological impact of ART on human immunodeficiency virus (HIV) RNA suppression in this middle-income country has not been well evaluated. We estimate first-line ART effectiveness in a large Brazilian cohort and examine the socio-demographic, behavioral, clinical and structural factors associated with virologic suppression.

Methods: Virologic suppression on first-line ART at 6, 12, and 24 months from start of ART was defined as having a viral load measurement ≤400 copies/mL without drug class modification and/or discontinuation. Drug class modification and/or discontinuation were defined based on the class of a particular drug. Quasi-Poisson regression was used to quantify the association of factors with virologic suppression.

Results: From January 2000 through June 2010, 1311 patients started first-line ART; 987 (75%) patients used NNRTI-based regimens. Virologic suppression was achieved by 77%, 76% and 68% of patients at 6, 12 and 24 months, respectively. Factors associated with virologic suppression at 12 months were: >8 years of formal education (compared to <4 years, risk ratio (RR) 1.13, 95% confidence interval (95% CI) 1.03-1.24), starting ART in 2005-2010 (compared to 2000-2004, RR 1.25 95% CI 1.15-1.35), and clinical trial participation (compared to no participation, RR 1.08 95% CI 1.01-1.16). Also at 12 months, women showed less virologic suppression compared to heterosexual men (RR 0.90 95% CI 0.82-0.99). For the 24-month endpoint, in addition to higher education, starting ART in the later period, and clinical trial participation, older age and an NNRTI-based regimen were also independently associated with virologic suppression.

Conclusions: Our results show that in Brazil, a middle-income country with free access to treatment, over three-quarters of patients receiving routine care reached virologic suppression on first-line ART by the end of the first year. Higher education, more recent ART initiation and clinical trial participation were associated with improved outcomes both for the 12-month and the 24-month endpoints, suggesting that further studies are needed to understand what aspects relating to these factors lead to higher virologic suppression.

Keywords: HIV/AIDS, Antiretroviral treatment, Effectiveness, Cohort study, Rio de Janeiro, Brazil

Background

Since the beginning of the HIV/AIDS epidemic, Brazil's response has been both timely and inclusive, addressing prevention as well as treatment. A noteworthy moment was the decision to provide highly active antiretroviral therapy (ART) for all patients in need in 1996. With over 15 years of universal access to ART and almost 300,000 patients receiving ART, Brazil's HIV treatment program stands alone in its universal coverage of all in need compared to other middle-income or resource-limited countries [1]. Despite the enormous publicity it has received, evaluations of Brazil's HIV treatment program are limited. Studies have indicated that morbidity and mortality from HIV infection has fallen since the introduction of ART [2-4]. However, studies evaluating the impact of ART in suppressing HIV viral load, i.e. its effectiveness within the routine care provided through the public health system (the Unified Health System) of Brazil are scarce.

* Correspondence: paula.luz@ipec.fiocruz.br
[1]Instituto de Pesquisa Clínica Evandro Chagas, Fundação Oswaldo Cruz, Rio de Janeiro, Brasil
Full list of author information is available at the end of the article

The efficacy of new drugs is assessed in short-term randomized clinical trials usually conducted in selected populations which frequently exclude participants with concurrent opportunistic diseases, substance abuse and/or psychiatric comorbidities [5]. As such, results from clinical trials are often not generalizable to all treated individuals who might be part of a clinical cohort or to longer-term outcomes [6]. Understanding ART effectiveness within the routine care setting is crucial to guide the evolution of the Brazilian HIV Treatment program. In this study, we evaluated first-line ART effectiveness for patients starting therapy from 2000 to 2010, as well as the factors that correlate with virologic suppression in a large urban cohort in Rio de Janeiro, Brazil.

Methods

The IPEC clinical cohort

This study was conducted at the Evandro Chagas Clinical Research Institute, Oswaldo Cruz Foundation (IPEC/FIOCRUZ), one of the largest infectious disease research centers in Brazil, where care has been provided to HIV/AIDS patients since the beginning of the AIDS epidemic in Brazil in 1986. An observational, longitudinal, clinical database is maintained on patients receiving primary and specialized outpatient and inpatient HIV care at the clinic; it includes socio-demographic, behavioral, clinical and therapeutic information. Details of the HIV/AIDS clinical cohort can be found elsewhere [7,8]. The IPEC Institutional Review Board reviewed and approved this study.

Study population and definitions

All patients who started first-line ART between January 1, 2000 and June 30, 2010 were included and follow-up information included data through September 30, 2011. Though combination ART became available in mid-1996, we specifically excluded 1996-1999 because it was a period characterized by non-standardized combinations as well as continued exposure to mono or dual therapy, which were kept in the prior to 2000 guidelines as alternative first-line regimens. ART was defined as two nucleoside reverse transcriptase inhibitors (NRTI) in combination with one non-nucleoside reverse transcriptase inhibitor (NNRTI) or one protease inhibitor (PI). Drug class modification and/or discontinuation were defined based on the class of a particular drug. A patient who started a first-line NNRTI-based regimen, for example, was assumed to have modified and/or discontinued the regimen if it was changed to a PI-based regimen or if the NNRTI was discontinued. NRTI modifications and/or discontinuations were not considered since these could be due to reasons unrelated to a drug-class failure. For the years 2000-2010, ART guidelines were consistent regarding first-line ART with NNRTI-based regimens cited as preferred and PI-based regimens as alternative options.

First-line ART effectiveness

First-line ART effectiveness was defined as having HIV viral load ≤ 400 copies/mL and no drug class modification and/or discontinuation. Deaths from AIDS-related causes were considered as failures. Because the limit of detection of viral load assays used throughout the study period varied from ≤400 copies/mL to ≤50 copies/mL, we used the ≤400 copies/mL threshold for the entire study period for consistency.

We examined virologic outcomes at 6, 12, and 24 months from first-line ART initiation. Window periods were defined for each time point as 5-9 months, 9-15 months, and 21-27 months, respectively. Within each window, the viral load measurement occurring closest to the target time point (either before or after) was chosen. Drug class modification and/or discontinuations were evaluated for the entire period from the start of first-line ART until the upper limit of each window period.

Missing data

The IPEC Cohort has a validated algorithm for identification of deaths which has been previously described [8,9]. In addition, since IPEC provides outpatient and inpatient care, as well as a multidisciplinary team including a cadre of clinical specialties coupled with pharmaceutical care, the rate of loss-to-follow-up is low (4.1/100 person-years). Absence of laboratory measurements is most frequently a result of insufficient infrastructure to support the CD4/viral load monitoring needed for all patients on ART. As such, we evaluated the impact of missing viral load measurements on first-line ART effectiveness by examining both best and worst-case scenarios. In the best case scenario, missing viral load data were assumed as suppression. Alternatively, in the worst-case scenario, missing viral loads were imputed as failures.

Immunologic response

We examined CD4 counts 6, 12, and 24 months from ART initiation. Window periods were, as for viral loads, defined for each time point as 5-9 months, 9-15 months, and 21-27 months. Within each window, the CD4 count occurring closest to the target time point (either before or after) was chosen.

Statistical analyses

First-line ART effectiveness was calculated as the probability (95% CI) of viral suppression at 6, 12 and 24 months after ART initiation. The impact of socio-demographic, behavioral, clinical and structural factors on virologic suppression at 12 and 24 months was estimated using a quasi-Poisson regression model; this corrected for variance estimation and allowed for the estimation of relative risks. We chose the use of quasi-Poisson models since the data showed overdispersion (i.e. the variance was greater than the mean; this would be contrary to the assumption of the Poisson model which assumes that the variance is equal to the mean) and because log-binomial regression models did not converge. The final model included variables found to be significant at a threshold p-value of 0.05, as well as factors known to be clinically relevant or that were shown to modify the effect of a covariate in the adjusted model. We also examined the impact of missing viral load measurements on the final model by re-estimating the parameters while assuming the worst-case and best-case scenarios. R software version 2.15.2 (www.r-project.org) was used for all statistical analyses.

Results

Study population

From January 2000 through June 2010, 1,311 patients started first-line ART; 40% were ≥40 years old (Table 1). Among men, men who have sex with men (MSM) predominated as the HIV risk exposure category; 9.8% of the study population reported injection drug use (IDU) or other modes of HIV risk exposure. Half of the cohort had over 8 years of education. Sixty-four percent of the patients had three years or less since their first positive HIV test; 494 (37.7%) had a pre-treatment CD4 count ≤200 cells/μL (overall median 222/μL, IQR:105-322 cells/μL), and 466 (35.5%) had a pre-treatment viral load >100,000 copies/mL. The majority of patients started a first-line NNRTI-based regimen (987, 75.3%). Seventy percent of patients started their first-line regimens in the calendar period 2005-2010. Just over one-third of patients started first-line ART within a clinical trial conducted at IPEC.

Among the 987 patients who started an NNRTI-based regimen, efavirenz (EFV) was used by 93.3% (921/987); the most frequent EFV-based combination was zidovudine (AZT) + lamivudine (3TC) + EFV (590/921, 64.1%), followed by tenofovir (TDF) + 3TC + EFV or TDF + emtricitabine (FTC) + EFV (252/921, 27.4%). Among the 324 patients who started a PI-containing regimen, the majority used a boosted PI (197/324, 60.8%). The most frequent boosted PI was ritonavir-boosted lopinavir LPV/r (93/197, 47.2%) followed by ritonavir-boosted atazanavir ATV/r (62/197, 31.4%). Among those who started a non-boosted PI regimen (127/324, 39.2%), 65.4% (83/127) started with ATV. The frequency of boosted PI prescriptions was 47.8% (54/113) for the calendar year 2000-04 and 67.7% (143/211) for 2005-10.

First-line ART effectiveness

Overall first-line ART effectiveness, inclusive only of those with viral load data, was 76.9%, 76.1% and 67.9% at 6, 12 and 24 months (Table 2, top section). When assuming the best-case scenario including all patients, ART effectiveness increased to 82.8%, 80.8% and 77.0% at 6, 12 and 24 months. Inclusive of all patients, the worse-case scenario produced ART effectiveness rates of 57.5%, 61.2% and 48.6% at 6, 12 and 24 months. First-line ART effectiveness at each time point was consistently higher for those using an NNRTI-based regimen compared to a PI-based regimen (Table 2, middle section). Increased effectiveness was also observed for those who started first-line ART in 2005-2010 compared to those who started in 2000-2004 (Table 2, bottom section).

CD4 counts

Median CD4 counts for the entire cohort significantly increased with the progression of the time points evaluated (Figure 1). At baseline, the median CD4 count was 221/μL whereas at 6, 12 and 24 months, it was 338/μL, 375/μL and 448/μL. These improvements correspond to a median CD4 count increase from baseline of 107/μL, 151/μL and 242/μL at 6, 12, and 24 months.

Factors associated with virologic suppression

In the adjusted model for the 12-month endpoint, gender/risk category, education, calendar year of ART initiation and participation in a clinical trial all remained independently associated with virologic suppression (Table 3). Compared to heterosexual men, women were less likely to be virologically suppressed (RR 0.90 95% CI 0.82-0.99). Having over eight years of formal education resulted in improved virologic suppression (RR 1.13 95% CI 1.03-1.24), compared to less than four years of formal education. Increased virologic suppression was also associated with starting ART in 2005-2010 (RR 1.25 95% CI 1.15-1.35) compared to starting in 2000-2004. Participation in a clinical trial versus not was associated with increased virologic suppression (RR 1.08 95% CI 1.01-1.16).

In the adjusted model for the 24-month endpoint, age, gender/risk category, education, type of ART regimen, calendar year of ART initiation, and clinical trial participation remained independently associated with virologic suppression (Table 3). Virologic suppression was associated with older age (RR for ≥40 years old 1.12 95% CI 1.00-1.26, compared to < 30 years old), and there was a trend toward greater virologic suppression among MSM compared to heterosexual men (RR 1.11 95% CI 0.98-1.27). Again, women compared to heterosexual men were less likely to be virologically suppressed, although this estimate did not reach statistical significance. Virologic suppression remained associated with first-line NNTRI-based regimen (RR 1.17 95% CI 1.05-1.31, compared to PI-based regimen), calendar year 2005-10 (RR 1.14 95% CI 1.03-1.27, compared to 2000-2004), and participation in a clinical trial (RR 1.12 95% CI 1.02-1.23).

Table 1 Baseline socio-demographic, behavioral, clinical and structural characteristics at first-line antiretroviral therapy (ART) initiation (IPEC Clinical Cohort, 2000 to 2010)

Total		1311
Age		
	Mean (SD)	37.1 (9.9)
	< 30	355 (27.1)
	30-39	446 (34.0)
	≥ 40	510 (38.9)
Race		
	Non-white	621 (47.4)
	White	690 (52.6)
Gender/Risk category[a]		
	Women	432 (33.0)
	Heterosexual men	327 (24.9)
	MSM	423 (32.3)
	IDU/Other	129 (9.8)
Years of formal education		
	< 4	277 (21.1)
	4-8	380 (29.0)
	> 8	654 (49.9)
Years since HIV + test		
	<= 3	836 (63.8)
	> 3	475 (36.2)
Pre-treatment CD4 count/μL[b]		
	Mean (SD)	233 (184)
	<= 200	494 (37.7)
	201-350	392 (29.9)
	> 350	208 (15.9)
	Missing	217 (16.6)
Pre-treatment HIV viral load copies/mL[c]		
	<= 100000	532 (40.6)
	> 100000	466 (35.5)
	Missing	313 (23.9)
Concurrent AIDS defining illness[d]		
	No	1013 (77.3)
	Yes	298 (22.7)
Hepatitis B/C co-infection[e]		
	No	1270 (96.9)
	Yes	41 (3.1)
ART regimen[f]		
	PI-based	324 (24.7)
	NNRTI-based	987 (75.3)
Calendar year of ART initiation		
	2000-2004	392 (29.9)
	2005-2009	919 (70.1)

Table 1 Baseline socio-demographic, behavioral, clinical and structural characteristics at first-line antiretroviral therapy (ART) initiation (IPEC Clinical Cohort, 2000 to 2010) *(Continued)*

Started ART in clinical trial		
	No	856 (65.3)
	Yes	455 (34.7)

SD: standard deviation, HIV: human immunodeficiency virus, PI: protease inhibitor, NNRTI: non-nucleoside reverse transcriptase inhibitor.
[a]Gender and reported mode of HIV exposure were categorized jointly into women, men who have sex with men (MSM), heterosexual men, and injection drug users (IDU, men and women) and other reported modes of HIV exposure (men and women). Individuals reporting both injection drug use and other modes of HIV exposure were categorized as IDU.
[b]Measurement closest to the date of start of ART up to 30 days after.
[c]Measurement closest to the date of start of ART up to 7 days after.
[d]Defined as the presence of any Centers for Disease Control and Prevention (CDC) 1993 disease from 90 days prior to up to 30 days after start of ART.
[e]Chronic Hepatitis B infection was defined as persistence of a positive HBsAg for more than six months without a subsequent negative HBsAg; chronic Hepatitis C infection was defined as a confirmed positive anti-HCV detected at least six months from the first test.
[f]Patients starting Integrase inhibitor-based regimens were too few and thus excluded (7 individuals with start of ART in 2010).
Unless otherwise stated, number (percentages) are shown.

The impact of missing viral load measurements on the adjusted models (Table 4) showed that the direction of the association of each variable with the 12-month and the 24-month outcomes remained the same for both the best case and worst case scenarios.

Discussion

In this large cohort study of HIV-infected patients in Rio de Janeiro, Brazil, we estimated ART effectiveness for patients cared for between 2000 and 2010. We found that ART effectiveness at 6 months was 77% among patients with viral load results and no drug class modification and/or discontinuation. Using an intent-to-continue-treatment approach, that is, a less stringent criterion compared to that of the present study, the ART-CC cohort reported an estimate of 76% of undetectable viral load 6 months after ART initiation [10]. For the 12-month time point, our estimate of 61% for ART effectiveness when assuming missing data equals failure is consistent with that reported in a systematic review of clinical trials and cohort studies that employed the same approach to evaluating first-line ART efficacy (57-66% [11-13]). In line with our results, Barth et al., in a study conducted in rural South Africa, found 55% effectiveness using the same intent-to-treat approach [14]. It is important to consider the calendar period, the stringency of study definitions and the availability of one pill once-daily regimens, all factors that could partially explain diverging suppression rates in other cohort studies when compared to our findings [5,6,10,11,13-23].

We showed in a stratified analysis that ART effectiveness was higher for NNRTI-based regimens. These

Table 2 Effectiveness of first-line antiretroviral therapy at 6, 12, and 24 months from start of antiretroviral therapy (ART) stratified by regimen and calendar year

		6 months	12 months	24 months
Overall		N (%)	N (%)	N (%)
	For patients with HIV VL	754/980 (76.9)	802/1054 (76.1)	637/938 (67.9)
	Best-case scenario[a]	1085/1311 (82.8)	1059/1311 (80.8)	1010/1311 (77.0)
	Worst-case scenario[b]	754/1311 (57.5)	802/1311 (61.2)	637/1311 (48.6)
Stratified by type of ART regimen				
NNRTI-based				
	For patients with HIV VL	583/740 (78.8)	603/784 (76.9)	503/711 (70.7)
	Best-case scenario	830/987 (84.1)	806/987 (81.7)	779/987 (78.9)
	Worst-case scenario	583/987 (59.1)	603/987 (61.1)	503/987 (51.0)
PI-based				
	For patients with HIV VL	171/240 (71.3)	199/270 (73.7)	134/227 (59.0)
	Best-case scenario	255/324 (78.7)	253/324 (78.1)	231/324 (71.3)
	Worst-case scenario	171/324 (52.8)	199/324 (61.4)	134/324 (41.4)
Stratified by calendar year of ART initiation				
2000-2004				
	For patients with HIV VL	157/252 (62.3)	188/297 (63.3)	171/287 (59.6)
	Best-case scenario	297/392 (75.8)	283/392 (72.2)	276/392 (70.4)
	Worst-case scenario	157/392 (40.1)	188/392 (48.0)	171/392 (43.6)
2005-2010				
	For patients with HIV VL	597/728 (82.0)	614/757 (81.1)	466/651 (71.6)
	Best-case scenario	788/919 (85.7)	776/919 (84.4)	734/919 (79.9)
	Worst-case scenario	597/919 (65.0)	614/919 (66.8)	466/919 (50.7)

HIV: human immunodeficiency virus, VL: viral load, PI: protease inhibitor, NNRTI: non-nucleoside reverse transcriptase inhibitor.
[a]Best-case scenario assumes missing viral load data as suppression.
[b]Worst-case scenario assumes missing viral loads data as failures.

findings corroborate results from clinical trials and cohort studies that demonstrate greater effectiveness of NNRTI-based regimens, in particular, of efavirenz-based regimens [11,19,24]. In the adjusted analysis, however, the NNRTI-based regimen was found to be independently associated with virologic suppression solely at the 24-month endpoint; as such, when other factors were taken into account the regimens were not significantly different. LPV/r was the most frequently prescribed PI, as recommended by the Brazilian HIV Treatment Guidelines, which may explain the poorer outcomes observed with PI-based regimens, as opposed to the comparable effectiveness shown in AIDS Clinical Trials Group (ACTG5202), when boosted atazanavir was the PI comparator [25]. Of note, 39% of the patients in our cohort who started a PI-based regimen started on a non-boosted PI, of which 65% were

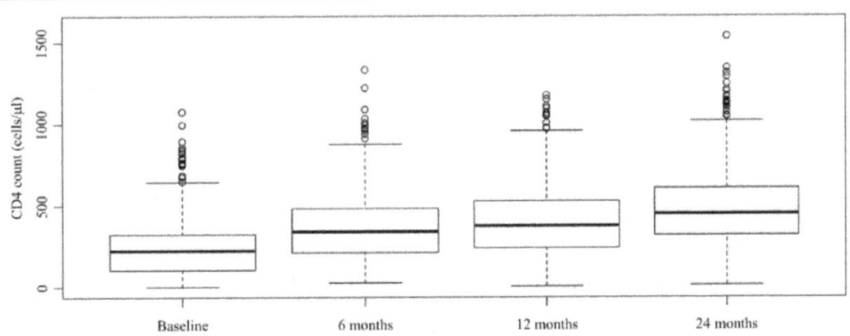

Figure 1 Box plot of CD4 count distribution at baseline and 6, 12, and 24 months after antiretroviral therapy initiation. Pair-wise comparisons of baseline measurement with 6-, 12-, and 24-month time points indicate statistically significant differences (Wilcoxon paired test).

Table 3 Unadjusted and adjusted relative risks (95% confidence intervals) for first-line antiretroviral therapy effectiveness at 12 and 24 months (IPEC cohort, 2000 to 2010)

		12 months		24 months	
		Unadjusted RR (95% CI)	Adjusted RR (95% CI)	Unadjusted RR (95% CI)	Adjusted RR (95% CI)
Age					
	< 30	Ref.		Ref.	Ref.
	30-39	0.99 (0.91, 1.08)		1.05 (0.93, 1.18)	1.06 (0.94, 1.19)
	>=40	1.04 (0.95, 1.13)		1.09 (0.98, 1.22)	**1.12 (1.00, 1.26)**
Race					
	Non-white	Ref.		Ref.	
	White	**1.07 (1.00, 1.14)**		1.05 (0.97, 1.15)	
Gender/Risk category[a]					
	Women	**0.89 (0.82, 0.98)**	**0.90 (0.82, 0.99)**	0.92 (0.82, 1.03)	0.94 (0.84, 1.06)
	Heterosexual men	Ref.	Ref.	Ref.	Ref.
	MSM	1.05 (0.97, 1.15)	1.02 (0.93, 1.12)	1.11 (0.99, 1.25)	1.11 (0.98, 1.25)
	IDU/Other	1.02 (0.90, 1.16)	1.02 (0.89, 1.16)	0.93 (0.78, 1.11)	0.95 (0.79, 1.13)
Education					
	< 4 years	Ref.	Ref.	Ref.	Ref.
	4-8 years	1.06 (0.96, 1.17)	1.07 (0.96, 1.18)	1.12 (0.98, 1.28)	1.13 (0.99, 1.29)
	> 8 years	**1.16 (1.06, 1.27)**	**1.13 (1.03, 1.24)**	**1.17 (1.04, 1.32)**	**1.14 (1.00, 1.29)**
Years since HIV + test					
	<= 3	Ref.		Ref.	
	> 3	0.97 (0.90, 1.04)		0.94 (0.86, 1.03)	
Baseline CD4 cell count[b]					
	<= 200	Ref.		Ref.	
	201-350	1.05 (0.97, 1.14)		1.01 (0.91, 1.12)	
	> 350	1.09 (0.99, 1.20)		1.11 (0.97, 1.26)	
	Missing	0.92 (0.83, 1.03)		1.01 (0.88, 1.15)	
Baseline HIV viral load[c]					
	<= 100000	Ref.		Ref.	
	> 100000	1.00 (0.93, 1.08)		1.03 (0.93, 1.14)	
	Missing	0.95 (0.87, 1.04)		0.99 (0.88, 1.11)	
Concurrent ADI[d]					
	No	Ref.		Ref.	
	Yes	1.06 (0.98, 1.16)		1.06 (0.95, 1.18)	
Hepatitis B/C co-infection[e]					
	No	Ref.		Ref.	
	Yes	1.16 (0.95, 1.43)		1.07 (0.83, 1.39)	
Initial ART regimen[f]					
	PI-based	Ref.		Ref.	Ref.
	NNRTI-based	1.04 (0.96, 1.13)		**1.20 (1.08, 1.34)**	**1.17 (1.05, 1.31)**
Calendar year of ART initiation					
	2005-2010	**1.28 (1.18, 1.39)**	**1.25 (1.15, 1.35)**	**1.20 (1.09, 1.33)**	**1.14 (1.03, 1.27)**
	2000-2004	Ref.	Ref.	Ref.	Ref.

Table 3 Unadjusted and adjusted relative risks (95% confidence intervals) for first-line antiretroviral therapy effectiveness at 12 and 24 months (IPEC cohort, 2000 to 2010) *(Continued)*

Started ART in clinical trial				
No	Ref.	Ref.	Ref.	Ref.
Yes	**1.10 (1.03, 1.18)**	**1.08 (1.01, 1.16)**	**1.14 (1.04, 1.25)**	**1.12 (1.02, 1.23)**

Bold numbers indicate statistically significant results.
HIV: human immunodeficiency virus, VL: viral load, PI: protease inhibitor, NNRTI: non-nucleoside reverse transcriptase inhibitor.
[a]Gender and reported mode of HIV exposure were categorized jointly into women, men who have sex with men (MSM), heterosexual men, and injection drug users (IDU, men and women) and other reported modes of HIV exposure (men and women). Individuals reporting both injection drug use and other modes of HIV exposure were categorized into IDU.
[b]Measurement closest to the date of start of ART up to 30 days after.
[c]Measurement closest to the date of start of ART up to 7 days after.
[d]Defined as the presence of any Centers for Disease Control and Prevention (CDC) 1993 ADI at 90 days prior to up to 30 days after start of ART.
[e]Chronic Hepatitis B infection was defined as persistence of a positive HBsAg for more than six months without a subsequent negative HBsAg; chronic Hepatitis C infection was defined as a confirmed positive anti-HCV detected at least six months from the first test.
[f]Patients starting Integrase inhibitor-based regimens were too few and thus excluded (7 individuals with start of ART in 2010).

atazanavir-based. It is well known that drug regimens including non-boosted PIs have poorer outcomes compared to other ART strategies [26]. The ACTG A5175 PEARLS trial, which was conducted in both high-income and low-middle-income settings, found non-boosted atazanavir to be inferior to efavirenz-based regimens [27]. Thus, the use of non-boosted PI-based regimens could partially explain the differences in ART effectiveness between our study and these trial findings.

Our study covered a time span of 11 years which allowed us to evaluate ART effectiveness in two periods, namely 2000-2004 and 2005-2010. Both the crude estimates and

Table 4 Adjusted relative risks (95% confidence intervals) for first-line antiretroviral (ART) effectiveness at 12 and 24 months when assuming best-case (missing as success) and worst-case scenarios (missing as failure) (IPEC cohort, 2000 to 2010)

	12 months			24 months		
	RR (95% CI) Missing excluded	RR (95% CI) Missing = Success	RR (95% CI) Missing = Failure	RR (95% CI) Missing excluded	RR (95% CI) Missing = Success	RR (95% CI) Missing = Failure
Age						
< 30				Ref.	Ref.	Ref.
30-39				1.06 (0.94, 1.19)	1.01 (0.94, 1.09)	1.15 (0.99, 1.33)
> = 40				1.12 (1.00, 1.26)	1.04 (0.97, 1.13)	1.24 (1.07, 1.44)
Gender/Risk category						
Women	0.90 (0.82, 0.99)	0.93 (0.87, 1.00)	0.87 (0.77, 0.98)	0.94 (0.84, 1.06)	0.94 (0.87, 1.02)	0.98 (0.84, 1.14)
Heterosexual men	Ref.	Ref.	Ref.	Ref.	Ref.	Ref.
MSM	1.02 (0.93, 1.12)	1.03 (0.96, 1.11)	0.98 (0.87, 1.10)	1.11 (0.98, 1.25)	1.08 (0.99, 1.17)	1.05 (0.90, 1.22)
IDU/Other	1.02 (0.89, 1.16)	1.03 (0.94, 1.14)	0.89 (0.75, 1.05)	0.95 (0.79, 1.13)	0.97 (0.87, 1.09)	0.87 (0.70, 1.09)
Education						
< 4 years	Ref.	Ref.	Ref.	Ref.	Ref.	Ref.
4-8 years	1.07 (0.96, 1.18)	1.05 (0.97, 1.13)	1.05 (0.93, 1.20)	1.13 (0.99, 1.29)	1.06 (0.98, 1.16)	1.18 (1.00, 1.39)
> 8 years	1.13 (1.03, 1.24)	1.08 (1.01, 1.17)	1.16 (1.03, 1.30)	1.14 (1.00, 1.29)	1.07 (0.99, 1.16)	1.21 (1.03, 1.41)
Initial ART regimen						
PI-based				Ref.	Ref.	Ref.
NNRTI-based				1.17 (1.05, 1.31)	1.09 (1.02, 1.17)	1.21 (1.05, 1.39)
Calendar year of ART initiation						
2005-2009	1.25 (1.15, 1.35)	1.14 (1.08, 1.22)	1.34 (1.21, 1.49)	1.14 (1.03, 1.27)	1.11 (1.03, 1.19)	1.08 (0.95, 1.23)
2000-2004	Ref.	Ref.	Ref.	Ref.	Ref.	Ref.
Started ART in clinical trial						
No	Ref.	Ref.	Ref.	Ref.	Ref.	Ref.
Yes	1.08 (1.01, 1.16)	1.05 (0.99, 1.11)	1.10 (1.00, 1.21)	1.12 (1.02, 1.23)	1.04 (0.98, 1.11)	1.24 (1.10, 1.39)

the adjusted analyses showed that the more recent calendar period was associated with increased ART effectiveness. This finding most likely results from the availability, more recently, of regimens with improved drug combinations, drugs with better tolerability and dosing convenience and, as a result, improved treatment adherence [28].

We found that clinical trial participation was independently associated with virologic suppression at 12 and 24 months from start of ART, corroborating other published results [29,30]. Notably, in contrast to routine care, clinical trial participants are more intensively followed, adherence to study visits and drugs is monitored, drug toxicities are closely sought, and access to medical appointments is facilitated. For the time points evaluated in this study, clinical trial participants had significantly fewer missing viral load measurements. We believe these results highlight the need for more vigilant monitoring within the routine care provided by Brazil's Unified Health System in order to improve ART effectiveness. Additionally, a comparative analysis of the procedures carried out in routine care versus the clinical trial setting could shed light into the most important aspects of trial participation that lead to increased ART effectiveness. Further studies are also needed to evaluate the long-term benefits of clinical trial participation, given that at the end of the trials patients are fully incorporated into routine care.

Two socio-demographic factors (older age and higher education level) were found to be independently associated with increased ART effectiveness, and there was a trend toward increased virologic suppression for one behavioral factor (MSM HIV risk exposure). Regarding older age, our findings corroborate results from other cohort studies that have found increased ART effectiveness among older individuals [31,32]. Likewise, improved virologic response among those with more years of formal education has also been reported in studies from both Brazil and the United States [33,34]. Older age and higher education are likely correlated with a better understanding of the importance and value of ART and, consequently, better treatment adherence [35,36]. We also found that MSM, compared to heterosexual men, had increased ART effectiveness. In our study population, MSM was linked to higher education, as 69% of the MSM reported > 8 years of formal education while only 38% of the women and heterosexual men reported this same level of education. In the multivariate model for the 12-month endpoint, women were found to have decreased ART effectiveness. In other studies that considered ART discontinuations as failures, men showed improved ART outcomes when compared to women [37]. Moreover, several clinical trials [38] and observational studies [7,39,40] have described a higher frequency of ART-related adverse events among women compared to men. In our cohort, we have previously reported that the hazard of ART modification or discontinuation for women is 1.67 times the hazard for men within the first year of treatment [7]. For Brazil, these findings highlight the need to focus interventions aiming to improve ART outcomes among young, less educated heterosexual men and women, and to address specific issues particularly among women including ART tolerability and competing caretaking priorities.

Our study has several limitations. One is the substantial fraction of missing viral load measurements. We addressed this limitation by conducting sensitivity analyses which allowed us to generate upper and lower limits for the ART effectiveness estimates. We also evaluated the impact of the missing viral loads on the adjusted analysis by modeling both best- and worst-case scenarios. These modeling exercises generated results which are similar to those obtained when the missing data were excluded. In contrast, CD4 counts were not imputed and did suffer from a somewhat smaller degree of missing data, and therefore care is needed when extrapolating from these results.

In summary, we have shown that in Brazil, a middle-income country universal access to care and treatment, virologic suppression on first-line ART was achieved by over three-quarters of patients receiving routine care in a public facility. We also studied factors associated with virologic suppression at 12- and 24 months since ART initiation and found that higher education, more recent ART initiation and clinical trial participation were associated with improved outcomes. To translate these findings into applicable interventions to improve ART outcomes, the specifics relating to the factors leading to higher virologic suppression need to be further studied.

Competing interests

The authors declare no conflict of interest.

Authors' contributions

SWC contributed to the conception and design of the study, acquired the data, and drafted the manuscript. PML contributed to the conception and design of the study, and drafted the manuscript. LV contributed to the conception and design of the study, and performed the statistical analysis. TT and LC acquired and revised the data. KAF participated in the study's design, discussed the results, helped to draft and revise the manuscript for important intellectual content. VGV participated in the study's design and coordination and helped to draft the manuscript. RPW participated in the study's design, discussed the results, helped to draft and revise the manuscript for important intellectual content. BG contributed to the conception and design of the study, coordinated efforts, drafted and revised the manuscript for important intellectual content. All authors read and approved the final manuscript.

Funding sources

BG acknowledges funding from the National Council of Technological and Scientific Development (CNPq) and the Research Funding Agency of the State of Rio de Janeiro (FAPERJ). PML acknowledges funding from the National Council of Technological and Scientific Development (CNPq) and the Research Funding Agency of the State of Rio de Janeiro (FAPERJ). KAF and RPW acknowledge funding from National Institute of Allergy and Infectious Diseases (NIAID, R01 AI058736, R01 AI093269).

Author details

[1]Instituto de Pesquisa Clínica Evandro Chagas, Fundação Oswaldo Cruz, Rio de Janeiro, Brasil. [2]Departamento de Matemática e Estatística, Universidade Federal do Estado do Rio de Janeiro, Rio de Janeiro, Brasil. [3]The Divisions of Infectious Disease and General Medicine, and the Medical Practice Evaluation Center, Department of Medicine, Massachusetts General Hospital and the Harvard University Center for AIDS Research, Harvard Medical School, Boston, MA, U.S.A.

References

1. Alves SDAS, Freitas C, Pascom ARP, Pereira GF, Pinto AP, da Silva FVN, Ravasi G, for The Brazilian Ministry of Health, Health Surveillance Secretariat, Department of STD, AIDS and Viral Hepatitis: **Progress Report on the Brazilian Response to HIV/AIDS (2010–2011).** In *Book Progress Report on the Brazilian Response to HIV/AIDS (2010–2011).* 2012.
2. Guerreiro MF, Kerr-Pontes LR, Mota RS, Franca MC Jr, Tavora FF, Caminha I: **Survival of adult AIDS patients in a reference hospital of a metropolitan area in Brazil.** *Revista de saude publica* 2002, **36**:278–284.
3. Marins JR, Jamal LF, Chen SY, Barros MB, Hudes ES, Barbosa AA, Chequer P, Teixeira PR, Hearst N: **Dramatic improvement in survival among adult Brazilian AIDS patients.** *AIDS* 2003, **17**:1675–1682.
4. Campos DP, Ribeiro SR, Grinsztejn B, Veloso VG, Valente JG, Bastos FI, Morgado MG, Gadelha AJ: **Survival of AIDS patients using two case definitions, Rio de Janeiro, Brazil, 1986–2003.** *AIDS* 2005, **19**(Suppl 4):S22–26.
5. Fletcher CV: **Translating efficacy into effectiveness in antiretroviral therapy: beyond the pill count.** *Drugs* 2007, **67**:1969–1979.
6. Samaranayake A, Chen MY, McNeil J, Read TR, Hocking JS, Bradshaw CS, Fairley CK: **Definitions of antiretroviral treatment failure for measuring quality outcomes.** *HIV medicine* 2010, **11**:427–431.
7. Cardoso SW, Grinsztejn B, Velasque L, Veloso VG, Luz PM, Friedman RK, Morgado M, Ribeiro SR, Moreira RI, Keruly J, Moore RD: **Incidence of modifying or discontinuing first HAART regimen and its determinants in a cohort of HIV-infected patients from Rio de Janeiro, Brazil.** *AIDS Res Hum Retroviruses* 2010, **26**:865–874.
8. Grinsztejn B, Luz PM, Pacheco AG, Santos DV, Velasque L, Moreira RI, Guimaraes MR, Nunes EP, Lemos AS, Ribeiro SR, Campos DP, Vitoria MA, Veloso VG: **Changing mortality profile among HIV-infected patients in Rio de Janeiro, Brazil: shifting from AIDS to non-AIDS related conditions in the HAART era.** *PLoS One* 2013, **8**:e59768.
9. Pacheco AG, Saraceni V, Tuboi SH, Moulton LH, Chaisson RE, Cavalcante SC, Durovni B, Faulhaber JC, Golub JE, King B, Schechter M, Harrison LH: **Validation of a hierarchical deterministic record-linkage algorithm using data from 2 different cohorts of human immunodeficiency virus-infected persons and mortality databases in Brazil.** *American Journal of epidemiology* 2008, **168**:1326–1332.
10. May M, Sterne JA, Sabin C, Costagliola D, Justice AC, Thiebaut R, Gill J, Phillips A, Reiss P, Hogg R, Ledergerber B, D'Arminio Monforte A, Schmeisser N, Staszewski S, Egger M, Antiretroviral Therapy Cohort C: **Prognosis of HIV-1-infected patients up to 5 years after initiation of HAART: collaborative analysis of prospective studies.** *Aids* 2007, **21**:1185–1197.
11. Bartlett JA, Fath MJ, Demasi R, Hermes A, Quinn J, Mondou E, Rousseau F: **An updated systematic overview of triple combination therapy in antiretroviral-naive HIV-infected adults.** *Aids* 2006, **20**:2051–2064.
12. Carr A, Amin J: **Efficacy and tolerability of initial antiretroviral therapy: a systematic review.** *Aids* 2009, **23**:343–353. discussion 355–346.
13. Ivers LC, Kendrick D, Doucette K: **Efficacy of antiretroviral therapy programs in resource-poor settings: a meta-analysis of the published literature.** *Clinical infectious diseases: an official publication of the Infectious Diseases Society of America* 2005, **41**:217–224.
14. Barth RE, van der Meer JT, Hoepelman AI, Schrooders PA, van de Vijver DA, Geelen SP, Tempelman HA: **Effectiveness of highly active antiretroviral therapy administered by general practitioners in rural South Africa.** *European journal of clinical microbiology & infectious diseases: official publication of the European Society of Clinical Microbiology* 2008, **27**:977–984.
15. Mocroft A, Devereux H, Kinloch-de-Loes S, Wilson D, Madge S, Youle M, Tyrer M, Loveday C, Phillips AN, Johnson MA: **Immunological, virological and clinical response to highly active antiretroviral therapy treatment regimens in a complete clinic population. Royal Free Centre for HIV Medicine.** *Aids* 2000, **14**:1545–1552.
16. Elliott JH, Lynen L, Calmy A, De Luca A, Shafer RW, Zolfo M, Clotet B, Huffam S, Boucher CA, Cooper DA, Schapiro JM: **Rational use of antiretroviral therapy in low-income and middle-income countries: optimizing regimen sequencing and switching.** *Aids* 2008, **22**:2053–2067.
17. Perez-Elias MJ, Moreno A, Casado JL, Dronda F, Antela A, Lopez D, Quereda C, Navas E, Hermida JM, Del Sol E, Moreno S: **Observational study to evaluate clinical outcomes after first-line efavirenz-or lopinavir-ritonavir-based HAART in treatment-naive patients.** *Journal of the International Association of Physicians in AIDS Care* 2009, **8**:308–313.
18. Elzi L, Erb S, Furrer H, Ledergerber B, Cavassini M, Hirschel B, Vernazza P, Bernasconi E, Weber R, Battegay M, Swiss HIVCS: **Choice of Initial Combination Antiretroviral Therapy in Individuals With HIV Infection: Determinants and Outcomes.** *Archives of internal medicine* 2012, **172**:1313–1321.
19. Taniguchi T, Grubb JR, Nurutdinova D, Onen NF, Shacham E, Donovan M, Overton ET: **Efavirenz outperforms boosted atazanavir among treatment-naive HIV-1-infected persons in routine clinical care.** *Journal of the International Association of Providers of AIDS Care* 2013, **12**:138–141.
20. Mugavero MJ, May M, Ribaudo HJ, Gulick RM, Riddler SA, Haubrich R, Napravnik S, Abgrall S, Phillips A, Harris R, Gill MJ, de Wolf F, Hogg R, Gunthard HF, Chene G, D'Arminio Monforte A, Guest JL, Smith C, Murillas J, Berenguer J, Wyen C, Domingo P, Kitahata MM, Sterne JA, Saag MS, Team ACTGD, Team ACTGS, team ACTGS, Antiretroviral Cohort C: **Comparative effectiveness of initial antiretroviral therapy regimens: ACTG 5095 and 5142 clinical trials relative to ART-CC cohort study.** *Journal of acquired immune deficiency syndromes* 2011, **58**:253–260.
21. May MT, Hogg RS, Justice AC, Shepherd BE, Costagliola D, Ledergerber B, Thiebaut R, Gill MJ, Kirk O, van Sighem A, Saag MS, Navarro G, Sobrino-Vegas P, Lampe F, Ingle S, Guest JL, Crane HM, D'Arminio Monforte A, Vehreschild JJ, Sterne JA, Antiretroviral Therapy Cohort C: **Heterogeneity in outcomes of treated HIV-positive patients in Europe and North America: relation with patient and cohort characteristics.** *International journal of epidemiology* 2012, **41**:1807–1820.
22. Fox MP, Cutsem GV, Giddy J, Maskew M, Keiser O, Prozesky H, Wood R, Hernan MA, Sterne JA, Egger M, Boulle A, Ie DEASAc: **Rates and predictors of failure of first-line antiretroviral therapy and switch to second-line ART in South Africa.** *Journal of acquired immune deficiency syndromes* 2012, **60**:428–437.
23. Fielding KL, Charalambous S, Stenson AL, Pemba LF, Martin DJ, Wood R, Churchyard GJ, Grant AD: **Risk factors for poor virological outcome at 12 months in a workplace-based antiretroviral therapy programme in South Africa: a cohort study.** *BMC infectious diseases* 2008, **8**:93.
24. Riddler SA, Haubrich R, DiRienzo AG, Peeples L, Powderly WG, Klingman KL, Garren KW, George T, Rooney JF, Brizz B, Lalloo UG, Murphy RL, Swindells S, Havlir D, Mellors JW, Team ACTGSA: **Class-sparing regimens for initial treatment of HIV-1 infection.** *The New England journal of medicine* 2008, **358**:2095–2106.
25. Daar ES, Tierney C, Fischl MA, Sax PE, Mollan K, Budhathoki C, Godfrey C, Jahed NC, Myers L, Katzenstein D, Farajallah A, Rooney JF, Pappa KA, Woodward WC, Patterson K, Bolivar H, Benson CA, Collier AC, Team ACTGSA: **Atazanavir plus ritonavir or efavirenz as part of a 3-drug regimen for initial treatment of HIV-1.** *Annals of internal medicine* 2011, **154**:445–456.
26. Lichterfeld M, Wohrmann A, Schmeisser N, Fatkenheuer G, Salzberger B, Wyen C, Schmitz K, Sauerbruch T, Rockstroh JK: **Superior virological efficacy of ritonavir-boosted protease inhibitor regimens compared to single protease inhibitor therapy.** *European journal of medical research* 2003, **8**:56–60.
27. Campbell TB, Smeaton LM, Kumarasamy N, Flanigan T, Klingman KL, Firnhaber C, Grinsztejn B, Hosseinipour MC, Kumwenda J, Lalloo U, Riviere C, Sanchez J, Melo M, Supparatpinyo K, Tripathy S, Martinez AI, Nair A, Walawander A, Moran L, Chen Y, Snowden W, Rooney JF, Uy J, Schooley RT, De Gruttola V, Hakim JG, ACTG Pstot: **Efficacy and safety of three antiretroviral regimens for initial treatment of HIV-1: a randomized clinical trial in diverse multinational settings.** *PLoS medicine* 2012, **9**:e1001290.
28. Marconi VC, Grandits GA, Weintrob AC, Chun H, Landrum ML, Ganesan A, Okulicz JF, Crum-Cianflone N, O'Connell RJ, Lifson A, Wortmann GW, Agan BK, Infectious Disease Clinical Research Program HIVWG: **Outcomes of highly active antiretroviral therapy in the context of universal access to healthcare: the U. S. Military HIV Natural History Study.** *AIDS research and therapy* 2010, **7**:14.
29. Hansen AB, Gerstoft J, Kirk O, Mathiesen L, Pedersen C, Nielsen H, Jensen-Fangel S, Sorensen HT, Obel N: **Unmeasured confounding**

caused slightly better response to HAART within than outside a randomized controlled trial. *Journal of clinical epidemiology* 2008, **61**:87–94.

30. Lopez-Martinez A, O'Brien NM, Caro-Vega Y, Crabtree-Ramirez B, Sierra-Madero J: **Different baseline characteristics and different outcomes of HIV-infected patients receiving HAART through clinical trials compared with routine care in Mexico.** *Journal of acquired immune deficiency syndromes* 2012, **59**:155–160.
31. Bosch RJ, Bennett K, Collier AC, Zackin R, Benson CA: **Pretreatment factors associated with 3-year (144-week) virologic and immunologic responses to potent antiretroviral therapy.** *Journal of acquired immune deficiency syndromes* 2007, **44**:268–277.
32. Greenbaum AH, Wilson LE, Keruly JC, Moore RD, Gebo KA: **Effect of age and HAART regimen on clinical response in an urban cohort of HIV-infected individuals.** *AIDS* 2008, **22**:2331–2339.
33. Tuboi SH, Harrison LH, Sprinz E, Albernaz RK, Schechter M: **Predictors of virologic failure in HIV-1-infected patients starting highly active antiretroviral therapy in Porto Alegre, Brazil.** *Journal of acquired immune deficiency syndromes* 2005, **40**:324–328.
34. Zaragoza-Macias E, Cosco D, Nguyen ML, Del Rio C, Lennox J: **Predictors of success with highly active antiretroviral therapy in an antiretroviral-naive urban population.** *AIDS research and human retroviruses* 2010, **26**:133–138.
35. Hinkin CH, Hardy DJ, Mason KI, Castellon SA, Durvasula RS, Lam MN, Stefaniak M: **Medication adherence in HIV-infected adults: effect of patient age, cognitive status, and substance abuse.** *Aids* 2004, **18**(Suppl 1):S19–25.
36. Silverberg MJ, Leyden W, Horberg MA, DeLorenze GN, Klein D, Quesenberry CP Jr: **Older age and the response to and tolerability of antiretroviral therapy.** *Archives of internal medicine* 2007, **167**:684–691.
37. Currier J, Averitt Bridge D, Hagins D, Zorrilla CD, Feinberg J, Ryan R, Falcon R, Tennenberg A, Mrus J, Squires K, Group GS: **Sex-based outcomes of darunavir-ritonavir therapy: a single-group trial.** *Annals of internal medicine* 2010, **153**:349–357.
38. Squires KE, Johnson M, Yang R, Uy J, Sheppard L, Absalon J, McGrath D: **Comparative gender analysis of the efficacy and safety of atazanavir/ritonavir and lopinavir/ritonavir at 96 weeks in the CASTLE study.** *The Journal of antimicrobial chemotherapy* 2011, **66**:363–370.
39. Collazos J, Asensi V, Carton JA: **Sex differences in the clinical, immunological and virological parameters of HIV-infected patients treated with HAART.** *Aids* 2007, **21**:835–843.
40. d'Arminio Monforte A, Lepri AC, Rezza G, Pezzotti P, Antinori A, Phillips AN, Angarano G, Colangeli V, De Luca A, Ippolito G, Caggese L, Soscia F, Filice G, Gritti F, Narciso P, Tirelli U, Moroni M: **Insights into the reasons for discontinuation of the first highly active antiretroviral therapy (HAART) regimen in a cohort of antiretroviral naive patients. I.CO.N.A. Study Group. Italian Cohort of Antiretroviral-Naive Patients.** *Aids* 2000, **14**:499–507.

23

Population-based human immunodeficiency virus 1 drug resistance profiles among individuals who experienced virological failure to first-line antiretroviral therapy in Henan, China during 2010–2011

Jia Liu[1], Yasong Wu[2], Wenjie Yang[1], Xiujuan Xue[1], Guoqing Sun[1], Chunhua Liu[1], Suian Tian[1], Dingyong Sun[1], Qian Zhu[1] and Zhe Wang[1*]

Abstract

Background: In Henan, China, first-line antiretroviral treatment (ART) was implemented early in a large number of treatment-experienced patients who were more likely to have a drug resistance. Therefore, we investigated the human immunodeficiency virus (HIV)-1 drug resistance profiles among patients in Henan who experienced virological failure to ART.

Method: A cross-sectional survey was administered in 10 major epidemic cities from May 2010 to October 2011. Adult patients who experienced virological failure (virus load ≥1,000 copies/mL) with >1 year of first-line antiretroviral treatment consented to provide blood for genotype resistance testing. The clinical and demographic data were obtained from the patients' medical records. Logistic regression analysis was performed to determine the factors associated with ≥1 significant drug resistance mutation.

Results: We included 3,235 patients with integral information and valid genotypic resistance data. The city, age, CD4 counts, virus load, treatment duration, and World Health Organization stage were associated with drug resistance, and 64.76% of patients acquired drug resistance. The nucleoside reverse transcriptase inhibitor (NRTI), non-(N)NRTI, and protease inhibitor resistance mutations were found in 50.26, 63.12, and 1.30% of subjects, respectively. Thymidine analogue mutations, NNRTI and even multidrug resistance complex were quite common in this patient cohort.

Conclusion: Multiple and complex patterns of HIV-1 drug resistance mutations were identified among individuals who experienced virological failure to first-line ART in Henan, China during 2010–2011. Therefore, timely virological monitoring, therapy adjustments, and more varieties of drugs and individualized treatment should be immediately considered in this patient population.

Keywords: HIV, Drug resistance, First-line antiretroviral therapy, Virological failure

Background

Continuous improved antiretroviral therapy (ART) has been one of the most significant breakthroughs in human immunodeficiency virus (HIV)/acquired immune deficiency syndrome (AIDS) prevention and control over the past 30 years because of its outstanding effect on reducing AIDS mortality and morbidity [1, 2], ameliorating quality of life, and preventing HIV-1 infection [3]. However, the emergence of HIV drug resistance is inevitable following the large-scale rollout of ART. The enhanced resistance to first-line antiretroviral drugs has led to

*Correspondence: wangzhe@hncdc.com.cn
[1] Henan Center for Disease Control and Prevention, Zhengzhou, Henan, China
Full list of author information is available at the end of the article

persistent viral replication that impairs patients' immunological and clinical status, and the accumulation of resistance mutations after continuing a failing regimen may compromise the second-line therapy [4]. To maximize the long-term effectiveness of first-line ART regimens and to ensure the sustainability of ART programs, it is essential to minimize the further spread of HIV drug resistance. The World Health Organization (WHO) recommends that the scale-up of HIV ART should always be accompanied by a robust assessment of drug resistance emergence [5].

The Chinese government initiated the China Comprehensive AIDS Response program to provide free HIV treatment in 2002, which rapidly scaled up the National Free Antiretroviral Therapy Program. Subsequently, drug resistance surveillance in different areas was attempted, and the popularization of drug resistance monitoring was performed in 2010. The Henan Province has always drawn concern because of the extensive spread of HIV among former plasma donors and the earlier initiation of the National Free ART Program with a large number of ART patients [6, 7]. Numerous HIV drug resistance studies with heterogeneous designs, defined areas, and methods have been performed in China with small populations from Henan [8–11]; however, until recently, few studies have illuminated the typical prevalence and pattern of HIV drug resistance in the Henan Province. Therefore, we assessed the HIV-1 drug resistance profile among first-line ART patients in Henan who experienced virological failure.

Method

Study design

The administration of ART, delivery of antiviral drugs, adherence education, and collection of plasma specimens mainly depended on the local centers for disease control and prevention (CDC) and the community clinics in the Henan Province. The CD4 cell counts were measured twice and virus load were measured once 1 year by a local CDC and Henan CDC, and the results were provided to treating physicians and the national HIV/AIDS case reporting system. All the cases of HIV/AIDS in China are reported via the national HIV/AIDS case reporting system. Records in this system include identity and demographic information, HIV testing results, the self-reported transmission route, and health status information. Base data for this study was derived from this system. For the purpose of this study, virological failure patients (defined as having an HIV virus load of ≥1,000 copies/mL) underwent genotypic drug resistance testing and the results were also provided to treating physicians and the national HIV/AIDS case reporting system.

Ethics statement

Written consent was obtained from patients to participate in the China's routine HIV/AIDS surveillance program and the regular administration of the national ART program, and parental consent was also obtained on behalf of the participants aged less than 18 years. Since the data and the samples used in this study were collected as a function of surveillance program above, no additional informed consent was required. This study was reviewed and approved by the Institutional Review Board of the Henan CDC.

Participants

According to the aforementioned conditions, first-line ART-virological failure patients (aged ≥15 years) were selected if the virus load was ≥1,000 copies/mL with >1 year of treatment from May 2010 to October 2011 in 10 cities that held the highest HIV-1 epidemic in the Henan Province. The patients could not followed or refused to give samples were not included. The first-line ART regimens consisted of two nucleoside reverse transcriptase inhibitors (NRTIs): (azidothymidine [AZT] or stavudine [D4T]) + (didanosine [DDI] or lamivudine [3TC]) and one non-(N)NRTIs: (nevirapine [NVP] or efavirenz [EFV]). AZT, D4T, DDI, and NVP are generically produced in China, whereas 3TC and EFV are branded drugs that became available in 2005.

Laboratory tests

The CD4 cell counts were measured using flow cytometry by the local CDCs. The plasma HIV-1 virus load was tested by the local city and Henan CDCs using the Abbott Real-Time HIV-1 assay (Abbott Molecular Inc., Des Plaines, IL, USA), NucliSENS EasyQ-EasyMag HIV-1 assay (bioMerieux, Marcy l'Etoile, France), or Cobas AmpliPrep-Cobas TaqMan HIV-1 assay (Roche Diagnostics, Mannheim, Germany). Samples with a virus load of ≥1,000 copies/mL underwent HIV-1 drug resistance genotyping using an in-house method developed by the national core laboratories as described in previous studies [12, 13]. A fragment of the HIV-1 pol gene (protease, amino acids 1–99, and part of the reverse transcriptase amino acids 1–252) was bulk-sequenced from the plasma ribonucleic acid (RNA). The resulting fragment was analyzed for subtype, drug resistance mutations and drug susceptibility using the Stanford HIV Drug Resistance Database (http://hivdb.stanford.edu).

Data analysis

The demographic variables were analyzed using descriptive statistics, and the risk factors for developing HIV drug resistance were analyzed using logistic regression. Variables associated with resistance in the univariate analyses (p value <0.05) and those clinically meaningful were included in the multivariable regression model. The tests were two-sided, and a p-value <0.05 indicated statistical significance. All the statistical analyses were performed using SPSS, version 19.0 (IBM Corp., Armonk, NY, USA).

Result

Demographic characteristics

In our study, 4,020 individuals were investigated and sampled, which included 23 non-Henan, 154 dual-tested. Moreover, 81 patients with incomplete information and 527 with a fragmentary sequence were excluded, leaving 3,235 subjects in the final analysis (Table 1). The following five cities accounted for a substantially larger proportion: Zhumadian (22.97%), Kaifeng (19.07%), Shangqiu (18.89%), Zhoukou (17.25%), and Nanyang (11.16%) (Figure 1). Of the 3,235 patients, 63.37% were aged 31–50 years, 52.49% were male, 82.87% were married, 90.11% reported former plasma donors as the route of HIV infection, 39.54% had WHO stage II HIV disease, 51.56% had been treated for >6 years, 27.02% have CD4 counts ≥350 cells/μL, 58.83% have virus load in between 3 and 4 log copies/ml. All the 3235 individuals were B subtypes. ART was initialized with AZT/D4T + DDI + NVP/EFV in 1,428 subjects (44.14%), with AZT/D4T + 3TC + NVP/EFV in 1,170 (36.17%). The regimen that included DDI was substituted with a regimen that included 3TC after 2005 when it was widely available.

Risk factors associated with genotypic human immunodeficiency virus drug resistance

Exploratory logistic regression analysis was performed to assess the factors that were significantly associated with resistance (Table 1). According to the univariate logistic regression model, eight potential factors correlated with HIV drug resistance. In the multivariate model, the following six factors had correlations: the city (patients in Xinyang had the highest level of drug resistances, 79.27%); age (patients in <30 years group had the highest level of drug resistance, 78.65%); CD4 counts (patients in <50 cells/μL group had the highest level of drug resistance, 71.01%); Virus load (patients in 3-4 log copies/ml group had the highest level of drug resistance, 67.47%); WHO stage (patients in WHO stage III group had the highest level of drug resistance, 66.63%); and treatment duration (patients in 5–6 years group had the highest level of drug resistance, 72.81%).

Pattern and frequency of predicted HIV drug resistance mutations

At least one significant HIV drug resistance mutation was identified in 2,095 (64.76%) patients, according to the Stanford HIV Drug Resistance Database. The frequency of NNRTI, NRTI, and PI resistance mutations were 63.12, 50.26, and 1.30%, respectively. In this study, 42.60% of patients had both NRTI and NNRTI resistance mutations, 7.67% had NRTI but not NNRTI, and 20.53% had NNRTI but not NRTI resistance mutations (Figure 2).

M184 V/I (35.64%) emerged as the most common NRTI resistance mutation, followed by thymidine analogue mutations (TAMs): T215Y/F (27.17%), M41L (18.39%), D67 N (12.21%), K70R/E/G (10.20%), L210 W (10.17%), and K219E/Q (10.02%). The prevalence of >1 TAMs was 42.32%. Furthermore, the prevalence of M184 V/I + TAMs was 21.36%, TAMs-1 (M41L, L210 W, and T215Y) was 8.96%, and TAMs-2 (D67 N, K70R, T215F, and K219Q) was 4.61%. Fifty-one (1.58%) and thirteen (0.40%) patients had the K65R/N and Q151 M complex, respectively. Among the NNRTI resistance mutations, K103 N (34.84%) was the most common NNRTI, followed by Y181C/V/I (22.04%) and G190A/S/E (18.24%) (Table 2).

Estimated susceptibility to various antiretroviral drugs

Mutational patterns were used to estimate the drug susceptibility in patients based on the Stanford University HIV Drug Resistance Database (Figure 3). Of the 40.93 and 40.90% subjects in this cohort had an estimated resistance against 3TC and FTC; 35–37% against ABC, AZT, D4T, and DDI; and 26.89% against TDF. There was a comparatively high prevalence of an estimated resistance to EFV and NVP, which reached 62–63%, and 0.62% of the subjects had a resistance to lopinavir.

Discussion

ART has expanded in Henan during the last decade, and the continued success of ART programs will require an understanding of the profiles of HIV drug resistance among individuals in whom the treatment has failed. This study's findings demonstrated the presence of HIV drug resistance among individuals from the Henan Province of China (2010–2011) in whom the first-line therapy had virologically failed.

In the early years, the magnitude of the focus was on former plasma donors, however, with the change of the HIV epidemic, sexual intercourse has been the focus of HIV/AIDS control and prevention, which has attracted substantial resources [14–17]. This study had a large number of subjects, and 90.11% of the virological failure population accounted for former plasma donors. This finding indicates that these people also currently occupy an important position in the ART programs; thus, measurements such as virology surveillance, drug resistance monitoring, therapy adjustments, and related social security need to be ensured.

Table 1 The subjects' characteristic and the factors associated with at least one human immunodeficiency virus (HIV) drug resistance mutation

Variable	Number (%)	HIV drug resistance (%)	Crude OR (95% CI)	P-value	Adjusted OR (95% CI)	P-value
City						
Zhumadian	743 (22.97)	481 (64.74)				
Zhengzhou	81 (2.50)	38 (46.91)	0.5 (0.3,0.8)	0.00	0.8 (0.5,1.4)	0.49
Kaifeng	617 (19.07)	329 (53.32)	0.6 (0.5,0.8)	0.00	0.7 (0.6,0.9)	0.01
Jiaozuo	48 (1.48)	26 (54.17)	0.6 (0.4,1.2)	0.14	0.8 (0.4,1.6)	0.59
Zhoukou	558 (17.25)	352 (63.08)	0.9 (0.7,1.2)	0.54	1.1 (0.9,1.5)	0.33
Pingdingshan	13 (0.40)	11 (83.33)	3.0 (0.7,13.6)	0.16	3.1 (0.7,14.8)	0.15
Luohe	121 (3.74)	85 (70.25)	1.3 (0.8,2.0)	0.24	1.7 (1.1,2.8)	0.02
Shangqiu	611 (18.89)	440 (72.01)	1.4 (1.1,1.8)	0.00	1.5 (1.2,1.9)	0.00
Nanyang	361 (11.16)	268 (74.24)	1.6 (1.2,2.1)	0.00	1.9 (1.4,2.5)	0.00
Xinyang	82 (2.53)	65 (79.27)	2.1 (1.2,3.6)	0.01	2.4 (1.3,4.4)	0.00
Age						
≤30	89 (2.75)	70 (78.65)				
31–50	2,050 (63.37)	1,295 (63.17)	0.5 (0.3,0.8)	0.00	0.5 (0.2,0.8)	0.01
>50	1,096 (33.88)	730 (66.61)	0.5 (0.3,0.9)	0.02	0.5 (0.3,0.9)	0.03
Gender						
Female	1,537 (47.51)	1,011 (65.78)				
Male	1,698 (52.49)	1,084 (63.84)	0.9 (0.8,1.1)	0.25		
Married						
No	2,681 (82.87)	1,737 (64.79)				
Yes	554 (17.13)	358 (64.62)	1.0 (0.8,1.2)	0.94		
HIV transmission route						
FPD	2,915 (90.11)	1,909 (65.49)				
Sexual intercourse	238 (7.36)	139 (58.40)	0.7 (0.6,1.0)	0.03	1.1 (0.8,1.5)	0.71
Mother-to-Child	24 (0.74)	22 (91.67)	5.8 (1.4,24.7)	0.02	3.3 (0.7,16.6)	0.14
Other	58 (1.79)	25 (43.10)	0.4 (0.2,0.7)	0.00	0.8 (0.4,1.4)	0.36
CD4						
≥350	874 (27.02)	536 (61.33)				
200–349	1,112 (34.37)	718 (64.57)	0.9 (0.7,1.1)	0.20	0.9 (0.7,1.2)	0.52
50–199	1,011 (31.25)	672 (66.47)	1.3 (1.0,1.7)	0.03	1.4 (1.1,1.9)	0.01
<50	238 (7.36)	169 (71.01)	1.9 (1.3,2.7)	0.00	2.6 (1.7,4.0)	0.00
Virus load						
>4log	1,332 (41.47)	811 (60.89)				
3–4log	1,903 (58.83)	1,284 (67.47)	1.4 (1.1,1.9)	0.01	1.6 (1.1,2.0)	0.01
Initial ART regimen						
AZT/D4T + DDI + EFV/NVP	1,428 (44.14)	975 (68.28)				
AZT/D4T + 3TC + EFV/NVP	1,170 (36.17)	714 (61.03)	0.7 (0.6,0.9)	0.00	1.0 (0.8,1.2)	0.85
Other regimens	637 (19.69)	406 (63.74)	0.8 (0.7,1.0)	0.04	0.9 (0.8,1.2)	0.61
WHO stage						
I	635 (19.63)	382 (60.16)				
II	1,279 (39.54)	829 (64.82)	1.2 (1.0,1.5)	0.05	1.1 (0.9,1.4)	0.32
III	860 (26.58)	573 (66.63)	1.3 (1.1,1.6)	0.01	1.4 (1.0,1.7)	0.01
IV	226 (6.99)	146 (64.60)	1.2 (0.9,1.7)	0.24	1.4 (1.0,1.9)	0.08
No information	235 (7.26)	165 (70.21)	1.6 (1.1,2.2)	0.01	0.9 (0.6,1.3)	0.63
Duration of ART (year)						
7–	930 (28.75)	650 (70.49)				
6–	738 (22.81)	502 (68.02)	0.9 (0.7,1.1)	0.41	0.9 (0.7,1.1)	0.24
5–	331 (10.23)	241 (72.81)	1.2 (0.9,1.5)	0.32	0.9 (0.7,1.2)	0.60

Table 1 continued

Variable	Number (%)	HIV drug resistance (%)	Crude OR (95% CI)	P-value	Adjusted OR (95% CI)	P-value
4–	264 (8.16)	182 (68.94)	1.0 (0.7,1.3)	0.77	0.7 (0.5,1.0)	0.05
3–	253 (7.82)	171 (67.59)	0.9 (0.7,1.2)	0.48	0.6 (0.4,0.9)	0.00
2–	289 (8.93)	183 (63.32)	0.7 (0.6,1.0)	0.04	0.5 (0.4,0.7)	0.00
1–	430 (13.29)	166 (38.60)	0.3 (0.2,0.3)	0.00	0.2 (0.1,0.2)	0.00

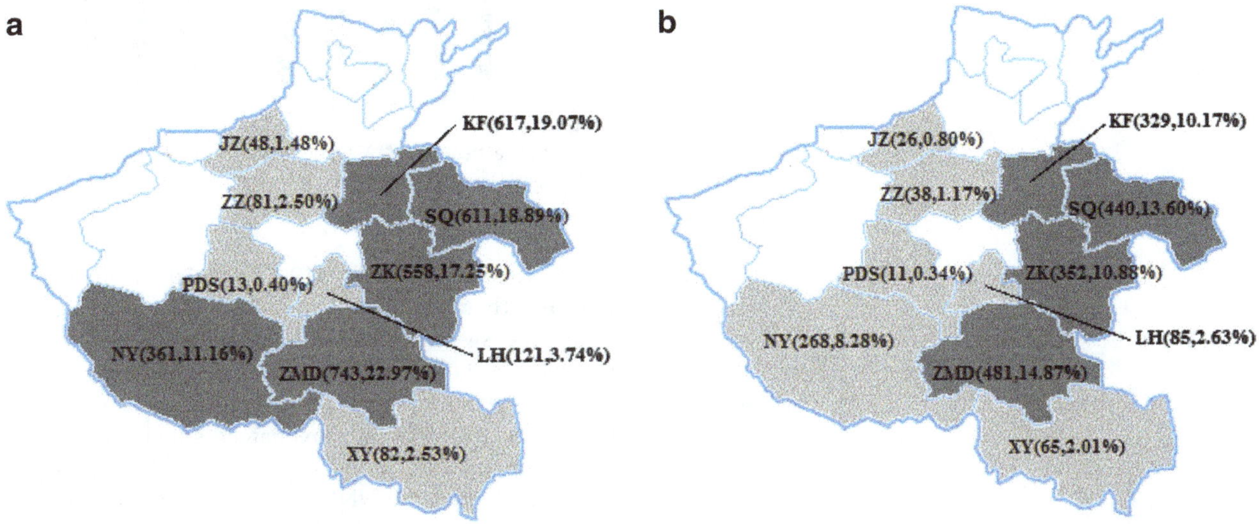

Figure 1 The geographical distribution of subjects according to the cities analyzed in this study. **a** The geographical distribution of treatment failures. **b** The geographical distribution of drug resistance genotypes detected. The abbreviation of city names are ZMD (Zhumadian), ZZ(Zhengzhou), KF(Kaifeng), JZ(Jiaozuo), ZK(Zhoukou), PDS(Pingdingshan), LH(Luohe), SQ(Shangqiu), NY(Nanyang), XY(Xinyang). The *number* and *percentage* in the brackets are the absolute number of subjects and the percent in the 3235 individuals. *Heavy gray*, cities with >10% of subjects; *light gray*, cities with <10% of subjects.

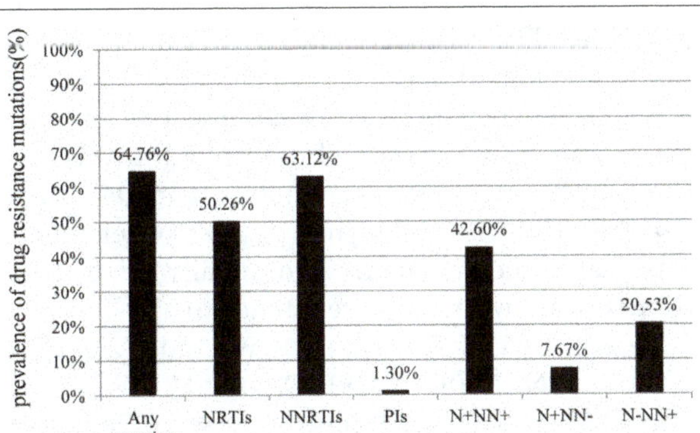

Figure 2 The prevalence of predicted human immunodeficiency virus 1 drug resistance mutations in different drug classes among individuals experiencing virological failure to first-line antiretroviral treatment in Henan, China during 2010–2011. *N+NN+* the existence of both nucleoside reverse transcriptase inhibitor (NRTI) and non-(N) NRTI resistance mutation, *N+NN−* the existence of NRTI but not NNRTI resistance mutations, *N-NN+* the existence of NNRTI but not NRTI resistance mutations.

The prevalence of HIV drug resistance is not constant across Henan. Zhumadian, Kaifeng, Shangqiu, Nanyang, and Xinyang have assembled a great deal of resources in the field of HIV/AIDS control and prevention because of their high HIV epidemic [14]. Compared to Zhumadian, multivariate analysis showed that Shangqiu, Nanyang, and Xinyang were associated with a higher likelihood of drug resistance mutations, whereas Kaifeng was not. Similarly, the other five cities also have the disconcordance phenomenon. These findings clarified that the scale of epidemic and resource focus on HIV/AIDS control and prevention has no direct correlation with the development of HIV drug resistance; however like other study had set forth, the local ART programmatic factors play a significant role [10]. Patients with low CD4 counts (below 200 cells/μL) and long-time treatment(over 4-years) were at the high risk of HIV drug resistance in this study that can be easily understood. The lower virus load(3–4 log copies/ml other than >4 log copies/ml) were correlated

Table 2 Frequency of the predicted human immunodeficiency virus drug resistance mutations

Resistance mutation (n = 3,235)	No. of patients (%)
NRTI mutation	
M184V/I	1,153 (35.64)
T215Y/F	879 (27.17)
M41L	595 (18.39)
D67N	395 (12.21)
K70R/E/G	330 (10.20)
L210 W	329 (10.17)
K219E/Q	324 (10.02)
L74I/V	118 (3.65)
V75I/M	110 (3.40)
Q151 M	93 (2.87)
A62 V	74 (2.29)
F116Y	67 (2.07)
K65R/N	51 (1.58)
F77L	30 (0.93)
Y115F	9 (0.28)
≥1TAM	1,369 (42.32)
TAM-1	290 (8.96)
TAM-2	149 (4.61)
TAM-1/TAM-2	10 (0.31)
Q151 M complex	13 (0.40)
M184 V/I + TAMs	691 (21.36)
NNRTI mutation	
K103 N/S	1,127 (34.84)
Y181C/V/I	713 (22.04)
G190A/S/E	590 (18.24)
K101E/P	247 (7.64)
V108I	225 (6.96)
V106A/M	177 (5.47)
Y188L/C/H	140 (4.33)
F227L/C	121 (3.74)
K238T	117 (3.62)
V179D/E/F	93 (2.87)
P225H	63 (1.95)
A98G	53 (1.64)
L100I	11 (0.34)
P236L	1 (0.03)
PI mutation	
M46I/L	22 (0.68)
V82F	11 (0.34)

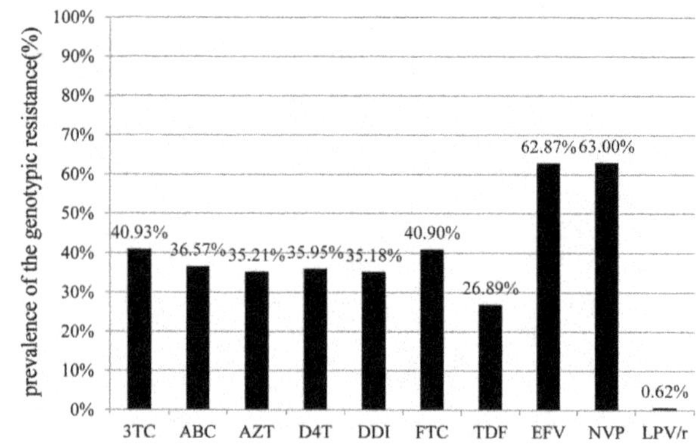

Figure 3 Prevalence of the genotypic resistance against different antiretroviral treatment (ART) drugs among individuals experiencing virological failure to first-line ART in Henan, China during 2010–2011.

to the high risk of HIV drug resistance mainly because of the HIV drug resistance strains were defective virus, and it probably have a lower capability of replication [4, 18].

NNRTIs have a low genetic barrier to resistance. Therefore, a single mutation is often sufficient for causing resistance to the currently recommended first generation of NNRTIs, NVP, or EFV [19, 20], which is why the second-line therapy did not include NNRTIs. Henan initiated the switch to second-line ART in patients who experienced failure with the first-line treatment in 2009. In this study, the prevalence of NNRTI resistance mutations (63.12%) was approximately equal to the total resistance mutations (64.76%). In addition, 20.53% of the patients had the NNRTI resistance mutations without NRTI, while only 7.67% had NRTI without NNRTI. Lastly, the prevalence of estimated resistance against EFV (62.87%) and NVP (63.00%) was both high with no significant different. All of these findings illustrated that the NNRTI resistance was more pervading than NRTI in ART failure patients. Therefore, it is just and reasonable for the government to perform second-line ART.

As expected, M184 V/I was the most commonly detected NRTI resistance mutation, which was also found in previous studies [21, 22], and this was followed by a high frequency of TAMs. A comparative amount of TAMs-1 and TAMs-2 were also detected in this study. TAMs confer cross-resistance to AZT and D4T as well as to most NRTIs in varying degrees when enough TAMs have accumulated. Additionally, two typical TAM pathways with a high resistance to all NRTIs were discovered: TAM-1 (M41L, L210W, and T215Y) and TAM-2 (D67N, K70R, K219E/Q, and T215F) [23–25]. Fewer K65R and Q151M complexes were detected in the study, mainly because they were apt to other subtypes and regimens [26, 27]. The Q151M complexes and K65R were also resistance mutations to multiple or even all of the NRTIs. The Q151M complex confers resistance to all NRTIs, except for TDF [28], and K65R confers resistance to D4T and TDF and possibly also to 3TC/FTC, DDI, and ABC [29]. Among patients with a detectable HIV RNA at 12 months, the HIV drug resistance was primarily due to M184V and NNRTI mutations. Complex mutation patterns, including the TAMs, K65R, and multinucleoside mutations, are prevalent among cases of treatment failure that were identified by clinical or immunologic methods as a result of the accumulation of drug resistance [21, 22]. The accumulation of drug resistance depends on the frequency of monitoring [30] and belated regimen adjustment. Thus, the duration of virologic failure must be somewhat longer than it should be because of the delayed virology surveillance or therapy adjustment in Henan during 2010–2011. Meanwhile, as Figure 3 shows, 35–40% of patients showed an estimated resistance against most NRTIs with 40.39 and 26.89% against 3TC and TDF, respectively. Since the second-line ART consists of two NRTIs (usually 3TC and TDF) and one PI, all of these findings suggest that a considerable amount of patients in Henan may already be compromised to second-line ART, indicating that approaches to more newer drugs with different mechanisms and individualized treatment should be considered sooner.

The emergence of transmitted HIV drug resistance can be anticipated, because such a large quantity of individuals acquired HIV drug resistance in this population-based survey. Recently, a moderate level of prevalence for transmitted HIV drug resistance has been reported in Henan [31]. More active monitoring strategies, such as conducting drug resistance testing prior to the initiation of ART should be performed as recommended by WHO in developed countries [32, 33].

Drug resistance mutations were undetected in 35.26% of patients among this treatment failure cohort, a significant proportion of individuals without mutations for treatment failure has also been reported in all similarity studies [5]. This probably because HIV drug resistance presented in some patients as minority variants (lower than 10–20% of the virus population) that may pass undetected by Sanger sequencing method [18], and non-adherence or treatment interruption must be another etiology of treatment failure without drug resistance. This study has gaps in knowledge on adherence, and we were not able to determine the duration of virological failure by using a cross-sectional survey. In view of these limitations, a further study needs to be conducted to provide sufficient evidence for evaluating a more precise and comprehensive profile of drug resistance among ART failures in Henan.

Conclusion

In conclusion, long-term ART roll-out leads to a comparatively high prevalence of HIV drug resistance among individuals who have experienced virological failure to first-line ART in Henan during 2010–2011, indicating a magnitude of former plasma donors. Multiple mutations and complex patterns have been identified, which may cause a growing number of those being treated with second-line therapy with partial or no activity. Performing routine drug resistance surveillance programs and timely therapy adjustment, especially among former plasma donors, ensuring access to new kinds of drugs, and initiating individualized treatment must be a priority in order to preserve programmatic treatment success in long-life therapy.

Data and materials availability Sequences generated for this study were deposited in the national AIDS treatment database of China.

Authors' contributions

JL wrote the paper. JL and ZW conceived and designed the study. JL, WY, DS and QZ performed the statistical analysis. JL and YW performed the experiments. JL and YW carried out staff training and quality management. JL, XX, GS, CL and ST conducted research at sites. All authors read and approved the final manuscript.

Author details

[1] Henan Center for Disease Control and Prevention, Zhengzhou, Henan, China.
[2] Chinese Center for Disease Control and Prevention, Beijing, China.

Acknowledgements

The authors wish to express their appreciation to the staff from the Zhumadian, Zhengzhou, Kaifeng, Jiaozuo, Zhoukou, Pingdingshan, Luohe, Shangqiu, Nanyang, Xinyang CDCs for their efforts and assistance with this study. We also wish to acknowledge the four national central laboratories (Shanghai Municipal CDC, Chinese Medical University Center for AIDS Research, Institute of Microbiology and Epidemiology of the Chinese Academy of Military Medical Sciences and State Key Laboratory for Infectious Disease Prevention and Control of National Center for AIDS/STD Control and Prevention) in China for their help with the HIV-1 genotypic drug resistance testing.

Competing interests

The authors declare that they have no competing interests.

References

1. Antiretroviral Therapy Cohort C (2008) Life expectancy of individuals on combination antiretroviral therapy in high-income countries: a collaborative analysis of 14 cohort studies. Lancet 372(9635):293–299. doi:10.1016/S0140-6736(08)61113-7
2. Bor J, Herbst AJ, Newell ML, Barnighausen T (2013) Increases in adult life expectancy in rural South Africa: valuing the scale-up of HIV treatment. Science 339(6122):961–965. doi:10.1126/science.1230413
3. Cohen MS, Chen YQ, McCauley M, Gamble T, Hosseinipour MC, Kumarasamy N et al (2011) Prevention of HIV-1 infection with early antiretroviral therapy. N Engl J Med 365(6):493–505. doi:10.1056/NEJMoa1105243
4. Iyidogan P, Anderson KS (2014) Current perspectives on HIV-1 antiretroviral drug resistance. Viruses 6(10):4095–4139. doi:10.3390/v6104095
5. WHO (2012) WHO HIV drug resistance report 2012. World Health Organazation, Geneva
6. He N, Detels R (2005) The HIV epidemic in China: history, response, and challenge. Cell Res 15(11–12):825–832. doi:10.1038/sj.cr.7290354
7. Zhang F, Haberer JE, Wang Y, Zhao Y, Ma Y, Zhao D et al (2007) The Chinese free antiretroviral treatment program: challenges and responses. AIDS 21(Suppl 8):S143–S148. doi:10.1097/01.aids.0000304710.10036.2b

8. Sun J, Ma L, Yu X, Huang Y, Yuan L, Shao Y (2009) Replication and drug resistant mutation of HIV-1 subtype B' (Thailand B) variants isolated from HAART treatment individuals in China. Virol J. 6:201. doi:10.1186/1743-422X-6-201
9. Ma L, Huang J, Xing H, Yuan L, Yu X, Sun J et al (2010) Genotypic and phenotypic cross-drug resistance of harboring drug-resistant HIV type 1 subtype B' strains from former blood donors in central Chinese provinces. AIDS Res Hum Retroviruses 26(9):1007–1013. doi:10.1089/aid.2009.0252
10. Xing H, Ruan Y, Li J, Shang H, Zhong P, Wang X et al (2013) HIV drug resistance and its impact on antiretroviral therapy in Chinese HIV-infected patients. PLoS One 8(2):e54917. doi:10.1371/journal.pone.0054917
11. Zhang M, Shang M, Yang W, Chen J, Wang Z, Shang H (2014) Treatment effect and drug-resistant mutations in chinese AIDS patients switching to second-line antiretroviral therapy. PLoS One 9(10):e110259. doi:10.1371/journal.pone.0110259
12. Zhong P, Pan Q, Ning Z, Xue Y, Gong J, Zhen X et al (2007) Genetic diversity and drug resistance of human immunodeficiency virus type 1 (HIV-1) strains circulating in Shanghai. AIDS Res Hum Retroviruses 23(7):847–856. doi:10.1089/aid.2006.0196
13. Liao L, Xing H, Shang H, Li J, Zhong P, Kang L et al (2010) The prevalence of transmitted antiretroviral drug resistance in treatment-naive HIV-infected individuals in China. J Acquir Immune Defic Syndr 53(Suppl 1):S10–S14. doi:10.1097/QAI.0b013e3181c7d363
14. Li N, Wang Z, Sun D, Zhu Q, Sun G, Yang W et al (2010) HIV among plasma donors and other high-risk groups in Henan, China. J Acquir Immune Defic Syndr. 53(Suppl 1):S41–S47. doi:10.1097/QAI.0b013e3181c7d717
15. Zhang F, Dou Z, Ma Y, Zhang Y, Zhao Y, Zhao D et al (2011) Effect of earlier initiation of antiretroviral treatment and increased treatment coverage on HIV-related mortality in China: a national observational cohort study. Lancet Infect Dis 11(7):516–524. doi:10.1016/S1473-3099(11)70097-4
16. Liu J, Qu B, Ezeakile MC, Zhang Y, Liang S (2013) Factors associated with HIV infection among men who have sex with men in Henan Province, China: a cross-sectional study. BMC Public Health 13:356. doi:10.1186/1471-2458-13-356
17. Zhang L, Chow EP, Jing J, Zhuang X, Li X, He M et al (2013) HIV prevalence in China: integration of surveillance data and a systematic review. Lancet Infect Dis 13(11):955–963. doi:10.1016/S1473-3099(13)70245-7
18. Halvas EK, Aldrovandi GM, Balfe P, Beck IA, Boltz VF, Coffin JM et al (2006) Blinded, multicenter comparison of methods to detect a drug-resistant mutant of human immunodeficiency virus type 1 at low frequency. J Clin Microbiol 44(7):2612–2614. doi:10.1128/JCM.00449-06
19. Balzarini J (2004) Current status of the non-nucleoside reverse transcriptase inhibitors of human immunodeficiency virus type 1. Curr Top Med Chem 4(9):921–944
20. De Clercq E (2004) Non-nucleoside reverse transcriptase inhibitors (NNRTIs): past, present, and future. Chem Biodivers 1(1):44–64. doi:10.1002/cbdv.200490012
21. Barth RE, van der Loeff MF, Schuurman R, Hoepelman AI, Wensing AM (2010) Virological follow-up of adult patients in antiretroviral treatment programmes in sub-Saharan Africa: a systematic review. Lancet Infect Dis 10(3):155–166. doi:10.1016/S1473-3099(09)70328-7
22. Hosseinipour MC, Gupta RK, Van Zyl G, Eron JJ, Nachega JB (2013) Emergence of HIV drug resistance during first- and second-line antiretroviral therapy in resource-limited settings. J Infect Dis 207(Suppl 2):S49–S56. doi:10.1093/infdis/jit107
23. Marcelin AG, Delaugerre C, Wirden M, Viegas P, Simon A, Katlama C et al (2004) Thymidine analogue reverse transcriptase inhibitors resistance mutations profiles and association to other nucleoside reverse transcriptase inhibitors resistance mutations observed in the context of virological failure. J Med Virol 72(1):162–165. doi:10.1002/jmv.10550
24. Miller MD (2004) K65R, TAMs and tenofovir. AIDS Rev 6(1):22–33
25. Cozzi-Lepri A, Ruiz L, Loveday C, Phillips AN, Clotet B, Reiss P et al (2005) Thymidine analogue mutation profiles: factors associated with acquiring specific profiles and their impact on the virological response to therapy. Antivir Ther 10(7):791–802
26. Sunpath H, Wu B, Gordon M, Hampton J, Johnson B, Moosa MY et al (2012) High rate of K65R for antiretroviral therapy-naive patients with subtype C HIV infection failing a tenofovir-containing first-line regimen. AIDS 26(13):1679–1684. doi:10.1097/QAD.0b013e328356886d
27. Tang MW, Rhee SY, Bertagnolio S, Ford N, Holmes S, Sigaloff KC et al (2013) Nucleoside reverse transcriptase inhibitor resistance mutations associated with first-line stavudine-containing antiretroviral therapy: programmatic implications for countries phasing out stavudine. J Infect Dis 207(Suppl 2):S70–S77. doi:10.1093/infdis/jit114
28. Maeda Y, Venzon DJ, Mitsuya H (1998) Altered drug sensitivity, fitness, and evolution of human immunodeficiency virus type 1 with pol gene mutations conferring multi-dideoxynucleoside resistance. J Infect Dis 177(5):1207–1213
29. Sungkanuparph S, Manosuthi W, Kiertiburanakul S, Saekang N, Pairoj W, Chantratita W (2008) Prevalence and risk factors for developing K65R mutations among HIV-1 infected patients who fail an initial regimen of fixed-dose combination of stavudine, lamivudine, and nevirapine. J Clin Virol 41(4):310–313. doi:10.1016/j.jcv.2007.12.015
30. De Luca A, Prosperi M, Bracciale L (2010) Resistance considerations in sequencing of antiretroviral therapy in low-middle income countries with currently available options. Curr Opin HIV AIDS 5(1):27–37. doi:10.1097/COH.0b013e328333ad45
31. Li L, Sun G, Liang S, Li J, Li T, Wang Z et al (2013) Different distribution of HIV-1 subtype and drug resistance were found among treatment naive individuals in Henan, Guangxi, and Yunnan province of China. PLoS One 8(10):e75777. doi:10.1371/journal.pone.0075777
32. Gazzard BG, Anderson J, Babiker A, Boffito M, Brook G, Brough G et al (2008) British HIV Association Guidelines for the treatment of HIV-1-infected adults with antiretroviral therapy 2008. HIV Med. 9(8):563–608. doi:10.1111/j.1468-1293.2008.00636.x
33. Bartmeyer B, Kuecherer C, Houareau C, Werning J, Keeren K, Somogyi S et al (2010) Prevalence of transmitted drug resistance and impact of transmitted resistance on treatment success in the German HIV-1 Seroconverter Cohort. PLoS One 5(10):e12718. doi:10.1371/journal.pone.0012718

24

Disease progression of HIV-1 infection in symptomatic and asymptomatic seroconverters in Osaka, Japan

Dai Watanabe[1*], Sachiko Suzuki[1], Misa Ashida[1], Yuka Shimoji[2], Kazuyuki Hirota[1], Yoshihiko Ogawa[1], Keishiro Yajima[1], Daisuke Kasai[1], Yasuharu Nishida[1], Tomoko Uehira[1] and Takuma Shirasaka[1]

Abstract

Background: Estimates of the interval from HIV-1 infection to disease progression may be affected by selection bias, and data concerning asymptomatic early seroconverters are limited. We examined the interval until disease progression in HIV-1 seroconverters in whom the timing of infection could be estimated within 1 year before diagnosis.

Methods: Subjects included newly diagnosed patients at Osaka National Hospital between 2003 and 2010 who had either (1) symptomatic acute HIV-1 infection with a negative or intermediate reaction on Western blotting and a positive reaction on an HIV RNA test (symptomatic acute group) or (2) a positive reaction on Western blotting at diagnosis and a <1-year interval from the last negative HIV test until the first positive test. The latter was divided into symptomatic recent or asymptomatic recent groups based on the presence or absence, respectively, of any transient fever between the last negative and first positive tests. Disease progression was defined as a fall in the CD4 count to <350 cells/microL on 2 consecutive tests, the start of anti-HIV therapy, or the onset of AIDS-indicator diseases. Information was retrospectively collected from medical records.

Results: Subjects included 210 patients: 91 in the symptomatic acute group, 72 in the symptomatic recent group, and 47 in the asymptomatic recent group. In the symptomatic acute (0.8 years) and symptomatic recent (2.2 years) groups, the Kaplan-Meier estimate of median interval until disease progression was significantly shorter than that in the asymptomatic recent group (2.9 years). Multivariate analysis by Cox's proportional hazards test showed that the symptomatic acute group (vs. asymptomatic recent group: hazard ratio: 1.93; 95% confidence interval: 1.14–3.36; $p = 0.0140$) and a baseline CD4 count of <400 cells/microL (hazard ratio: 3.88; 95% confidence interval: 2.57–5.96; $p < 0.0001$) were independent prognostic factors associated with early disease progression.

Conclusions: Symptomatic seroconversion was associated with early disease progression. Furthermore, the estimated median interval until the CD4 count was <350 cells/microL was only 2.9 years even in patients with asymptomatic seroconversion. These results suggest the importance of early diagnosis in early seroconverters.

Keywords: HIV-1 infection, Seroconverters, Disease progression

* Correspondence: dai@onh.go.jp
[1]AIDS Medical Center, National Hospital Organization Osaka National Hospital, 2-1-14 Hoenzaka, Chuo-ku, Osaka City, Osaka 540-0006, Japan
Full list of author information is available at the end of the article

Background

Studies in the late 1980s reported that the asymptomatic phase persisted for about 10 years in patients infected with human immunodeficiency virus (HIV)-1 [1-4]. However, various observational studies and meta-analyses have indicated that the baseline CD4-positive T-lymphocyte count (CD4 cell count) of the patients infected with HIV-1 in recent years is lower than that in previous studies, and that the plasma HIV-1-RNA level at the set point is higher [5-10], suggesting the possibility that HIV-1 has become more virulent and the asymptomatic phase has been shorter [11,12].

After primary infection with HIV-1, symptoms such as fever, lymph node swelling, and headache appear in 40%–90% of patients [13]. Fever is the most common symptom related to primary HIV-1 infection [14-16]. A cohort study involving patients with symptomatic acute HIV-1 infection is one way to observe and evaluate the spontaneous course of HIV-1 infection. However, there are some limitations regarding observational studies involving patients with symptomatic acute HIV-1 infection. In these patients, the disease progression is more rapid than in those with asymptomatic acute HIV-1 infection [17-20]. In addition, the severity of acute HIV-1 infection is also associated with disease progression [15,16,18]. Therefore, the spontaneous history in patients with symptomatic acute HIV-1 infection does not always reflect that of HIV-1 infection overall. In a cohort study involving early HIV-1 seroconverters, the proportion of patients with symptoms was also high, suggesting the presence of a selection bias [12,18].

With the appearance of new anti-HIV drugs and an accumulation of evidence, it has been recommended that antiretroviral therapy (ART) should be introduced in patients with a high CD4-positive T lymphocyte count (CD4 cell count). In Japanese guidelines, the CD4 cell count cutoff for the start of ART also increased from 200 to 350 cells/μL in 2008 and then to 500 cells/μL in 2013. However, the estimated interval from HIV infection until the CD4 cell count decreases to 350 cells/μL is still important for evaluating the timing of ART initiation. Concerning recent reports [5,16,20-27] of the estimated interval until disease progression, limitations of selection bias may be present as described above. In addition, data concerning asymptomatic early seroconverters are limited. We therefore focused on the characteristics of HIV-1 seroconverters both with and without symptoms related to primary HIV-1 infection. In this study, patients newly diagnosed based on positive reactions on Western blotting were investigated. Those in whom the timing of HIV-1 infection could be estimated to have been within 1 year before the HIV-1 infection diagnosis were divided into 2 groups with respect to the presence or absence of a history of fever between the last negative and first positive tests. We examined the characteristics by comparing the clinical course between these 2 groups and patients diagnosed with symptomatic acute HIV-1 infection.

Results

Patient groups

Of 1199 patients newly diagnosed with HIV-1 infection between 2003 and 2010 at the National Hospital Organization Osaka National Hospital, in 210, the timing of HIV-1 infection could be estimated within 1 year before their diagnosis. Ninety-five symptomatic patients had a negative or intermediate reaction detected on Western blotting at the time of HIV-1 infection diagnosis, and the polymerase chain reaction (PCR) method showed a positive reaction. Of these, 4 were diagnosed with chronic infection based on the changes in the Western blotting results, clinical course, and absence of a recent risk of infection. Therefore, 91 were diagnosed with symptomatic acute HIV infection (symptomatic acute group). In 119 patients, a positive reaction was detected on Western blotting at the time of HIV-1 infection diagnosis and the interval from the last negative test until the first positive test was ≤1 year (recent group). Of these, 72 reported having a transient fever between the last negative and first positive tests (symptomatic recent group). The other 47 patients were assigned to the asymptomatic recent group.

Patient characteristics and comparisons among symptomatic acute, symptomatic recent, and asymptomatic recent groups

Patient characteristics are shown in Table 1. The demographic and clinical characteristics of the subjects were compared among the symptomatic acute, symptomatic recent, and asymptomatic recent groups. There were no differences in the age or estimated route of infection among these 3 groups. In the symptomatic acute and symptomatic recent groups, the proportion of patients diagnosed in the late phase (2007–2010) was higher than that of patients diagnosed in the early phase (2003–2006). In the symptomatic recent group, 46 patients (64%) consulted a hospital for fever between the last negative and first positive tests. However, no HIV test was performed in any patient. The interval from the last negative test until the first positive test was compared between the symptomatic recent and asymptomatic recent groups. In the former (median 7.1 months), it was significantly shorter than in the latter (median 10.1 months), suggesting that a diagnosis of HIV infection was made earlier in the symptomatic recent group. Information regarding HIV-1 subtype was available in 111 of 210 participants. The most common subtype was B (n = 108), followed by CRF_01AE (n = 3). The

Table 1 Demographic and clinical characteristics of participants

Characteristic	Symptomatic acute group	Symptomatic recent group	Asymptomatic recent group	p value
Number of participants	91	72	47	
Age at first visit (y), median [IQR]	33 [28–38]	30 [25–35]	31 [24–36]	0.0841
Men, n (%)	91 (100%)	69 (97%)	47 (100%)	0.0387
Estimated route of transmission, n (%)				
Homosexual	79 (87%)	66 (92%)	43 (92%)	0.3234
Heterosexual	9 (10%)	6 (8%)	2 (4%)	
Unknown	3 (3%)	0 (0%)	2 (4%)	
HIV-1 subtype				
B	41 (45%)	40 (56%)	27 (57%)	0.0983
CRF01_AE	0 (0%)	1 (1%)	2 (4%)	
Not determined	50 (55%)	31 (43%)	18 (38%)	
Nationality, n (%)				
Japanese	89 (98%)	70 (97%)	47 (100%)	0.3490
Other	2 (2%)	2 (2%)	0 (0%)	
Calendar year at diagnosis, (%)				
2007–2010	65 (71%)	45 (63%)	20 (43%)	0.0044
2003–2006	26 (29%)	27 (37%)	27 (57%)	
Medical exam between last negative and first positive test, n (%)				
No	3 (3%)	26 (36%)	47 (100%)	<0.0001
Outpatient	28 (31%)	36 (50%)	0 (0%)	
Hospitalization	60 (66%)	10 (14%)	0 (0%)	
Interval between last negative and first positive test (mo), median [IQR]		7.1 [4.1–10.2]	10.1 [6.1–11.7]	0.0472
Baseline CD4 cell count (cells/μL), median [IQR]	359 [243–464]	353 [257–481]	445 [353–526]	0.0323
Percentage of patients with CD4 cell count <400 cells/μL, n (%)	54 (59%)	43 (60%)	15 (31%)	0.0035
Baseline HIV-1 RNA level (copies/mL), median [IQR]	470000 [52000–270000]	32000 [6900–74800]	21000 [12000–66000]	<0.0001
Percentage of patients with HIV-1 RNA level ≥50000 copies/mL, n (%)	69 (76%)	26 (36%)	14 (30%)	<0.0001

Abbreviation: IQR, interquartile range

percentage of patients with subtype B HIV-1 infection was not statistically different among the symptomatic acute, symptomatic recent, and asymptomatic recent groups (Table 1) and was not changed from the early phase (2003–2006, 55%) to the late phase (2007–2010, 49%) ($p = 0.1900$).

Comparison of baseline CD4 cell count and plasma HIV-1 RNA level

We examined the CD4 cell count and viral level on the initial consultation. Overall, the median CD4 cell count and plasma HIV-1 RNA level were 383 cells/μL and 51,900 copies/mL, respectively. The proportion of patients with a CD4 cell count of <400 cells/μL and that of patients with a plasma HIV-1-RNA level of ≥50,000 copies/mL are presented in Table 1. In the symptomatic acute and symptomatic recent groups, the proportions of patients with a baseline CD4 cell count of <400 cells/μL were higher than that in the asymptomatic recent group (symptomatic acute vs. asymptomatic recent: $p < 0.01$; symptomatic recent vs. asymptomatic recent: $p < 0.01$). Furthermore, the proportion of patients with a baseline plasma HIV-1-RNA level of ≥50,000 copies/mL was the highest in the symptomatic acute group among the 3 groups (symptomatic acute vs. asymptomatic recent: $p < 0.001$; symptomatic acute vs. symptomatic recent: $p < 0.001$).

Estimated interval from HIV-1 infection until disease progression

We examined the interval from the estimated timing of infection until disease progression. Twelve patients enrolled in a clinical study, in whom ART was started regardless of their CD4 cell counts, were excluded from the analysis. Of the 198 patients, 119 met the criteria for disease progression during the follow-up period (median 0.78 years). Of these, 96 patients showed a CD4 cell count of <350 cells/μL on 2 consecutive tests. In the other 19 patients who had a CD4 cell count of <350 cells/μL on at least 1 test, ART was started (9 in the acute symptomatic phase and 6 in the chronic asymptomatic phase) or AIDS-indicator diseases were diagnosed before the above criterion was met. In the remaining 4, although the CD4 cell count did not reach <350 cells/μL on either test, ART was started for prevention of partner infection, HBV infection, thrombocytopenia, and HIV infection-related malaise in each patient. In the symptomatic acute group, in only one of the patients with a CD4 cell count of <350 cells/μL on the first and second tests did the CD4 cell count return to ≥350 cells/μL within the next 3 months. Using the Kaplan-Meier method, we estimated the interval from the estimated timing of infection until disease progression. In the cohort overall, the median interval until disease progression was 1.9 years. In the symptomatic acute, symptomatic recent, and asymptomatic recent groups, it was 0.8, 2.2, and 2.9 years, respectively (Figure 1), showing significant differences (symptomatic acute vs. symptomatic recent: $p < 0.001$; symptomatic acute vs. asymptomatic recent: $p < 0.001$; symptomatic recent vs. asymptomatic recent: $p < 0.05$). Using Cox's proportional hazards model, we investigated factors involved in early disease progression (Table 2). On univariate analysis, a baseline CD4 cell count of <400 cells/μL, and belonging to the symptomatic acute group were significant factors. Multivariate analysis showed that the baseline CD4 cell count and belonging to the symptomatic acute group were independent factors. To verify the results of multivariate analysis, we conducted subgroup analysis by stratification of the CD4 cell count on the initial consultation (Figure 2). In the symptomatic acute group, disease progression was observed in the early stage regardless of the baseline CD4 cell count. However, the interval until disease progression was similar between the symptomatic recent and asymptomatic recent groups through stratification. These results showed that the interval from HIV infection until disease progression was associated with the CD4 cell count on the initial consultation, a diagnosis of acute HIV infection, and fever suggestive of primary infection with HIV-1 and that the former 2 were independent factors.

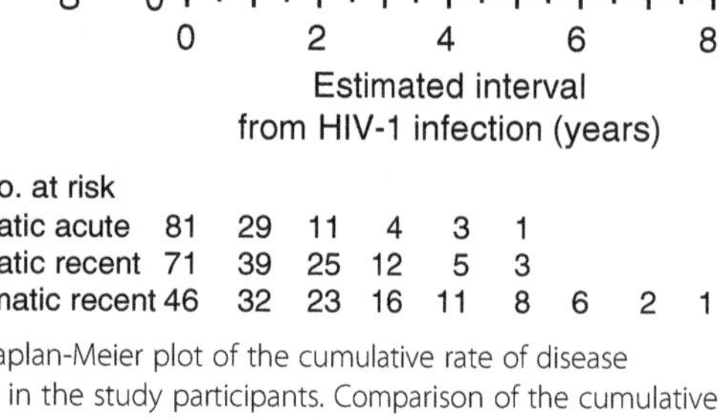

No. at risk								
Symptomatic acute	81	29	11	4	3	1		
Symptomatic recent	71	39	25	12	5	3		
Asymptomatic recent	46	32	23	16	11	8	6	2	1

Figure 1 Kaplan-Meier plot of the cumulative rate of disease progression in the study participants. Comparison of the cumulative rate of disease progression among the symptomatic acute, symptomatic recent, and asymptomatic recent groups.

Discussion

This study was conducted in HIV-1 seroconverters in Osaka (Japan) in whom the timing of infection could be estimated within 1 year before diagnosis. Initially, as important observation points, disease progression was noted in the early stage in symptomatic HIV-1 seroconverters. In those diagnosed in the acute stage of HIV-1, the median interval until disease progression was only 0.8 years (Figure 1). Although some studies have estimated the interval from infection until the CD4 cell count reaches <350 cells/μL in patients with acute HIV-1 infection [5,16,20-24,26,27], it is difficult to compare the results among different cohorts due to differences in the definition of acute HIV-1 infection and disease progression or patient background. However, similar median intervals have been reported from Japan (<1 year) [16], Holland (<1 year) [24], and Germany (8.3 months) [26], although some reports showed longer median intervals than this report does [5,20,21,23,27]. The reasons suggested for early disease progression include host-related factors such as genetic background, route of infection, and social background; viral factors such as subtype and escape mutations; and the possibility of a selection bias in which severe-status patients were predominantly enrolled in the study [28,29]. The mechanism of early disease progression remains to be clarified, but it must be considered that disease progression is rapid in patients with symptomatic acute HIV-1 infection.

Even in patients without primary infection symptoms (asymptomatic recent group), the median interval from infection until disease progression was 2.9 years. In a large-scale observational study involving 18,495 seroconverters, the interval from infection until the CD4 cell count reached <350 cells/μL was estimated to be 4.19 years [25]. However, approximately 50% of the study subjects had been diagnosed with HIV-1 infection before 1996. The subjects included patients with symptomatic acute HIV infection. Therefore, although the interval from infection until the CD4 cell count reached <350 cells/μL is longer than what we report here, a

Table 2 Association with early disease progression in early HIV-1 seroconverters

	Univariate results			Multivariate results		
	HR	95% CI	p value	HR	95% CI	p value
Age (≥40 vs. <40)	1.21	0.73–1.93	0.4411	1.25	0.75–2.00	0.3739
Calendar year at diagnosis (2007–2010 vs. 2003–2006)	1.36	0.93–2.03	0.1170	1.26	0.83–1.93	0.2823
With baseline CD4 cell count <400 cells/μL	4.02	2.70–6.08	<0.0001	3.88	2.57–5.96	<0.0001
Group						
Asymptomatic recent group	1			1		
Symptomatic recent group	1.62	0.97–2.74	0.0621	1.12	0.67–1.93	0.6772
Symptomatic acute group	2.95	1.79–4.99	<0.0001	1.93	1.14–3.36	0.0140

Abbreviations: HR, hazard ratio; CI, confidence interval.

direct comparison between the previous report [25] and ours is not possible.

Of the 119 patients with positive reactions on Western blotting at the time of HIV-1 infection diagnosis, symptoms possibly related to primary infection with HIV-1 were observed in 72. However, this figure may include an error. Although patients were questioned about a history of fever at the initial consultation, fever is not always related to primary HIV-1 infection. Furthermore, we cannot rule out the possibility that some patients could not recollect the appearance of symptoms related to primary infection and were assigned to the asymptomatic recent group. However, when analyzing the HIV-1 RNA level (Table 1) and interval from infection until disease progression (Figure 1), the symptomatic acute and asymptomatic recent groups showed opposite characteristics. Those of the symptomatic recent group were intermediate between the other 2 groups. Based on these results, we believe the majority of participants were assigned to the correct groups. Several possibilities may explain why the symptomatic acute and symptomatic recent groups showed different disease progression. One possible reason is the difference in disease severity because the proportion of patients who were hospitalized in the symptomatic acute group was higher than that in the symptomatic recent group (Table 1). However, we cannot exclude the possibility that recall bias, as mentioned above, may have affected this difference.

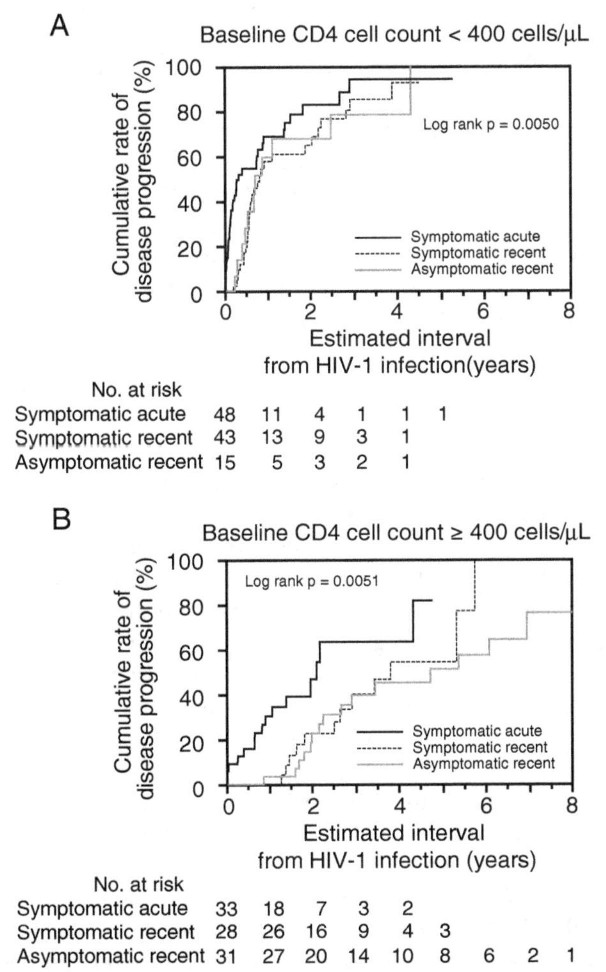

Figure 2 Kaplan-Meier plot of the cumulative rate of disease progression stratified with the CD4 cell count. **(A)** Patients with a CD4 cell count of <400 cells/μL on the initial consultation. **(B)** Patients with a baseline CD4 cell count of 400 cells/μL or more.

As shown in Table 1, the interval from the last negative test until the first positive test in the symptomatic recent group was significantly shorter than in the symptomatic recent group. This suggests the possibilities that the development of fever motivated those who recognize the risk of HIV-1 infection to undergo voluntary HIV testing and that the true seroconversion date with symptomatic seroconverters would be closer to the date of the first positive test rather than the date of the last negative test. These possibilities were also indicated by the recent report estimating the date of infection for HIV-1 infected patients using the HIV-1-specific immunoglobulin G (IgG) levels measured by the IgG-capture BED-enzyme immunoassay [30].

A limitation of this study is that it was a retrospective analysis involving a limited number of patients in a single institution. We are also aware of possible limitations of selection and recall biases in this study. Selection of the patients with fever related to the primary HIV-1 infection could be a potential source of selection bias. However, the data presented in this study are consistent with the results of previous studies. Patients diagnosed with acute HIV-1 infection showed disease progression in the early stage. Fever related to primary HIV-1 infection encouraged patients undergo HIV testing. Additionally, disease progression may be observed within a relatively short period even in asymptomatic early-infection patients.

Conclusions

Symptomatic HIV-1 seroconversion was associated with early disease progression, especially in patients with symptomatic acute HIV-1 infection, with a median interval until disease progression of only 0.8 years. Furthermore, the estimated median period during which the CD4 cell count was <350 cells/μL was only 2.9 years even in patients with asymptomatic seroconversion. These results suggest the importance of early diagnosis in early HIV-1 seroconverters.

Methods

Case selection

This study was conducted at the National Hospital Organization Osaka National Hospital, a major hospital for HIV infection in Japan, located in the center of Osaka. Subjects included newly diagnosed patients with HIV-1 infection who consulted this hospital for the first time between 2003 and 2010 and who met 1 of the following 2 criteria: (1) a negative or intermediate reaction detected on Western blotting at the time of HIV-1 infection diagnosis and a positive PCR, leading to a diagnosis of symptomatic acute HIV-1 infection (symptomatic acute group) or (2) a positive reaction detected on Western blotting at the time of HIV-1 infection diagnosis and a <1-year interval from the final negative HIV test until the first positive HIV test (recent groups). The protocol of this study was approved by the Ethics Review Board of the National Hospital Organization Osaka National Hospital (Approval No. 0913).

Measurement of the CD4 cell count, plasma HIV-1 RNA level, and Western blotting

The CD4 cell count was measured by flow cytometry using the single-platform method. Peripheral blood (100 μL) was incubated with 10 μL of CYTO-STAT tetraCHROME reagent (Beckmann Coulter, Miami, FL) containing CD45-FITC/CD4-RD1/CD8-ECD/CD3-PC5 monoclonal antibodies. After erythrocyte hemolysis and cell fixation with the whole blood lysing reagent Kit (Beckmann Coulter), 100 μL of Flow-Count fluorospheres were added to the sample, and the absolute CD45 + CD3 + CD4 + CD8− cell counts were measured using a Cytomics FC500 system (Beckmann Coulter). The plasma HIV-1 RNA level was determined using the reverse-transcription PCR method (COBAS AMPLICOR HIV-1 test or COBAS TaqMan HIV-1 test; Roche Molecular Diagnostics, Branchburg, NJ). The CD4 cell count and plasma HIV-1 RNA level were measured at 1- to 4-month intervals. For Western blotting for HIV-1, LAV Blot I (Bio-Rad Laboratories, Hercules, CA) was used. Interpretation of the results was performed according to the criteria established by the World Health Organization.

Definition of the symptomatic acute, symptomatic recent, and asymptomatic recent groups and comparison of clinical information on the initial consultation among the groups

The symptomatic acute group was defined as described above. Patients meeting conditions for both the symptomatic acute and recent groups were assigned to the symptomatic acute group. In the recent group, any self-reported history of a transient fever was investigated at the initial consultation in our hospital. Fever was defined as a body temperature of 38°C or higher. When a definitive diagnosis of a disease that causes fever was made, the patient was excluded from a history of fever. Patients who recollected having a transient fever between the last negative and first positive tests for HIV infection were assigned to the symptomatic recent group, and those who did not were assigned to the asymptomatic recent group. Information on the age, sex, nationality, estimated route of infection, year of diagnosis, previous hospital consultations, CD4 cell count, and plasma HIV-1 RNA level was collected from medical records and compared among the 3 groups.

Estimation of the timing of HIV-1 infection and interval from infection until disease progression

In the symptomatic acute group, the timing of infection was estimated to be 1 month before a diagnosis of HIV-1 infection was made. In the recent groups, the midpoint between the last negative and first positive tests was regarded as the estimated timing of infection. The timing of disease progression was defined as the earliest date on which the CD4 cell count was less than 350 cells/μL on 2 consecutive tests conducted at more than 1 month apart, the start of ART, or the onset of an AIDS-indicator disease. In patients in whom the annual frequency of testing for the CD4 cell count and plasma HIV-1 RNA level became <3, follow-up was completed on the final day of testing. The interval from the estimated timing of infection until disease progression was calculated using the Kaplan-Meier method. For significance tests, the log-rank test was performed. When there was a significant difference, adjustment was conducted using Holm's correction, and multiple tests were performed. For multivariate analysis, Cox's proportional hazards analysis was carried out. With respect to individual factors, the hazard ratio, 95% confidence interval, and p-value were calculated.

Statistical analysis

For 3×2 cross-table tests, the χ^2 test was used. When there was a significant difference, adjustment was conducted using Holm's method, and multiple tests were performed. To compare the results among the 3 groups, analysis was conducted using Kruskal-Wallis one-way analysis of variance by ranks. The Kaplan-Meier method, log-rank test, and Cox's proportional hazards test were performed, as described above. For statistical analysis, JMP version 10.0.0 software (SAS Institute, Cary, NC) was used. A p-value of <0.05 was regarded as significant.

Competing interests

The authors declare that they have no competing interests.

Authors' contributions

DW and TS participated in the study design and coordination; TS, TU, DW, YN, DK, KY, YO, KH, YS, MA, and SS managed the patients and collected the data; and DW wrote the paper. All authors read and approved the final manuscript.

Acknowledgements

This work was supported by a Grant-in-Aid for Clinical Research from the National Hospital Organization to TS and a Grant-in-Aid for AIDS research from the Ministry of Health, Labor, and Welfare of Japan to DW (H24-AIDS-S-002).

Author details

[1]AIDS Medical Center, National Hospital Organization Osaka National Hospital, 2-1-14 Hoenzaka, Chuo-ku, Osaka City, Osaka 540-0006, Japan. [2]Department of Nursing, National Hospital Organization Osaka National Hospital, Osaka, Japan.

References

1. Medley GF, Anderson RM, Cox DR, Billard L. Incubation period of AIDS in patients infected via blood transfusion. Nature. 1987;328:719–21.
2. Lui KJ, Darrow WW, Rutherford 3rd GW. A model-based estimate of the mean incubation period for AIDS in homosexual men. Science. 1988;240:1333–5.
3. Bacchetti P, Moss AR. Incubation period of AIDS in San Francisco. Nature. 1989;338:251–3.
4. Munoz A, Wang MC, Bass S, Taylor JM, Kingsley LA, Chmiel JS, et al. Acquired immunodeficiency syndrome (AIDS)-free time after human immunodeficiency virus type 1 (HIV-1) seroconversion in homosexual men. Multicenter AIDS Cohort Study Group. Am J Epidemiol. 1989;130:530–9.
5. Gras L, Geskus RB, Jurriaans S, Bakker M, van Sighem A, Bezemer D, et al. Has the rate of CD4 cell count decline before initiation of antiretroviral therapy changed over the course of the Dutch HIV epidemic among MSM? PLoS One. 2013;8, e64437.
6. Herbeck JT, Muller V, Maust BS, Ledergerber B, Torti C, Di Giambenedetto S, et al. Is the virulence of HIV changing? A meta-analysis of trends in prognostic markers of HIV disease progression and transmission. AIDS. 2012;26:193–205.
7. Muller V, Maggiolo F, Suter F, Ladisa N, De Luca A, Antinori A, et al. Increasing clinical virulence in two decades of the Italian HIV epidemic. PLoS Pathog. 2009;5, e1000454.
8. Gras L, Jurriaans S, Bakker M, van Sighem A, Bezemer D, Fraser C, et al. Viral load levels measured at set-point have risen over the last decade of the HIV epidemic in the Netherlands. PLoS One. 2009;4, e7365.
9. Crum-Cianflone N, Eberly L, Zhang Y, Ganesan A, Weintrob A, Marconi V, et al. Is HIV becoming more virulent? Initial CD4 cell counts among HIV seroconverters during the course of the HIV epidemic: 1985–2007. Clin Infect Dis. 2009;48:1285–92.
10. Dorrucci M, Rezza G, Porter K, Phillips A, Concerted Action on Seroconversion to A, Death in Europe C. Temporal trends in postseroconversion CD4 cell count and HIV load: the Concerted Action on Seroconversion to AIDS and Death in Europe Collaboration, 1985–2002. J Infect Dis. 2007;195:525–34.
11. Rangsin R, Chiu J, Khamboonruang C, Sirisopana N, Eiumtrakul S, Brown AE, et al. The natural history of HIV-1 infection in young Thai men after seroconversion. J Acquir Immune Defic Syndr. 2004;36:622–9.
12. Rangsin R, Piyaraj P, Sirisanthana T, Sirisopana N, Short O, Nelson KE. The natural history of HIV-1 subtype E infection in young men in Thailand with up to 14 years of follow-up. AIDS. 2007;21 Suppl 6:S39–46.
13. Kahn JO, Walker BD. Acute human immunodeficiency virus type 1 infection. N Engl J Med. 1998;339:33–9.
14. Sued O, Miro JM, Alquezar A, Claramonte X, Garcia F, Plana M, et al. Primary human immunodeficiency virus type 1 infection: clinical, virological and immunological characteristics of 75 patients (1997–2003). Enferm Infecc Microbiol Clin. 2006;24:238–44.
15. Lavreys L, Baeten JM, Chohan V, McClelland RS, Hassan WM, Richardson BA, et al. Higher set point plasma viral load and more-severe acute HIV type 1 (HIV-1) illness predict mortality among high-risk HIV-1-infected African women. Clin Infect Dis. 2006;42:1333–9.
16. Nakamura H, Teruya K, Takano M, Tsukada K, Tanuma J, Yazaki H, et al. Clinical symptoms and courses of primary HIV-1 infection in recent years in Japan. Intern Med. 2011;50:95–101.
17. Lindback S, Brostrom C, Karlsson A, Gaines H. Does symptomatic primary HIV-1 infection accelerate progression to CDC stage IV disease, CD4 count below 200 x 10(6)/l, AIDS, and death from AIDS? BMJ. 1994;309:1535–7.
18. Vanhems P, Lambert J, Cooper DA, Perrin L, Carr A, Hirschel B, et al. Severity and prognosis of acute human immunodeficiency virus type 1 illness: a dose–response relationship. Clin Infect Dis. 1998;26:323–9.
19. Ghosn J, Deveau C, Chaix ML, Goujard C, Galimand J, Zitoun Y, et al. Despite being highly diverse, immunovirological status strongly correlates with clinical symptoms during primary HIV-1 infection: a cross-sectional study based on 674 patients enrolled in the ANRS CO 06 PRIMO cohort. J Antimicrob Chemother. 2010;65:741–8.
20. Socias ME, Sued O, Laufer N, Lazaro ME, Mingrone H, Pryluka D, et al. Acute retroviral syndrome and high baseline viral load are predictors of rapid HIV progression among untreated Argentinean seroconverters. J Int AIDS Soc. 2011;14:40.
21. Investigators ST, Fidler S, Porter K, Ewings F, Frater J, Ramjee G, et al. Short-course antiretroviral therapy in primary HIV infection. N Engl J Med. 2013;368:207–17.
22. Hogan CM, Degruttola V, Sun X, Fiscus SA, Del Rio C, Hare CB, et al. The setpoint study (ACTG A5217): effect of immediate versus deferred antiretroviral therapy on virologic set point in recently HIV-1-infected individuals. J Infect Dis. 2012;205:87–96.
23. Sucupira MC, Sanabani S, Cortes RM, Giret MT, Tomiyama H, Sauer MM, et al. Faster HIV-1 disease progression among Brazilian individuals recently infected with CXCR4-utilizing strains. PLoS One. 2012;7, e30292.
24. Grijsen ML, Steingrover R, Wit FW, Jurriaans S, Verbon A, Brinkman K, et al. No treatment versus 24 or 60 weeks of antiretroviral treatment during primary HIV infection: the randomized Primo-SHM trial. PLoS Med. 2012;9, e1001196.
25. Lodi S, Phillips A, Touloumi G, Geskus R, Meyer L, Thiebaut R, et al. Time from human immunodeficiency virus seroconversion to reaching CD4+ cell count thresholds <200, <350, and <500 Cells/mm(3): assessment of need following changes in treatment guidelines. Clin Infect Dis. 2011;53:817–25.
26. Koegl C, Wolf E, Hanhoff N, Jessen H, Schewe K, Rausch M, et al. Treatment during primary HIV infection does not lower viral set point but improves CD4 lymphocytes in an observational cohort. Eur J Med Res. 2009;14:277–83.
27. Goujard C, Bonarek M, Meyer L, Bonnet F, Chaix ML, Deveau C, et al. CD4 cell count and HIV DNA level are independent predictors of disease progression after primary HIV type 1 infection in untreated patients. Clin Infect Dis. 2006;42:709–15.
28. Langford SE, Ananworanich J, Cooper DA. Predictors of disease progression in HIV infection: a review. AIDS Res Ther. 2007;4:11.

29. Lewden C, Thiebaut R, Boufassa F, Coulibaly A, Malateste K, Seng R, et al. Comparison of early CD4 T-cell count in HIV-1 seroconverters in Cote d'Ivoire and France: the ANRS PRIMO-CI and SEROCO cohorts. J Acquir Immune Defic Syndr. 2010;53:260–5.
30. Skar H, Albert J, Leitner T. Towards estimation of HIV-1 date of infection: a time-continuous IgG-model shows that seroconversion does not occur at the midpoint between negative and positive tests. PLoS One. 2013;8, e60906.

Permissions

All chapters in this book were first published in AIDS R&T, by BioMed Central; hereby published with permission under the Creative Commons Attribution License or equivalent. Every chapter published in this book has been scrutinized by our experts. Their significance has been extensively debated. The topics covered herein carry significant findings which will fuel the growth of the discipline. They may even be implemented as practical applications or may be referred to as a beginning point for another development.

The contributors of this book come from diverse backgrounds, making this book a truly international effort. This book will bring forth new frontiers with its revolutionizing research information and detailed analysis of the nascent developments around the world.

We would like to thank all the contributing authors for lending their expertise to make the book truly unique. They have played a crucial role in the development of this book. Without their invaluable contributions this book wouldn't have been possible. They have made vital efforts to compile up to date information on the varied aspects of this subject to make this book a valuable addition to the collection of many professionals and students.

This book was conceptualized with the vision of imparting up-to-date information and advanced data in this field. To ensure the same, a matchless editorial board was set up. Every individual on the board went through rigorous rounds of assessment to prove their worth. After which they invested a large part of their time researching and compiling the most relevant data for our readers.

The editorial board has been involved in producing this book since its inception. They have spent rigorous hours researching and exploring the diverse topics which have resulted in the successful publishing of this book. They have passed on their knowledge of decades through this book. To expedite this challenging task, the publisher supported the team at every step. A small team of assistant editors was also appointed to further simplify the editing procedure and attain best results for the readers.

Apart from the editorial board, the designing team has also invested a significant amount of their time in understanding the subject and creating the most relevant covers. They scrutinized every image to scout for the most suitable representation of the subject and create an appropriate cover for the book.

The publishing team has been an ardent support to the editorial, designing and production team. Their endless efforts to recruit the best for this project, has resulted in the accomplishment of this book. They are a veteran in the field of academics and their pool of knowledge is as vast as their experience in printing. Their expertise and guidance has proved useful at every step. Their uncompromising quality standards have made this book an exceptional effort. Their encouragement from time to time has been an inspiration for everyone.

The publisher and the editorial board hope that this book will prove to be a valuable piece of knowledge for researchers, students, practitioners and scholars across the globe.

List of Contributors

Tesfaye Berhe and Amanuel Amare
Department of Neurology, Addis Ababa University, Addis Ababa, Ethiopia

Yilma Melkamu
School of Public Health, Addis Ababa University, Addis Ababa, Ethiopia

Gita Ramjee and Brodie Daniels
HIV Prevention Research Unit, South African Medical Research Council, 123 Jan Hofmeyr Road, Westville, Durban 3629, South Africa

Gita Ramjee
London School of Hygiene and Tropical Medicines, Keppel Street,London WC1E, 7HT, UK

Assefa Missaye
Dessie regional laboratory, Amhara regional state, Northeast Ethiopia

Mulat Dagnew
Department of Medical Microbiology, School of Biomedical and Laboratory Sciences, College of Medicine and Health Sciences, University of Gondar, Gondar, Ethiopia

Abebe Alemu and Agersew Alemu
Department of Medical Parasitology, School of Biomedical and Laboratory Sciences, College of Medicine and Health Sciences, University of Gondar, Gondar, Ethiopia

Desta Kassa, Gebremedhin Gebremichael, Yodit Alemayehu and Tsehaynesh Messele
Infectious and non-infectious diseases research directorate, Ethiopian Health and Nutrition Research Institute (EHNRI), Addis Ababa, Ethiopia

Desta Kassa and Debbie van Baarle
Department of Internal Medicine and Infectious Diseases and Department of Immunology, University Medical Center Utrecht, Utrecht, The Netherlands

Dawit Wolday
Medical Biotech Laboratory, Addis Ababa, Ethiopia

Erick M Bosire and Michael M Gicheru
Department of Zoological Science, Kenyatta University, Nairobi, Kenya

Anthony K Nyamache
Department of Plant and Microbial Sciences, Kenyatta University, Nairobi, Kenya

Samoel A Khamadi, Raphael W Lihana and Vincent Okoth
Kenya Medical Research Institute, Centre for Viral Research, Nairobi, Kenya

Veronica Wambui, Edward Muge, Peter Kinyanjui and Elijah M Songok
Department of Biochemistry, University of Nairobi, Nairobi 30197-00100, Kenya

Michael Kiptoo, Joyceline Kinyua, Irene Odera, Raphael Lihana and Elijah M Songok
Centre for Virus Research, Kenya Medical Research Institute, Nairobi 54848-00200, Kenya

Peter Muiruri
Comprehensive Care Centre, Kenyatta National Hospital, Nairobi 2146-00202, Kenya

Vasudev R Rao, Arthur P Ruiz and Vinayaka R Prasad
Department of Microbiology and Immunology, Albert Einstein College of Medicine, 1300 Morris Park Avenue, Bronx, NY 10461, USA

Janet Michel, Richard Lessells and Marie-Louise Newell
Africa Centre for Health and Population Studies, University of KwaZulu-Natal, Somkhele, Mtubatuba, KwaZulu-Natal 3935, South Africa

Marie-Louise Newell
Faculty of Medicine, University of Southampton, Southampton, UK

Christina Matlakala
University of South Africa, Preller St., Pretoria 0002, South Africa

Rene English
Health Systems Trust, Westville, South Africa

Johannes Prottengeier
Department of Anesthesiology, Erlangen University Hospital, Krankenhausstrasse 12, 91054 Erlangen, Germany

Eleni Koutsilieri and Carsten Scheller
Institute of Virology and Immunobiology, University of Würzburg, Würzburg, Germany

Laura Fernández-Sender, Carlos Alonso-Villaverde, Anna Rull, Esther Rodríguez-Gallego, Marta Riera-Borrull, Anna Hernández-Aguilera, Jordi Camps, Raúl Beltrán-Debón, Gerard Aragonès and Jorge Joven
Unitat de Recerca Biomèdica, Hospital Universitari Sant Joan, Institut d'Investigació Sanitaria Pere Virgili (IISPV), Universitat Rovira i Virgili, Reus, Spain, carrer Sant Llorenç 21, Reus 43201, Spain

Carlos Alonso-Villaverde
Servei de Medicina Interna, Hospital Sant Pau i Santa Tecla, carrer Rambla Vella 14, Tarragona 43003, Spain

Javier A Menendez
Translational Research Laboratory, Catalan Institute of Oncology (ICO) and Girona Biomedical Research Institute (IdIBGi), Avda de França s/n 17007, Girona, Spain

Thanyawee Puthanakit, Umaporn Siangphoe, Tulathip Suwanlerk, Wasana Prasitsuebsai, Naris Waranawat and Jintanat Ananworanich
The HIV Netherlands Australia Thailand Research Collaboration (HIV-NAT), Bangkok, Thailand

Thanyawee Puthanakit
Department of Pediatrics, Faculty of Medicine, Chulalongkorn University, Bangkok, Thailand

Gonzague Jourdain
Institut de Recherche pour le Développement (IRD), UMI 174, Program for HIV Prevention and Treatment, Department of Medical Technology, Faculty of Associated Medical Sciences, Chiang Mai University, Chiang Mai, Thailand

Piyarat Suntarattiwong
Queen Sirikit National Institute of Child Health, Bangkok, Thailand

Kulkanya Chokephaibulkit and Wasana Prasitsuebsai
Department of Pediatrics, Faculty of Medicine Siriraj Hospital, Mahidol University, Bangkok, Thailand

Virat Sirisanthana
Research Institute for Health Sciences, Chiang Mai University, Chiang Mai, Thailand

Pope Kosalaraksa
Department of Pediatrics, Faculty of Medicine, Khon Kaen University, Khon Kaen, Thailand

Witaya Petdachai
Petchburi Hospital, Petchburi, Thailand

Rawiwan Hansudewechakul
Chiang Rai Regional Hospital, Chiang Rai, Thailand

Jintanat Ananworanich
South East Asia Research Collaboration with Hawaii, Hawaii, Thailand
Department of Medicine, Faculty of Medicine, Chulalongkorn University, Bangkok, Thailand

Monica Basso, Marzia Franzetti, Renzo Scaggiante, Andrea Sattin, Carlo Mengoli, Marta Fiscon, Giorgio Palù and Saverio Giuseppe Parisi
Department of Molecular Medicine, University of Padova, Via Gabelli 63, 35100 Padova, Italy

Mario Cruciani
Center of Community & Medicine and HIV Outpatient Clinic, Verona, Italy

Wing Young Nicola Man, Angela Kellys, Heather Worth, Andrew Frankland and Patti Shih
School of Public Health and Community Medicine, UNSW Medicine, University of New South Wales, Sydney, Australia

Wing Young Nicola Man
Faculty of Health Sciences, University of Sydney, Sydney, New South Wales, Australia

Angela Kelly, Martha Kupul, Agnes Mek, Barbara Kepa, Rebecca Emori, Frances Akuani, Brenda Cangah, Lucy Walizopa, Lawrencia Pirpir, Somu Nosi and Peter M Siba
Sexual & Reproductive Health Unit, Papua New Guinea Institute of Medical Research, Goroka, Papua New Guinea

Uduak Okomo, Toyin Togun, Francis Oko and Assan Jaye
Medical Research Council (UK) Laboratories, Atlantic Road, Fajara, Banjul, The Gambia

Kevin Peterson
Institute of Tropical Medicine, Nationalestraat 155, 2000, Antwerp, Belgium

Assan Jaye
WAPHIR Network, Universite Cheikh Anta Diop Laboratoire de Bacteriologie Virologie, Hopital A. le Dantec, 30 Avenue Pasteur, Dakar, Senegal

Gero Hütter, Christian Blüthgen and Harald Klüter
Institute of Transfusion Medicine and Immunology, Medical Faculty Mannheim, Heidelberg University; German Red Cross Blood Service Baden-Württemberg- Hessen, Mannheim, Germany

Gero Hütter
Cellex GmbH, Dresden, Germany

Martin Neumann
Medical Department III (Hematology, Oncology), Charité Campus Benjamin Franklin, Berlin, Germany

Mark Reinwald and Daniel Nowak
Medical Department III (Hematology, Oncology), University Medical Centre Mannheim, Heidelberg University, Heidelberg, Germany

Lawrence Mbuagbaw, Pierre Ongolo-Zogo and David Yondo
Centre for Development of Best Practices in Health (CDBPH), Yaoundé Central Hospital, Avenue Henri Dunant, Messa, Yaoundé, Cameroon

Lawrence Mbuagbaw, Lehana Thabane, Stephen Noorduyn and Marek Smieja
Department of Clinical Epidemiology and Biostatistics, McMaster University, Hamilton, ON, Canada

Lehana Thabane
Biostatistics Unit, Father Sean O'Sullivan Research Centre, St Joseph's Healthcare, Hamilton, ON, Canada

Marek Smieja
St. Joseph's Healthcare Hamilton, Hamilton, ON, Canada

Lisa Dolovich
Department of Family Medicine, McMaster University, McMaster Innovation Park, Hamilton, ON, Canada

Zulfa Abrahams, Joel A Dave and Naomi S Levitt
Division of Diabetic Medicine and Endocrinology, Department of Medicine, University of Cape Town, Cape Town, South Africa

Gary Maartens
Division of Clinical Pharmacology, Department of Medicine, University of Cape Town, Cape Town, South Africa

Maia Lesosky
Department of Medicine, University of Cape Town, Cape Town, South Africa

Charlotte M Verolet
Department of Pediatrics, Children's Hospital-University Hospitals of Geneva, 6 Rue Willy-Donzé, 1211 Geneva 14, Switzerland

Cécile Delhumeau-Cartier, Marlène Sartori and Alexandra Calmy
HIV Unit, Department of Infectious Diseases, University Hospitals of Geneva, 4, Rue Gabrielle-Perret-Gentil, 1211 Geneva 4, Switzerland

Laurence Toutous Trellu
Department of Dermatology and Venerology, University Hospitals of Geneva, 4, Rue Gabrielle-Perret-Gentil, 1211 Geneva 4, Switzerland

Marlène Sartori and Simona Toma
Department of Psychiatric Diseases, University Hospitals of Geneva, 4, Rue Gabrielle-Perret-Gentil, 1211 Geneva 4, Switzerlands

Sophie Zawadynski
Department of Nuclear Medicine, University Hospitals of Geneva, 4, Rue Gabrielle-Perret-Gentil, 1211 Geneva 4, Switzerland

Minerva Becker
Department of Radiology, University Hospitals of Geneva, 4, Rue Gabrielle-Perret-Gentil, 1211 Geneva 4, Switzerland

Enos Bernasconi
Department of Infectious Diseases, Hospital of Lugano, Via Tesserete 46, 6900 Lugano, Switzerland

Tomohiro Kotaki, Siti Qamariyah Khairunisa, Adiana Mutamsari Witaningrum, Muhammad Qushai Yunifiar M, Septhia Dwi Sukartiningrum, Retno Pudji Rahayu, Nasronudin and Masanori Kameoka
Institute of Tropical Disease, Indonesia-Japan Collaborative Research Center for Emerging and Re-emerging Infectious Diseases, Airlangga University, Surabaya, Indonesia

Tomohiro Kotaki and Masanori Kameoka
Center for Infectious Diseases, Kobe University Graduate School of Medicine, Hyogo, Japan

Nasronudin
Faculty of Medicine, Airlangga University, Surabaya, Indonesia

Muhammad Noor Diansyah
Airlangga University Teaching Hospital, Surabaya, Indonesia

Masanori Kameoka
Department of International Health, Kobe University Graduate School of Health Sciences, Hyogo, Japan

Rajshree Thapa, Archana Amatya and Durga Prasad Pahari
Institute of Medicine, Maharajgunj Medical Campus, Tribhuwan University, Kathmandu, Nepal

Kiran Bam
James P Grant School of Public Health, BRAC University, Dhaka, Bangladesh

M Sophia Newman
Independent Scholar, Chicago, IL, USA

John Rubaihayo, Nazarius M Tumwesigye and Joseph Konde-Lule
Department of Epidemiology and Biostatistics, School of Public Health, College of Health Sciences, Makerere University, Kampala, Uganda

John Rubaihayo
Department of Public Health, School of Health Sciences, Mountains of the Moon University, Fort Portal, Uganda

Sandra W Cardoso, Paula M Luz, Luciane Velasque, Thiago Torres, Lara Coelho, Valdilea G Veloso and Beatriz Grinsztejn
Instituto de Pesquisa Clínica Evandro Chagas, Fundação Oswaldo Cruz, Rio de Janeiro, Brasil

Luciane Velasque
Departamento de Matemática e Estatística, Universidade Federal do Estado do Rio de Janeiro, Rio de Janeiro, Brasil

Kenneth A Freedberg and Rochelle P Walensky
The Divisions of Infectious Disease and General Medicine, and the Medical Practice Evaluation Center, Department of Medicine, Massachusetts General Hospital and the Harvard University Center for AIDS Research, Harvard Medical School, Boston, MA, U.S.A

Jia Liu, Wenjie Yang, Xiujuan Xue, Guoqing Sun, Chunhua Liu, Suian Tian, Dingyong Sun, Qian Zhu and Zhe Wang
Henan Center for Disease Control and Prevention, Zhengzhou, Henan, China

Yasong Wu
Chinese Center for Disease Control and Prevention, Beijing, China

Dai Watanabe, Sachiko Suzuki, Misa Ashida, Kazuyuki Hirota, Yoshihiko Ogawa, Keishiro Yajima, Daisuke Kasai, Yasuharu Nishida, Tomoko Uehira and Takuma Shirasaka
AIDS Medical Center, National Hospital Organization Osaka National Hospital, 2-1-14 Hoenzaka, Chuo-ku, Osaka City, Osaka 540-0006, Japan

Yuka Shimoji
Department of Nursing, National Hospital Organization Osaka National Hospital, Osaka, Japan

Index

www.ingramcontent.com/pod-product-compliance
Lightning Source LLC
LaVergne TN
LVHW080717210926
848485LV00003B/479